Anatomy, Physiology and Clinical Applications of Pupil

Anatomy, Physiology and Clinical Applications of Pupil

Editor: Kameron Sommer

AMERICAN
MEDICAL PUBLISHERS
www.americanmedicalpublishers.com

AMERICAN
MEDICAL PUBLISHERS
www.americanmedicalpublishers.com

Cataloging-in-Publication Data

Anatomy, physiology and clinical applications of pupil / edited by Kameron Sommer.
p. cm.
Includes bibliographical references and index.
ISBN 978-1-63927-871-8
1. Pupil (Eye). 2. Pupil (Eye)--Diseases. 3. Pupil (Eye)--Anatomy. 4. Pupil (Eye)--Physiology.
5. Pupil (Eye)--Diseases--Treatment. 6. Ophthalmology. I. Sommer, Kameron.
RE46 .A53 2023
617.7--dc23

American Medical Publishers,
41 Flatbush Avenue,
1st Floor, New York,
NY 11217, USA

ISBN 978-1-63927-871-8 (Hardback)

Contents

Preface

Pupil refers to a black hole located in the center of the iris that permits light to enter the eye and strike the retina. Light rays entering the pupil are either absorbed directly by the tissues inside the eye or absorbed after diffuse reflections within the eye that generally miss exiting the narrow pupil. This makes the pupil appear black. Pupil reacts to stimuli such as contraction in response to near fixation and brightness, and dilation as a response to mental effort and arousal. The pupil's image seen from the outside is referred to as entrance pupil. It does not exactly correspond to the location and size of the physical pupil as it is magnified by the cornea. Pupil testing can expose severe neuro-ophthalmic and retinal disease and thereby must be incorporated in the eye examination. This book unfolds the innovative studies on the pupil. It aims to serve as a resource guide for students and experts alike and contribute to the growth of the research on the anatomy, physiology and clinical applications of pupil.

The researches compiled throughout the book are authentic and of high quality, combining several disciplines and from very diverse regions from around the world. Drawing on the contributions of many researchers from diverse countries, the book's objective is to provide the readers with the latest achievements in the area of research. This book will surely be a source of knowledge to all interested and researching the field.

In the end, I would like to express my deep sense of gratitude to all the authors for meeting the set deadlines in completing and submitting their research chapters. I would also like to thank the publisher for the support offered to us throughout the course of the book. Finally, I extend my sincere thanks to my family for being a constant source of inspiration and encouragement.

Editor

1

Both a Gauge and a Filter: Cognitive Modulations of Pupil Size

R. Becket Ebitz[1*] *and Tirin Moore*[2,3]

[1] Department of Neuroscience and Center for Magnetic Resonance Research, University of Minnesota, Minneapolis, MN, United States, [2] Department of Neurobiology, Stanford University School of Medicine, Stanford, CA, United States, [3] Howard Hughes Medical Institute, Seattle, WA, United States

***Correspondence:**
R. Becket Ebitz
rebitz@gmail.com

Over 50 years of research have established that cognitive processes influence pupil size. This has led to the widespread use of pupil size as a peripheral measure of cortical processing in psychology and neuroscience. However, the function of cortical control over the pupil remains poorly understood. Why does visual attention change the pupil light reflex? Why do mental effort and surprise cause pupil dilation? Here, we consider these functional questions as we review and synthesize two literatures on cognitive effects on the pupil: how cognition affects pupil light response and how cognition affects pupil size under constant luminance. We propose that cognition may have co-opted control of the pupil in order to filter incoming visual information to optimize it for particular goals. This could complement other cortical mechanisms through which cognition shapes visual perception.

Keywords: pupil light response (PLR), pupil size, visual perception, attention, pupil light reflex, decision-making, exploration

INTRODUCTION

The first filter through which the visual world passes is the pupil. We use the word "filter" because the pupil is not a passive window unto the world. The pupil is constantly changing size as the musculature of the iris constricts and dilates. These adjustments have consequences for the amount of light that hits the retina, but also for the quality of our percepts of the visual world—how we see the world and, by extension, interact with it.

We can read a remarkable amount of information about people's cognitive processing through their pupils. For example, the pupil dilates in response to attractive social partners (1, 2). This is such an important interpersonal signal that women in the Middle Ages used belladonna (a dangerous poison) to dilate their pupils in order to attract partners. Of course, belladonna would also have consequences for the user's perception. This is because it produces pupil dilation, which increases optical aberrations (3–6). By scattering photons of light, these aberrations add positional noise in terms of where light hits the retina, thereby reducing high spatial frequency information and effectively rendering the visual world in softer focus. In photography, soft focus is frequently used to produce a youthful and romantic glow (7, 8). Thus, it is possible then that pupil dilation signals attraction to other humans and amplifies attraction by rendering social partners in a softer, more attractive focus.

Attraction is not the only mental process that influences the size of the pupil. Pupil size scales with mental effort (9, 10), surprise (11, 12), attention (13–15), and abstract goal states such as exploration (16–18). As tools for measuring pupil size become more readily available, pupil size is increasingly being used as a non-invasive peripheral index of cognitive processes. It is tempting to think of these modulations as simply a fortunate byproduct of a cognitive process of interest.

However, it is also possible that cognitive modulations of the pupil have a function. They may be an adaptive motor response generated by that cognitive process. Just as attraction increases pupil dilation, which, in turn, may render a more attractive world, it is possible that cognition adjusts pupil size in order to produce specific changes in our visual percepts. There is certainly evidence that cognitive processes shape visual processing via other mechanisms. For example, there are rich descending projections from prefrontal to visual cortex which change information processing and visual representations (19). Cognition also controls where we position our fovea—that is, which points of the visual scene we acquire high spatial frequency information about (20–22). In both cases, cognition acts to enhance and emphasize visual features that are relevant to that cognitive process: it optimizes perception toward its own ends.

In this review, we first discuss possible functions of cognitive modulations of the pupil light response—a pupil reflex arc that is essential for light adaptation. Then, we apply this same functional framework to consider the effect that spontaneous or cognitive fluctuations in pupil size may have on visual perception. We build an intuition for these effects by briefly reviewing how the aperture was used to produce different qualities of images in early art photography. However, we caution that much additional work is necessary to determine the extent to which physiological changes in pupil size affect gaze and perception. Ultimately, the goal of this review is to highlight these open questions and identify next steps for research on the perceptual consequences of pupil size.

ATTENTION AND THE PUPIL LIGHT RESPONSE

The pupillary light reflex (PLR; **Figure 1B**) is the first and most fundamental mechanism for light adaptation in the brain. When a focal or global luminance change occurs, the pupil constricts (23). This constriction is generally thought to serve a protective function, preventing photoreceptor fatigue and transient blindness when luminance increases (23). The PLR is mediated through a subcortical reflex pathway. Luminance information from the retina is relayed to the midbrain pretectal nucleus, which in turn projects to the Edinger-Westphal nucleus, which signals the pupillary sphincter to contract (23, 24). However, the subcortical reflex pathway is not the only pathway by which visual information can influence the pupil response to increasing luminance. For example, in the absence of direct retinal input to the pretectum—when the subcortical pathway is eliminated—a small pupillary light response can still be observed. Moreover, postgeniculate, cortical lesions can impair normal pupil light responses, though these effects are smaller than the consequences of eliminating the subcortical pathway (25–27). Thus, the pupil light reflex is only one small part of a larger PLR, some of which is mediated by cortical processing.

The existence of cortical influences raises the possibility that higher-order visual or even cognitive processes could shape the PLR. Indeed, there is empirical evidence for this view. For example, we know that the PLR is reduced during performance of a competing task (30), suggesting that it could be subject to resource limitations (31). Studies linking the PLR specifically to changes in visual processing go back at least as far as the 1940s. For example, in 1948, a binocular rivalry study examined the PLR evoked by illuminating one eye. They found that the PLR was larger when the visual input to that eye was dominating perception, compared to when it was not (32). This result was soon replicated (33) and other studies began finding that the PLR depended on visual processing in other ways. For example, a stimulus detection study found that the PLR was absent for probes reported as not seen (34) and a presaccadic processing study found that the likelihood of evoking a PLR was suppressed before a saccade (35)—following a similar time course as the presaccadic suppression of visual perception [also see (36)]. One unifying interpretation of these observations is the idea that the PLR is modulated by visual attention. This is because attention is strongly linked to ocular dominance (37, 38), target detection (39), and saccadic preparation (40–44).

However, it was not until much later that studies began to explicitly test the idea that the PLR is modulated by selective visual attention (13–15, 29, 45). For example, instructions to attend to a bright stimulus enhance the PLR to that stimulus, while instructions to attend away diminish PLR magnitude (13, 15). The PLR also tracks trial-by-trial variability in the selective attention paid to an evoking probe [**Figures 1A,C**; (14, 29)]. Preparing an oculomotor response to a probe location, which is known to recruit visual spatial attention (41, 43), also enhances the PLR to that probe (14, 29, 46, 47). Together, these results showed that the PLR scales with visual attention regardless of whether it is endogenously cued (13, 15), exogenously cued (14, 29, 48), and or recruited by saccadic preparation [**Figure 1D**; (14, 29, 46, 47)].

It seems plausible that attention-related modulations of the PLR would require cortical control. But what is the source of this control? The pretectal nucleus receives input from the frontal eye field (FEF), an area within prefrontal cortex (49–51), and the lateral intraparietal cortex (52). These regions are causally implicated in selective attention (53, 54) and saccadic control (55–59). Moreover, we have previously found that microstimulation of the FEF is sufficient to bidrectionally modulate the gain of the PLR [**Figure 2**; (28)]. Thus, the PLR may be subject to prefrontal control by the same region causally responsible for shaping visual perception in the service of attention (19). Because of these studies, a strong argument can be made that the PLR is a valid, implicit, peripheral measure of selective visual attention. That is, (1) it is modulated by the same cognitive and presaccadic processes involved in selective visual attention (13–15, 29, 47, 48) and (2) it is modulated by the same neural perturbations that cause other correlates of selective visual attention, such as changes in extrastriate cortex (13, 28). Thus, the PLR is a powerful new way to measure selective attention in circumstances in which it was not previously possible (60). However, the use of the PLR as an implicit index of attention should not preclude the possibility that these modulations have a function.

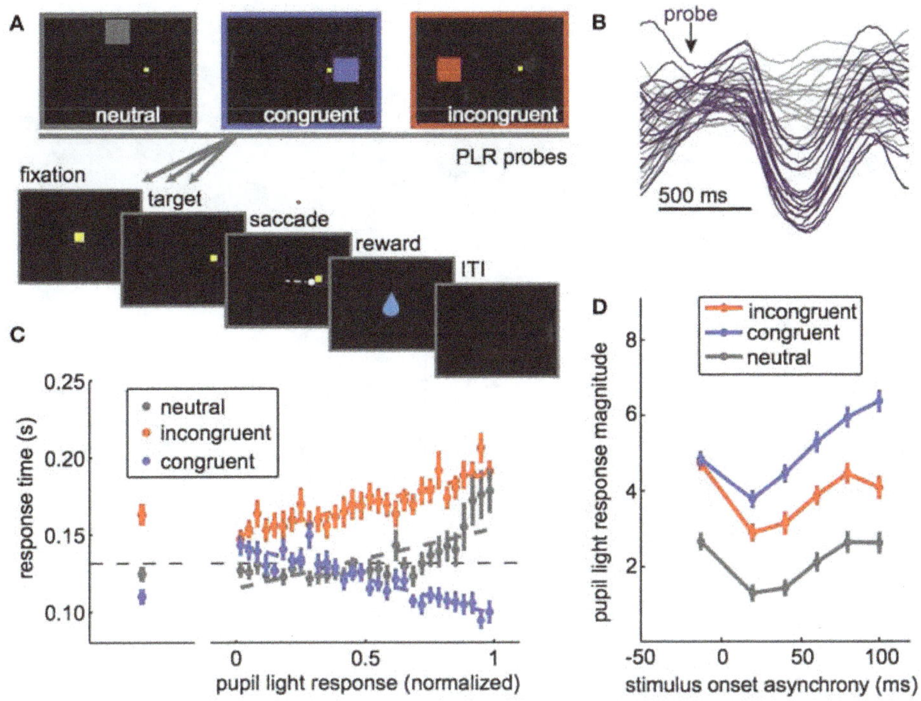

FIGURE 1 | The PLR is correlated with stimulus attention and PLR magnitude can be used to probe the dynamics of visuospatial attention. **(A)** The PLR distraction task. In this task, PLR-evoking probes are presented in one of three locations relative to a rewarded target: above fixation, away from all possible target locations ("neutral"), on the same side as the rewarded target ("congruent"), or in the opposite hemifield from the rewarded target ("incongruent"). PLR probes were presented both before and at various latencies after target onset. **(B)** Some example pupil traces [data from Ebitz and Moore (28)] showing the characteristic light-evoked constriction after an evoking probe (purple) compared to sham-probe trials (gray). **(C)** Left: Response time effects of PLR probes in each location. Congruent probes sped response times, while incongruent ones slowed response time. Neutral probes had little impact on response time. Right: The evoked PLR strongly predicted the extent to which that probe would capture attention, as measured by response time effects of the probes. **(D)** PLR magnitude (bigger = more constriction) as a function of the timing of the PLR probe. If the probe was presented before the rewarded target (negative stimulus onset asynchrony), there was no difference between congruent and incongruent probes. All PLRs were suppressed to probes presented immediately after the rewarded target. Then, as monkeys began to prepare a saccade to the rewarded target, congruent probes PLRs (blue) were enhanced relative to both incongruent (red) and neutral (gray). Figures modified from Ebitz et al. (14) and Ebitz (29) under a Creative Commons Attribution license and with permission from copyright holders.

Possible Functions of Attentional Modulations of the Pupil Light Response

The first and most often cited function of the pupil light reflex is for light adaptation. Perhaps one function of the attentional modulations of the PLR is to allow light adaptation across saccades (14, 28, 46). We know that selective attention is an integral part of saccade planning (41, 43), so perhaps attentional modulations of the PLR play a presaccadic role. In natural vision, two sequential saccades may target regions that differ in luminance by several orders of magnitude (61). Anticipatory light adaptation could be useful because the pupil requires hundreds of milliseconds to constrict (62). Initializing this process before a saccade would give the pupil time to begin to constrict before a bright target is foveated—ensuring that the pupil is at least partially constricted before the retina is oriented toward a bright eccentric target. Indeed, one elegant study found that the luminance information at the target of an upcoming eye movement is integrated into the PLR before the saccade begins (47), consistent with presaccadic processes. By accelerating the constriction of the aperture for the target of an upcoming saccade, attentional modulation of the PLR could improve the efficiency of visual scanning by adapting the pupil across luminance gradients found in natural vision. Of course, any advantage in scanning efficiency is theoretical and, if empirically observable at all, may be quite small (47).

An alternative, and perhaps complimentary, hypothesis is that attentional modulations of the PLR may play a role in optimizing visual acuity across light intensities (4, 46). In this view, attentional modulations of the PLR may act to optimize visual acuity for the attended stimulus. This is because decreasing pupil size both limits the light hitting the retina (63), and improves visual acuity by reducing various optical aberrations (3–6). As there is background noise in our photoreceptor output (64, 65), there is a natural tradeoff, gated by the pupil, between visual acuity and the signal to noise ratio of the selected visual signal (66). Decreasing incoming drive by decreasing pupil size could bury a visual signal in the noise floor—unless that visual signal is sufficiently bright. By allowing attention to enhance the pupil constriction evoked by bright signals—beyond what would be

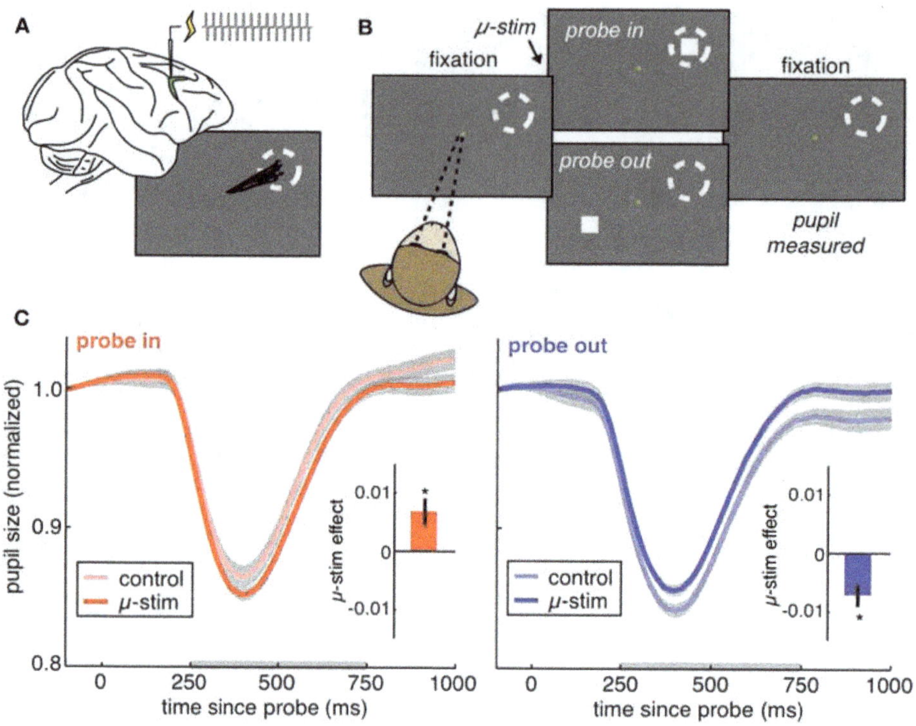

FIGURE 2 | The PLR is bidirectionally modulated by cortical stimulation. **(A)** The frontal eye fields (green) are a part of prefrontal cortex responsible for directing gaze and attention. Injecting current into the frontal eye fields produces repeated saccades to the same location in space (the "response field," dotted circle). Stimulating at very low currents ("microstimulation") directs covert visual attention to the response field without moving the eye. **(B)** The PLR stimulation task. Rhesus monkeys hold fixation while PLR-evoking light probes are flashed on the screen. On some trials, microstimulation is delivered in order to direct covert visual attention to one of the two possible probe locations. **(C)** The pupil light response from an example session on trials where the probe was flashed in the stimulated response field (left), our outside of the stimulated field (right). Pale colors = no stimulation control trials. Saturated colors = stimulation was delivered. Inset) Difference between control and stimulation trials across all sessions. *$p < 0.05$. Figures modified from Ebitz and Moore (28), reproduced under a Creative Commons Attribution license.

evoked by the stimulus if attention was directed elsewhere—the eye could take advantage of the greater acuity that is possible when the incoming signal is brighter (**Figure 3**).

An important caveat to this argument is that attentional enhancements of the PLR likely have only subtle, small effects on visual acuity. These modulations enhance pupil constriction on the order of a tenth of a millimeter, which would produce negligible changes in acuity for eyes with normal or corrected-to-normal vision [though changes in acuity would certainly be larger in eyes with refractive errors; (3)]. Nevertheless, it remains unclear whether such small changes in pupil size would be sufficient to produce substantive changes in visual acuity during natural vision in primates today.

This question of magnitude is important because prefrontal control over a brainstem reflex requires long-range connections that seem costly to evolve and maintain. Shouldn't they confer some substantive benefit in order to have been selected for by evolution? It is important to note that a substantive benefit to perception in primates today is not necessary for either evolving attentional modulations of the pupil light reflex or for these modulations to have a function today. First, it is plausible that attentional modulations of the PLR are an exaptation (67)—a byproduct of evolution that was not selected for directly. In this view, these modulations could have evolved via a noisy selection process operating on some other, related competency, such as for prefrontal control over other brainstem circuits. Once evolved, exaptations nevertheless can be co-opted to serve some function, such as improving visual acuity during natural vision in the myopic eye. Second and alternatively, it is possible that attentional modulations of the pupil light response are vestigial: a competency that was selected for when it did confer a substantive benefit and maintained because it does not substantially hinder fitness. If the frequency of refractive errors has reduced over primate evolution, then it is possible that some ancestral nervous system evolved attentional modulations of the pupil light reflex at a time when they did provide substantive perceptual benefits, though these benefits have become smaller over time as the primate eye became increasingly emmetropic. Differentiating between these possibilities will require comparative studies. However, in either case observing attentional modulations of the pupil in the primate eye today does not imply or require that these modulations were selected for directly. It may imply that they did not hinder fitness enough to be selected against—perhaps because they work synergistically, rather than competitively, with other mechanisms for light adaptation or for improving visual acuity with attention.

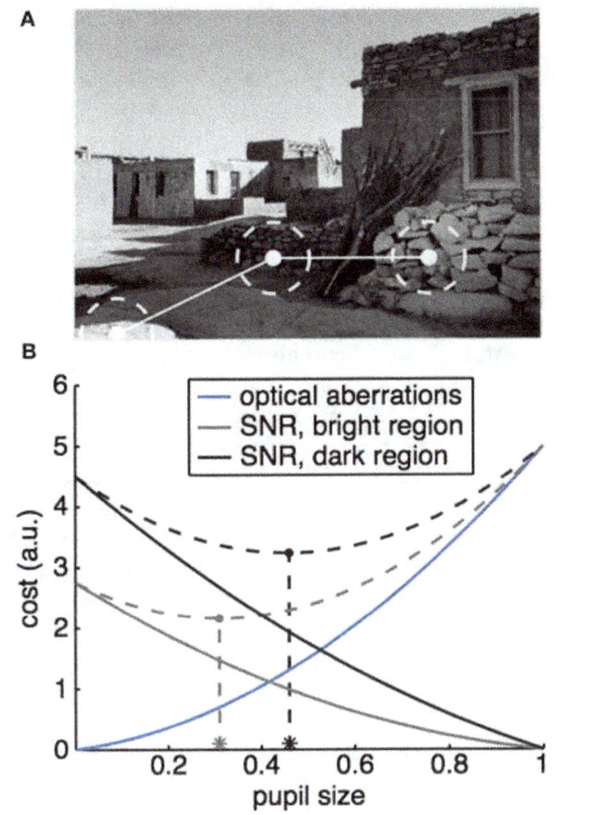

FIGURE 3 | A potential role for the PLR in optimizing acuity in natural vision. **(A)** Natural scenes have luminance gradients, such that successive saccades can target regions with very different brightness (Image: Ansel Adams, "Acoma Pueblo. [National Historic Landmark, New Mexico]," U.S. National Archives, identifier #519836). **(B)** Cartoon illustrating how a tradeoff between signal to noise and optical aberrations could produce different optimal pupil sizes for different luminance regions. The effect of optical aberrations on vision (costs, solid blue line) increase as a function of pupil size. A larger pupil also increases the amount of light passing through, which means that the signal to noise ratio (SNR) would also increase as a function of pupil size, producing a decreasing cost for vision as a function of pupil size (solid gray and black lines). Because luminance varies across the scene, different regions would have different intrinsic signal levels, which would interact with pupil size to determine the costs (compare solid gray and black lines). To find the optimal pupil size across these two conditions, we can calculate the total costs due to both SNR and optical aberrations (dotted gray lines), then find the pupil size that minimizes these total costs (asterisks).

COGNITION AND PUPIL SIZE UNDER CONSTANT LUMINANCE

In addition to modulating the PLR, covertly reorienting selective attention could also cause a transient pupil constriction. A small pupil constriction is observed following subtle equiluminant changes in stimuli, including changes in color, spatial frequency, structure, and motion (68–71). [This is in contrast to an arousing or alerting response to a highly salient stimulus, which produces pupil dilation, rather than constriction (72, 73)] However, these same subtle changes in stimuli also transiently capture and reorient selective visual attention (74, 75). These reorienting pupil constrictions depend on visual processing in the cortex: they are not observed in cortical blindness (68), where the visual signals in cortex are significantly reduced (76). Of course, reorienting pupil constrictions are quite transient—decaying within about 2 s after the evoking stimulus—but they could still permit a transient improvement in acuity, locked to the moment when a change in stimulus structure is capturing selective, spatial attention. Of course, future work is necessary to determine whether this pupil onset response is specifically related to reorienting selective visual attention toward a stimulus on a display, or if it is instead mediated by other mechanisms, such as a generalized alerting or arousal response.

Other cognitive processes produce sustained decreases in pupil size. For example, during a learning task, commitments to a behavioral policy are associated with sustained pupil constriction (11). Similarly, the pupil under constant luminance is smaller on trials following both errors of task performance and task conflict in a well-learned task (77). Together, these results suggest that pupil size may be tonically smaller when humans and other primates are committed to executing a well-learned behavioral task, rather than learning about a changing environment (11, 17, 78) or struggling to perform a difficult task (1, 9, 79).

Learning and task difficulty are not the only mental processes associated with *larger* pupil sizes. Instead, the pupil size increases with a diversity of cognitive processes including surprise (11, 12), motivation (80), emotion (81, 82), exploration (17), and many other cognitive processes that have been reviewed extensively elsewhere (9, 83). One interpretation of these effects is that the pupil simply increases in size with autonomic arousal—that modulations of autonomic arousal are some final common outcome of all of these cognitive processes (77). Indeed, pupil size covaries with other measures of autonomic arousal, including changes in skin conductance (79, 81) and activity in the locus coeruleus (84). Another interpretation of these results is that pupil size is larger any time a behavioral change is needed (i.e., when a surprising or arousing experience suggests that it is important to adapt behavior). In this view, pupil size under constant luminance and related cognitive or neural processes may track the balance between behavioral stability and flexibility (85–90). There is certainly some evidence in favor of the view that pupil size predicts changes in core components of flexibility, including behavioral variability (14, 77, 91) and learning (11, 17, 78). Moreover, neurons in the dorsal anterior cingulate, a part of the brain thought to be responsible for regulating the balance between stability and flexibility (88, 92–94) also encode information about or predict changes in pupil size (29, 77, 84, 95, 96). However, future work is necessary to determine whether there are pupil-linked changes in the behavioral and neural mechanisms that support flexibility and/or stability [e.g., (97, 98)].

In many studies, pupil size under constant luminance is used as a peripheral index of autonomic arousal (79, 81), noradrenergic tone (12, 91, 99–101), control states (77, 99), or changes in cortical processing (77, 102–105). Because of its utility in these applications, pupil size can be implicitly treated as a by-product of the process of interest, rather than a motoric consequence of these processes. However, it is also possible that these modulations of pupil size have some adaptive function in their own right. To address this possibility, we will next consider what effect changes in pupil size might have on information processing via examining how the aperture has been used in photography.

The Photographer's Aperture

The optics of a camera and the human eye are certainly not the same. For example, the camera is not foveal, and modern camera lenses are corrected for many of the optical aberrations that plague the eye. However, we can still build an intuition for the functional consequences of changing pupil size by looking at historical photographs. This is because we, as viewers, operate on these photographs, much as we operate on the visual world around us. We decide where to saccade within these images based on some combination of the visual salience within the image and our top down goals or beliefs about what is important (21). The power of the photographer is to change how we view the veridical world—by shaping how the viewer perceives and interacts with the visual scene (7, 106, 107). Our suggestion here is that the brain operates the aperture of our eye to just such an end.

In the introduction, we discussed how larger apertures produce softer-focus images by increasing optical aberrations. This occurs because large apertures allow greater scattering of photons from adjacent sources. This is more pronounced when the plane of focus is even slightly misaligned with the sensors [i.e., the photographers' film or our eye's photoreceptors; (3)]. Of course, camera optics have improved substantially since the technology was first developed in the early nineteenth century and modern digital cameras often eliminate these aberrations in software. This means that today, photographers predominantly adjust their aperture to set the depth of field of a photograph. A large aperture produces a narrow depth of field, where much of the scene is out of focus. A small aperture, conversely, produces a deep depth of field, where the fine detail is preserved across a range of distances. However, in historical photographic images, we can still see how photographers adjusted the aperture in order to enhance or eliminate optical aberrations in order to achieve different goals over time.

A large aperture produces a soft focus. That is, it reduces the fine, high-spatial frequency detail in the image, emphasizing larger forms at the expense of detail (**Figure 4A**). This type of aesthetic was exemplified in the images produced by "Pictorialist" photographers in the late nineteenth and early twentieth centuries (8, 108). Pictorialism was perhaps the first stylistic tradition in fine art photography, marking the transition of the camera from a mechanical device to a medium for artistic expression (106, 108). To separate this new form of photography from other, more technical uses, Pictorialists such as Alfred Horsley Hinton (106) sought to produce images that went beyond the "faithful and perfect delineation [...] toward which Science and mechanics have striven in photography" (p. 5). Instead, Hinton described his goal to produce an image that captured the impression of a scene, noting "if the impression made upon me by the original scene was a very powerful one, then most probably I should have been unconscious of and be blind to petty details" (p. 7). Toward this end Hinton sought to capture "a general outline or by the portrayal of the chief items only" (p. 7) where "detail and crisp outlines [may be] intentionally subdued" (p. 8), and sharp lines are sacrificed for a depth of tones, an infinite gradation that makes objects appear to glow (106).

Pictorialist photographers used a range of techniques to produce these images. For example, in his 1917 manual on photography, Paul L. Anderson highlighted the benefits of selecting "a lens possessing all possible errors," which gives, "as a result of its optical defects, a very soft and pleasing quality of definition" (p. 37). Anderson also described how the photographer could enhance these effects: "by the use of an aperture larger than normal it is possible to obtain greater diffusion, thus aiding in the suggestion of mystery, a suggestion which is of importance in any work of art" (p. 52). Many pictorialist photographers continued to work with large apertures and soft-focus lenses, long after the development of lenses corrected for various optical aberrations. This was particularly pronounced in Hollywood, where photographers and cinematographers continued to produce Pictorialism-inspired images for several decades after aberration-corrected lenses, "anastigmat" lenses, had been developed in the 1890's (7, 8, 109). These photographers produced the iconic images that we think of when we imagine female Hollywood icons the 1920's and 30's (8).

Starting in the 1920's and 1930's, however, many photographers began experimenting with precisely the opposite choice: using small apertures to produce images that engaged the viewer with detail. This became the Purist or objectivist photography movement (109). At the forefront of movement was Ansel Adams, perhaps the best-known American landscape photographer (**Figure 4B**). To achieve his engulfing views of the natural world, Adams used the smallest apertures that were available. This choice of aperture was so central to his process that he later formed a gallery and working group in Oakland, California under precisely this name [Group f/64; (109)]. Another member of this group was Edward Weston, a major master of 20th century photography. Weston used precisely the same techniques—long exposures with the smallest possible apertures—to produce richly detailed and absorbing images. In a 1930 essay declaring his disdain for the Pictorialists ("if they had no camera [they] would be third rate, or worse, painters"), Weston passionately described what he felt to be the true best-use of photography (107). The camera can "enable one to see through the eye, augmenting the eye, seeing more than the eye sees, exaggerating details, recording surfaces, textures that the human hand could not render with the most skill and labor." The photograph "contains no lines in the painter's sense, but is entirely made up of tiny particles. The extreme fineness of these particles gives a special tension to the image, and when that tension is destroyed the integrity of the photograph is destroyed."

The transition from Pictorialism to Purism in photography is clearly a far cry from what our pupils are doing as they transition from dilation and constriction. For example, the photographic apertures used to produce **Figures 4A,B** would have differed in size by more than the physiological range of the pupil—and certainly more than any cognitive modulation of the pupil. But,

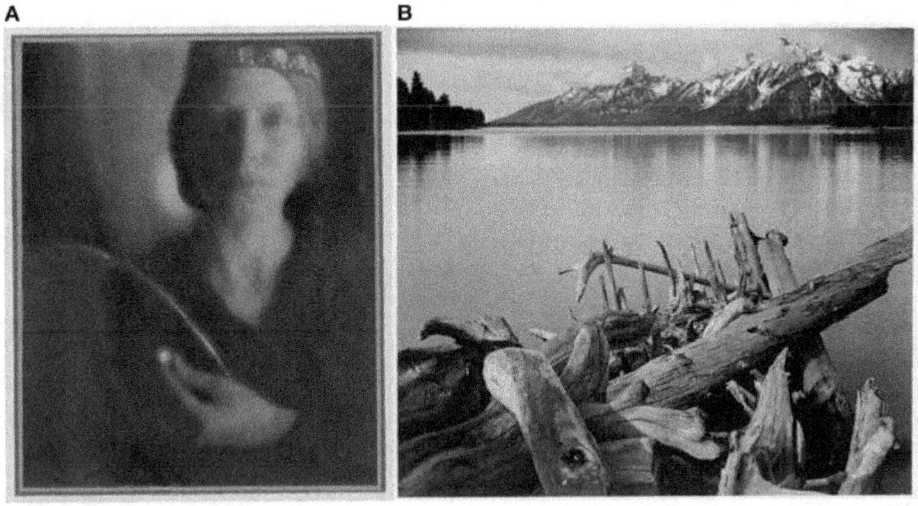

FIGURE 4 | Example images from the Pictorialist and Purist photographic traditions. **(A)** "The Firefly," A photograph in the Pictorialist style by George Seeley, 1911. (Source: Getty Museum, identifier: #84.XM.163.1). Note the soft focus and lack of high spatial frequency detail. **(B)** A photograph in the Purist style by Ansel Adams. "Jackson Lake, with Teton Ridge in the background." Taken for the National Park Service, circa 1933–1942. Note the increase in fine, high spatial frequency detail. (Source: U.S. National Archives, identifier: #519909).

perhaps these images have value as a caricature of the effects of pupil size on perception: these images enhance and emphasize the effects of aperture size on our image of the world around us. Moreover, by looking at how we interact with these images as a viewer—and by thinking about what information is coded in the high spatial frequency channels that were enhanced in purism and discarded in pictorialism—we might be able to gain some insights into what, if any, function cognitive modulations of the pupil could serve.

Possible Perceptual and Oculomotor Effects of Pupil Size

Small pupils would bias visual representations toward the purist tradition—emphasizing the fine detail and high spatial frequency information of the visual world. In a sense then, the pupil constriction caused by attention-capturing changes in stimuli (68–71) would mirror the known effects of attention on visual acuity (110) and contrast sensitivity (111). This is because, by decreasing defocus, smaller pupils necessarily increase visual acuity and sensitivity for the fine-grained contrast gradations typical of attention tasks (3–6). (Of course, larger pupils might increase contrast sensitivity for larger spatial scales, because they could increase the signal to noise ratio of vision by allowing more light to hit the retina).

Although there are clear parallels between the pupil constriction observed at attentional reorienting and the effects of pupil constriction on vision, several caveats must be noted. First, the perceptual consequences of attention and pupil size differ in space. *Selective* visual attention only improves contrast sensitivity and visual acuity only for a selected region in visual space (110–113). Conversely, any change in pupil size is necessarily a *global* effect. Thus, pupil constriction at attentional capture can provide a global compliment to ongoing, local perceptual processes. Second, the perceptual consequences of attention and pupil size also differ in magnitude. Attention improves visual acuity on the order of several arc minutes (114). For individuals with normal (20/20) vision, the change in pupil size that would be required to produce the equivalent change in visual acuity would be larger than the physiological range of the pupil (3). Of course, the perceptual effects of small reductions in pupil diameter can produce arc minute changes in visual acuity in myopic or astigmatic individuals (3). Thus, effects of pupil constriction on vision complement and may work synergistically with other known effects of attention on vision.

What consequences would increasing the fine detail in a visual representation have for gaze and perception? In natural vision, high spatial frequency information scales with proximity, such that closer objects and features contain finer details (115). Given that this information carries forward through the visual system to preferentially attract gaze (20, 21, 116, 117), enhancing the representation of this information by any means—including decreasing pupil size—could help to bias perception and gaze toward nearby objects, rather than distant ones. Indeed, pupil constriction is a fundamental component of the near response. That is, when we do focus on a nearby object, a triad of oculomotor effects occurs: the eyes converge, the lenses accommodate, and the pupils constrict (118, 119). Of course, future work is necessary to determine whether changes in pupil size on the order of these cognitive influences can produce perceptual biases of sufficient magnitude to modulate gaze.

The idea that the pupil constriction component of the pupil near response could function to focus gaze on nearby objects seems at odds with the observation that small apertures are used to produce a deeper depth of field in modern photography. A small aperture allows the region of focus to extend further both toward and away from the viewer (**Figure 5**). This implies that there would be more high spatial frequency information when pupils are small across both nearby and distant locations—not just in the current plane of focus. Of course, this would not change the fact that nearby objects contain more high-spatial frequency information, so increasing depth of field could still bias gaze toward nearby objects. It is also important to note that while there is substantial evidence that decreasing pupil size (<4 or 5 mm) does narrow the eye's depth-of-field (120, 121), the effects of pupil size on depth-of-field in the eye are not necessarily as straightforward as they are in a modern digital camera. For example, depth-of-field in our visual systems is also substantially affected by optical aberrations that are eliminated in these cameras, there are modulatory effects of both neural and retinal processing (121), and there is evidence that increasing pupil size (e.g., from 4 to 6 mm) can narrow, rather than deepen depth-of-field (121). Moreover, because blur is important for estimating depth (122, 123), it is possible that the function of any deepened depth of field with small pupil size is to reduce this depth information when it is unnecessary—such as in near-work tasks. Ultimately, future work is needed to determine how pupil size affects perception and gaze in three dimensional environments.

In higher level vision—visual representations of objects or social partners—high spatial frequency information often carries a disproportionate amount of information about the identity of that visual target (124–127). Moreover, there is evidence that changing goals could change the spatial frequency information that we prioritize for processing (128, 129). For example, human observers tend to rely on high spatial frequency information to discriminate facial identities (125, 127, 130) or to differentiate objects within broader conceptual categories [i.e., breeds of dogs (125) or the identity of a specific toy (126)]. Enhancing high spatial frequency information could help the viewer to individuate objects, perhaps even along task-relevant dimensions. Of course, this is a strong prediction—that decreasing pupil size would increase individuation of faces and objects—and empirical studies are needed to determine whether cognitive modulations of pupil size are of sufficient magnitude to produce this kind of change.

If decreasing pupil size draws gaze to nearby objects, increasing pupil size might have the opposite effect reducing the drive to look at proximate objects by eliminating the high-spatial frequency information that may partially drive this bias (20, 21, 115–117). It is intriguing to note that this could focus gaze on regions with large changes in contrast across low spatial frequencies for two reasons. First, it would reduce the encoding (and thus salience) of competing high spatial frequency information. Second, it could potentially increase contrast sensitivity at low spatial frequencies by allowing more light into the eye. By allowing more photons to hit the retina, large pupils could increase the signal-to-noise ratio of vision—effectively increasing the perception of contrast at any spatial scale that is larger than the scale of dilation-induced defocus. Additional work is necessary to determine how pupil size affects contrast sensitivity at various spatial scales. However, there is some evidence for the view that pharmacological perturbations that increase pupil size do bias gaze toward regions where

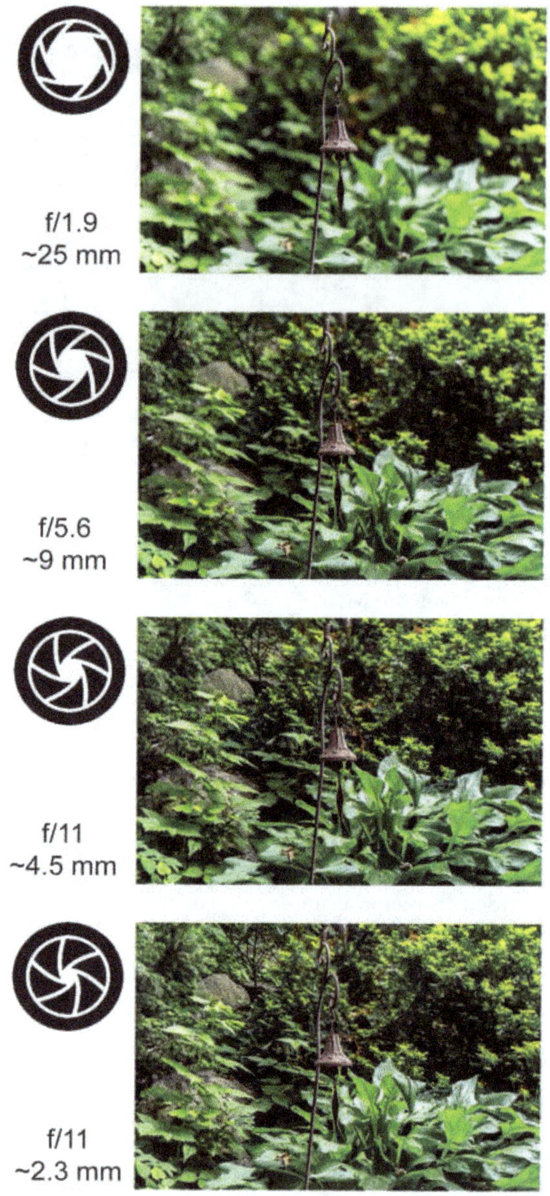

FIGURE 5 | The effects of aperture size on depth of field. (Top to bottom) The effects of decreasing aperture size on defocus in three dimensions in a modern digital camera. The large aperture increases the sense of depth in the top photographs, but the small aperture increases the high spatial frequency information in the bottom photographs. Note that the range of aperture sizes used here is larger than the physiological range of the pupil (which is only 2–8 mm) and these images were corrected for optical aberrations by processing in the camera (Photo credit: Boris Oicherman).

contrast varies substantially across large regions in space (131, 132), though it remains unclear whether these effects are mediated by changes in pupil size or by changes in neural activity (14, 29).

Other perceptual consequences of reducing high spatial frequency information may be to bias perception toward global, categorical, and configural properties of the visual world (133, 134). We know that low spatial frequency information is sufficient, and indeed more useful than high spatial frequency information, in rapidly perceiving the gist of a scene (135). This implies that observers with larger pupils might focus more on global properties of a scene, rather than the specific details. In object perception, pupil dilation might decrease information about object or face identity in favor of type, mimicking the effects of disrupting high spatial frequency information in images (124–127). This could make it easier to represent a figure according to more abstract classes—such as whether an object is a car or an animal—rather than according to fine grain distinctions between different animals (136). Finally, large pupils could also aid in estimating the three dimensional configuration of a scene—that is, the distance between ourselves and some salient cue. This is because blur is a salient depth cue, useful for estimating distances in three dimensions (122, 123), and it also increases as the depth of field decreases with large pupil sizes (**Figure 5**).

Given the link between pupil size and autonomic arousal, an increase in configural processing with large pupil sizes could certainly be adaptive. Much as sympathetic arousal quickens heart rate and shifts blood flow to skeletal muscles, perhaps it also changes our visual filter in order to more rapidly and accurate differentiate between trees and tigers and estimate their distance from ourselves, without regard for the texture or individual identity of either. This could also help with generalizing learned associations to members of a broader class. For example, if your previous experiences with tigers have been particularly arousing, perhaps it is best that those memories generalize across all big cats. It is probably a waste of limited neural resources to even represent the specific details of any given tiger!

Of course, it is also possible that cognitive modulations of the pupil are not large enough to produce any substantial perceptual change, given the modern primate eye. This is an empirical question that can be addressed psychophysically, either through combining pharmacological dilation with artificial pupils or through filtering images to match the putative effects of plausible changes in pupil size. However, even if cognitive modulations of the pupil are not sufficiently large to produce perceptual changes in the normal primate eye today, this does not preclude the possibility that they either evolved in an ancestral eye, where they did produce adaptive perceptual changes. Their continued existence today may simply imply that they did not hinder fitness enough to be selected against—perhaps because they work synergistically, rather than competitively, with other mechanisms for biasing perceptual processing according to pupil-linked goals or brain states.

DIRECTIONS FOR FUTURE RESEARCH ON PERCEPTION, GAZE, AND PUPIL SIZE

Much of the above is a speculative juxtaposition of the known optical consequences of pupil size and the effects of various image manipulations on natural image viewing. In particular, we have noted that more work is needed to determine the precise magnitude of any effect of pupil size on perception and any perceptual effects on gaze and behavior. Although pupil size necessarily gates spatial frequency and blur information, to our knowledge, few studies have looked at how pupil size influences gaze and visual perception. In part, this is because naturally-occurring fluctuations in pupil size are inexorably linked with changes in autonomic arousal (79, 81), noradrenergic tone (12, 91, 99–101), control states (77, 99), and cortical processing (77, 102–105). Any of these processes could produce changes in gaze, visual processing, or task performance via mechanisms other than pupil size.

Of course, the converse is also true: without knowing the effects of pupil size on gaze, visual processing, and task performance, we cannot ascribe behavioral correlates of pupil size to changes in arousal, norepinephrine, control states, or cortical processing. This is because any behavioral correlates of pupil size—even those that seem deeply cognitive *primafacie*—could be due to the effects of pupil size on perception, rather than a latent state that is indexed by pupil size.

Changes in low-level perceptual cues can have substantial consequences for higher-order cognitive processes. For example, there is certainly some evidence that the spatial frequency of vision is consequential for higher order cognitive processes, including as memory and decision-making. One thoughtful study reported that small pupil size at encoding was associated with better recognition memory for objects (137). Does this mean that pupil-linked mechanisms such as arousal, norepinephrine, control states, or cortical processing underlie recognition memory? There are two pieces of evidence that suggest otherwise. First, this study also noted that subjects with smaller pupils also made more frequent, shorter direction fixations when viewing the objects. These patterns of gaze predicted future recognition memory just as well as pupil size did. We know from other studies that these gaze patterns mimic the effects of increasing high spatial frequency information in an image (116) and that high spatial frequency information is important for object recognition (138). Thus, it is entirely possible that the increase in recognition memory in this study was mediated by a change in the way the pupil filtered the visual world. Second, if pupil size indexed some brain state that was optimized for memory encoding, it should have the same relationship with recognition memory, regardless of what kind of information was being encoded. Yet, small pupils at encoding may only predict better recognition memory for objects (137). Small pupils are associated with *poorer* recognition for faces (139). This is striking because low—not high—spatial frequency information is essential for encoding faces (140–142). Thus, during object encoding, smaller pupils would preserve the high spatial frequency information that is important for object recognition—drawing attention *toward* the critical stimulus dimensions. However, during face encoding, smaller pupils would preserve the high spatial frequency information that competes with the important low spatial frequency cues—in this case, drawing attention *away* from the critical stimulus dimensions.

Mnemonic encoding is not the only cognitive process that can be gated by perception or the effects of perception on gaze and attention. For example, we know that gaze is sufficient to shape economic (143) and social (144) decision-making. Perhaps this occurs because gaze gates value signals in higher order decision-making regions (145). This suggests that changes in fixations patterns propagate through decision processes to shape behavior. By systematically reducing the high spatial frequency information, pupil size could bias gaze, and therefore decisions away from high spatial frequency targets. For example, we previously found that pupil size predicted decisions to look at large (~15° visual angle) images of conspecific faces, rather than small (<1°) rewarded targets [**Figures 6A,B**; (14, 77)]. We interpreted this as a change in monkeys' susceptibility to distraction, but it is entirely possible that this susceptibility was mediated by a change in the monkeys' percept of the visual display. Perhaps their larger pupils simply deemphasized the visual salience of the small rewarded target (29). In a natural environment, this shift in perception could mean the difference between decisions to forage at a local patch (which is necessarily richer in high-spatial frequency information by virtue of its proximity) or decisions to explore more distant opportunities.

Much more work is necessary to establish what effect pupil size has on gaze and attention, much less on higher order cognitive processes like memory and decision-making. This is a substantial need because, as we have just illustrated, it can be tempting to think of pupil size as an *index* of a latent brain state, but it remains possible that pupil size could *cause* changes in perception that then influence cognition via shaping attention or gaze.

Because of these potential confounds, building a taxonomy of the direct behavioral effects of pupil size is an essential precondition for the use of the pupil as an index of any cognitive or neural state. First, it is important to determine how spatial frequency information changes across pupil size. One promising approach might be to have human subjects report their percepts of ambiguous images, that contain differing objects or scenes in parametrically varied frequency channels (128). This would allow a quantitative description how pupil size sets the spatial frequencies that are prioritized for processing. Second, it is necessary to determine whether any neural and/or behavioral correlates of pupil-linked states can be replicated by filtering the display to enhance or suppress these frequency channels. An alternative and perhaps complementary approach might be to dilate the pupils with mydriatic agents (such as the tropicamide and the phenylephrine), then use an artificial "pupil" to determine whether manipulating pupil size was, by itself, sufficient to replicate any behavioral effects (66). Addressing these two questions will be essential for both understanding the perceptual consequences of pupil size and for establishing the circumstances in which pupil size does simply index a latent mental state.

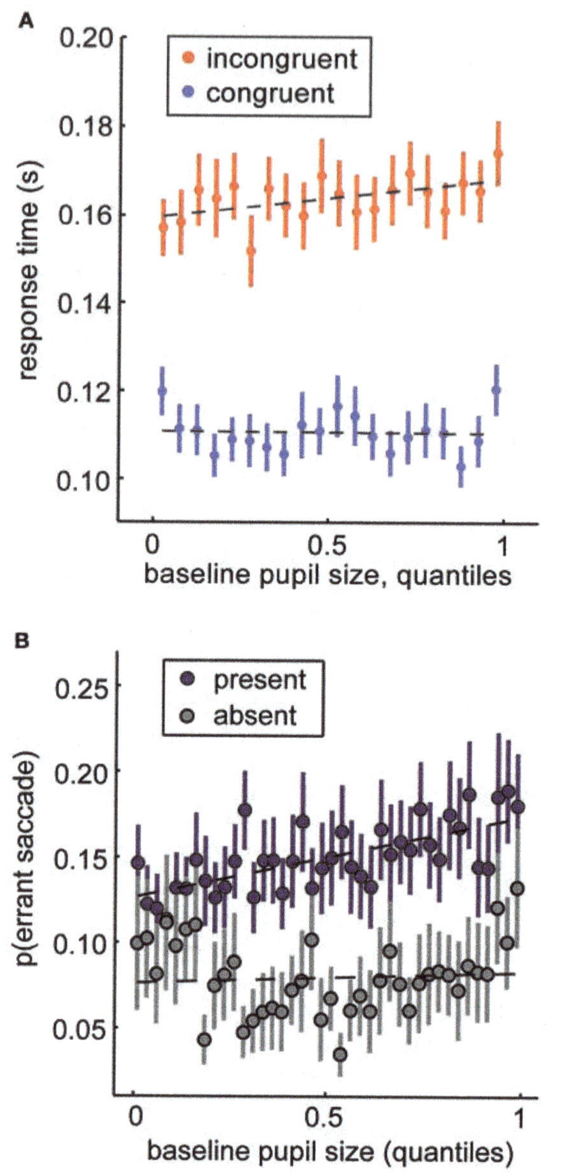

FIGURE 6 | Baseline pupil size under constant luminance predicts changes in attentional priorities. **(A)** In the distraction task (**Figure 1A**), large, salient distractors are presented in conflict with a rewarded target. Monkeys are faster for congruent distractors and slower for incongruent distractors (**Figure 1C**). Increasing pupil size magnifies these effects: attention is more affected by the distractors when pupil size is large. **(B)** In the same task, we can also measure the probability that monkeys would make an "errant saccade" to a task-irrelevant distractor, rather than a rewarded target (these trials were excluded from analysis in **A**). Errant saccade likelihood increases as a function of pupil size at fixation. Panel **(A)** is modified from Ebitz et al. (14) and is reproduced under a Creative Commons Attribution license. Panel **(B)** is modified from Ebitz and Platt (77) with permission from Cell Press and Elsevier.

DISCUSSION

Our central hypothesis is that cognitive modulations of the pupil may be functional, rather than epiphenomenal. To illustrate this perspective, we first discussed the attentional modulation of the pupil light reflex. Previously, we reported that these modulations can be qualitatively reproduced by electrically stimulating part of the prefrontal cortex involved in directing visual spatial attention (28). This suggests that the brain somehow evolved prefrontal control over a brainstem pupil reflex—a motif that seems costly to evolve and/or maintain had it not conferred some adaptive benefit. We highlighted two potential functions this descending control might have, but cautioned that more work is necessary to determine the magnitude of these effects on visual acuity, sensitivity, and light adaptation.

Next, we posited that the pupil may act to filter the visual world—to emphasize some visual features while suppressing others. We highlighted high spatial frequency information as the primary type of information that would be preserved when pupils are small, but suppressed when they are large. This is because optical aberrations—which cause blur and defocus at fine spatial scales—increase as the pupil gets larger. This means that when the pupil is large, the visual world is rendered with a Pictorialist brush: defocus and blur are maximal. Conversely, when the pupil is small, the visual world is rendered in the Purist tradition: rich with detailed, high spatial frequency information.

We have argued that blur and defocus are ideal in circumstances where processing larger forms—e.g., the class of an object, the gist of a scene—is most beneficial. It seems to us that these circumstances are precisely the ones in which pupil size is at its largest—the circumstances where rapid decision-making and generalization across classes are perhaps the most useful for our survival. High spatial frequency information, conversely, is the currency of visual attention, where the selective processing of this fine grained information is critical for individuating targets by recognizing differences in the fine details that differ between them.

AUTHOR CONTRIBUTIONS

RE and TM formulated the hypothesis and wrote the manuscript.

FUNDING

This work was funded by the National Eye Institute (R01-EY014924 to TM and 5T32-EY020485 to RE) and the National Institute of Mental Health (F32-MH102049).

ACKNOWLEDGMENTS

We would like to thank Michael Platt, R. Alison Adcock, Boris Oicherman, and David Ebitz for invaluable discussions. **Figure 6B** is reprinted from Ebitz and Platt (77), Copyright (2015), with permission from Cell Press and Elsevier.

REFERENCES

1. Hess EH. Attitude and pupil size. *Sci Am.* (1965) 212:46–55.
2. Rieger G, Savin-Williams RC. The eyes have it: sex and sexual orientation differences in pupil dilation patterns. *PLoS ONE* (2012) 7:e40256. doi: 10.1371/journal.pone.0040256
3. Atchison DA, Smith G, Efron N. The effect of pupil size on visual acuity in uncorrected and corrected myopia. *Am J Optom Physiol Opt.* (1979) 56:315–23. doi: 10.1097/00006324-197905000-00006
4. Campbell FW, Gregory AH. Effect of size of pupil on visual acuity. *Nature* (1960) 187:1121. doi: 10.1038/1871121c0
5. Liang J, Williams DR. Aberrations and retinal image quality of the normal human eye. *J Opt Soc Am A* (1997) 14:2873. doi: 10.1364/JOSAA.14.002873
6. Walsh G, Charman WN. The effect of pupil centration and diameter on ocular performance. *Vision Res.* (1988) 28:659–65. doi: 10.1016/0042-6989(88)90114-9
7. Anderson P. *Pictorial Photography; Its Principles and Practice.* Philadelphia; London: J. B. Lippincott company (1917).
8. Keating P. From the portrait to the close-up: gender and technology in still photography and Hollywood cinematography. *Cine J.* (2006) 45:90–108. doi: 10.1353/cj.2006.0034
9. Goldwater BC. Psychological significance of pupillary movements. *Psychol Bull.* (1972) 77:340–55.
10. Kahneman D, Beatty J. Pupil diameter and load on memory. *Science* (1966) 154:1583–5. doi: 10.1126/science.154.3756.1583
11. O'Reilly JX, Schüffelgen U, Cuell SF, Behrens TE, Mars RB, Rushworth MF. Dissociable effects of surprise and model update in parietal and anterior cingulate cortex. *Proc Natl Acad Sci USA.* (2013) 110:E3660–9. doi: 10.1073/pnas.1305373110
12. Preuschoff K, t Hart BM, Einhauser W. Pupil dilation signals surprise: evidence for noradrenaline's role in decision making. *Front Neurosci.* (2011) 5:115. doi: 10.3389/fnins.2011.00115
13. Chin-An, W., and Munoz, D. P. Neural basis of location-specific pupil luminance modulation. *Proc. Natl. Acad. Sci. U.S.A.* 115:10446–51. doi: 10.1073/pnas.1809668115
14. Ebitz RB, Pearson JM, Platt ML. Pupil size and social vigilance in rhesus macaques. *Front Neurosci.* (2014) 8:100. doi: 10.3389/fnins.2014.00100
15. Mathôt S, Van der Linden L, Grainger J, Vitu F. The pupillary light response reveals the focus of covert visual attention. *PLoS ONE* (2013) 8:e78168. doi: 10.1371/journal.pone.0078168
16. Algermissen J, Bijleveld E, Jostmann NB, Holland RW. Explore or reset? Pupil diameter transiently increases in self-chosen switches between cognitive labor and leisure in either direction. *BioRxiv* (2018) 379214. doi: 10.1101/379214
17. Jepma M, Nieuwenhuis S. Pupil diameter predicts changes in the exploration–exploitation trade-off: evidence for the adaptive gain theory. *J Cogn Neurosci.* (2011) 23:1587–96. doi: 10.1162/jocn.2010.21548
18. Pajkossy P, Sz Holl Hosi Á, Demeter G, Racsmány M. Tonic noradrenergic activity modulates explorative behavior and attentional set shifting: evidence from pupillometry and gaze pattern analysis. *Psychophysiology* (2017) 54:1839–54. doi: 10.1111/psyp.12964
19. Squire RF, Noudoost B, Schafer RJ, Moore T. Prefrontal contributions to visual selective attention. *Annu Rev Neurosci.* (2013) 36:451–66. doi: 10.1146/annurev-neuro-062111-150439
20. Henderson JM. Human gaze control during real-world scene perception. *Trends Cogn Sci.* (2003) 7:498–504. doi: 10.1016/j.tics.2003.09.006
21. Itti L, Koch C. Computational modelling of visual attention. *Nat Rev Neurosci.* (2001) 2:194–203. doi: 10.1038/35058500
22. Oliva A, Torralba A, Castelhano MS, Henderson JM. Top-down control of visual attention in object detection. In: *IEEE Proceedings of the International Conference on Image Processing, Vol. I, IEEE* (2003) p. 253–6.
23. Loewenfeld IE, Lowenstein O. *The Pupil: Anatomy, Physiology, and Clinical Applications.* Woburn, MA: Butterworth-Heinemann Medical (1993).
24. Magoun HW, Atlas D, Hare WK, Ranson SW. The afferent path of the pupillary light reflex in the monkey. *Brain* (1936) 59:234–49. doi: 10.1093/brain/59.2.234
25. Papageorgiou E, Ticini LF, Hardiess G, Schaeffel F, Wiethoelter H, Mallot HA, et al. The pupillary light reflex pathway Cytoarchitectonic probabilistic maps in hemianopic patients. *Neurology* (2008) 70:956–63. doi: 10.1212/01.wnl.0000305962.93520.ed
26. Wilhelm BJ, Wilhelm H, Moro S, Barbur JL. Pupil response components: studies in patients with Parinaud's syndrome. *Brain* (2002) 125:2296–307.
27. Wilhelm H, Wilhelm B, Petersen D, Schmidt U, Schiefer U. Relative afferent pupillary defects in patients with geniculate and retrogeniculate

lesions. *Neuro Ophthalmol.* (1996) 16:219–24. doi: 10.3109/01658109609 044629
28. Ebitz RB, Moore T. Selective modulation of the pupil light reflex by microstimulation of prefrontal cortex. *J Neurosci.* (2017) 37:5008–18. doi: 10.1523/JNEUROSCI.2433-16.2017
29. Ebitz RB. *Determinants of Distractibility in the Rhesus Macaque*. Ph.D. Thesis. Duke University (2013).
30. Steinhauer SR, Condray R, Kasparek A. Cognitive modulation of midbrain function: task-induced reduction of the pupillary light reflex. *Int J Psychophysiol.* (2000) 39:21–30. doi: 10.1016/S0167-8760(00)00119-7
31. Broadbent DE. *Perception and Communication*. London: Pergamon (1958).
32. Bárány EH, Halldén U. Phasic inhibition of the light reflex of the pupil during retinal rivalry. *J Neurophysiol.* (1948) 11:25–30.
33. Lowe SW, Ogle KN. Dynamics of the pupil during binocular rivalry. *Arch Ophthalmol.* (1966) 75:395–403.
34. Hakerem GAD, Sutton S. *Pupillary response at visual threshold. Nature* (1966) 212:485–6. doi: 10.1038/212485a0
35. Zuber BL, Stark L, Lorber M. Saccadic suppression of the pupillary light reflex. *Exp Neurol.* (1966) 14:351–70. doi: 10.1016/0014-4886(66)90120-8
36. Benedetto A, Binda P. Dissociable saccadic suppression of pupillary and perceptual responses to light. *J Neurophysiol.* (2015) 115:1243–51. doi: 10.1152/jn.00964.2015
37. Mitchell JF, Stoner GR, Reynolds JH. Object-based attention determines dominance in binocular rivalry. *Nature* (2004) 429:410–3. doi: 10.1038/nature02584
38. Stoner GR, Mitchell JF, Fallah M, Reynolds JH. Interacting competitive selection in attention and binocular rivalry. *Prog Brain Res.* (2005) 149:227–34. doi: 10.1016/S0079-6123(05)49016-0
39. Posner MI, Snyder CR, Davidson BJ. Attention and the detection of signals. *J Exp Psychol Gen.* (1980) 109:160–74. doi: 10.1037/0096-3445.109.2.160
40. Deubel H, Schneider WX. Saccade target selection and object recognition: evidence for a common attentional mechanism. *Vision Res.* (1996) 36:1827–37. doi: 10.1016/0042-6989(95)00294-4
41. Hoffman JE, Subramaniam B. The role of visual attention in saccadic eye movements. *Percept Psychophys.* (1995) 57:787–95. doi: 10.3758/BF03206794
42. Moore T, Armstrong KM, Fallah M. Visuomotor origins of covert spatial attention. *Neuron* (2003) 40:671–83. doi: 10.1016/S0896-6273(03)00716-5
43. Rizzolatti G, Riggio L, Dascola I, Umiltá C. Reorienting attention across the horizontal and vertical meridians: evidence in favor of a premotor theory of attention. *Neuropsychologia* (1987) 25:31–40.
44. Steinmetz NA, Moore T. Eye movement preparation modulates neuronal responses in area V4 when dissociated from attentional demands. *Neuron* (2014) 83:496–506. doi: 10.1016/j.neuron.2014.06.014
45. Binda P, Murray SO. Spatial attention increases the pupillary response to light changes. *J Vis.* (2015) 15:1. doi: 10.1167/15.2.1
46. Mathôt S, Van der Stigchel S. New light on the mind's eye: the pupillary light response as active vision. *Curr Dir Psychol Sci.* (2015) 24:374–8. doi: 10.1177/0963721415593725
47. Mathôt S, van der Linden L, Grainger J, Vitu F. The pupillary light response reflects eye-movement preparation. *J Exp Psychol Hum Percept Perform.* (2015) 41:28–35. doi: 10.1037/a0038653
48. Mathôt S, Dalmaijer E, Grainger J, Van der Stigchel S. The pupillary light response reflects exogenous attention and inhibition of return. *J Vis.* (2014) 14:7. doi: 10.1167/14.14.7
49. Huerta MF, Krubitzer LA, Kaas JH. Frontal eye field as defined by intracortical microstimulation in squirrel monkeys, owl monkeys, and macaque monkeys: I. *Subcortical connections. J Comp Neurol.* (1986) 253:415–39. doi: 10.1002/cne.902530402
50. Künzle H, Akert K. Efferent connections of cortical, area 8 (frontal eye field) in Macaca fascicularis. A reinvestigation using the autoradiographic technique. *J Comp Neurol.* (1977) 173:147–63.
51. Leichnetz GR. Connections between the frontal eye field and pretectum in the monkey: an anterograde/retrograde study using HRP gel and TMB neurohistochemistry. *J Comp Neurol.* (1982) 207:394–402.
52. Leichnetz GR. Connections of the medial posterior parietal cortex (area 7m) in the monkey. *Anat Rec.* (2001) 263:215–36. doi: 10.1002/ar.1082
53. Bisley JW, Goldberg ME. Neuronal activity in the lateral intraparietal area and spatial attention. *Science* (2003) 299:81–6. doi: 10.1126/science.1077395
54. Moore T, Fallah M. Control of eye movements and spatial attention. *Proc Natl Acad Sci USA.* (2001) 98:1273–6. doi: 10.1073/pnas.98.3.1273
55. Bruce CJ, Goldberg ME, Bushnell MC, Stanton GB. Primate frontal eye fields. II Physiological and anatomical correlates of electrically evoked eye movements. *J Neurophysiol.* (1985) 54:714–34.
56. Goldberg ME, Bisley J, Powell KD, Gottlieb J, Kusunoki M. The role of the lateral intraparietal area of the monkey in the generation of saccades and visuospatial attention. *Ann NY Acad Sci.* (2002) 956:205–15. doi: 10.1111/j.1749-6632.2002.tb02820.x
57. Schall JD, Hanes DP. Neural basis of saccade target selection in frontal eye field during visual search. *Nature* (1993) 366:467. doi: 10.1038/366467a0
58. Schiller PH, Tehovnik EJ. Neural mechanisms underlying target selection with saccadic eye movements. *Prog Brain Res.* (2005) 149:157–71. doi: 10.1016/S0079-6123(05)49012-3
59. Schiller PH, Sandell JH, Maunsell JH. The effect of frontal eye field and superior colliculus lesions on saccadic latencies in the rhesus monkey. *J Neurophysiol.* (1987) 57:1033–49. doi: 10.1152/jn.1987.57.4.1033
60. Binda P, Murray SO. Keeping a large-pupilled eye on high-level visual processing. *Trends Cogn Sci.* (2015) 19:1–3. doi: 10.1016/j.tics.2014.11.002
61. Frazor RA, Geisler WS. Local luminance and contrast in natural images. *Vision Res.* (2006) 46:1585–98. doi: 10.1016/j.visres.2005.06.038
62. Clarke RJ, Zhang H, Gamlin PD. Characteristics of the pupillary light reflex in the alert rhesus monkey. *J Neurophysiol.* (2003) 89:3179–89. doi: 10.1152/jn.01131.2002
63. De Groot SG, Gebhard JW. Pupil size as determined by adapting luminance. *JOSA* (1952) 42:492–5. doi: 10.1364/JOSA.42.000492
64. Barlow HB. Retinal noise and absolute threshold. *JOSA* (1956) 46:634–9. doi: 10.1364/JOSA.46.000634
65. Baylor DA, Nunn BJ, Schnapf JL. The photocurrent, noise and spectral sensitivity of rods of the monkey Macaca fascicularis. *J Physiol.* (1984) 357:575–607. doi: 10.1113/jphysiol.1984.sp015518
66. Schurman DL. Effects of an artificial pupil in visual perception. *Psychon Sci.* (1968) 11:57.
67. Gould SJ, Vrba ES. Exaptation—a missing term in the science of form. *Paleobiology* (1982) 8:4–15. doi: 10.1017/S0094837300004310
68. Barbur JL, Harlow AJ, Sahraie A. Pupillary responses to stimulus structure, colour and movement. *Ophthalmic Physiol Opt.* (1992) 12:137–41. doi: 10.1111/j.1475-1313.1992.tb00276.x
69. Gamlin PD, Zhang H, Harlow A, Barbur JL. Pupil responses to stimulus color, structure and light flux increments in the rhesus monkey. *Vision Res.* (1998) 38:3353–8. doi: 10.1016/S0042-6989(98)00096-0
70. Kardon R. Pupillary light reflex. *Curr Opin Ophthalmol.* (1995) 6:20–6. doi: 10.1097/00055735-199512000-00004
71. Sahraie A, Barbur JL. Pupil response triggered by the onset of coherent motion. *Graefes Arch Clin Exp Ophthalmol.* (1997) 235:494–500. doi: 10.1007/BF00947006
72. Sokolov EN. Higher nervous functions: The orienting reflex. *Annu Rev Physiol.* (1963) 25:545–80.
73. Wang C-A, Boehnke SE, White BJ, Munoz DP. Microstimulation of the monkey superior colliculus induces pupil dilation without evoking saccades. *J Neurosci.* (2012) 32:3629–36. doi: 10.1523/JNEUROSCI.5512-11.2012
74. Abrams RA, Christ SE. Motion onset captures attention. *Psychol Sci.* (2003) 14:427–32. doi: 10.1111/1467-9280.01458
75. Yantis S, Hillstrom AP. Stimulus-driven attentional capture: evidence from equiluminant visual objects. *J Exp Psychol Hum Percept Perform.* (1994) 20:95. doi: 10.1037/0096-1523.20.1.95
76. Schmid MC, Mrowka SW, Turchi J, Saunders RC, Wilke M, Peters AJ, et al. Blindsight depends on the lateral geniculate nucleus. *Nature* (2010) 466:373. doi: 10.1038/nature09179
77. Ebitz RB, Platt ML. Neuronal activity in primate dorsal anterior cingulate cortex signals task conflict and predicts adjustments in pupil-linked arousal. *Neuron* (2015) 85:628–40. doi: 10.1016/j.neuron.2014.12.053
78. Nassar MR, Rumsey KM, Wilson RC, Parikh K, Heasly B, Gold JI. Rational regulation of learning dynamics by pupil-linked arousal systems. *Nat Neurosci.* (2012) 15:1040–6. doi: 10.1038/nn.3130

79. Kahneman D, Tursky B, Shapiro D, Crider A. Pupillary, heart rate, and skin resistance changes during a mental task. *J Exp Psychol.* (1969) 79:164–7. doi: 10.1037/h0026952
80. Bijleveld E, Custers R, Aarts H. The unconscious eye opener: pupil dilation reveals strategic recruitment of resources upon presentation of subliminal reward cues. *Psychol Sci.* (2009) 20:1313–5. doi: 10.1111/j.1467-9280.2009.02443.x
81. Bradley MM, Miccoli L, Escrig MA, Lang PJ. The pupil as a measure of emotional arousal and autonomic activation. *Psychophysiology* (2008) 45:602–7. doi: 10.1111/j.1469-8986.2008.00654.x
82. Partala T, Surakka V. Pupil size variation as an indication of affective processing. *Int J Hum Comput Stud.* (2003) 59:185–98. doi: 10.1016/S1071-5819(03)00017-X
83. Laeng B, Sirois S, Gredebäck G. Pupillometry: a window to the preconscious? *Perspect Psychol Sci.* (2012) 7:18–27. doi: 10.1177/1745691611427305
84. Joshi S, Li Y, Kalwani RM, Gold JI. Relationships between pupil diameter and neuronal activity in the locus coeruleus, colliculi, and cingulate cortex. *Neuron* (2016) 89:221–34. doi: 10.1016/j.neuron.2015.11.028
85. Aston-Jones G, Cohen JD. An integrative theory of locus coeruleus-norepinephrine function: adaptive gain and optimal performance. *Annu Rev Neurosci.* (2005) 28:403–50. doi: 10.1146/annurev.neuro.28.061604.135709
86. Bouret S, Sara SJ. Network reset: a simplified overarching theory of locus coeruleus noradrenaline function. *Trends Neurosci.* (2005) 28:574–82. doi: 10.1016/j.tins.2005.09.002
87. Cools R, Robbins TW. Chemistry of the adaptive mind. *Philos Trans R Soc Lond Math Phys Eng Sci.* (2004) 362:2871–88. doi: 10.1098/rsta.2004.1468
88. Tervo DG, Proskurin M, Manakov M, Kabra M, Vollmer A, Branson K, et al. Behavioral variability through stochastic choice and its gating by anterior cingulate cortex. *Cell* (2014) 159:21–32. doi: 10.1016/j.cell.2014.08.037
89. Ueltzhöffer K, Armbruster-Genç DJ, Fiebach CJ. Stochastic dynamics underlying cognitive stability and flexibility. *PLoS Comput Biol.* (2015) 11:e1004331. doi: 10.1371/journal.pcbi.1004331
90. Musslick S, Jang SJ, Shvartsman M, Shenhav A, Cohen JD. Constraints associated with cognitive control and the stability-flexibility dilemma. *Proceedings of the 40th Annual Meeting of the Cognitive Science Society.* Madison, WI: Cognitive Science Society (2018) p. 806–11.
91. Einhäuser W, Stout J, Koch C, Carter O. Pupil dilation reflects perceptual selection and predicts subsequent stability in perceptual rivalry. *Proc Natl Acad Sci USA.* (2008) 105:1704–9. doi: 10.1073/pnas.0707727105
92. Ebitz RB, Hayden BY. Dorsal anterior cingulate: a Rorschach test for cognitive neuroscience. *Nat Neurosci.* (2016) 19:1278–9. doi: 10.1038/nn.4387
93. Kolling N, Wittmann MK, Behrens TE, Boorman ED, Mars RB, Rushworth MF. Value, search, persistence and model updating in anterior cingulate cortex. *Nat Neurosci.* (2016) 19:1280–5. doi: 10.1038/nn.4382
94. Shenhav A, Cohen JD, Botvinick MM. Dorsal anterior cingulate cortex and the value of control. *Nat Neurosci.* (2016) 19:1286–91. doi: 10.1038/nn.4384
95. Costa VD, Rudebeck PH. More than meets the eye: the relationship between pupil size and locus coeruleus activity. *Neuron* (2016) 89:8–10. doi: 10.1016/j.neuron.2015.12.031
96. Critchley HD, Tang J, Glaser D, Butterworth B, Dolan RJ. Anterior cingulate activity during error and autonomic response. *Neuroimage* (2005) 27:885–95. doi: 10.1016/j.neuroimage.2005.05.047
97. Ebitz RB, Albarran E, Moore T. Exploration disrupts choice-predictive signals and alters dynamics in prefrontal cortex. *Neuron* (2018) 97:450–61.e9. doi: 10.1016/j.neuron.2017.12.007
98. Ebitz RB, Sleezer BJ, Jedema HP, Bradberry CW, Hayden BY. Exploratory noise governs both flexibility and spontaneous errors and is regulated by cocaine. *BioRxiv* (2018) 328872. doi: 10.1101/328872
99. Gilzenrat MS, Nieuwenhuis S, Jepma M, Cohen JD. Pupil diameter tracks changes in control state predicted by the adaptive gain theory of locus coeruleus function. *Cogn Affect Behav Neurosci.* (2010) 10:252–69. doi: 10.3758/CABN.10.2.252
100. Koss MC. Pupillary dilation as an index of central nervous system α2-adrenoceptor activation. *J Pharmacol Methods* (1986) 15:1–19. doi: 10.1016/0160-5402(86)90002-1
101. Reimer J, McGinley MJ, Liu Y, Rodenkirch C, Wang Q, McCormick DA, et al. Pupil fluctuations track rapid changes in adrenergic and cholinergic activity in cortex. *Nat Commun.* (2016) 7:13289. doi: 10.1038/ncomms13289
102. Engel TA, Steinmetz NA, Gieselmann MA, Thiele A, Moore T, Boahen K. Selective modulation of cortical state during spatial attention. *Science* (2016) 354:1140–4. doi: 10.1126/science.aag1420
103. McGinley MJ, David SV, McCormick DA. Cortical membrane potential signature of optimal states for sensory signal detection. *Neuron* (2015) 87:179–92. doi: 10.1016/j.neuron.2015.05.038
104. McGinley MJ, Vinck M, Reimer J, Batista-Brito R, Zagha E, Cadwell CR, et al. Waking state: rapid variations modulate neural and behavioral responses. *Neuron* (2015) 87:1143–61. doi: 10.1016/j.neuron.2015.09.012
105. Reimer J, Froudarakis E, Cadwell CR, Yatsenko D, Denfield GH, Tolias AS. Pupil fluctuations track fast switching of cortical states during quiet wakefulness. *Neuron* (2014) 84:355–62. doi: 10.1016/j.neuron.2014.09.033
106. Hinton AH. *Practical Pictorial Photography: Practical Instructions in the Application of Photography to Artistic Ends.* London: Hazell, Watson & Viney, Ltd. (1898).
107. Weston E. Photography—not pictorial. *Camera Craft* (1930) 37:313–20.
108. Bunnell PC. Pictorial photography. *Rec Art Mus Princet Univ.* (1992) 51:11–2.
109. Hammond A. Ansel Adams and objectivism: making a photograph with group f/64. *Hist Photogr.* (1998) 22:169–78. doi: 10.1080/03087298.1998.10443873
110. Yeshurun Y, Carrasco M. Spatial attention improves performance in spatial resolution tasks. *Vision Res.* (1999) 39:293–306.
111. Carrasco M, Ling S, Read S. Attention alters appearance. *Nat Neurosci.* (2004) 7:308. doi: 10.1038/nn1194
112. Reynolds JH, Pasternak T, Desimone R. Attention increases sensitivity of V4 neurons. *Neuron* (2000) 26:703–14. doi: 10.1016/S0896-6273(00)81206-4
113. Williford T, Maunsell JH. Effects of spatial attention on contrast response functions in macaque area V4. *J Neurophysiol.* (2006) 96:40–54. doi: 10.1152/jn.01207.2005
114. Carrasco M, Williams PE, Yeshurun Y. Covert attention increases spatial resolution with or without masks: Support for signal enhancement. *J Vis.* (2002) 2:4. doi: 10.1167/2.6.4
115. Torralba A, Oliva A. Statistics of natural image categories. *Netw Comput Neural Syst.* (2003) 14:391–412. doi: 10.1088/0954-898X_14_3_302
116. Mannan SK, Ruddock KH, Wooding DS. The relationship between the locations of spatial features and those of fixations made during visual examination of briefly presented images. *Spat Vis.* (1996) 10:165–88.
117. Mannan SK, Ruddock KH, Wooding DS. Fixation patterns made during brief examination of two-dimensional images. *Perception* (1997) 26:1059–72. doi: 10.1068/p261059
118. Mays LE, Gamlin PD. Neuronal circuitry controlling the near response. *Curr Opin Neurobiol.* (1995) 5:763–8.
119. Myers GA, Stark L. Topology of the near response triad. *Ophthalmic Physiol Opt.* (1990) 10:175–81. doi: 10.1111/j.1475-1313.1990.tb00972.x
120. Charman WN, Whitefoot H. Pupil diameter and the depth-of-field of the human eye as measured by laser speckle. *Opt Acta Int J Opt.* (1977) 24:1211–6. doi: 10.1080/713819479
121. Marcos S, Moreno E, Navarro R. The depth-of-field of the human eye from objective and subjective measurements. *Vision Res.* (1999) 39:2039–49. doi: 10.1016/S0042-6989(98)00317-4
122. Mather G. The use of image blur as a depth cue. *Perception* (1997) 26:1147–58. doi: 10.1068/p261147
123. O'Shea RP, Govan DG, Sekuler R. Blur and contrast as pictorial depth cues. *Perception* (1997) 26:599–612.
124. Collin CA, Mcmullen PA. Subordinate-level categorization relies on high spatial frequencies to a greater degree than basic-level categorization. *Percept Psychophys.* (2005) 67:354–64. doi: 10.3758/BF03206498
125. Gao X, Maurer D. A comparison of spatial frequency tuning for the recognition of facial identity and facial expressions in adults and children. *Vision Res.* (2011) 51:508–19. doi: 10.1016/j.visres.2011.01.011
126. Norman J, Ehrlich S. Spatial frequency filtering and target identification. *Vision Res.* (1987) 27:87–96. doi: 10.1016/0042-6989(87)90145-3

127. Vuilleumier P, Armony JL, Driver J, Dolan RJ. Distinct spatial frequency sensitivities for processing faces and emotional expressions. *Nat Neurosci.* (2003) 6:624–31. doi: 10.1038/nn1057
128. Oliva A, Schyns PG. Coarse blobs or fine edges? Evidence that information diagnosticity changes the perception of complex visual stimuli. *Cognit Psychol.* (1997) 34:72–107. doi: 10.1006/cogp.1997.0667
129. Shulman GL, Wilson J. Spatial frequency and selective attention to local and global information. *Perception* (1987) 16:89–101. doi: 10.1068/p160089
130. Fiorentini A, Maffei L, Sandini G. The role of high spatial frequencies in face perception. *Perception* (1983) 12:195–201. doi: 10.1068/p120195
131. Ebitz RB, Watson KK, Platt ML. Oxytocin blunts social vigilance in the rhesus macaque. *Proc Natl Acad Sci USA.* (2013) 110:11630–5. doi: 10.1073/pnas.1305230110
132. Guastella AJ, Mitchell PB, Dadds MR. Oxytocin increases gaze to the eye region of human faces. *Biol Psychiatry* (2008) 63:3–5. doi: 10.1016/j.biopsych.2007.06.026
133. Ginsburg AP. Visual form perception based on biological filtering. In: L. Spillman and B. R. Wooten, editors. *Sensory Experience, Adaptation, and Perception.* Hillsdale, NJ: Lawrence Erlbaum Associates, Inc. (1984) p. 53–72.
134. Kauffmann L, Ramanoël S, Peyrin C. The neural bases of spatial frequency processing during scene perception. *Front Integr Neurosci.* (2014) 8:37. doi: 10.3389/fnint.2014.00037
135. Oliva A, Schyns PG. Diagnostic colors mediate scene recognition. *Cognit Psychol.* (2000) 41:176–210. doi: 10.1006/cogp.1999.0728
136. Ashtiani MN, Kheradpisheh SR, Masquelier T, Ganjtabesh M. Object categorization in finer levels relies more on higher spatial frequencies and takes longer. *Front Psychol.* (2017) 8:1261. doi: 10.3389/fpsyg.2017.01261
137. Kafkas A, Montaldi D. Recognition memory strength is predicted by pupillary responses at encoding while fixation patterns distinguish recollection from familiarity. *Q J Exp Psychol.* (2011) 64:1971–89. doi: 10.1080/17470218.2011.588335
138. Olds ES, Engel SA. Linearity across spatial frequency in object recognition. *Vis Res.* (1998) 38:2109–18.
139. Goldinger SD, Papesh MH. Pupil dilation reflects the creation and retrieval of memories. *Curr. Dir. Psychol. Sci.* (2012) 21:90–5. doi: 10.1177/0963721412436811
140. Gao Z, Bentin S. Coarse-to-fine encoding of spatial frequency information into visual short-term memory for faces but impartial decay. *J Exp Psychol Hum Percept Perform.* (2011) 37:1051–64. doi: 10.1037/a0023091
141. Tanaka JW, Sengco JA. Features and their configuration in face recognition. *Mem Cognit.* (1997) 25:583–92.
142. Wenger MJ, Townsend JT. Spatial frequencies in short-term memory for faces: a test of three frequency-dependent hypotheses. *Mem Cogn.* (2000) 28:125–42. doi: 10.3758/BF03211581
143. Armel KC, Beaumel A, Rangel A. Biasing simple choices by manipulating relative visual attention. *Judgm Decis Mak.* (2008) 3:396–403.
144. Shimojo S, Simion C, Shimojo E, Scheier C. Gaze bias both reflects and influences preference. *Nat Neurosci.* (2003) 6:1317–22. doi: 10.1038/nn1150
145. McGinty VB, Rangel A, Newsome WT. Orbitofrontal cortex value signals depend on fixation location during free viewing. *Neuron* (2016) 90:1299–311. doi: 10.1016/j.neuron.2016.04.045

2

Chromatic Pupillometry Methods for Assessing Photoreceptor Health in Retinal and Optic Nerve Diseases

A. V. Rukmini [1], Dan Milea [2,3] and Joshua J. Gooley [1]*

[1] Programme in Neuroscience and Behavioural Disorders, Centre for Cognitive Neuroscience, Duke-NUS Medical School, Singapore, Singapore, [2] Singapore National Eye Centre, Singapore Eye Research Institute, Singapore, Singapore, [3] The Ophthalmology and Visual Sciences Academic Clinical Programme (EYE-ACP), SingHealth and Duke-NUS, Singapore, Singapore

***Correspondence:**
Joshua J. Gooley
joshua.gooley@duke-nus.edu.sg

The pupillary light reflex is mediated by melanopsin-containing intrinsically-photosensitive retinal ganglion cells (ipRGCs), which also receive input from rods and cones. Melanopsin-dependent pupillary light responses are short-wavelength sensitive, have a higher threshold of activation, and are much slower to activate and de-activate compared with rod/cone-mediated responses. Given that rod/cone photoreceptors and melanopsin differ in their response properties, light stimuli can be designed to stimulate preferentially each of the different photoreceptor types, providing a read-out of their function. This has given rise to chromatic pupillometry methods that aim to assess the health of outer retinal photoreceptors and ipRGCs by measuring pupillary responses to blue or red light stimuli. Here, we review different types of chromatic pupillometry protocols that have been tested in patients with retinal or optic nerve disease, including approaches that use short-duration light exposures or continuous exposure to light. Across different protocols, patients with outer retinal disease (e.g., retinitis pigmentosa or Leber congenital amaurosis) show reduced or absent pupillary responses to dim blue-light stimuli used to assess rod function, and reduced responses to moderately-bright red-light stimuli used to assess cone function. By comparison, patients with optic nerve disease (e.g., glaucoma or ischemic optic neuropathy, but not mitochondrial disease) show impaired pupillary responses during continuous exposure to bright blue-light stimuli, and a reduced post-illumination pupillary response after light offset, used to assess melanopsin function. These proof-of-concept studies demonstrate that chromatic pupillometry methods can be used to assess damage to rod/cone photoreceptors and ipRGCs. In future studies, it will be important to determine whether chromatic pupillometry methods can be used for screening and early detection of retinal and optic nerve diseases. Such methods may also prove useful for objectively evaluating the degree of recovery to ipRGC function in blind patients who undergo gene therapy or other treatments to restore vision.

Keywords: pupillometry, pupillary light reflex, melanopsin, retina, blind, optic nerve, glaucoma, blue light

INTRODUCTION

The pupillary light reflex is routinely used to assess visual system function and optic nerve disease. As noted by the Greek physician Galen more than 1,800 years ago, poor vision is often characterized by a poor pupillary response to light (1). Until the end of the twentieth century, it was widely assumed that rod and cone photoreceptors that mediate image-forming vision were also responsible for the pupillary light reflex. In normally-sighted individuals, the threshold and spectral sensitivity of pupillary responses closely resembled visual responses (2–5), suggesting involvement of rod and cone photoreceptors. Additionally, pupillary light responses were abnormal in patients with loss of either rod or cone function (6, 7), and were altered in individuals with various forms of color-defective vision (8). Visual field defects were also generally well matched by pupillary field deficits using pupil perimetry (9). Together, these findings supported the conclusion that similar photoreceptor pathways were involved in the pupillary light reflex and image-forming vision. This view was turned on its head when it was discovered that the outer retina was not required for the pupil to respond to light.

Clyde Keeler's pioneering studies of "rodless mice" (gene symbol, *r*, or *rd*) in the 1920s foreshadowed work that led to the identification of photoreceptors in the inner retina. Keeler's *rd/rd* mice showed rapid loss of rods in early postnatal development, followed by secondary degeneration of cone photoreceptors (10). Despite showing behavioral and physiologic signs of blindness, these mice exhibited intact pupillary responses to light that were slower and lower in amplitude compared with normal mice (11). Keeler speculated that retinal ganglion cells or other cell types in the eye might be activated directly (12), but critics argued that *rd/rd* mice were not actually blind and that Keeler's observations could be explained by sparing of visual photoreceptors in the outer retina (13). Criticism of Keeler's work was addressed several decades later when *rd/rd* mice were crossed with *cl* mice, resulting in complete ablation of rods and cones. Pupillary light responses were intact in *rd/rd cl* mice (14), suggesting that a non-rod, non-cone photoreceptor in the mammalian eye was capable of mediating the pupillary light reflex. Similarly, *rd/rd cl* mice exhibited intact light-induced resetting of circadian rhythms and melatonin suppression (15, 16). In parallel, it was found that pupillary responses were preferentially spared in patients with impaired vision caused by mitochondrial disease (17, 18), and some blind patients with no light perception showed intact circadian and melatonin suppression responses to light (19). These studies provided evidence that visual and non-visual light responses were mediated by distinct photoreceptor pathways.

The discovery of intrinsically photosensitive retinal ganglion cells (ipRGCs) was a turning point in our understanding of the pupillary light reflex and other non-visual light responses. Although ipRGCs can be activated by rod and cone photoreceptors in the outer retina (20, 21), they contain the invertebrate-like opsin melanopsin (*Opn4*) which renders them directly photosensitive (20, 22, 23). Melanopsin cells project to the olivary pretectal nucleus to mediate the pupillary light reflex (22, 24, 25), as well as brain areas involved in circadian rhythms and sleep-wake regulation (22, 24, 26, 27). In mice, there are several types of melanopsin cells (named M1 to M6) that have been identified based on their morphology, central projections, electrophysiological response properties, and their role in different non-visual light responses (28, 29). The M1 ipRGCs in mice that express the transcription factor *Brn3b* project to the olivary pretectal nucleus and are thought to be necessary for the pupillary light reflex (25). Different types of melanopsin cells have also been described in macaques and humans (30, 31), but their role in different non-visual light responses is still under investigation. Melanopsin is required for pupillary light responses in blind mice (32, 33), but visual photoreceptors are capable of mediating the pupillary light reflex in melanopsin knockout mice (34). The pupillary light reflex and other non-visual light responses are abolished only when rod, cone, and melanopsin signaling pathways are disrupted simultaneously (32, 33). Selective ablation of the melanopsin-containing ipRGCs also severely attenuates pupillary responses to light (35), suggesting that most, if not all, light information from outer retinal photoreceptors to the olivary pretectal nucleus is channeled through a few thousand melanopsin cells that are distributed broadly across the retina (**Figure 1**). It remains possible, however, that conventional RGCs also provide input to the midbrain, either directly or indirectly, to modulate pupillary light responses.

Differences between rod/cone photoreceptors and melanopsin in their anatomic location and response properties has led to renewed interest in using the pupillary light reflex to detect loss of photoreceptor function in retinal and optic nerve diseases. Melanopsin cells are not required for sight in mice (35) and are insufficient to support image-forming vision in blind patients without a functional outer retina (19, 37). Pupillary light responses can be used to estimate damage to the afferent pathway involved in image-forming-vision, however, if the function of ipRGCs and conventional RGCs is similarly impaired by a given disease. Given that rods, cones, and melanopsin play different roles in mediating the pupillary light reflex (38, 39), light stimuli can be designed to stimulate preferentially one or more photoreceptor types, providing a read-out of their function. This serves as the basis for chromatic pupillometry (also termed color pupillometry or selective wavelength pupillometry), which refers to measuring pupillary responses to different wavelengths and intensities of light in order to differentiate rod, cone, and melanopsin-dependent contributions to the pupillary light reflex.

The goal of this article is to review how chromatic pupillometry methods can be used to detect loss of photoreceptor function in retinal and optic nerve diseases. In the first part of this article, we focus on research in humans demonstrating that rod/cone photoreceptors and melanopsin differ in their contributions to the pupillary light reflex. We discuss evidence that the wavelength, irradiance, and duration of a light stimulus can be manipulated to stimulate preferentially rod, cone, or melanopsin-dependent pupillary light responses. In the second part of this article, we review evidence that chromatic pupillometry methods, in particular those that measure pupillary responses to blue light vs. red light, can be used to detect loss of photoreceptor function in

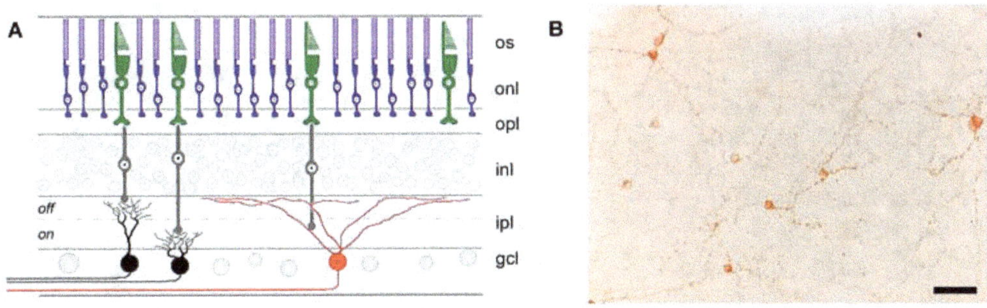

FIGURE 1 | Retinal location of different photoreceptor types. **(A)** Rods (blue) and cones (green) in the outer retina transmit light information via bipolar cells (gray) to retinal ganglion cells (RGCs) in the inner retina. RGCs that are involved in image-forming vision are not directly photosensitive (black), whereas RGCs involved in non-visual light responses (e.g., the pupillary light reflex) contain the photopigment melanopsin (red) and are intrinsically photosensitive. os, outer segments; onl, outer nuclear layer; opl, outer plexiform layer; inl, inner nuclear layer; ipl, inner plexiform layer; gcl, ganglion cell layer. **(B)** Melanopsin-containing RGCs (labeled immunohistochemically in brown) are distributed broadly and in small numbers across the retina, as shown in a flat-mount preparation of a rat retina (scale bar = 50 μm). Panel **(A)** was reproduced with permission from Berson (36). Panel **(B)** is a photomicrograph provided by the corresponding author, JG (Clifford Saper Laboratory, Beth Israel Deaconess Medical Center, Boston, MA).

diseases that primarily affect either the outer retina or the inner retina. We discuss protocols that use light flashes or short-duration light stimuli to assess the health of rod/cone photoreceptors and ipRGCs (e.g., based on the post-illumination pupillary response), as well as protocols in which pupillary constriction is measured during continuous exposure to light (e.g., stepwise changes in irradiance or ramp-up light exposures). Strengths and limitations of these chromatic pupillometry methods are discussed, with a view toward developing clinical protocols that can be used as part of a routine ophthalmic examination to assess the functional integrity of different photoreceptor types. Finally, we review potential future applications for chromatic pupillometry in screening for retinal diseases, and in monitoring disease progression and/or recovery.

PHOTORECEPTOR CONTRIBUTIONS TO THE PUPILLARY LIGHT REFLEX

Based on electrophysiological studies of ipRGCs in mice and macaques (20, 23), melanopsin-dependent responses differ markedly from those mediated by rod/cone photoreceptors. First, when synaptic transmission from the outer retina is blocked, the action spectrum for the intrinsically-driven (i.e., melanopsin-dependent) light response exhibits peak sensitivity to short-wavelength light in the blue portion of the visual spectrum ($\lambda_{max} \approx 480$ nm). Hence, the spectral maximum for melanopsin differs from human rods ($\lambda_{max} \approx 505$ nm) (40, 41) and short, medium, and long-wavelength cones (42–44). Second, melanopsin-dependent ipRGC responses to light are less sensitive than extrinsically-driven responses mediated by rods and cones. Therefore, the ipRGCs can be activated by outer retinal photoreceptors below the threshold of activation for the intrinsic, melanopsin-dependent light response. Third, melanopsin-dependent light responses of ipRGCs are slower and last longer, relative to rod/cone-dependent responses. The intrinsic response shows a longer response latency following light stimulus onset, and is sustained for as long as the light stimulus is presented. The intrinsic response also extends markedly after light offset unlike rod and cone signaling (20, 21, 23). As reviewed in the following sections, these response characteristics closely match those of the pupillary light reflex in humans, demonstrating complementary roles of outer retinal photoreceptors and melanopsin in mediating pupillary responses to light.

Melanopsin-Dependent Pupillary Responses Are Sensitive to Short-Wavelength Light

The identity of photoreceptors that contribute to the pupillary light reflex has been investigated by measuring the sensitivity of pupillary responses to light as a function of wavelength. In studies that have examined the minimum amount of light energy required to elicit a detectable change in size of the dark-adapted pupil, spectral responses to light flashes closely resemble the scotopic luminosity function ($\lambda_{max} \approx 500$–$510$) (2, 5, 45) (**Figure 2A**). If the effects of rod stimulation are masked by providing a background of blue light to render them insensitive, threshold spectral responses to monochromatic light stimuli are higher and closely match the photopic luminosity function ($\lambda_{max} \approx 555$ nm) (2, 45) (**Figure 2A**). These studies implicate rods and cones in mediating pupillary responses to short-duration light exposures. When the pupil is measured during exposure to continuous dim light (e.g., after 20–30 s of continuous light) below the threshold of color vision, pupillary responses are also matched well by the scotopic luminosity function (3, 4). In the photopic visual range, however, pupillary responses to continuous light are not well matched by either scotopic or photopic luminosity functions (**Figure 2B**). With the exception of one study (2), pupillary responses during continuous exposure to light were most sensitive to short-wavelength light ($\lambda_{max} \approx 480$–$500$ nm) (4, 39, 45, 46, 48). These findings are consistent with an important role for melanopsin in mediating the sustained

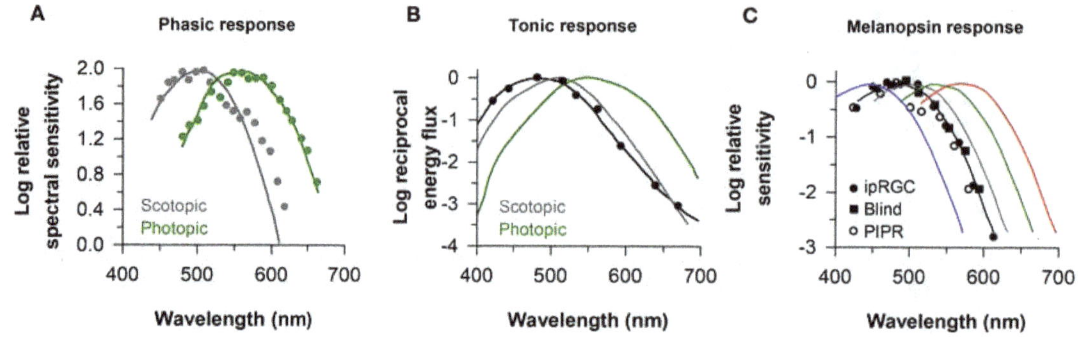

FIGURE 2 | Spectral responses of the pupillary light reflex. **(A)** The spectral sensitivity for pupillary responses to flashes of dim light (gray circles) and bright light on a rod-suppressing blue background (green circles) are shown for representative subjects. Spectral responses for the phasic pupillary light reflex closely resemble scotopic and photopic luminosity functions (gray and green lines, respectively). **(B)** The spectral sensitivity for the tonic pupillary light reflex during continuous exposure to light (black circles) is short-wavelength shifted (peak constriction, ≈ 490 nm) relative to scotopic and photopic luminosity functions (gray and green lines, respectively). **(C)** The spectral sensitivity of melanopsin-dependent responses (peak constriction, ≈ 480 nm) is shown for intrinsically-photosensitive retinal ganglion cells in macaques (ipRGCs, black circles), the pupillary light reflex in a blind individual with no light perception (Blind, black squares), and the sustained post-illumination pupillary light response in individuals with normal vision (PIPR, open circles). The spectral sensitivity of rod and cone photoreceptors is shown for comparison (rods, gray; S-cones, blue; M-cones, green; L-cones, red). Panel **(A)** is redrawn and modified with permission from (2); Panel **(B)** was redrawn and modified with permission from (46); Panel **(C)** was redrawn and modified with permission from (23), with data superimposed from (37) and (47).

(i.e., tonic) pupillary light reflex. As discussed below, however, detailed analyses of spectral responses suggest that rod and cone photoreceptors contribute substantially during the early part of a continuous light exposure, and outer retinal photoreceptors mediate the tonic pupillary light reflex at low irradiances (38, 39).

The response properties of melanopsin-dependent pupillary light responses can be studied in isolation in blind individuals with complete loss of visual function and degeneration of the outer retina, but with a relatively intact retinal ganglion cell layer (19, 37, 38, 49). In a blind woman with autosomal-dominant cone-rod dystrophy and no detectable rod or cone function (no light perception or electroretinography response, and no outer retina based on fundus photography and ocular coherence tomography), the action spectrum for the pupillary light reflex showed peak sensitivity to 476 nm light (**Figure 2C**). In a different blind individual with retinitis pigmentosa and no light perception, the spectral response for monochromatic exposures matched for corneal photon density (13 log photons/cm^2/s) exhibited peak sensitivity to 490 nm light (38). These results are consistent with action spectra for the pupillary light reflex in *rd/rd cl* mice with complete degeneration of the outer retina ($\lambda_{max} \approx 479$ nm) (14), and in macaques with synaptic blockade of signals from the outer retina ($\lambda_{max} \approx 479$ nm) (47). Moreover, spectral responses for the pupillary light reflex in blind individuals are similar to electrophysiological responses of ipRGCs of mice and macaques with blocked synaptic transmission from rods and cones ($\lambda_{max} \approx 484$ and 482 nm, respectively) (20, 23) (**Figure 2C**). In humans with normal vision, the action spectrum for the post-illumination pupillary response (i.e., sustained pupillary constriction after light exposure offset) also exhibits peak sensitivity to about 482 nm light (**Figure 2C**), suggesting that this response is driven predominantly by melanopsin (47, 50). Together, these findings in humans show that melanopsin-dependent pupillary responses are sensitive to short-wavelength blue light (i.e., $\lambda_{max} \approx 480$ nm).

Melanopsin-Dependent Pupillary Responses Are Less Sensitive to Light Than Rods and Cones

The relative sensitivity of rod, cone, and melanopsin-dependent ipRGC responses has been characterized *in vitro* in the retinae of macaques, which have trichromatic vision similar to humans (23). Following dark adaptation, rod-driven responses in ipRGCs are highly sensitive and can respond to light stimuli as low as 6–7 log quanta/cm^2/s, which is 4–5 log units below the threshold for (L + M) cone-mediated responses. By comparison, melanopsin-driven responses are about a log unit less sensitive than cones, with a threshold of activation of about 11–12 log quanta/cm^2/s (23). As reviewed in the previous section, rods mediate the pupillary light reflex at light intensities below the threshold of color discrimination, and cones contribute to phasic pupillary light responses in the photopic visual range. Decades before melanopsin was discovered, there was evidence that neither rods nor cones were necessary for pupillary constriction responses to bright light. In achromats without cone photoreceptor function, it was shown that the pupils could respond to light in a dose-dependent manner well beyond the point of rod saturation (51). After light adaptation, achromats also exhibited short-wavelength sensitivity ($\lambda_{max} \approx 490$ nm) to flashes of light within the photopic visual range (7), hence deviating substantially from responses in normally-sighted individuals ($\lambda_{max} \approx 555$ nm) (2, 45). In a patient with congenital stationary night blindness (Oguchi disease) with total loss of rod function, the sustained pupillary light reflex was severely impaired at low-to-moderate light intensities, but appeared relatively normal during exposure to bright light (6). With the benefit of hindsight, intact pupillary responses to high-irradiance light stimuli in patients with achromatopsia and Oguchi disease were likely due to stimulation of melanopsin.

The relative sensitivity of melanopsin-dependent pupillary light responses has been studied in a totally-visually blind individual with intact non-visual photoreception (37, 38). Based on irradiance-response curves to 480 nm light, pupillary constriction responses in the blind individual were preserved at higher irradiances, i.e., $\geq$13 log photons/cm^2/s measured at the cornea, but were severely attenuated compared with sighted individuals across most of the photopic range of vision (**Figure 3**). These results are consistent with findings in *rd/rd* mice and *rd/rd cl* mice in which pupillary light responses were reduced except at the highest irradiances tested (>13 log quanta/cm^2/s) (33, 34). In contrast, *Opn4* null mice show normal pupillary light responses at lower irradiances, but reduced responses to higher-intensity light stimuli (>13 log quanta/cm^2/s) (33, 34). The threshold for pupillary constriction in the blind individual ($\approx$11–12 log photons/cm^2/s) was also similar to results reported for pupillary light responses in mice that lack rod and cone function (34, 52), and in macaques in which rod and cone signaling was pharmacologically blocked (47). Together, these findings demonstrate that outer retinal photoreceptors are required for normal pupillary responses at low-to-moderate intensities of light, whereas melanopsin alone is sufficient to drive a normal pupillary light reflex in the presence of a bright, continuous light stimulus (especially blue light). Even in normally-sighted individuals, pupillary responses to bright light (using a criterion of a 75% maximum constriction response) are consistent with the spectral sensitivity of melanopsin, suggesting that melanopsin dominates the pupillary light reflex at high irradiances (39).

Melanopsin-Dependent Pupillary Responses to Light Are Slow and Sustained

The pupillary light reflex is often described as having phasic and tonic components. The phasic component refers to the transient, high-amplitude response that occurs in response to a light flash or at the beginning of a continuous light stimulus. By comparison, the tonic component refers to the sustained pupillary response that occurs during continuous exposure to light. To a large degree, phasic and tonic components of the pupillary light reflex reflect the contribution of rod/cone photoreceptors and melanopsin to ipRGC responses (20, 23). Rods and cones contribute strongly to ipRGC responses and pupillary constriction at the beginning of light exposure (e.g., over seconds to minutes), but their contribution declines substantially over time (23, 39, 53). After the phasic component of the pupillary light reflex, rods and melanopsin appear to contribute to sustained ipRGC and pupillary light responses (21, 23, 54). Consequently, there is a short-wavelength shift in spectral sensitivity over time during a continuous light stimulus, with responses to higher-irradiance light dominated by melanopsin (38, 39, 48). Studies using the silent substitution method have provided additional evidence that melanopsin contributes to sustained pupillary constriction in the photopic visual range, with lesser contributions from rods and/or (L + M) cones (55, 56). Consistent with a role for outer retinal photoreceptors in mediating the tonic component of the pupillary light reflex, sustained pupillary constriction can be driven by long-wavelength red light (631 nm; for at least 50 min) outside the range of sensitivity of melanopsin-dependent ipRGC responses (57).

The time-course of pupillary re-dilation after light stimulus offset also appears to have phasic and tonic components that are differentially influenced by rod/cone photoreceptors and melanopsin (38, 39). The pupil typically re-dilates rapidly (i.e., over the course of several seconds) toward its dark-adapted size after exposure to a light stimulus of low-to-moderate intensity (**Figure 4A**). In contrast, the pupil can show a sustained constriction response (i.e., over tens of seconds) after exposure to a high-intensity light stimulus (**Figure 4B**). The phasic component of pupillary re-dilation is absent or markedly delayed in blind humans and mice lacking a functional outer retina (38, 59), demonstrating that rods and cones contribute to the fast pupillary response after light stimulus offset. As shown in humans and in macaques, the sustained post-illumination pupillary response (PIPR) is driven predominantly by melanopsin and is sensitive to short-wavelength blue light (47). Consequently, a strong PIPR can be driven after the offset of a bright-blue light stimulus, whereas there is little or no PIPR after a red-light stimulus (**Figure 4B**). Notably, the PIPR in visually-normal individuals is much greater when the light stimulus is presented to the dark-adapted eye compared with an adapting background field, indicating that pre-exposure light conditions modulate the strength of the PIPR (60).

The sluggish response properties of melanopsin have been studied in detail in a blind individual without a functional outer retina (**Figure 5A**) (38). In the blind person, the pupil responded slowly to light stimulus onset, often taking several seconds to show a detectable response, with a response latency that decreased linearly with increasing light intensity. By comparison, the rapid pupillary light response in sighted individuals masked the slow contribution of melanopsin to the pupillary light reflex at the start of a continuous light exposure. After the pupil reached its minimal size in the blind individual, the melanopsin-dependent pupillary response was sustained, similar to the response in sighted individuals for a high-irradiance light stimulus. After light stimulus offset, however, the pupil in the blind participant re-dilated slowly compared with sighted individuals (**Figure 5A**), suggesting that the melanopsin-dependent PIPR was unmasked or enhanced in the absence of rod and cone function (61–63). Due to the slow time course of pupillary light responses in the blind individual, his pupil was unable to track an intermittent light stimulus (5 s on, 5 s off), whereas pupillary constriction and dilation responses were time-locked to each light and dark pulse in sighted individuals (**Figure 5B**). These findings suggest that rods and cones are superior to melanopsin at encoding rapid changes in light intensity (i.e., abrupt changes in light). Hence, rod/cone photoreceptors likely dominate phasic pupillary responses to the onset and offset of a light stimulus, whereas melanopsin can track low-contrast modulation of light intensity (64).

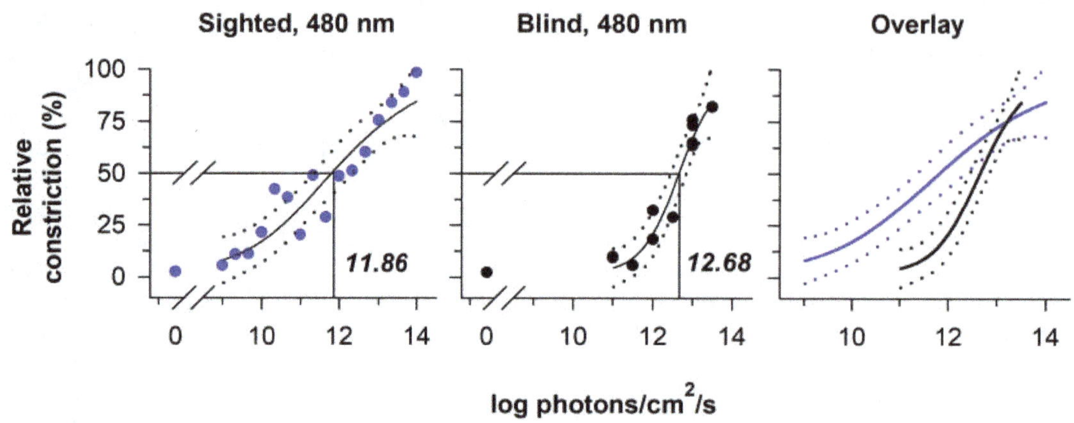

FIGURE 3 | The contribution of rod-cone photoreceptors and melanopsin to pupillary light responses is irradiance-dependent. Irradiance-response curves for the pupillary light reflex are shown for a continuously presented blue-light stimulus (480 nm; pupil measured from 90 to 120 s after light onset) in individuals with normal vision (blue circles, left panel) and in a blind individual with no light perception (black circles, middle panel). An overlay of the irradiance-response curves (right panel) shows reduced pupillary responses to lower-irradiance exposures in the blind individual, whereas the melanopsin-dependent response at the highest irradiances tested was comparable to sighted individuals. In each plot, the best-fit regression line is shown with 95% CIs (solid and dotted lines, respectively). Drop lines indicate the irradiance corresponding to a half-maximal pupillary constriction response. Data are replotted with permission from (38).

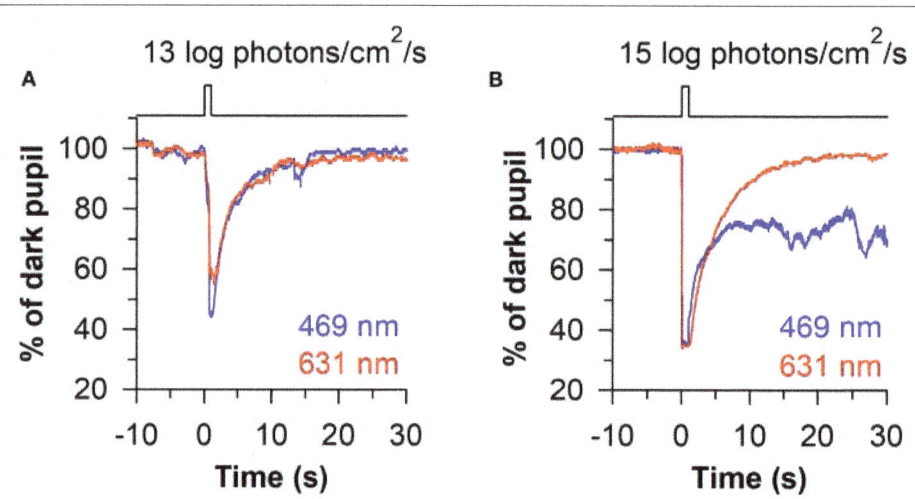

FIGURE 4 | Phasic and sustained pupillary responses to 1-s flashes of blue or red light. **(A)** Pupillary responses are shown for a representative individual exposed to a moderately-bright 1-s flash of either blue light or red light (469 or 631 nm; 13 log photons/cm^2/s). The pupil showed a transient high-amplitude constriction response after light onset, with fast re-dilation of the pupil after light offset. **(B)** In response to a high-intensity 1-s flash of light (15 log photons/cm^2/s), the transient pupillary constriction response was followed by a prolonged post-illumination pupillary light response (PIPR) to the blue light stimulus, but not the red light stimulus. The sustained PIPR is thought to be driven by slow-deactivation of melanopsin after light offset. The figure is replotted with permission from (58).

Summary of Photoreceptor Contributions to the Pupillary Light Reflex

Outer retinal photoreceptors and melanopsin contribute differentially to the pupillary light reflex. Melanopsin-dependent pupillary responses are short-wavelength sensitive compared with rod- and cone-mediated responses and have a higher threshold of activation. Additionally, rods and cones dominate the phasic component of pupillary responses after light stimulus onset and offset. In contrast, melanopsin-dependent responses are much slower and sustained, and dominate the tonic component of the pupillary light reflex during exposure to high-irradiance, continuous light stimuli. Rods can mediate the tonic pupillary light reflex at low-to-moderate light intensities, whereas the role of cones is uncertain. Following the offset of a high-intensity short-wavelength light stimulus, melanopsin dominates the slower component of the PIPR, resulting in a slower re-dilation of the pupil toward its dark-adapted size. These findings demonstrate that responses of rod/cone photoreceptors and melanopsin can be assessed differentially using the pupillary light reflex. This has given rise to chromatic pupillometry, in which the functional integrity of photoreceptors in the outer retina and inner retina

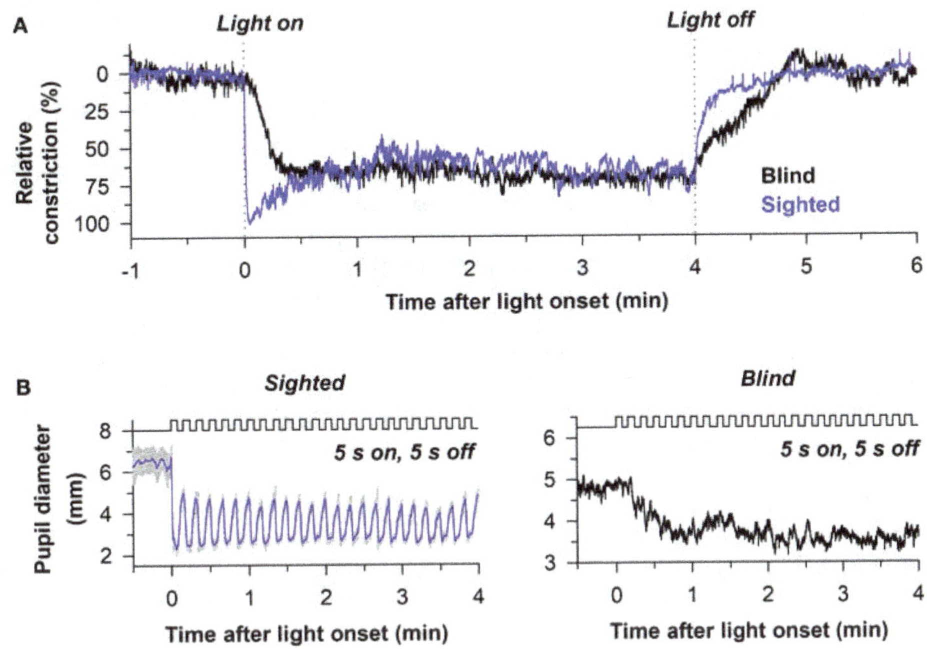

FIGURE 5 | Melanopsin-dependent pupillary responses are slower than rod/cone-dependent responses. **(A)** Representative pupillary light responses are shown for a sighted individual and a blind individual without rod and cone function. The pupil in the blind individual responded slowly after light onset and light offset, indicating that outer retinal photoreceptors are necessary for the phasic component of the pupillary light reflex. **(B)** In sighted individuals, the pupil could track an intermittent light stimulus (480 nm, 13 log photons/cm^2/s) with alternating periods of light and darkness (5 s of light, 5 s of darkness). By comparison, the pupil in the blind individual was unable to track the intermittent stimulus. Rather, the melanopsin-dependent pupillary response increased across several light pulses until reaching a steady response. Data are replotted with permission from (38).

can be examined using light stimuli that target rods, cones, or melanopsin.

CHROMATIC PUPILLOMETRY METHODS FOR ASSESSING RETINAL AND OPTIC NERVE DISEASES

Chromatic pupillometry methods exploit differences in response characteristics of rod/cone photoreceptors and melanopsin to assess damage to the outer retina and inner retina, respectively. Over the past decade, several types of light exposure protocols have been developed to assess the functional integrity of rods, cones, and ipRGCs. Most of these studies have compared pupillary responses to blue light and red light using light-emitting diodes, in order to isolate as best as possible the function of outer retinal photoreceptors vs. ipRGCs. Rod-mediated pupillary responses have the lowest threshold of activation, and hence low-irradiance blue light stimuli in the scotopic visual range can be used to test for rod function (e.g., dim light flashes after dark adaptation). Cone-mediated pupillary responses are less sensitive to light than rods and are preferentially sensitive to longer-wavelength light. Therefore, red light stimuli in the photopic visual range can be used to test for cone function (e.g., red light flashes after light adaptation). Melanopsin-dependent pupillary responses are the least sensitive to light and are preferentially sensitive to short-wavelength blue light. As such, high-irradiance blue light stimuli can be used to test for ipRGC function. Chromatic pupillometry protocols can be categorized broadly as those using short-duration light stimuli to assess photoreceptor health (e.g., light flashes or pulses), or those using continuously presented light stimuli (e.g., >30 s). Here, we review evidence that either of these approaches can be used to detect inner vs. outer retinal damage.

Chromatic Pupillometry Methods That use Short-Duration Light Stimuli

Assessing Photoreceptor Function Using 1-s Light Flashes

An important goal of chromatic pupillometry is to develop a standardized clinical protocol for assessing the health of retinal photoreceptors. Using a Ganzfeld system with full-field illumination of the eye (with the other eye covered with a patch), it was shown that a series of 1-s light exposures (470 nm blue light or 640 nm red light) could be used to assess rod, cone, and melanopsin contributions to the pupillary light reflex (60). Rod function was tested using a dim blue light stimulus after 10 min of dark adaptation (−3 or −2 log cd/m^2), cone function was tested using a bright red light stimulus under light adaptation with a rod-suppressing blue background (2.6 log cd/m^2 of red light on a background of 0.78 cd/m^2 of blue light), and melanopsin function was tested using a bright blue light stimulus after dark adaptation (2.6 log cd/m^2) and measured using the PIPR.

Pupillary responses under these lighting conditions were then compared between normally-sighted individuals and patients with either retinitis pigmentosa ($n = 5$) or Leber congenital amaurosis (LCA, $n = 3$). Consistent with loss of rod function and a higher threshold of activation for the pupillary light reflex (65, 66), patients with outer retinal disease showed weak or absent pupillary responses to the rod-weighted dim blue light stimulus, as well as attenuated responses to the cone-weighted red light stimulus (60). In contrast, the PIPR for the melanopsin-weighted stimulus appeared normal in patients with retinitis pigmentosa or LCA after dark adaptation. Interestingly, the PIPR was prolonged in patients with outer retinal disease compared with controls when bright blue light was presented on a blue background (2.6 log cd/m^2 of blue light on a background of 0.78 cd/m^2 of blue light), suggesting that light adaptation did not suppress melanopsin-dependent responses to the same extent as seen in healthy participants.

These findings were confirmed and extended using a similar light exposure protocol in patients with *CEP290*-associated LCA ($n = 6$), demonstrating reduced pupillary responses to rod- and cone-weighted light stimuli and an intact PIPR to the melanopsin-weighted stimulus after dark adaptation (**Figures 6A–C**) (67). Comparable results were obtained in another study in which pupillary responses were assessed in patients with LCA or early-onset severe retinal dystrophy ($n = 6$) caused by *RPE65* mutations (68), except that the PIPR measured after light offset for the bright blue light stimulus (percentage of constriction after 30 s) was greater in patients compared with controls. The ability of this protocol to detect selective loss of cone function has also been demonstrated in a pair of patients with mutations in the *CNGB3* gene, resulting in achromatopsia. In these patients, pupillary responses to rod- and melanopsin-weighted light stimuli were in the normal range, whereas pupillary responses were severely blunted for the cone-weighted light stimulus (68). In contrast, in patients with idiopathic intracranial hypertension ($n = 13$), which can result in ischemia of the optic nerve, pupillary responses were reduced for rod-, and melanopsin-weighted light stimuli, demonstrating reduced ipRGC transmission to the midbrain (69). In another study, patients with moderate-to-severe non-proliferative diabetic retinopathy (NPDR) showed normal pupillary responses to the rod-weighted light stimulus and reduced responses to the cone-weighted light stimulus (70). Patients with mild or moderate-to-severe NPDR also exhibited an attenuated PIPR in the melanopsin-weighted light condition, suggesting damage to both the outer and inner retina.

Pupillometry protocols have also been developed to assess the irradiance-dependent effects of blue and red light stimuli (1-s flashes) on the pupillary light reflex in patients with retinal or optic nerve disease. In such protocols, irradiance-response curves are constructed by exposing participants to a sequence of 1-s light flashes that increase in intensity over time, with each stimulus preceded by a period of darkness (or on a background of continuous light) to allow the pupil to re-dilate before the next stimulus is administered. Loss of rod or cone function can be inferred by reduced sensitivity to blue and red light stimuli compared with individuals with normal vision (i.e., a rightward shift in the irradiance-response curve), whereas impairment of the melanopsin-dependent ipRGC response can be assessed by the PIPR after exposure to high-intensity blue light. This method has been tested in patients with LCA ($n = 4$) using a Ganzfeld system, in which pupillary responses (i.e., peak pupillary constriction, normalized to the baseline pupil) to 1-s red light (640 nm) and blue light (467 nm) stimuli were measured over a 6 log unit range of intensities matched for photopic luminance (−4.0 to 2.0 log cd/m^2, increased in 0.5 log steps) (71). Patients with LCA exhibited decreased sensitivity to blue light with severely reduced pupillary responses for dim light stimuli (<-1.0 log cd/m^2), whereas pupillary responses were in the normal range for bright red light stimuli. These findings are consistent with degeneration of rods and loss of scotopic visual function, with sparing of cone-mediated responses. The PIPR for bright blue light (2.6 log cd/m^2) was also in the normal range in patients with LCA, which is consistent with intact retinal ganglion cell function. Comparable results were obtained in patients with autosomal dominant retinitis pigmentosa caused by a mutation in the *NR2E3* gene ($n = 9$; 1-s exposures blue light; −6.0 to 1 log cd/m^2 in 0.5 log unit steps), in which rod-dependent pupillary responses to blue light exhibited reduced sensitivity compared with healthy controls (72). Using a protocol in which red light flashes were presented on a background of rod-suppressing blue light (−1.0 to 1.5 log cd/m^2 of red light after 3 min of light adaptation to 0.78 log cd/m^2 of blue light), cone-weighted responses were in the normal range in patients with retinitis pigmentosa. The PIPR after exposure to bright blue light (2.6 log cd/m^2) was intact but marginally reduced in patients, indicating that function of the inner retina was largely preserved. Similar results were observed in patients with retinal dystrophy caused by enhanced S-cone syndrome ($n = 4$), in which autosomal recessive mutations in the *NR2E3* gene result in an overabundance of S-cones and reduced function of rods (73). In these patients, rod-dependent pupillary responses were undetectable and cone-dependent responses to red light were slightly attenuated, whereas pupillary responses to the melanopsin-weighted stimulus were in the normal range.

Irradiance-dependent responses to 1-s light flashes have also been examined in patients affected by various types of optic neuropathies. In patients with mild-to-moderate visual dysfunction due to hereditary optic neuropathy (HON; $n = 8$), dose-response curves to rod-weighted blue light stimuli (463 nm, −4.0 to −1.0 log cd/m^2 in 0.5 log unit steps with intervening dark periods) and cone-weighted red light stimuli (635 nm, 1.0 to 2.5 log cd/m^2 in 0.5 log unit steps on a background of 92 lux of light) were comparable to responses observed in healthy controls (74). The PIPR after exposure to bright blue light (2.3 log cd/m^2) in these patients was also in the normal range, indicating preserved melanopsin-dependent ipRGC function. In another study, pupillary responses were examined in 10 patients with Leber HON (LHON), having severe visual field loss and marked thinning of the retinal nerve fiber layer (RNFL), quantified with optical coherence tomography (OCT) (75). In these LHON patients, the phasic pupillary responses to blue light and red light stimuli (0, 1, 2, and 2.4 log cd/m^2) were reduced relative to healthy controls, but there was substantial overlap in

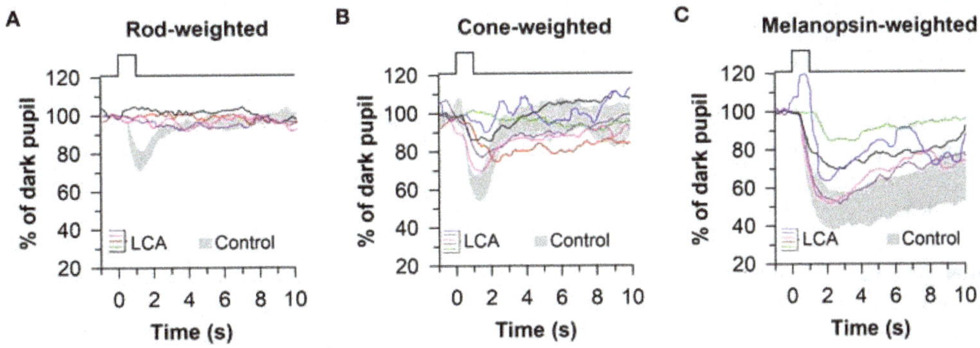

FIGURE 6 | Protocol for assessing photoreceptor health using 1-s light flashes. Pupillary responses were assessed in patients with Leber congenital amaurosis (LCA), using light stimuli designed to stimulate preferentially rods, cones, or melanopsin. **(A)** Pupillary responses to the rod-weighted light stimulus (465 nm, −3 log cd/m^2 after 10 min of dark adaptation) were non-recordable in LCA patients. **(B)** Responses to the cone-weighted light stimulus (642 nm, 1 log cd/m^2 on a blue background of 0.78 log cd/m^2) were reduced in LCA patients compared with healthy controls. **(C)** The post-illumination pupillary response to the melanopsin-weighted stimulus (2.6 log cd/m^2) was intact in LCA patients but the amplitude was reduced. Gray traces show the range of pupillary responses in the control group. The figure is redrawn and modified with permission from (67) .

responses between groups. The PIPR after exposure to bright blue light was also only modestly reduced in patients with LHON, suggesting that ipRGC function was preferentially spared relative to conventional retinal ganglion cells involved in image-forming vision. Similarly, in another study that measured the PIPR after a 1-s flash of bright blue light, the post-stimulus pupil size (at 6 s after light offset) was not different between HON patients (n = 11) and healthy controls (76).

Several studies have suggested that ipRGCs are resistant to neurodegeneration in mitochondrial optic neuropathies (i.e., LHON and autosomal dominant optic atrophy) (77–79), but they are vulnerable in other, more common types of optic neuropathies (i.e., patients with ischemic, inflammatory, or glaucomatous optic neuropathies). In a series of patients with anterior ischemic optic neuropathy (AION; n = 18) the sensitivity of pupillary responses to blue light (464 nm, −4.0 to −1.0 cd/m^2 in 0.5 log unit steps with intervening dark periods) and red light (635 nm, 1.0 to 2.5 log cd/m^2 in 0.5 log unit steps under light adaptation to 90 cd/m^2) was in the normal range, but the PIPR after exposure to bright blue light was impaired in eyes affected by AION, compared with contralaterally unaffected eyes and healthy control eyes (80). These findings indicate that ipRGCs are damaged following ischemic injury to the optic nerve. Several studies have also shown that the PIPR to a 1-s flash of short-wavelength light is impaired in patients with glaucomatous optic neuropathy compared with healthy controls (76, 81–84). Moreover, in glaucoma patients (n = 38), the magnitude of the PIPR (normalized pupil size measured 6 s after light offset) after exposure to a bright blue light stimulus (470 nm, 2.4 log cd/m^2) correlated with the magnitude of visual field loss assessed by standard automated perimetry (SAP), and RNFL thickness assessed by OCT (81). Similar results were obtained in another study in patients with glaucoma (n = 46) in which the consensual pupillary light reflex was assessed after monocular exposure to either a full-field or superonasal-quadrant light stimulus (464 nm, 2.9 log cd/m^2) (84). The PIPR amplitude (6 s after light offset) in glaucomatous eyes was associated with visual field deficits and RNFL thinning, suggesting that reduced melanopsin-dependent pupillary responses might be used as a proxy to estimate the loss of conventional retinal ganglion cells involved in image-forming vision.

Assessing ipRGC Function Using the PIPR After a 10-Second or 20-Second Light Stimulus

The melanopsin-dependent PIPR was first demonstrated in humans and macaques using a 10-s light stimulus protocol (47). Prior work had shown that macaque ipRGCs studied *in vitro* continued to fire long after the offset of a 10-s light exposure (23). Hence, subsequent clinical studies have also investigated the PIPR using a 10-s light stimulus, with average pupil size measured from 10 to 40 s after light offset. Using this approach, the consensual PIPR was characterized in healthy individuals (n = 45) after exposing the other eye to a bright blue light or red light stimulus, centered on the pupil in Maxwellian view (470 nm vs. 623 nm; retinal irradiance of 13 log quanta/cm^2/s with a fully-dilated pupil using a mydriatic agent) (85). Although there were substantial individual differences in the magnitude of pupillary constriction, all participants exhibited a sustained PIPR based on the change in pupil size after exposure to blue light relative to red light, adjusted for the percentage change in pupil size relative to the baseline pupil diameter (i.e., the net PIPR change, determined by subtracting the blue PIPR percentage value from the red PIPR percentage value). Similar methods have been used to examine ipRGC function in patients with glaucoma (86, 87). After exposure to 10 s of bright light (488 vs. 610 nm; corneal irradiance, 14.2 log quanta/cm^2/s), the net PIPR to blue light vs. red light was reduced in patients with advanced glaucoma (n = 11) compared with healthy controls (**Figures 7A,B**), but there was no difference in the PIPR between patients with early glaucoma (n = 14) and healthy controls (87). In another study, the net PIPR change in glaucoma patients (n = 16) after exposure to bright light (470 vs. 623 nm; retinal irradiance of 13 log quanta/cm^2/s) was linearly correlated with the magnitude of visual field loss (**Figure 7C**), demonstrating that ipRGC dysfunction in glaucoma is associated with disease severity (86). In patients with type 2 diabetes without diabetic retinopathy ($n = 7$), the PIPR to bright light (488 vs. 610 nm; corneal irradiance, 14.2 log quanta/cm^2/s) was also reduced and associated with the duration of diabetes (88), suggesting that ipRGC dysfunction may occur in diabetes prior to onset of visual loss. Similarly, in patients with age-related macular degeneration (AMD; $n = 2$), the PIPR to bright light (464 vs. 635 nm; corneal irradiance, 15 log photons/cm^2/s) was reduced in both early and advanced, neovascular AMD compared with controls (89).

In other studies, the PIPR to a bright 20-s light stimulus has been used to examine ipRGC function. In a patient with LHON with unilateral visual loss, sustained pupillary constriction after light offset (460 vs. 660 nm; 2.0 or 2.5 log cd/m^2) did not differ between the affected eye and the healthy eye, suggesting that ipRGC function was resistant to effects of the disease (90). In contrast, in patients with unilateral AION ($n = 10$), pupillary responses of the affected eye were reduced compared with the contralateral, non-affected eye, both during and after exposure to 20-s of bright light (470 vs. 660 nm; 2.5 log cd/m^2) (91). In patients with choroideremia ($n = 18$), which is characterized by progressive degeneration of the outer retina, the peak pupillary constriction response was also reduced during exposure to bright blue light or red light (463 vs. 643 nm; 100 lux), but the PIPR was intact and lasted longer compared with healthy individuals (92). Together, these results are consistent with studies that used 1-s light flashes (see previous section), showing that the PIPR is reduced in diseases that result in damage to ipRGCs, but remains largely intact in diseases that primarily affect the outer retina.

Chromatic Pupillometry Methods That use Continuously Presented Light

Assessing Photoreceptor Function Using Stepwise Increases in Light Intensity

The pupillary light reflex shows a phasic (i.e., transient) constriction response at the beginning of a continuous light stimulus, followed by a tonic (i.e., sustained) response that is lower in amplitude. Hence, deficits in outer retinal function can be assessed by the phasic response to a step of blue or red light, and deficits in inner retinal function can be assessed by the tonic pupillary response and the PIPR to high-intensity blue light. These response characteristics can be investigated using protocols in which the light intensity is increased stepwise over time. Using a Ganzfeld system to administer light to the eye continuously under mesopic conditions (with the non-stimulated eye covered), the direct pupillary response to a sequence of increasing blue or red light stimuli was measured over a 2 log unit range, with each light step presented for 13 s and matched for photopic luminance (467 and 640 nm; 0, 1, and 2 log cd/m^2; **Figure** 7) (93). The transient pupillary response was defined as the maximum constriction response measured within 180–500 ms after light onset, and the sustained pupillary response was defined as pupillary constriction at the 13th second of stimulation for each light step (with each measure adjusted for pre-stimulus pupil size). After characterizing pupillary responses in healthy individuals, this protocol was tested in a patient with retinitis pigmentosa with loss of rod function and reduced cone function based on electroretinography, a patient with achromatopsia in whom cone function was disrupted due to a mutation in the *CNGA3* gene, and a patient with unilateral AION with severe visual loss in the affected eye (93). The patient with retinitis pigmentosa showed deficits in phasic and tonic pupillary responses to the rod-weighted dim blue light stimulus, whereas the melanopsin-weighted response to bright blue light was in the normal range. Responses to moderate-to-bright red light were also attenuated, which is consistent with reduced cone function. In the achromat, pupillary responses to blue light were comparable to healthy controls, suggesting normal function of rods and melanopsin, whereas the cone-weighted response to red light was on the lower end of the normal range, perhaps due to activation of rods (see below). In the AION patient, pupillary responses in the affected eye were markedly reduced for all light stimuli, indicating reduced function of ipRGCs and their input from the outer retina.

This protocol was subsequently evaluated in a group of patients with retinitis pigmentosa ($n = 32$) (62), in whom the transient pupillary response to dim blue light (467 nm; 0 log cd/m^2) was defined as the rod-weighted light response, and the transient pupillary response to bright red light (640 nm; 2 log cd/m^2) was defined as the cone-weighted response. The melanopsin-dependent pupillary response was assessed by sustained pupillary constriction at the end of the bright blue light stimulus (467 nm; 2 log cd/m^2). Under these testing conditions, patients with a non-recordable or abnormal scotopic/photopic electroretinogram showed reduced transient pupillary responses to rod- and cone-weighted light stimuli, as well as a reduced tonic response to the melanopsin-weighted light stimulus. However, patients with retinitis pigmentosa showed a slower and more sustained PIPR after exposure to the melanopsin-weighted stimulus, as compared with patients with normal vision. Consistent with these findings, another study that used the same protocol found that patients with mutations in the *RPE65* gene ($n = 11$) exhibited reduced transient pupillary responses to rod- and cone-weighted light stimuli, a small reduction in sustained pupillary constriction during exposure to the melanopsin-weighted stimulus, and a prolonged PIPR after light offset compared with healthy controls (68). In a pair of achromats, pupillary responses were in the normal range for the rod-weighted stimulus, but were attenuated for the cone-weighted stimulus. The finding that achromats could still respond to red light is likely explained by activation of rods by the cone-weighted stimulus because total loss of cone function was confirmed in other experiments in the same individuals (68).

The stepwise pupillometry protocol has also been compared between patients with degeneration of the outer retina ($n = 23$; retinitis pigmentosa, LCA, corneoretinal dystrophy of Bietti, cone-rod dystrophy, or Stargardt disease) and optic nerve disease ($n = 13$; ischemic optic neuropathy or compression lesion of the optic nerve) (63). Pupillary constriction responses to rod-, cone-, and melanopsin-weighted light stimuli were reduced in patients with either outer or inner retinal disease compared with healthy controls (**Figures 8A,B**). However, the pupillary re-dilation response after blue-light offset was much slower in

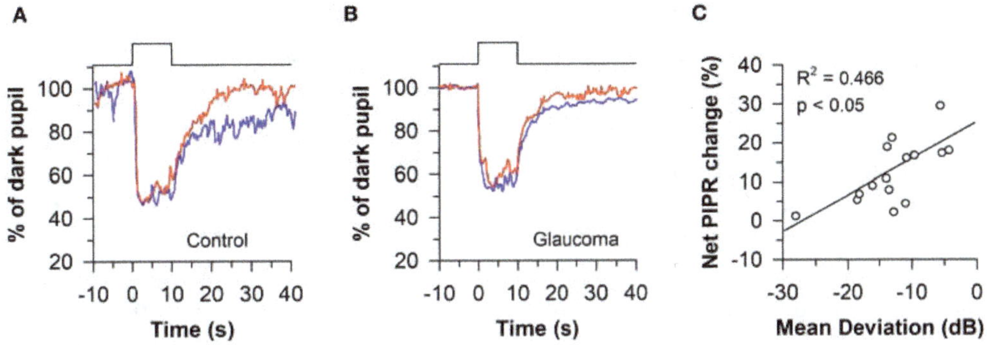

FIGURE 7 | Protocol for assessing melanopsin-dependent pupillary responses using the post-illumination pupillary light response (PIPR). The PIPR was assessed after exposure to 10 s of bright blue light or red light (488 or 610 nm; 14.2 log quanta/cm^2/s). **(A)** In individuals with normal vision, the PIPR to blue light was greater than the PIPR to red light for at least 30 s after light offset. **(B)** In patients with glaucoma, the PIPR to blue light was reduced relative to red light, indicating reduced light transmission from melanopsin-containing retinal ganglion cells. **(C)** In glaucomatous eyes, the net PIPR change (the difference in the PIPR to blue light vs. red light, adjusted for baseline pupil size) correlated with visual field loss assessed by Humphrey visual field mean deviation. Panels **(A,B)** are redrawn with permission from (87). Panel **(C)** is redrawn with permission from (86).

patients with outer retinal disease compared with patients with optic nerve disease or healthy controls, which is consistent with other studies in which the stepwise light protocol was used (62, 68). In contrast, most studies that have used a 1-s flash of blue light to elicit the PIPR have found a relatively normal response after light offset in patients with outer retinal disease (60, 67, 72, 73), with only one study reporting a greater PIPR relative to controls (68). The difference in the PIPR across light exposure protocols may be related to the pre-exposure lighting conditions. In the stepwise light protocol, patients are exposed to continuously presented light and hence the PIPR is measured after light adaptation. Similar to results using the stepwise light protocol, a prolonged time course of pupillary re-dilation has been observed in patients with outer retinal disease after the offset of a bright blue light stimulus lasting 20 s or longer (i.e., after light adaptation) (38, 92). Even for a 1-s flash of bright blue light, the PIPR has been shown to be extended in patients with retinitis pigmentosa or LCA if the stimulus is presented after light adaption, rather than dark adaption (60). Together, these studies suggest that the stepwise pupillometry protocol can be used to differentiate loss of outer retinal function vs. melanopsin-dependent ipRGC function, by measuring transient pupillary responses at the start of each light step and the PIPR after light adaptation.

Assessing Photoreceptor Function Using Ramp-Up Light Protocols

Given that rods and cones are more sensitive to light than the melanopsin-dependent ipRGC response, photoreceptors in the outer retina and inner retina can be activated sequentially by using a gradually increasing light stimulus (i.e., a ramp-up light protocol). Based on irradiance-response curves for the pupillary light reflex, damage to the outer retina can be assessed by reduced pupillary responses to light stimuli at lower irradiances, i.e., below the threshold of activation for the melanopsin-dependent pupillary response (low-to-moderate intensity blue light or moderate-to-high intensity red light). By comparison, damage to the inner retina can be detected by measuring the pupillary response during exposure to continuous, high-intensity blue light. This approach has been tested using a modified Ganzfeld system to administer a gradually-increasing blue or red light stimulus (469 or 631 nm; corneal irradiance from 7 to 14 log photons/cm^2/s) to one eye over a 2-min period (with the other eye covered), in order to construct irradiance-response curves for the direct pupillary light reflex (58). In patients with glaucoma ($n = 40$) with different stages of disease severity (Early, $n = 19$; Moderate, $n = 10$; Severe, $n = 11$), pupillary responses were impaired for the blue light stimulus at irradiances corresponding with the range of activation of the melanopsin-dependent response (>11.5 log photons/cm^2/s), and the difference between patients and healthy controls was greatest at the highest irradiances tested (**Figure 9A**). Pupillary responses in glaucoma patients were also reduced for the red light stimulus at moderate-to-high intensities of red light (>11.5 log photons/cm^2/s), suggesting reduced transmission from rod/cone photoreceptors to ipRGCs (**Figure 9B**). In contrast, the pupillary response in a patient with retinitis pigmentosa with no light perception was markedly reduced for the blue light stimulus at low-to-moderate light intensities (<13 log photons/cm^2/s), and there was no detectable response to the red light stimulus (**Figures 9A,B**), which is consistent with loss of rod and cone function (94). However, the amplitude of his pupillary constriction response was in the normal range for high intensity blue light, suggesting preserved melanopsin-dependent ipRGC function. In the glaucoma patients, the magnitude of pupillary constriction to high-irradiance blue light (>13.5 log photons/cm^2/s) was inversely correlated with Humphrey visual field mean deviation and optic disc cupping assessed using Heidelberg Retinal Tomography (**Figures 9C,D**) (58). These results suggest that ipRGC responses in glaucoma can be used to estimate damage to retinal ganglion cells that mediate image-forming vision.

In a later study, the ramp-up light exposure protocol was tested in a group of patients with early-stage glaucoma ($n = 46$;

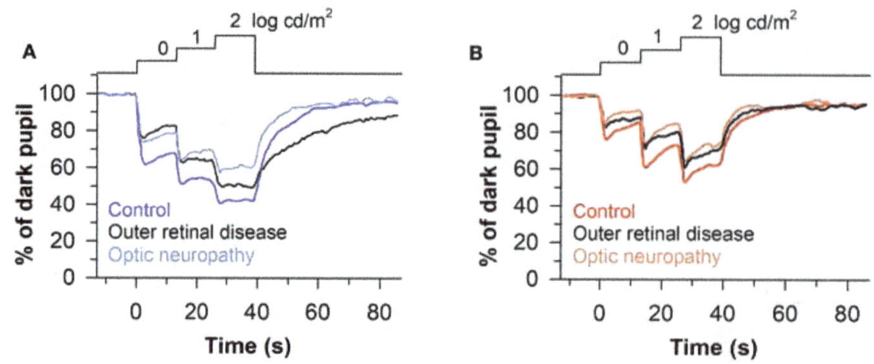

FIGURE 8 | Protocol for assessing photoreceptor health using stepwise increases in light intensity. Pupillary responses were assessed in patients with outer retinal disease or optic nerve disease, using blue and red light stimuli that were presented for 13 s in each step (467 or 640 nm; 0, 1, and 2 log cd/m^2). **(A)** Patients with outer retinal disease or optic nerve disease showed reduced pupillary light responses to each stepwise increase in blue light. However, the post-illumination pupillary light response after the last light step was prolonged only in patients with outer retinal disease. **(B)** Both groups of patients showed impaired pupillary responses to each stepwise increase in red light compared with controls, but there was no difference between groups in the PIPR. The figure is redrawn and modified with permission from (63).

visual field mean deviation of −6 dB or better on automated perimetry) (95). Pupillary light responses were reduced in patients compared with healthy controls at moderate-to-high intensities of blue and red light (>11.0 log photons/cm^2/s). In glaucomatous eyes, the maximum pupillary constriction amplitude correlated with RNFL thickness, but unsurprisingly, not with the amount of visual field loss. Hence, ipRGC dysfunction or cell loss can be detected in early stages of glaucoma and is associated with structural correlates of disease progression. In another study that used the ramp-up light protocol, patients with autosomal-dominant optic atrophy ($n = 5$) showed pupillary responses that were comparable to healthy controls (96), which is consistent with other studies that have found preserved ipRGC function in mitochondrial disease (77).

Summary of Chromatic Pupillometry Methods Used to Assess Photoreceptor Health

Chromatic pupillometry methods can detect dysfunction of photoreceptors in diseases affecting either the outer retina or the inner retina. Clinical protocols that measure pupillary responses to 1-s light flashes allow for testing of rod function using a dim blue light stimulus after dark adaption, while cone function can be tested using a moderate-to-bright red light stimulus under light adaptation. This approach has been used to demonstrate loss of rod and/or cone function in outer retinal disease (e.g., retinitis pigmentosa and LCA). Melanopsin-dependent ipRGC function can be assessed by measuring the PIPR after exposure to a bright blue light stimulus. The PIPR after dark adaptation is reduced in patients with optic nerve disease (e.g., glaucoma and AION), with the notable exception of mitochondrial disease (e.g., LHON and autosomal dominant optic atrophy) in which ipRGCs appear to be preferentially spared. In stepwise light protocols, the phasic pupillary response to light stimulus onset, which is dominated by rods/cones, is impaired in outer retinal disease. In contrast, the sustained pupillary response to bright blue light, which is dominated by melanopsin, is impaired in diseases affecting ipRGC function, whereas the subsequent PIPR is prolonged in patients with outer retinal disease. In protocols in which light intensity is increased gradually over time (ramp-up light protocol), the tonic pupillary light reflex is impaired during exposure to dim-to-moderate intensity blue light or red light in outer retinal disease, whereas sustained pupillary constriction to high-irradiance blue light is impaired in inner retinal disease. In glaucoma, melanopsin-dependent pupillary responses correlate with visual field loss and anatomic correlates of optic nerve damage, suggesting that pupillometry methods can be used to estimate the degree of damage to ipRGCs and conventional retinal ganglion cells.

LIMITATIONS AND CONSIDERATIONS OF CHROMATIC PUPILLOMETRY

Chromatic pupillometry is currently the only approach that can be used to assess rapidly the health of rods, cones, and melanopsin using a single light protocol. However, the contribution of outer retinal photoreceptors to phasic and tonic components of the pupillary light reflex is still not fully understood. Based on studies using the silent substitution method to selectively modulate the activity of different photoreceptor types, S-cones and M-cones may provide inhibitory input to ipRGCs that mediate the pupillary light reflex, whereas stimulation of L-cones and melanopsin induces pupillary constriction (55, 97, 98). A subset of melanopsin cells in the macaque retina has also been shown to exhibit an S-Off, (L+M)-On type of color-opponent receptive field (23). These findings have potential implications for interpreting the effects of blue light and red light stimuli on pupillary responses in chromatic pupillometry protocols, in which multiple photoreceptor types (i.e., rods, S-cones, M-cones, L-cones,

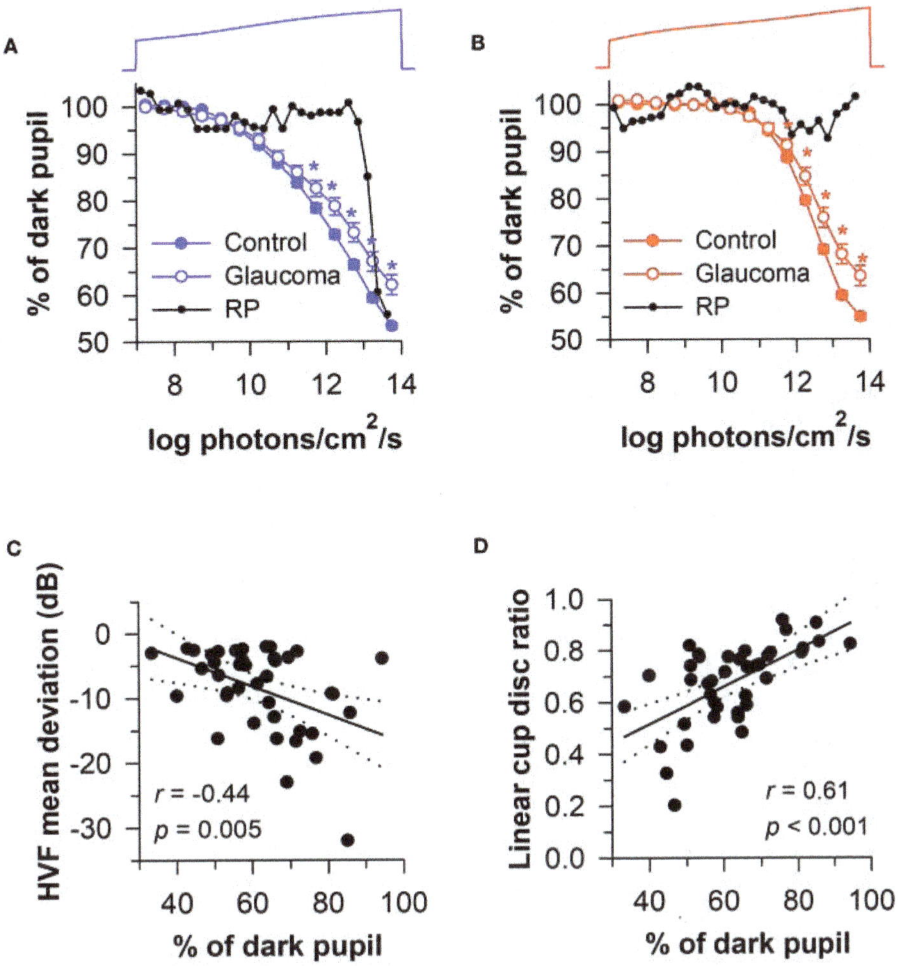

FIGURE 9 | Protocol for assessing photoreceptor health using a ramp-up light exposure. Pupillary responses to blue light or red light were assessed during exposure to a continuously presented light stimulus that was increased gradually over a 2-min period (469 or 631 nm; from 7 to 14 log photons/cm^2/s). **(A)** Pupillary responses to blue light were reduced in patients with glaucoma at higher irradiances compared with controls. In contrast, pupillary responses were reduced at dim-to-moderate light intensities in a patient with retinitis pigmentosa (RP) without rod/cone function, but were normal at the highest irradiances tested. **(B)** Pupillary responses to red light were also reduced in patients with glaucoma at higher irradiances, whereas there was no detectable response in the RP patient. In glaucomatous eyes, the magnitude of pupillary constriction during exposure to high-irradiance blue light (>13.5 log photons/cm^2/s) correlated with **(C)** visual field loss determined by Humphrey Visual Field (HVF) mean deviation, and **(D)** optic disc cupping determined by Heidelberg Retinal Tomography. In **(C,D)**, the linear regression line is shown with 95% CIs. Data for glaucoma patients are replotted and modified with permission from (58). Data for the RP patient are replotted and modified with permission from (94).

and melanopsin) may be activated simultaneously and interact in complex ways at the level of ipRGCs. Outer retinal photoreceptors and melanopsin also differ in their time-course of dark adaptation and light adaptation (39, 99). Therefore, pre-exposure lighting conditions (e.g., the duration of prior darkness or exposure to light) can influence results of chromatic pupillometry testing (100, 101). Differences in the distribution of rods, cones, and melanopsin-containing retinal ganglion cells in the retina also gives rise to regional differences in spatial summation and ipRGC responses to light (102, 103). This may have implications for chromatic pupillometry protocols that administer light to different parts of the visual field to assess retinal health, e.g., central-field, hemi-field, quadrant-field, or annular light stimulation (84, 104–106).

Although chromatic pupillometry methods can be used to localize damage to the outer retina or the inner retina, they do not provide information on the specific disease type. For example, similar deficits in pupillary light responses are observed between patients with retinitis pigmentosa and LCA, and between patients with glaucoma or AION. Therefore, additional ophthalmic tests are required to establish an accurate diagnosis and its underlying pathophysiology. Pupillary light responses are also impaired in non-ocular diseases that result in demyelination or degeneration of the optic nerve, or altered autonomic nervous system function. For example, phasic pupillary light responses and the PIPR are reduced in patients with multiple sclerosis or Parkinson's disease (107–109). Efferent pathway defects from the midbrain to the pupils can also give rise to impaired pupillary constriction responses despite intact photoreceptor responses (110, 111). Moreover, the PIPR is reduced in patients with Seasonal Affective Disorder (SAD) or non-seasonal depression (112, 113), in whom there are no pathological changes in optic nerve function. These observations may be related to effects of the number of daylight hours on the amplitude of the PIPR (113, 114), perhaps through modulation of melanopsin protein levels and/or the sensitivity of ipRGCs to light. Relatedly, genetic variation in the melanopsin gene modulates pupillary responses to bright blue light and risk of SAD (112, 115–117). The PIPR and other pupillary light responses are also influenced by circadian phase (118, 119), sleep deprivation (119), and some types of medication (120). Additionally, cortical visual pathways are thought to be involved in modulating pupillary light responses (121, 122). Collectively, these studies show that results of chromatic pupillometry testing are influenced not only by the stimulation of retinal photoreceptors, but also by other biological pathways and disease processes.

An important concern regarding the use of chromatic pupillometry is whether it is necessary to adjust for effects of aging on pupillary responses. In aging, decreased sympathetic activity and smaller pupil size (i.e., age-related miosis) are thought to contribute to reduced pupillary constriction responses to light (123). When pupillary responses are measured relative to the dark-adapted pupil size, however, there is little effect of age on the amplitude of pupillary constriction (85, 124, 125). Similarly, age-dependent yellowing of the lens, which reduces transmission of short-wavelength light, does not appear to affect melanopsin-dependent pupillary responses. Rather, baseline-adjusted pupillary light responses are similar between young and older adults (124, 125), and the magnitude of the PIPR to blue light vs. red light is preserved across adulthood (85, 126, 127). Moreover, there is no effect of mild cataract (125) or narrow irido-corneal angles (128) on spectral responses of the pupil, and no effect of refractive error on the PIPR (127). Together, these results indicate that melanopsin-dependent pupillary responses are relatively stable in healthy aging. The pupillary light reflex also shows good test-retest reliability when assessed in the same individuals over short time intervals (68, 129). However, pupillary light responses in healthy individuals show substantial between-subject differences (85, 93), and usually overlap with responses in patients with mild-to-moderate retinal or optic nerve disease. Therefore, further optimization of chromatic pupillometry protocols may be necessary to differentiate reliably individuals with normal health vs. those with retinal or optic nerve disease.

A challenge in interpreting and comparing chromatic pupillometry studies is that different methods have been applied for measuring and delivering light to the eyes. In this review, we report light stimuli as they were described in the original research articles in which different units of light measurement were used (lux, cd/m^2, and log photons/cm^2/s). Units based on the photopic luminosity function (e.g., lux or cd/m^2) are familiar to engineers and vision researchers, but should not be used for non-visual light responses including the pupillary light reflex (130). This is because it is well established that rods and melanopsin (not only cones) contribute to pupillary light responses in the photopic visual range, including sustained pupillary constriction and the PIPR. Instead, researchers should be encouraged to report either the power distribution (μW/cm^2) or photon density (log photons/cm^2/s) of their light stimulus, and/or calculate the α-opic illuminance values (α-opic lux) to provide an estimate of the effective illuminance for each of the 5 human photopigments. Doing so will make it easier to replicate experimental conditions across studies and to interpret the relative contribution of different photopigments to pupillary responses. Different types of light delivery systems have also been used in chromatic pupillometry studies. Most studies have administered light using a Ganzfeld system, or directed light through the pupil in Maxwellian view. While Ganzfeld systems are relatively easy to build and implement in pupillometry studies, the retinal illuminance is limited and cannot be specified by the experimenter for different stimulus conditions. In Maxwellian view, a high retinal illuminance field can be readily obtained and the size of the entry pupil can be controlled, but these systems require precise alignment of the eye, which is often achieved by using a bite bar to stabilize the participant's eye position (131). Hence, there are trade-offs that must be taken into consideration when choosing the type of light delivery system used for chromatic pupillometry.

Another challenge in comparing pupillometry studies is that different methods have been used for measuring pupillary responses. Some studies have measured the direct pupillary light reflex while covering the other eye (i.e., the pupil of the stimulated eye is recorded), whereas other studies have measured the consensual pupillary light reflex (i.e., the stimulated eye is dilated with a mydriatic agent and the pupil of the non-stimulated eye is recorded). Because the consensual light response is greater when the pupil of the stimulated eye is dilated, rather than constricted (132), the size of the pupil exposed to light must be taken into consideration when interpreting results of chromatic pupillometry. Additionally, many different types of pupillary response metrics have been used in chromatic pupillometry studies. For example, there are several metrics that have been used to quantify the PIPR, including the 6-s PIPR, area under the curve, re-dilation velocity, and the plateau of the PIPR based on the best-fit exponential model of the data. Some of these measures may be better than others at capturing the melanopsin-dependent component of the PIPR vs. the mixed contribution of rods/cones and melanopsin during the early phase of pupillary re-dilation. The reliability of these PIPR metrics has been shown to differ in healthy participants, with lower coefficients of variation for the 6-s PIPR and the plateau of the PIPR (50). Hence, some PIPR metrics are likely better than others, and this may also depend on the type of disease being examined. The PIPR amplitude also varies by stimulus duration, with shorter light stimuli (1 s) producing larger responses than longer light stimuli (10 or 30 s) (50). As such, a PIPR testing paradigm that utilizes a 1-s light stimulus and either a 6-s or plateau PIPR metric might prove most useful in clinical applications, as remains to be tested. Moving forward, researchers using chromatic pupillometry should strive to develop a set of consensus standards for light stimuli and pupillary response metrics that can be used to readily compare results across different studies and types of disease.

FUTURE APPLICATIONS OF CHROMATIC PUPILLOMETRY METHODS

Early detection of retinal and optic nerve diseases is important for treating and preventing loss of vision. However, gradual loss of peripheral vision can go unnoticed for years. For example, patients with glaucoma often seek treatment after substantial and irreversible damage to the optic nerve has occurred. Based on results of chromatic pupillometry testing, patients with early-stage glaucoma show deficits in pupillary responses to bright blue light compared with healthy controls (84, 95). Such findings raise the possibility that pupillometry testing could be used to screen for early optic nerve dysfunction. An advantage of chromatic pupillometry methods is that they can be readily incorporated into portable testing systems for population screening. For example, chromatic pupillometry devices could be used in a polyclinic setting or in geriatric clinics to identify patients with suspected retinal or optic nerve disease. Such patients could then be directed to undergo a comprehensive ophthalmic examination to determine the origin of their impaired pupillary light response. Additionally, chromatic pupillometry methods can potentially be used in patients who have difficulty communicating or who are unable to follow procedures for visual field testing. Following diagnosis of the underlying condition, chromatic pupillometry testing could be used periodically to track progression of the disease and effects of treatment.

The pupillary light reflex can be used to test for intact melanopsin-dependent ipRGC responses in patients who are blind. Notably, a standard penlight examination is inadequate for this purpose, with results that are often unreliable (133). For example, pupillary light responses were studied extensively in a pair of blind patients with no light perception who were previously described as having no detectable pupillary light response based on penlight examination by an ophthalmologist (37, 38). Clinical testing of optic nerve function should therefore include conditions that are appropriate for assessing melanopsin-dependent responses, i.e., exposure to high-irradiance blue light on a background of darkness. In the future, this may be especially important for identifying blind patients with intact optic nerve function who should be considered as candidates for gene therapy trials to restore vision (see below). Additionally, melanopsin-dependent pupillary light responses could be used as a surrogate measure for other responses mediated by ipRGCs (119, 134, 135), in order to screen for blind patients with intact circadian photoreception who should expose themselves to light-dark cues to entrain to the 24-h solar day. Chromatic pupillometry methods can also be used to assess photoreceptor health in veterinary medicine, as demonstrated in dogs with sudden acquired retinal degeneration syndrome and optic nerve disease (136–138).

With the development of technologies for restoring vision in blind individuals, there is a need for standard clinical tests that can be used to help select suitable candidates and to estimate the degree of recovery of non-visual photoreception after treatment. Chromatic pupillometry methods may be useful for testing photoreceptor health in degenerative diseases (e.g., retinitis pigmentosa and LCA), in which mutations in photoreceptor-specific or non-photoreceptor-specific cells in the retina result in rod cell death, followed by loss of cones. Given that retinal ganglion cells and other retinal neuronal cell types can survive for long periods after blindness, vision can be partially restored by rendering the remaining cells photosensitive. This can potentially be achieved by surgically-implanted subretinal prostheses that can electrically stimulate retinal ganglion cells, injection of small-molecule photoswitches to bestow light sensitivity to retinal ganglion cells, and gene therapy to express light-regulated ion channels, transporters, or receptors (e.g., melanopsin or microbial opsins) in retinal neurons. These approaches have been tested in blind mice, demonstrating restoration of some behavioral light responses, and improved pupillary responses to light at low-to-moderate intensities (139–143). Similarly, gene therapy has been used to treat LCA in blind mice with impaired ability to regenerate visual photopigments (by restoring function of lecithin:retinol acyl transferase), which resulted in increased sensitivity of the pupillary light reflex by about 2.5 log units (144).

Parallel findings have been reported for *RPE65*-associated LCA in humans, in whom viral delivery of the normal *RPE65* gene to the retina resulted in sustained improvement of subjective and objective measures of vision (145, 146), as well as an increase in sensitivity of pupillary responses to light that lasted for at least 3 years after follow-up. These studies demonstrate that gene therapy for restoring vision also results in improvement in the pupillary light reflex. In future studies, chromatic pupillometry protocols can potentially be used to quantify the degree of recovery of non-visual photoreceptor pathways in blind patients who undergo gene therapy or other treatments to restore vision.

In summary, chromatic pupillometry methods have the potential to improve detection and management of diseases affecting the retina or optic nerve. Previous studies have characterized the differential role of outer retinal photoreceptors and melanopsin in mediating the pupillary light reflex. This has led to development and testing of short-duration protocols for assessing pupillary responses in patients with retinal or optic nerve disease. Clinical studies have provided proof-of-concept that pupillometry can be used to localize loss of function to photoreceptors in the outer retina or inner retina in patients whose disease status was already known. We are now in the position to exploit these research findings to test prospectively the ability of chromatic pupillometry to detect abnormalities in ipRGC function. Future large-scale studies should therefore focus on optimizing, standardizing, and adapting chromatic pupillometry protocols for early detection of retinal and optic nerve diseases, and for monitoring disease progression or recovery after treatment.

AUTHOR CONTRIBUTIONS

AR, DM, and JG made substantial contributions to the conception and/or design of the work, acquisition, analysis, and interpretation of data, drafting and/or revising the manuscript critically for important intellectual content. AR, DM, and JG provided final approval of the version to be published and agree to be accountable for all aspects of the work in ensuring that questions related to the accuracy or integrity of any part of the work are appropriately investigated and resolved.

FUNDING

This work was supported by the Duke-NUS Signature Research Program funded by the Agency for Science, Technology and Research, Singapore, and the Ministry of Health, Singapore; the National Medical Research Council, Singapore (NMRC/NIG/1000/2009 and NMRC/CIRG/1401/2014); the Singapore National Eye Centre Health Research Endowment Fund, Singapore (R1005/20/2013); and the Biomedical Research Council, Singapore (01-TCRP-2010 and TCR0101674).

ACKNOWLEDGMENTS

We thank research coordinators at the Singapore Eye Research Institute for their assistance in carrying out some of the studies described in this review article.

REFERENCES

1. Bremner FD. Pupil assessment in optic nerve disorders. *Eye* (2004) 18:1175–81. doi: 10.1038/sj.eye.6701560
2. Alpern M, Campbell FW. The spectral sensitivity of the consensual light reflex. *J Physiol.* (1962) 164:478–507.
3. Laurens H. Studies on the relative physiologial value of spectral lights. *Am J Physiol Legacy Content* (1923) 64:97–119. doi: 10.1152/ajplegacy.1923.64.1.97
4. Wagman IH, Gullberg JE. The relationship between monochromatic light and pupil diameter. The low intensity visibility curve as measured by pupillary measurements. *Am J Physiol Legacy Content* (1942) 137:769–78. doi: 10.1152/ajplegacy.1942.137.4.769
5. Schweitzer NJ, Bouman MA. Differential threshold measurements on the light reflex of the human pupil. *AMA Arch Ophthalmol.* (1958) 59:541–50. doi: 10.1001/archopht.1958.00940050097012
6. Doesschate JT, Alpern M. Response of the pupil to steady-state retinal illumination: contribution by cones. *Science* (1965) 149:989–91. doi: 10.1126/science.149.3687.989
7. Koeppe ER, Alexandridis E. Pupil light reflex and Purkinje displacement. *Bericht uber die Zusammenkunft Deutsche Ophthalmologische Gesellschaft* (1968) 68:278–81.
8. Hedin A. Pupillomotor spectral sensitivity in normals and colour defectives. *Acta Ophthalmol.* (1978) 137:1–83.
9. Kardon RH, Kirkali PA, Thompson HS. Automated pupil perimetry. Pupil field mapping in patients and normal subjects. *Ophthalmology* (1991) 98:485–95; discussion 95-6.
10. Pittler SJ, Keeler CE, Sidman RL, Baehr W. PCR analysis of DNA from 70-year-old sections of rodless retina demonstrates identity with the mouse rd defect. *Proc Natl Acad Sci USA.* (1993) 90:9616–9.
11. Keeler CE. Iris movements in blind mice. *Am J Physiol.* (1927) 81:6.
12. Keeler CE. Blind mice. *J Exp Zool.* (1928) 51:495–508. doi: 10.1002/jez.1400510404
13. Hopkins AE. Vision in mice with "rodless" retinae. *Zeitschrift vergleichende Physiol.* (1927) 6:345–60. doi: 10.1007/bf00339260
14. Lucas RJ, Douglas RH, Foster RG. Characterization of an ocular photopigment capable of driving pupillary constriction in mice. *Nat Neurosci.* (2001) 4:621–6. doi: 10.1038/88443
15. Lucas RJ, Freedman MS, Munoz M, Garcia-Fernandez JM, Foster RG. Regulation of the mammalian pineal by non-rod, non-cone, ocular photoreceptors. *Science* (1999) 284:505–7.
16. Freedman MS, Lucas RJ, Soni B, von Schantz M, Munoz M, David-Gray Z, et al. Regulation of mammalian circadian behavior by non-rod, non-cone, ocular photoreceptors. *Science* (1999) 284:502–4.
17. Wakakura M, Yokoe J. Evidence for preserved direct pupillary light response in Leber's hereditary optic neuropathy. *Br J Ophthalmol.* (1995) 79:442–6.
18. Bremner FD, Tomlin EA, Shallo-Hoffmann J, Votruba M, Smith SE. The pupil in dominant optic atrophy. *Invest Ophthalmol Visual Sci.* (2001) 42:675–8.
19. Czeisler CA, Shanahan TL, Klerman EB, Martens H, Brotman DJ, Emens JS, et al. Suppression of melatonin secretion in some blind patients by exposure to bright light. *N Engl J Med.* (1995) 332:6–11. doi: 10.1056/nejm199501053320102
20. Berson DM, Dunn FA, Takao M. Phototransduction by retinal ganglion cells that set the circadian clock. *Science* (2002) 295:1070–3. doi: 10.1126/science.1067262
21. Wong KY, Dunn FA, Graham DM, Berson DM. Synaptic influences on rat ganglion-cell photoreceptors. *J Physiol.* (2007) 582(Pt 1):279–96. doi: 10.1113/jphysiol.2007.133751
22. Hattar S, Liao HW, Takao M, Berson DM, Yau KW. Melanopsin-containing retinal ganglion cells: architecture, projections, and intrinsic photosensitivity. *Science* (2002) 295:1065–70. doi: 10.1126/science.1069609
23. Dacey DM, Liao HW, Peterson BB, Robinson FR, Smith VC, Pokorny J, et al. Melanopsin-expressing ganglion cells in primate retina signal colour and irradiance and project to the LGN. *Nature* (2005) 433:749–54. doi: 10.1038/nature03387
24. Gooley JJ, Lu J, Fischer D, Saper CB. A broad role for melanopsin in nonvisual photoreception. *J Neurosci.* (2003) 23:7093–106.
25. Chen SK, Badea TC, Hattar S. Photoentrainment and pupillary light reflex are mediated by distinct populations of ipRGCs. *Nature* (2011) 476:92–5. doi: 10.1038/nature10206
26. Gooley JJ, Lu J, Chou TC, Scammell TE, Saper CB. Melanopsin in cells of origin of the retinohypothalamic tract. *Nat Neurosci.* (2001) 4:1165. doi: 10.1038/nn768
27. Hattar S, Kumar M, Park A, Tong P, Tung J, Yau KW, et al. Central projections of melanopsin-expressing retinal ganglion cells in the mouse. *J Compar Neurol.* (2006) 497:326–49.
28. Li JY, Schmidt TM. Divergent projection patterns of M1 ipRGC subtypes. *J Compar Neurol.* (2018) 526:2010–8. doi: 10.1002/cne.24469
29. Quattrochi LE, Stabio ME, Kim I, Ilardi MC, Michelle Fogerson P, Leyrer ML, et al. The M6 cell: a small-field bistratified photosensitive retinal ganglion cell. *J Compar Neurol.* (2019) 527:297–311. doi: 10.1002/cne.24556
30. Hannibal J, Christiansen AT, Heegaard S, Fahrenkrug J, Kiilgaard JF. Melanopsin expressing human retinal ganglion cells: subtypes, distribution, and intraretinal connectivity. *J Compar Neurol.* (2017) 525:1934–61. doi: 10.1002/cne.24181
31. Liao HW, Ren X, Peterson BB, Marshak DW, Yau KW, Gamlin PD, et al. Melanopsin-expressing ganglion cells on macaque and human retinas

form two morphologically distinct populations. *J Compar Neurol.* (2016) 524:2845–72. doi: 10.1002/cne.23995

32. Hattar S, Lucas RJ, Mrosovsky N, Thompson S, Douglas RH, Hankins MW, et al. Melanopsin and rod-cone photoreceptive systems account for all major accessory visual functions in mice. *Nature* (2003) 424:76–81. doi: 10.1038/nature01761
33. Panda S, Provencio I, Tu DC, Pires SS, Rollag MD, Castrucci AM, et al. Melanopsin is required for non-image-forming photic responses in blind mice. *Science* (2003) 301:525–7. doi: 10.1126/science.1086179
34. Lucas RJ, Hattar S, Takao M, Berson DM, Foster RG, Yau KW. Diminished pupillary light reflex at high irradiances in melanopsin-knockout mice. *Science* (2003) 299:245–7. doi: 10.1126/science.1077293
35. Guler AD, Ecker JL, Lall GS, Haq S, Altimus CM, Liao HW, et al. Melanopsin cells are the principal conduits for rod-cone input to non-image-forming vision. *Nature* (2008) 453:102–5. doi: 10.1038/nature06829
36. Berson DM. Strange vision: ganglion cells as circadian photoreceptors. *Trends Neurosci.* (2013) 26:314–20. doi: 10.1016/S0166-2236(03)00130-9
37. Zaidi FH, Hull JT, Peirson SN, Wulff K, Aeschbach D, Gooley JJ, et al. Short-wavelength light sensitivity of circadian, pupillary, and visual awareness in humans lacking an outer retina. *Curr Biol.* (2007) 17:2122–8. doi: 10.1016/j.cub.2007.11.034
38. Gooley JJ, Ho Mien I, St Hilaire MA, Yeo SC, Chua EC, van Reen E, et al. Melanopsin and rod-cone photoreceptors play different roles in mediating pupillary light responses during exposure to continuous light in humans. *J Neurosci.* (2012) 32:14242–53. doi: 10.1523/JNEUROSCI.1321-12.2012
39. McDougal DH, Gamlin PD. The influence of intrinsically-photosensitive retinal ganglion cells on the spectral sensitivity and response dynamics of the human pupillary light reflex. *Vis Res.* (2010) 50:72–87. doi: 10.1016/j.visres.2009.10.012
40. Wald G. Human Vision and the spectrum. *Science* (1945) 101:653–8. doi: 10.1126/science.101.2635.653
41. Wald G, Brown PK. Human Rhodopsin. *Science* (1958) 127:222–6.
42. Shlaer S, Smith EL, Chase AM. Visual acuity and illumination in different spectral regions. *J Gen Physiol.* (1942) 25:553–69.
43. Brown PK, Wald G. Visual pigments in single rods and cones of the human retina. *Science* (1964) 144:45–52.
44. Abramov I, Gordon J. Color vision in the peripheral retina. I. Spectral sensitivity. *J Optical Soc Am.* (1977) 67:195–202.
45. Alexandridis E, Koeppe ER. The spectral sensitivity of retinal photoreceptors conducting the pupillary light reflex in humans. *Albrecht Graefes Archiv klinische experimentelle Ophthalmol.* (1969) 177:136–51.
46. Bouma H. Size of the static pupil as a function of wavelength and luminosity of the light incident on the human eye. *Nature* (1962) 193:690–1.
47. Gamlin PD, McDougal DH, Pokorny J, Smith VC, Yau KW, Dacey DM. Human and macaque pupil responses driven by melanopsin-containing retinal ganglion cells. *Vis Res.* (2007) 47:946–54. doi: 10.1016/j.visres.2006.12.015
48. Mure LS, Cornut PL, Rieux C, Drouyer E, Denis P, Gronfier C, et al. Melanopsin bistability: a fly's eye technology in the human retina. *PLoS ONE* (2009) 4:e5991. doi: 10.1371/journal.pone.0005991
49. Klerman EB, Shanahan TL, Brotman DJ, Rimmer DW, Emens JS, Rizzo JF III, et al. Photic resetting of the human circadian pacemaker in the absence of conscious vision. *J Biol Rhythms* (2002) 17:548–55. doi: 10.1177/0748730402238237
50. Adhikari P, Zele AJ, Feigl B. The Post-Illumination Pupil Response (PIPR). *Invest Ophthalmol Visual Sci.* (2015) 56:3838–49. doi: 10.1167/iovs.14-16233
51. Alpern M, Ohba N, Birndorf L. Can the response of the iris to light be used to break the code of the second cranial nerve in man? In: Janisse MP, editor. *Pupillary Dynamics and Behavior.* Boston, MA: Springer US (1974). p. 9–38.
52. Do MT, Kang SH, Xue T, Zhong H, Liao HW, Bergles DE, et al. Photon capture and signalling by melanopsin retinal ganglion cells. *Nature* (2009) 457:281–7. doi: 10.1038/nature07682
53. Lall GS, Revell VL, Momiji H, Al Enezi J, Altimus CM, Guler AD, et al. Distinct contributions of rod, cone, and melanopsin photoreceptors to encoding irradiance. *Neuron* (2010) 66:417–28. doi: 10.1016/j.neuron.2010.04.037
54. Wong KY. A retinal ganglion cell that can signal irradiance continuously for 10 hours. *J Neurosci.* (2012) 32:11478–85. doi: 10.1523/JNEUROSCI.1423-12.2012
55. Tsujimura S, Ukai K, Ohama D, Nuruki A, Yunokuchi K. Contribution of human melanopsin retinal ganglion cells to steady-state pupil responses. *Proc Biol Sci.* (2010) 277:2485–92. doi: 10.1098/rspb.2010.0330
56. Vienot F, Bailacq S, Rohellec JL. The effect of controlled photopigment excitations on pupil aperture. *Ophthal Physiol Optics* (2010) 30:484–91. doi: 10.1111/j.1475-1313.2010.00754.x
57. Ho Mien I, Chua EC, Lau P, Tan LC, Lee IT, Yeo SC, et al. Effects of exposure to intermittent versus continuous red light on human circadian rhythms, melatonin suppression, and pupillary constriction. *PLoS ONE* (2014) 9:e96532. doi: 10.1371/journal.pone.0096532
58. Rukmini AV, Milea D, Baskaran M, How AC, Perera SA, Aung T, et al. Pupillary responses to high-irradiance blue light correlate with glaucoma severity. *Ophthalmology* (2015) 122:1777–85. doi: 10.1016/j.ophtha.2015.06.002
59. Kostic C, Crippa SV, Martin C, Kardon RH, Biel M, Arsenijevic Y, et al. Determination of rod and cone influence to the early and late dynamic of the pupillary light response. *Invest Ophthalmol Visual Sci.* (2016) 57:2501–8. doi: 10.1167/iovs.16-19150
60. Park JC, Moura AL, Raza AS, Rhee DW, Kardon RH, Hood DC. Toward a clinical protocol for assessing rod, cone, and melanopsin contributions to the human pupil response. *Invest Ophthalmol Visual Sci.* (2011) 52:6624–35. doi: 10.1167/iovs.11-7586
61. Markwell EL, Feigl B, Smith SS, Zele AJ. Circadian modulation of the intrinsically photosensitive (melanopsin) retinal ganglion cell driven pupil light response. *Invest Ophthalmol Visual Sci.* (2010) 51:671. doi: 10.1177/0748730409343767
62. Kardon R, Anderson SC, Damarjian TG, Grace EM, Stone E, Kawasaki A. Chromatic pupillometry in patients with retinitis pigmentosa. *Ophthalmology* (2011) 118:376–81. doi: 10.1016/j.ophtha.2010.06.033
63. Leon L, Crippa SV, Borruat FX, Kawasaki A. Differential effect of long versus short wavelength light exposure on pupillary re-dilation in patients with outer retinal disease. *Clin Exp Ophthalmol.* (2012) 40:e16–24. doi: 10.1111/j.1442-9071.2011.02665.x
64. Barrionuevo PA, Nicandro N, McAnany JJ, Zele AJ, Gamlin P, Cao D. Assessing rod, cone, and melanopsin contributions to human pupil flicker responses. *Invest Ophthalmol Visual Sci.* (2014) 55:719–27. doi: 10.1167/iovs.13-13252
65. Aleman TS, Jacobson SG, Chico JD, Scott ML, Cheung AY, Windsor EA, et al. Impairment of the transient pupillary light reflex in Rpe65(-/-) mice and humans with leber congenital amaurosis. *Invest Ophthalmol Visual Sci.* (2004) 45:1259–71.
66. Jacobson SG, Cideciyan AV, Aleman TS, Sumaroka A, Roman AJ, Swider M, et al. Human retinal disease from AIPL1 gene mutations: foveal cone loss with minimal macular photoreceptors and rod function remaining. *Invest Ophthalmol Visual Sci.* (2011) 52:70–9. doi: 10.1167/iovs.10-6127
67. Collison FT, Park JC, Fishman GA, McAnany JJ, Stone EM. Full-field pupillary light responses, luminance thresholds, and light discomfort thresholds in CEP290 leber congenital amaurosis patients. *Invest Ophthalmol Visual Sci.* (2015) 56:7130–6. doi: 10.1167/iovs.15-17467
68. Lorenz B, Strohmayr E, Zahn S, Friedburg C, Kramer M, Preising M, et al. Chromatic pupillometry dissects function of the three different light-sensitive retinal cell populations in RPE65 deficiency. *Invest Ophthalmol Visual Sci.* (2012) 53:5641–52. doi: 10.1167/iovs.12-9974
69. Park JC, Moss HE, McAnany JJ. The pupillary light reflex in idiopathic intracranial hypertension. *Invest Ophthalmol Visual Sci.* (2016) 57:23–9. doi: 10.1167/iovs.15-18181
70. Park JC, Chen YF, Blair NP, Chau FY, Lim JI, Leiderman YI, et al. Pupillary responses in non-proliferative diabetic retinopathy. *Sci Rep.* (2017) 7:44987. doi: 10.1038/srep44987
71. Kawasaki A, Munier FL, Leon L, Kardon RH. Pupillometric quantification of residual rod and cone activity in leber congenital amaurosis. *Arch Ophthal* (2012) 130:798–800. doi: 10.1001/archophthalmol.2011.1756

72. Kawasaki A, Crippa SV, Kardon R, Leon L, Hamel C. Characterization of pupil responses to blue and red light stimuli in autosomal dominant retinitis pigmentosa due to NR2E3 mutation. *Invest Ophthalmol Visual Sci.* (2012) 53:5562–9. doi: 10.1167/iovs.12-10230
73. Collison FT, Park JC, Fishman GA, Stone EM, McAnany JJ. Two-color pupillometry in enhanced S-cone syndrome caused by NR2E3 mutations. *Documenta Ophthalmol Adv Ophthalmol.* (2016) 132:157–66. doi: 10.1007/s10633-016-9535-0
74. Kawasaki A, Collomb S, Leon L, Munch M. Pupil responses derived from outer and inner retinal photoreception are normal in patients with hereditary optic neuropathy. *Exp Eye Res.* (2014) 120:161–6. doi: 10.1016/j.exer.2013.11.005
75. Moura AL, Nagy BV, La Morgia C, Barboni P, Oliveira AG, Salomao SR, et al. The pupil light reflex in Leber's hereditary optic neuropathy: evidence for preservation of melanopsin-expressing retinal ganglion cells. *Invest Ophthalmol Visual Sci.* (2013) 54:4471–7. doi: 10.1167/iovs.12-11137
76. Munch M, Leon L, Collomb S, Kawasaki A. Comparison of acute non-visual bright light responses in patients with optic nerve disease, glaucoma and healthy controls. *Sci Rep.* (2015) 5:15185. doi: 10.1038/srep15185
77. La Morgia C, Ross-Cisneros FN, Sadun AA, Hannibal J, Munarini A, Mantovani V, et al. Melanopsin retinal ganglion cells are resistant to neurodegeneration in mitochondrial optic neuropathies. *Brain* (2010) 133(Pt 8):2426–38. doi: 10.1093/brain/awq155
78. Ba-Ali S, Lund-Andersen H. Pupillometric evaluation of the melanopsin containing retinal ganglion cells in mitochondrial and non-mitochondrial optic neuropathies. *Mitochondrion* (2017) 36:124–9. doi: 10.1016/j.mito.2017.07.003
79. Georg B, Ghelli A, Giordano C, Ross-Cisneros FN, Sadun AA, Carelli V, et al. Melanopsin-expressing retinal ganglion cells are resistant to cell injury, but not always. *Mitochondrion* (2017) 36:77–84. doi: 10.1016/j.mito.2017.04.003
80. Tsika C, Crippa SV, Kawasaki A. Differential monocular vs. binocular pupil responses from melanopsin-based photoreception in patients with anterior ischemic optic neuropathy. *Sci Rep.* (2015) 5:10780. doi: 10.1038/srep10780
81. Gracitelli CP, Duque-Chica GL, Moura AL, Nagy BV, de Melo GR, Roizenblatt M, et al. A positive association between intrinsically photosensitive retinal ganglion cells and retinal nerve fiber layer thinning in glaucoma. *Invest Ophthalmol Visual Sci.* (2014) 55:7997–8005. doi: 10.1167/iovs.14-15146
82. Gracitelli CPB, Duque-Chica GL, Moura ALdA, Roizenblatt M, Nagy BV, de Melo GR, et al. Relationship between daytime sleepiness and intrinsically photosensitive retinal ganglion cells in glaucomatous disease. *J Ophthalmol.* (2016) 2016:1–9. doi: 10.1155/2016/5317371
83. Kelbsch C, Maeda F, Strasser T, Blumenstock G, Wilhelm B, Wilhelm H, et al. Pupillary responses driven by ipRGCs and classical photoreceptors are impaired in glaucoma. *Graefes Arch Clin Exp Ophthalmol.* (2016) 254:1361–70. doi: 10.1007/s00417-016-3351-9
84. Adhikari P, Zele AJ, Thomas R, Feigl B. Quadrant field pupillometry detects melanopsin dysfunction in glaucoma suspects and early glaucoma. *Sci Rep.* (2016) 6:33373. doi: 10.1038/srep33373
85. Kankipati L, Girkin CA, Gamlin PD. Post-illumination pupil response in subjects without ocular disease. *Invest Ophthalmol Visual Sci.* (2010) 51:2764–9. doi: 10.1167/iovs.09-4717
86. Kankipati L, Girkin CA, Gamlin PD. The post-illumination pupil response is reduced in glaucoma patients. *Invest Ophthalmol Visual Sci.* (2011) 52:2287–92. doi: 10.1167/iovs.10-6023
87. Feigl B, Mattes D, Thomas R, Zele AJ. Intrinsically photosensitive (melanopsin) retinal ganglion cell function in glaucoma. *Invest Ophthalmol Visual Sci.* (2011) 52:4362–7. doi: 10.1167/iovs.10-7069
88. Feigl B, Zele AJ, Fader SM, Howes AN, Hughes CE, Jones KA, et al. The post-illumination pupil response of melanopsin-expressing intrinsically photosensitive retinal ganglion cells in diabetes. *Acta Ophthalmol.* (2012) 90:e230–4. doi: 10.1111/j.1755-3768.2011.02226.x
89. Feigl B, Zele AJ. Melanopsin-expressing intrinsically photosensitive retinal ganglion cells in retinal disease. *Optometry Vision Sci.* (2014) 91:894–903. doi: 10.1097/OPX.0000000000000284
90. Kawasaki, Herbst, Sander, Milea. Selective wavelength pupillometry in Leber hereditary optic neuropathy. *Clin Experiment Ophthalmol.* (2010) 38:322–4. doi: 10.1111/j.1442-9071.2010.02212.x
91. Herbst K, Sander B, Lund-Andersen H, Wegener M, Hannibal J, Milea D. Unilateral anterior ischemic optic neuropathy: chromatic pupillometry in affected, fellow non-affected and healthy control eyes. *Front Neurol.* (2013) 4:52. doi: 10.3389/fneur.2013.00052
92. Ba-Ali S, Christensen SK, Sander B, Rosenberg T, Larsen M, Lund-Andersen H. Choroideremia: melanopsin-mediated postillumination pupil relaxation is abnormally slow. *Acta Ophthalmol.* (2017) 95:809–14. doi: 10.1111/aos.13394
93. Kardon R, Anderson SC, Damarjian TG, Grace EM, Stone E, Kawasaki A. Chromatic pupil responses: preferential activation of the melanopsin-mediated versus outer photoreceptor-mediated pupil light reflex. *Ophthalmology* (2009) 116:1564–73. doi: 10.1016/j.ophtha.2009.02.007
94. Rukmini AV. *Assessment of Photoreceptor Function Using the Pupillary Light Reflex.* Singapore: National University of Singapore (2016).
95. Najjar RP, Sharma S, Atalay E, Rukmini AV, Sun C, Lock JZ, et al. Pupillary responses to full-field chromatic stimuli are reduced in patients with early-stage primary open-angle glaucoma. *Ophthalmology* (2018). doi: 10.1016/j.ophtha.2018.02.024
96. Loo JL, Singhal S, Rukmini AV, Tow S, Amati-Bonneau P, Procaccio V, et al. Multiethnic involvement in autosomal-dominant optic atrophy in Singapore. *Eye* (2017) 31:475–80. doi: 10.1038/eye.2016.255
97. Spitschan M, Jain S, Brainard DH, Aguirre GK. Opponent melanopsin and S-cone signals in the human pupillary light response. *Proc Natl Acad Sci USA.* (2014) 111:15568–72. doi: 10.1073/pnas.1400942111
98. Woelders T, Leenheers T, Gordijn MCM, Hut RA, Beersma DGM, Wams EJ. Melanopsin- and L-cone-induced pupil constriction is inhibited by S- and M-cones in humans. *Proc Natl Acad Sci USA.* (2018) 115:792–7. doi: 10.1073/pnas.1716281115
99. Wong KY, Dunn FA, Berson DM. Photoreceptor adaptation in intrinsically photosensitive retinal ganglion cells. *Neuron* (2005) 48:1001–10. doi: 10.1016/j.neuron.2005.11.016
100. Wang B, Shen C, Zhang L, Qi L, Yao L, Chen J, et al. Dark adaptation-induced changes in rod, cone and intrinsically photosensitive retinal ganglion cell (ipRGC) sensitivity differentially affect the pupil light response (PLR). *Graefes Arch Clin Exp Ophthalmol.* (2015) 253:1997–2005. doi: 10.1007/s00417-015-3137-5
101. Joyce DS, Feigl B, Zele AJ. The effects of short-term light adaptation on the human post-illumination pupil response. *Invest Ophthalmol Visual Sci.* (2016) 57:5672–80. doi: 10.1167/iovs.16-19934
102. Joyce DS, Feigl B, Zele AJ. Melanopsin-mediated post-illumination pupil response in the peripheral retina. *J Vis.* (2016) 16:5. doi: 10.1167/16.8.5
103. Park JC, McAnany JJ. Effect of stimulus size and luminance on the rod-, cone-, and melanopsin-mediated pupillary light reflex. *J Vis.* (2015) 15:3. doi: 10.1167/15.3.13
104. Ortube MC, Kiderman A, Eydelman Y, Yu F, Aguilar N, Nusinowitz S, et al. Comparative regional pupillography as a noninvasive biosensor screening method for diabetic retinopathy. *Invest Ophthalmol Visual Sci.* (2013) 54:9–18. doi: 10.1167/iovs.12-10241
105. Lei S, Goltz HC, Chandrakumar M, Wong AM. Full-field chromatic pupillometry for the assessment of the postillumination pupil response driven by melanopsin-containing retinal ganglion cells. *Invest Ophthalmol Visual Sci.* (2014) 55:4496–503. doi: 10.1167/iovs.14-14103
106. Lei S, Goltz HC, Chandrakumar M, Wong AM. Test-retest reliability of hemifield, central-field, and full-field chromatic pupillometry for assessing the function of melanopsin-containing retinal ganglion cells. *Invest Ophthalmol Visual Sci.* (2015) 56:1267–73. doi: 10.1167/iovs.14-15945
107. Salter AR, Conger A, Frohman TC, Zivadinov R, Eggenberger E, Calabresi P, et al. Retinal architecture predicts pupillary reflex metrics in MS. *Mult Scler.* (2009) 15:479–86. doi: 10.1177/1352458508100503
108. Meltzer E, Sguigna PV, Subei A, Beh S, Kildebeck E, Conger D, et al. Retinal architecture and melanopsin-mediated pupillary response characteristics: a putative pathophysiologic signature for the retino-hypothalamic tract in multiple sclerosis. *JAMA Neurol.* (2017) 74:574–82. doi: 10.1001/jamaneurol.2016.5131

109. Joyce DS, Feigl B, Kerr G, Roeder L, Zele AJ. Melanopsin-mediated pupil function is impaired in Parkinson's disease. *Sci Rep.* (2018) 8:7796. doi: 10.1038/s41598-018-26078-0
110. Kawasaki AK. Diagnostic approach to pupillary abnormalities. *CONTINUUM Lifelong Learn Neurol.* (2014) 20:1008–22. doi: 10.1212/01.CON.0000453306.42981.94
111. Wilhelm H. Disorders of the pupil. *Handbook Clin Neurol.* (2011) 102:427–66. doi: 10.1016/b978-0-444-52903-9.00022-4
112. Roecklein K, Wong P, Ernecoff N, Miller M, Donofry S, Kamarck M, et al. The post illumination pupil response is reduced in seasonal affective disorder. *Psychiat Res.* (2013) 210:150–8. doi: 10.1016/j.psychres.2013.05.023
113. Berman G, Muttuvelu D, Berman D, Larsen JI, Licht RW, Ledolter J, et al. Decreased retinal sensitivity in depressive disorder: a controlled study. *Acta Psychiatr Scand.* (2018) 137:231–40. doi: 10.1111/acps.12851
114. Munch M, Ladaique M, Roemer S, Hashemi K, Kawasaki A. Melanopsin-mediated acute light responses measured in winter and in summer: seasonal variations in adults with and without cataracts. *Front Neurol.* (2017) 8:464. doi: 10.3389/fneur.2017.00464
115. Roecklein KA, Rohan KJ, Duncan WC, Rollag MD, Rosenthal NE, Lipsky RH, et al. A missense variant (P10L) of the melanopsin (OPN4) gene in seasonal affective disorder. *J Affect Disord.* (2009) 114:279–85. doi: 10.1016/j.jad.2008.08.005
116. Lee SI, Hida A, Tsujimura S, Morita T, Mishima K, Higuchi S. Association between melanopsin gene polymorphism (I394T) and pupillary light reflex is dependent on light wavelength. *J Physiol Anthropol.* (2013) 32:16. doi: 10.1186/1880-6805-32-16
117. Higuchi S, Hida A, Tsujimura S, Mishima K, Yasukouchi A, Lee SI, et al. Melanopsin gene polymorphism I394T is associated with pupillary light responses in a dose-dependent manner. *PLoS ONE* (2013) 8:e60310. doi: 10.1371/journal.pone.0060310
118. Zele AJ, Feigl B, Smith SS, Markwell EL. The circadian response of intrinsically photosensitive retinal ganglion cells. *PLoS ONE* (2011) 6:e17860. doi: 10.1371/journal.pone.0017860
119. Munch M, Leon L, Crippa SV, Kawasaki A. Circadian and wake-dependent effects on the pupil light reflex in response to narrow-bandwidth light pulses. *Invest Ophthalmol Visual Sci.* (2012) 53:4546–55. doi: 10.1167/iovs.12-9494
120. Ba-Ali S, Sander B, Brondsted AE, Lund-Andersen H. Effect of topical anti-glaucoma medications on late pupillary light reflex, as evaluated by pupillometry. *Front Neurol.* (2015) 6:93. doi: 10.3389/fneur.2015.00093
121. Sahraie A, Trevethan CT, MacLeod MJ, Urquhart J, Weiskrantz L. Pupil response as a predictor of blindsight in hemianopia. *Proc Natl Acad Sci USA.* (2013) 110:18333–8. doi: 10.1073/pnas.1318395110
122. Maeda F, Kelbsch C, Strasser T, Skorkovska K, Peters T, Wilhelm B, et al. Chromatic pupillography in hemianopia patients with homonymous visual field defects. *Graefes Arch Clin Exp Ophthalmol.* (2017) 255:1837–42. doi: 10.1007/s00417-017-3721-y
123. Bitsios P, Prettyman R, Szabadi E. Changes in autonomic function with age: a study of pupillary kinetics in healthy young and old people. *Age Ageing* (1996) 25:432–8.
124. Daneault V, Vandewalle G, Hebert M, Teikari P, Mure LS, Doyon J, et al. Does pupil constriction under blue and green monochromatic light exposure change with age? *J Biol Rhythms* (2012) 27:257–64. doi: 10.1177/0748730412441172
125. Rukmini AV, Milea D, Aung T, Gooley JJ. Pupillary responses to short-wavelength light are preserved in aging. *Sci Rep.* (2017) 7:43832. doi: 10.1038/srep43832
126. Herbst K, Sander B, Lund-Andersen H, Broendsted AE, Kessel L, Hansen MS, et al. Intrinsically photosensitive retinal ganglion cell function in relation to age: a pupillometric study in humans with special reference to the age-related optic properties of the lens. *BMC Ophthalmol.* (2012) 12:4. doi: 10.1186/1471-2415-12-4
127. Adhikari P, Pearson CA, Anderson AM, Zele AJ, Feigl B. Effect of Age and Refractive Error on the Melanopsin Mediated Post-Illumination Pupil Response (PIPR). *Sci Rep.* (2015) 5:17610. doi: 10.1038/srep17610
128. Rukmini AV, Najjar RP, Atalay E, Sharma S, Lock JZ, Baskaran M, et al. Pupillary responses to light are not affected by narrow irido-corneal angles. *Sci Rep.* (2017) 7:10190. doi: 10.1038/s41598-017-10303-3
129. Herbst K, Sander B, Milea D, Lund-Andersen H, Kawasaki A. Test-retest repeatability of the pupil light response to blue and red light stimuli in normal human eyes using a novel pupillometer. *Front Neurol.* (2011) 2:10. doi: 10.3389/fneur.2011.00010
130. Lucas RJ, Peirson SN, Berson DM, Brown TM, Cooper HM, Czeisler CA, et al. Measuring and using light in the melanopsin age. *Trends Neurosci.* (2014) 37:1–9. doi: 10.1016/j.tins.2013.10.004
131. Burns SA, Webb RH. Optical Generation of the Visual Stimulus, Sections 5.1 to 5.15. In: Bass M, Mahajan VN, Optical Society of A, editors. *Handbook of Optics. 3, Vision and Vision Optics. 3rd ed.* New York, NY: McGraw-Hill (2010).
132. Nissen C, Sander B, Lund-Andersen H. The effect of pupil size on stimulation of the melanopsin containing retinal ganglion cells, as evaluated by monochromatic pupillometry. *Front Neurol.* (2011) 2:92. doi: 10.3389/fneur.2011.00092
133. Couret D, Boumaza D, Grisotto C, Triglia T, Pellegrini L, Ocquidant P, et al. Reliability of standard pupillometry practice in neurocritical care: an observational, double-blinded study. *Critical Care* (2016) 20:99. doi: 10.1186/s13054-016-1239-z
134. Higuchi S, Ishibashi K, Aritake S, Enomoto M, Hida A, Tamura M, et al. Inter-individual difference in pupil size correlates to suppression of melatonin by exposure to light. *Neurosci Lett.* (2008) 440:23–6. doi: 10.1016/j.neulet.2008.05.037
135. van der Meijden WP, Van Someren JL, Te Lindert BH, Bruijel J, van Oosterhout F, Coppens JE, et al. Individual differences in sleep timing relate to melanopsin-based phototransduction in healthy adolescents and young adults. *Sleep* (2016) 39:1305–10. doi: 10.5665/sleep.5858
136. Grozdanic SD, Matic M, Sakaguchi DS, Kardon RH. Evaluation of retinal status using chromatic pupil light reflex activity in healthy and diseased canine eyes. *Invest Ophthalmol Visual Sci.* (2007) 48:5178–83. doi: 10.1167/iovs.07-0249
137. Yeh CY, Koehl KL, Harman CD, Iwabe S, Guzman JM, Petersen-Jones SM, et al. Assessment of rod, cone, and intrinsically photosensitive retinal ganglion cell contributions to the canine chromatic pupillary response. *Invest Ophthalmol Visual Sci.* (2017) 58:65–78. doi: 10.1167/iovs.16-19865
138. Terakado K, Yogo T, Nezu Y, Harada Y, Hara Y, Tagawa M. Efficacy of the use of a colorimetric pupil light reflex device in the diagnosis of fundus disease or optic pathway disease in dogs. *J Veterinary Med Sci.* (2013) 75:1491–5. doi: 10.1292/jvms.12-0363
139. Lin B, Koizumi A, Tanaka N, Panda S, Masland RH. Restoration of visual function in retinal degeneration mice by ectopic expression of melanopsin. *Proc Natl Acad Sci USA.* (2008) 105:16009–14. doi: 10.1073/pnas.0806114105
140. De Silva SR, Barnard AR, Hughes S, Tam SKE, Martin C, Singh MS, et al. Long-term restoration of visual function in end-stage retinal degeneration using subretinal human melanopsin gene therapy. *Proc Natl Acad Sci USA.* (2017) 114:11211–6. doi: 10.1073/pnas.1701589114
141. Caporale N, Kolstad KD, Lee T, Tochitsky I, Dalkara D, Trauner D, et al. LiGluR restores visual responses in rodent models of inherited blindness. *Mol Ther.* (2011) 19:1212–9. doi: 10.1038/mt.2011.103
142. Polosukhina A, Litt J, Tochitsky I, Nemargut J, Sychev Y, De Kouchkovsky I, et al. Photochemical restoration of visual responses in blind mice. *Neuron* (2012) 75:271–82. doi: 10.1016/j.neuron.2012.05.022
143. Tang J, Qin N, Chong Y, Diao Y, Yiliguma, Wang Z, et al. Nanowire arrays restore vision in blind mice. *Nat Commun.* (2018) 9:786. doi: 10.1038/s41467-018-03212-0

144. Batten ML, Imanishi Y, Tu DC, Doan T, Zhu L, Pang J, et al. Pharmacological and rAAV gene therapy rescue of visual functions in a blind mouse model of Leber congenital amaurosis. *PLoS Med.* (2005) 2:e333. doi: 10.1371/journal.pmed.0020333

145. Bennett J, Wellman J, Marshall KA, McCague S, Ashtari M, DiStefano-Pappas J, et al. Safety and durability of effect of contralateral-eye administration of AAV2 gene therapy in patients with childhood-onset blindness caused by RPE65 mutations: a follow-on phase 1 trial. *Lancet* (2016) 388:661–72. doi: 10.1016/s0140-6736(16)30371-3

146. Maguire AM, High KA, Auricchio A, Wright JF, Pierce EA, Testa F, et al. Age-dependent effects of RPE65 gene therapy for Leber's congenital amaurosis: a phase 1 dose-escalation trial. *Lancet* (2009) 374:1597–605. doi: 10.1016/s0140-6736(09)61836-5

3

Baseline Pupil Diameter is not a Reliable Biomarker of Subjective Sleepiness

Inès Daguet[1], Didier Bouhassira[2] and Claude Gronfier[1]*

[1] Lyon Neuroscience Research Center, Waking Team, INSERM UMRS 1028, CNRS UMR 5292, Université Claude Bernard Lyon 1, Université de Lyon, Lyon, France, [2] INSERM U987, Centre d'Evaluation et de Traitement de la Douleur, Hôpital Ambroise Paré, Boulogne-Billancourt, France

***Correspondence:**
Claude Gronfier
claude.gronfier@inserm.fr

Sleepiness is commonly seen as reflecting the basic physiological need to sleep and is associated with physiological and neurobiological changes. Subjective evaluations of sleepiness, however, are neither representative of cognitive and physical performances, nor of physiological sleepiness. Finding a simple, rapid, and objective marker of sleepiness is essential in order to prevent errors and accidents, but this has remained largely unsuccessful. The aim of this study was to determine whether the baseline pupil diameter is a physiological biomarker of sleepiness at all times of day and to isolate the regulatory components involved. Twelve healthy men (20–29 years old) participated in a 56-h experimental protocol, including a 34-h constant routine paradigm with enforced wakefulness. This protocol was used in order to eliminate the potential influence of all environmental rhythms and reveal the endogenous circadian rhythmicity of two physiological measures: sleepiness and pupil diameter. Sleepiness was assessed subjectively every hour on a computerized 10 cm visual analog scale and pupil size was recorded every 2 h with a hand-held video-pupilometer. Our results revealed that subjective sleepiness increased linearly with time awake and displayed a circadian rhythm. Baseline pupil diameter showed a linear decrease with time spent awake as well as a circadian 24-h rhythm. This is the first evidence of a circadian variation of the baseline pupil size in a highly-controlled constant routine paradigm conducted in very dim light conditions. An overall negative correlation between the size of the pupil and the subjective level of sleepiness was observed. Analyzing the contribution of the two sleep regulation components in this correlation, we further showed: (1) a negative correlation between the homeostatic sleep pressure components, (2) a negative correlation between the circadian drives only during half of the 24 hours, corresponding to 62% of the biological day and 25% of the biological night. These results highlight that, due to the dual regulation of sleepiness by the homeostatic and circadian processes, baseline pupil diameter is an index of sleepiness only at certain times and therefore cannot be used as a systematic and reliable biomarker of sleepiness.

Keywords: pupil diameter, sleepiness, circadian rhythm, sleep pressure, constant routine

INTRODUCTION

Sleepiness reflects the basic physiological need to sleep, and is classically recognized by yawning, eye rubbing and nodding (1). These behavioral changes are generally associated with neurobiological correlates such as cognitive decrements, microsleep episodes and an increase in alpha and theta activity in the EEG signal (2). Sleepiness results from the combination of a homeostatic process and a circadian process (3, 4). The homeostatic drive (process S) increases with wakefulness and decreases during sleep. The circadian drive (process C) relies on the self-sustained rhythmic 24-h activity of the endogenous biological clock, located in the suprachiasmatic nucleus (SCN) of the hypothalamus. These two processes interact to control the timing of sleep and wakefulness. Interestingly, their seemingly paradoxical drive, i.e. the high homeostatic sleep pressure at the end of the day together with the concomitantly high circadian pressure promoting wakefulness, is crucial to consolidate wakefulness during daytime and sleep at night (4).

Monitoring sleepiness is crucial in order to prevent accidents in everyday life conditions; for example in monotonous jobs, when driving a vehicle, or during night work. Yet, the assessment of sleepiness is also essential in patients suffering from sleep disorders, in order to diagnose and monitor excessive sleepiness or to evaluate the efficiency of a treatment. Different technics based on the measurement of objective physiological responses such as heart rate, skin conductance, reaction time, sleep latency, or pupil variations have been tested to estimate the level of sleepiness (5, 6). In clinical practice, sleep tendency during the day is commonly assessed by two validated tests: the Multiple Sleep Latency Test (MSLT) and the Maintenance of Wakefulness Test (MWT). However, both tests take almost a day to be conducted and sometimes need to be scheduled months in advance in a sleep clinic. Therefore, the need for a faster and more convenient biomarker of sleepiness is undeniable (6).

The eye has been the target of numerous studies on sleepiness as the opening or closing of the eyelids is one of the major differences between the states of sleep and wake. Indeed, the first studies using pupillometry as a biomarker of sleepiness emerged in the 1950s (7–9) and several variables have been studied over the years (6, 10–12). For example, psychological pupillography has been used in order to measure the percentage of eyelid closure during a vigilance task (11). The Pupillary Unrest Index (PUI) of the Pupillographic Sleepiness Test (PST) has been used to detect spontaneous pupillary oscillations, by measuring infrared video pupillography in darkness (12). Similarly, baseline pupil diameters have been measured in darkness during wake and sleep (12, 13). At first sight, it seems that the baseline pupil diameter could be a good marker of sleepiness as the pupil is dilated during wake and constricted during REM sleep (13). During NREM sleep, pupil size oscillates between small and large pupil diameters reflecting sleep depth; the deeper the sleep, the more the pupil constricts.

The circuitry involved in the control of sleep engages the reticular activating system, which consists of several nuclei such as the ventral tegmental area, the raphe nuclei and the locus coeruleus (LC) (14, 15). Even though sleepiness is thought to be controlled by the same structures, the neural substrates involved have not been clearly identified. The parasympathetic drive has been shown to be higher during sleep stages than during relaxed wakefulness, suggesting an implication of the autonomic nervous system in sleepiness (16). Other mechanisms, such as adenosine have been proposed to participate in sleepiness and sleep pressure (17), by activating "sleep-active" neurons in the ventro-lateral preoptic area of the hypothalamus (VLPO).

Pupil diameter in constant darkness is regulated by the automatic nervous system; activation of the parasympathetic pathway induces pupil constriction whereas activation of the sympathetic pathway leads to pupil dilation (18). In everyday life, pupil size is strongly influenced by the ambient lighting. Light stimulates the classic photoreceptors (rods and cones) but also activates the recently discovered intrinsically photosensitive retinal ganglion cells (ipRGCs), also known as melanopsin-containing retinal ganglion cells. These ipRGCs axons constitute the retino-hypothalamic tract (RHT) and project, among other structures, to the olivary pretectal nucleus (OPN), a brain region involved in the control of the pupillary light reflex (PLR) (19).

In sleepy subjects who are in the dark, the pupil size decreases and large spontaneous oscillations, called sleepiness waves, appear (10, 20–23). The intensity of these sleepiness waves increases with the duration of sleep deprivation (24). On the opposite, in non-sleepy subjects, the pupil remains constantly dilated in darkness. When comparing the pupil diameter in sleep deprived and alert conditions in the same participants, the pupil size is significantly smaller in sleep deprivation conditions (25, 26). Similarly, a large pupil size is associated with high levels of cognitive effort (27). A relationship between pupil diameter and sleepiness has also been observed in pathologies such as narcolepsy, with narcoleptic patients, who suffer from excessive daytime sleepiness, showing smaller pupil diameters than healthy participants, both in ambient light and in darkness (28).

Despite the numerous studies that have examined the relationship between alertness and pupil diameter, discrepancies remain. Certain studies have identified an association between high sleepiness and small pupil size (20, 25, 27–29) whereas others have not observed such a correlation between the two responses, both for intra-individual (30) and inter-individual correlations (31). It is important to highlight that these pupillometry and sleepiness measures were conducted either in the morning, the afternoon, the evening, or at night, depending on the study. Surprisingly, and even though this could explain the disparity in the results, the time-of-day effect has rarely been taken into consideration, suggesting that the role of the circadian system, both in regulating sleepiness and possibly pupil diameter, has been forgotten in these analyses.

To the best of our knowledge, only three studies have looked at the time course of the pupil diameter over the 24 hours (23, 26, 32). Loving and collaborators (32) measured pupil diameter in healthy adults every 30 min during a 24-h episode of constant wakefulness (sleep deprivation protocol) in ambient red light (<100 lux) and showed no variation of pupil size, suggesting no relationship between sleep debt and pupil size. In a 27-h paradigm with an ultradian sleep/wake cycle (15 min nap opportunity every hour) with ambient light (80 lux), Ranzijn et al. (26) observed that the baseline pupil diameter became smaller with progressive sleep loss, but this variation was not correlated to subjective sleepiness. Wilhelm et al. (23) conducted a 30-h enforced wakefulness protocol in constant low light levels (2 cd/m^2) with measures every 2 h, and revealed a decrease in pupil diameter and an increase in subjective sleepiness as time spent awake increased. Nevertheless, no studies have analyzed how sleepiness and pupil size covary as a function of time of day.

The objective of our study was to determine whether the baseline pupil diameter is a physiological biomarker of sleepiness at all times of day and to isolate the regulatory components involved (homeostatic and circadian). We used the highly controlled constant routine procedure in healthy individuals to separate and investigate how these two processes correlate with pupil diameter at different times of day. We hypothesized that the relationship between pupil diameter and sleepiness is not linear, simply related to the homeostatic drive for sleep, but more complex than previously thought, and involving the circadian system.

MATERIALS AND METHODS

Participants

Twelve healthy men (20–29 years old, mean = 22.7 ± 3.3 years old; BMI = 21.8 ± 3.1 kg/m^2) were included in this study. Neurological, psychiatric and sleep disorders were excluded by physical examination and psychological questionnaires (Pittsburg Sleep Quality Index Questionnaire and Beck Depression Inventory) (33, 34). Participants had an intermediate chronotype (Horne and Ostberg Chronotype Questionnaire score between 31 and 69) and did no shift work, nor transmeridian travel during the previous 3 months (35). Participants had normal visual acuity (Landolt Ring Test and Monoyer scale), contrast vision (Functional Acuity Contrast Test) and color vision (Farnworth D-15 and Ishihara Color Test). All experimental procedures were carried out in accordance to the principles of the Declaration of Helsinki. The study was approved by the local Research Ethics Committee (CPP Lyon Sud-Est II) and participants provided written informed consent.

Study Design

Participants were instructed to maintain a regular sleep-wake schedule (bedtimes and waketimes within ± 30 min of self-targeted times) for 1–3 weeks before admission to the laboratory, and this was verified by wrist activity and light exposure recordings (ActTrust, Condor Instruments, São Paulo, Brazil). Subjects were then admitted to the laboratory for a 56-h experimental protocol (**Figure 1**) where they were maintained in an environment free from external time cues (clocks, television, smartphones, internet, visitors, sunlight, etc.). Subjects maintained contact with staff members specifically trained to avoid communicating time of day or the nature of the experimental conditions to the subjects. Participants arrived around 10:00 on the first day, they familiarized themselves with the laboratory environment, the low light levels (~0.5 lux), the equipment, and the measurements. A series of measurements were carried out until bedtime (participant's habitual bedtime), and an 8-h sleep episode was scheduled (constant darkness; recumbent position). This was followed by a 34-h constant routine protocol that started at the participant's usual waketime on day 2 and finished around 18:00 on day 3.

Constant Routine Protocol

A Constant Routine (CR) paradigm was used in order to reveal the endogenous circadian rhythmicity of different parameters. The CR is conducted under constant environmental conditions, in order to eliminate or distribute across the circadian cycle the physiological responses evoked by environmental or behavioral stimuli (i.e., sleeping, eating, changes in posture, light intensity variations) (36, 37). In practical terms, participants were asked to remain awake for 34 h with minimal physical activity, while lying in a semi-recumbent (45°) posture in bed. This posture was also maintained for urine samples and bowel movements. Room temperature (mean = 23°C ± 0.6) and ambient very dim halogen light remained constant. Light intensity was homogeneous in the room (~0.5 lux at the participant's eye level in all gaze directions). Participants were given small equicaloric snacks and fluids at hourly intervals, to maintain an equal nutritional caloric intake and stable hydration across the circadian cycle. Caloric requirements were calculated with use of the Wilmore nomogram to determine the basal metabolic rate and were adjusted upward by a 7% activity factor (38, 39). Fluid intake was calculated for each subject to account for the sedentary nature of the CR (38). A study staff member remained in the room with the participant at all times during the CR to monitor wakefulness and to ensure compliance to study procedures.

Sleepiness Evaluation

Sleepiness was assessed subjectively every hour on a computerized 10 cm visual analog scale (VAS) ranging from 0 (no sleepiness) to 10 (maximum sleepiness).

Pupillometry

Pupil size was recorded every 2 h with a hand-held monocular video-pupilometer (Neurolight, IDMed, Marseille, France). This device, placed at 25 mm from cornea surface, detected pupil margins under infrared illumination (two infrared LED lights with a peak at 880 nm) and continuously tracked the pupil diameter. The pupilometer was placed in front of the participant's left eye and held steadily by the experimenter (**Supplementary Figure 1**). The participant was asked to keep the left eye wide open (without blinking) and to look straight ahead. During the measurement, the experimenter could see the pupil on the screen of the device and check that the device was correctly placed on the participant's eye. This measurement was conducted in complete darkness as the right eyelid was closed and covered by the participant's hand and the left eye was covered by the device. Before each measurement, we also questioned the participant in order to ensure that the participant did not detect any ambient lighting. The baseline pupil diameter was detected over a 5 s segment in darkness (without adaptation), with a sampling rate of 62 Hz and was determined by calculating the median pupil diameter during the stable portion of this 5 s measurement. Pupil diameter was recorded in mm in the output file of the pupilometer. Pupil diameter was considered abnormal

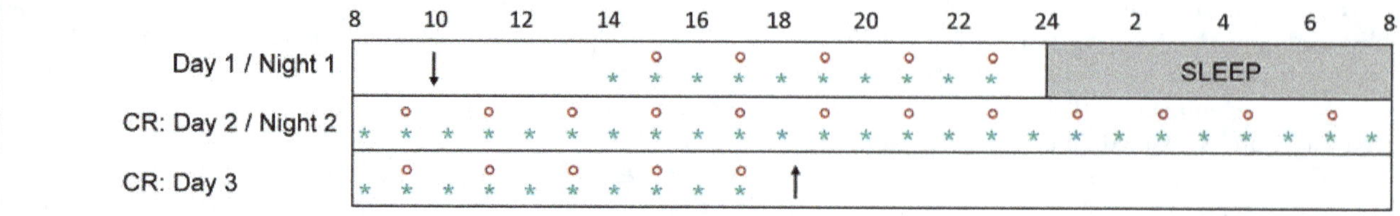

FIGURE 1 | Overview of the experimental protocol. After a habituation day (day 1) and an 8-h sleep episode, participants underwent a 34-h constant routine (CR: days 2 and 3). Subjective sleepiness was measured every hour (blue star) and pupil size was recorded every 2 h (red circle). Participants arrived around 10:00 on day 1 (down arrow) and left the protocol around 18:00 on day 3 (up arrow).

when values were above 9 mm or below 2 mm. Artifacts were defined when an absolute change between 2 samples (sampling rate of 62 Hz) was above 0.15 mm (which corresponds to a change of approximatively 9.3 mm per second).

Data Analysis

The sleepiness and pupil size measurements conducted during the first 2 h after waketime were removed from all analyses because sleep inertia has been shown to impair physiological responses such as alertness and cognitive function (40, 41). An outlier test was also applied on raw sleepiness and pupil diameter data, which identified no outliers in the datasets. To reduce inter-individual variability, all data were normalized by calculating individual z-scores (except for the analysis on raw values described in the **Supplementary Material**). For temporal analysis all values were plotted (32 values for sleepiness and 16 values for pupil size). For correlations, only half of the sleepiness values were used (measure every 2 h, starting 3 h after waketime), in order to have the same number of points for sleepiness and pupil size. After verification that data were normally distributed (Shapiro-Wilk test), Pearson correlations were computed between pupil diameter and sleepiness scores collected over the 34-h constant routine. To model the effect of time on the responses, the two main components regulating sleep (process S and process C) were modeled on the 34-h constant routine dataset. The homeostatic component (process S) of the data was regressed by a linear model on z-score transformed values (after removal of the sinusoidal trend): $f(time) = y0 + a \times time$. Circadian rhythmicity (process C) was determined on linearly detrended z-score values using a sinusoidal regression model: $f\,(time) = mesor + amplitude \times \cos(2\pi \times \frac{time}{tau} + \text{phase})$; Tau (circadian period) was constrained between 23.5 and 24.5 h (42, 43). Statistics were computed with *R* (Version 3.5.1, 2018-04-23, R Foundation for Statistical Computing, Vienna, Austria) and *SigmaPlot* (Version 12.0, Systat Software, San Jose, CA). Results were considered significant for $p < 0.05$.

RESULTS

Correlation Between Baseline Pupil Diameter and Subjective Sleepiness

To determine if there was an overall association between the size of the pupil and the level of subjective sleepiness during the 34-h constant routine protocol, all 16 values of all 12 participants were plotted on the same graph. The analysis on raw values revealed no correlation between subjective sleepiness and pupil diameter ($p = 0.23$; **Supplementary Figure 2**). In order to reduce inter-individual variability, all future analyses were conducted on normalized data (z-score calculation). Indeed, the negative correlation between pupil diameter and sleepiness is illustrated on **Figure 2**; the higher the sleepiness level, the lower the pupil diameter ($R^2 = 0.09$; $p \leq 0.0001$; **Figure 2**). In order to separate the potentially different relationships between pupil size and sleepiness during daytime and during nighttime, data were segregated into 4 time-episodes: CR daytime 2 (first 16 h of the constant routine protocol, corresponding to habitual daytime), CR nighttime 2 (next 8 h of the protocol, corresponding to habitual nighttime), CR daytime 3 (last 10 h of the protocol, corresponding to the first 10 h of habitual daytime after a full night of sleep deprivation) and CR daytimes 2 and 3 combined (habitual daytime over 2 days). The same correlation analysis was conducted on each of these epochs. No correlations between pupil size and sleepiness were observed for CR daytime 2, CR nighttime 2, nor CR daytime 3 respectively (**Figures 3A–C** respectively). When CR daytime 2 and CR daytime 3 were pooled together, a negative correlation appeared, suggesting that the time of day is a factor that needs to be taken into consideration ($R^2 = 0.17$; $p \leq 0.0001$; **Figure 3D**).

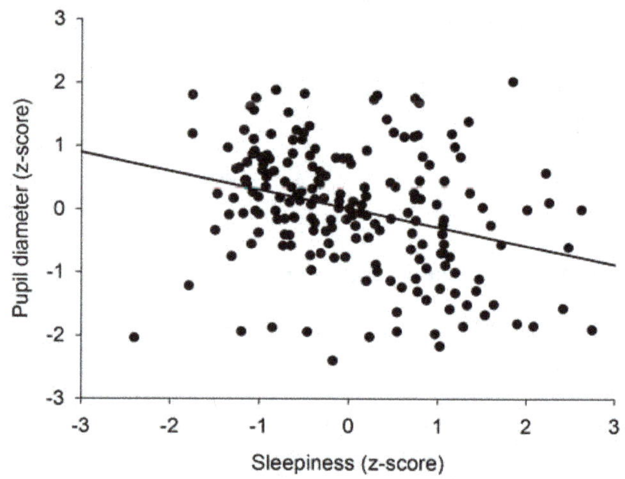

FIGURE 2 | Correlation between individual baseline pupil diameter and individual subjective sleepiness ($R^2 = 0.09$; $p \leq 0.0001$).

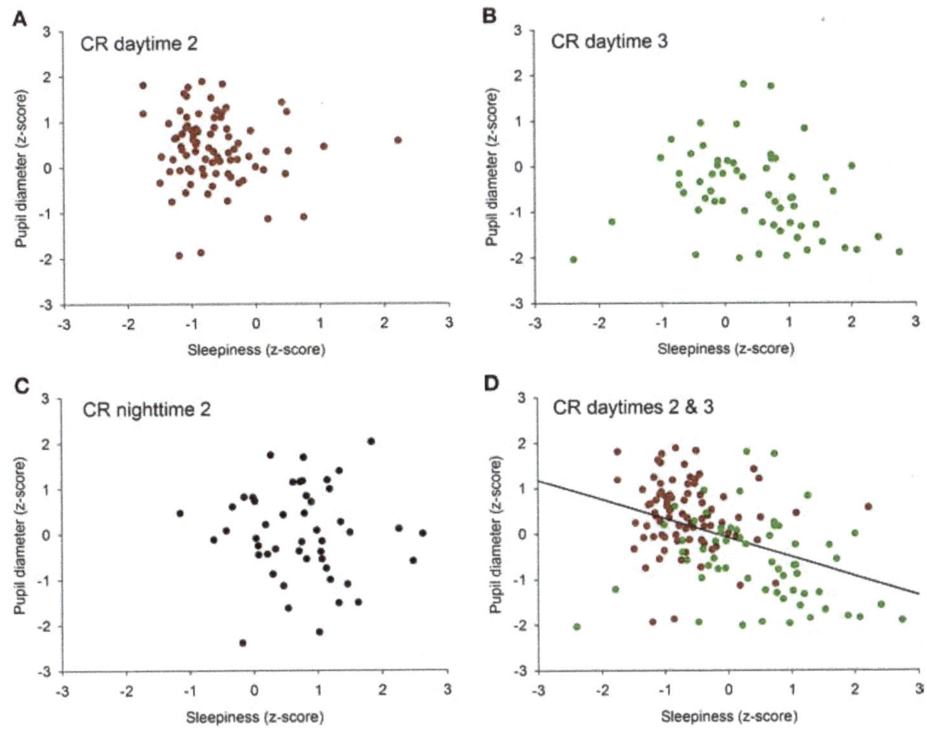

FIGURE 3 | Correlation between individual baseline pupil diameter and individual subjective sleepiness. **(A)** CR daytime 2 (first 16 h of the constant routine protocol), no correlation ($p = 0.34$). **(B)** CR daytime 3 (last 10 h of the protocol), no correlation ($p = 0.07$). **(C)** habitual nighttime, no correlation ($p = 0.78$). **(D)** habitual daytime (CR daytime 2 and CR daytime 3 pooled together), negative correlation ($R^2 = 0.17$; $p \leq 0.0001$).

Effect of Time-of-day on Subjective Sleepiness

To further investigate the relationships between sleepiness and baseline pupil diameter, we analyzed the mechanisms responsible for their respective time course. Sleepiness was evaluated subjectively every hour during the 34-h constant routine (**Figure 4A**) and raw sleepiness values ranged from 0 to 10 cm with a mean of 3.6 ± 2.6 cm on the VAS. Two models were fitted on the data in order to model the two components of sleep regulation: a linear trend modeling homeostatic sleep pressure and a sinusoidal component modeling the circadian drive. First, a significant linear fit was observed, confirming that sleepiness increases with time spent awake ($R^2 = 0.78$; $p \leq 0.0001$; **Figure 4B**). Second, after removal of the homeostatic trend, a sinusoidal regression significantly modeled the data, with a peak of sleepiness at 04:30 and a trough at 16:30 ($R^2 = 0.80$; $p \leq 0.0001$; **Figure 4C**).

Effect of Time-of-day on Baseline Pupil Size

Pupil diameter was measured every 2 h throughout the whole 34-h constant routine (**Figure 5A**) and raw pupil size values ranged from 5.8 to 8.7 mm with a mean of 7.4 ± 0.7 mm. A statistically significant linear regression was found between pupil diameter and time elapsed since waketime ($R^2 = 0.69$; $p \leq 0.0001$; **Figure 5B**). Pupil size decreases as time spent awake increases. Moreover, a statistically significant sinusoidal fit was found on linearly detrended data, with the largest pupil size at 22:30 and the smallest at 10:30 ($R^2 = 0.91$; $p \leq 0.001$; **Figure 5C**).

Separation of the Two Sleep Regulatory Components: Process S and Process C

We previously showed that the time course of sleepiness and pupil size are influenced by two components (homeostatic sleep pressure and circadian variation). We have isolated each component in order to observe, on one hand, the correlation between the linear processes of sleepiness and pupil size (**Figure 6A**) and, on the other hand, the correlation between the sinusoidal processes of these responses (**Figure 6B**). First, the homeostatic models of sleepiness and pupil size, illustrated on **Figure 6A**, showed that these responses covaried linearly but negatively. The pupil diameter decreased with time awake whereas sleepiness increased, partly explaining the negative correlation between the two responses observed in **Figure 2**. Indeed, we found a significant negative correlation between the linear processes of sleepiness and pupil size, revealing that sleepiness was high when the pupil size was small ($R^2 = 0.06$; $p \leq 0.001$; **Figure 7**). Second, **Figure 6B** showed that the circadian drives of sleepiness and pupil diameter did not covary in phase (maximum pupil size at 22:30 and maximum sleepiness at 04:30.), with a 6-h phase-lag between the two rhythms. This

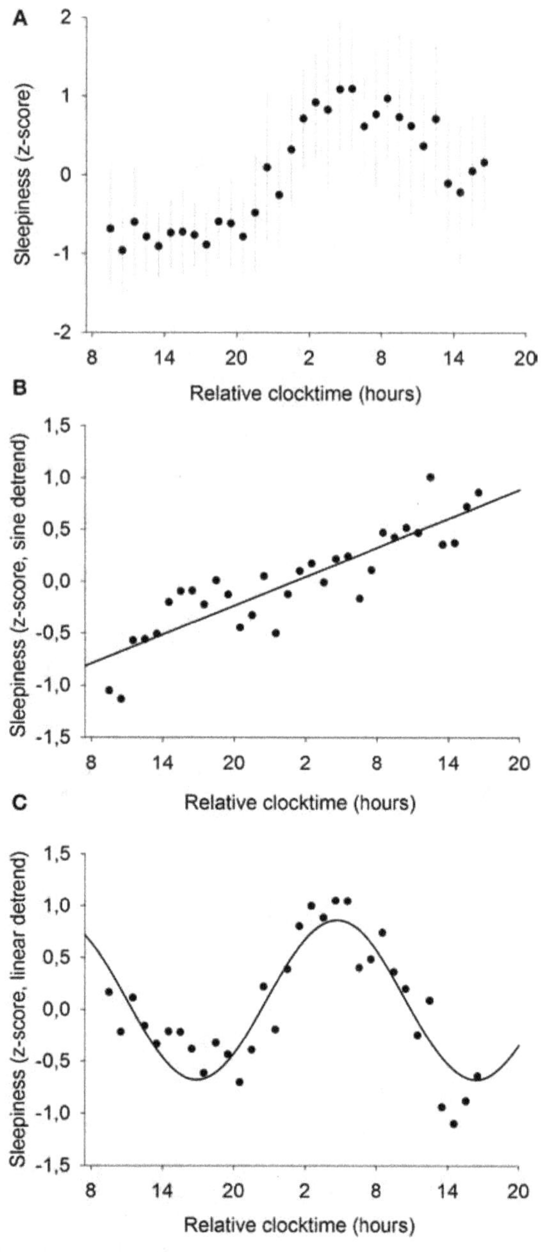

FIGURE 4 | Mean subjective sleepiness ($n = 12$). **(A)** normalized data (mean ± SD). **(B)** linear regression, after removal of the sinusoidal trend. Sleepiness increases with time spent awake ($R^2 = 0.78$; $p \leq 0.0001$). **(C)** sinusoidal regression, after removal of the linear trend; ($R^2 = 0.80$; $p \leq 0.0001$).

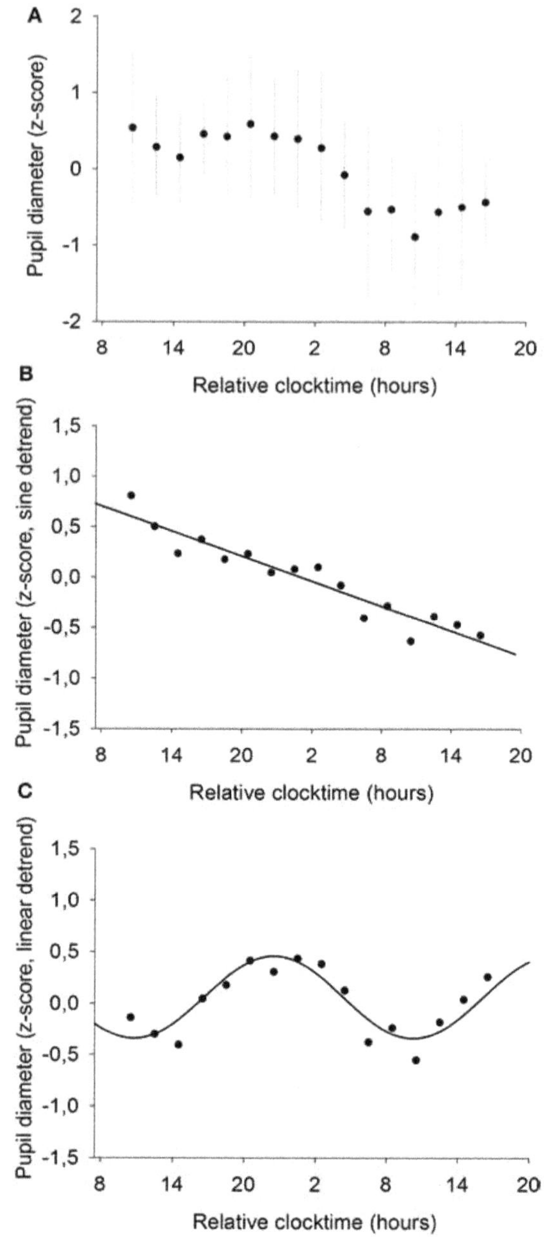

FIGURE 5 | Mean baseline pupil diameter ($n = 12$). **(A)** normalized data (mean ± SD). **(B)** linear regression, after removal of the sinusoidal trend. Pupil size decreases with time spent awake ($R^2 = 0.69$; $p \leq 0.0001$). **(C)** sinusoidal regression, after removal of the linear trend ($R^2 = 0.91$; $p \leq 0.001$).

lag allowed us to identify two different segments of time over the 24 hours: (1) the times of day when both responses vary in the same direction (both decrease or both increase) and (2) the times of day when they vary in opposite directions (one decreases when the other increases). The correlation between the circadian drives were therefore analyzed over the entire constant routine and during these two segments of time. We found a negative correlation between pupil size and sleepiness over the whole 24 hours ($R^2 = 0.03$; $p \leq 0.02$; **Figure 8A**) and also specifically when the two curves varied in the same direction (yellow shaded areas; between 4:30 and 10:30 and between 16:30 and 22:30; $R^2 = 0.09$; $p \leq 0.005$; **Figure 8B**). However, no correlation was found when they varied in opposite directions (pink shaded areas; between 10:30 and 16:30 and between 22:30 and 4:30; **Figure 8C**). These results demonstrate the presence of an association between the circadian drives for pupil size and sleepiness only during half of the 24-h day (in the morning and in the evening), or during 62% of the biological day and 25% of the biological night.

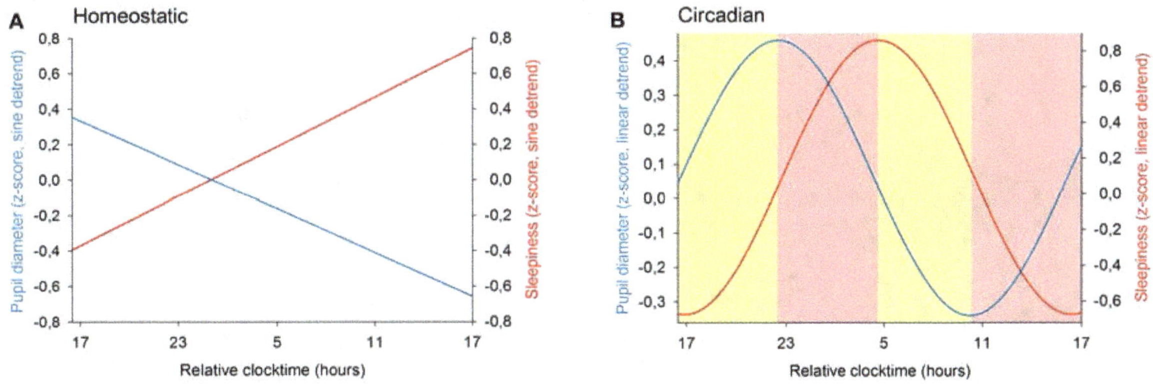

FIGURE 6 | Modeling of the two components of sleep regulation on baseline pupil diameter (blue line) and on sleepiness (red line) illustrated over a 24-h segment. **(A)** linear models of the effect of homeostatic sleep pressure on pupil size and sleepiness (after sinusoidal detrend). **(B)** sinusoidal components modeling the circadian drive on pupil size and sleepiness (after linear detrend). The yellow shaded areas correspond to the episodes of time where the circadian components of pupil diameter and of sleepiness vary in the same direction. The pink shaded areas correspond to the episodes of time where the responses change in opposite directions.

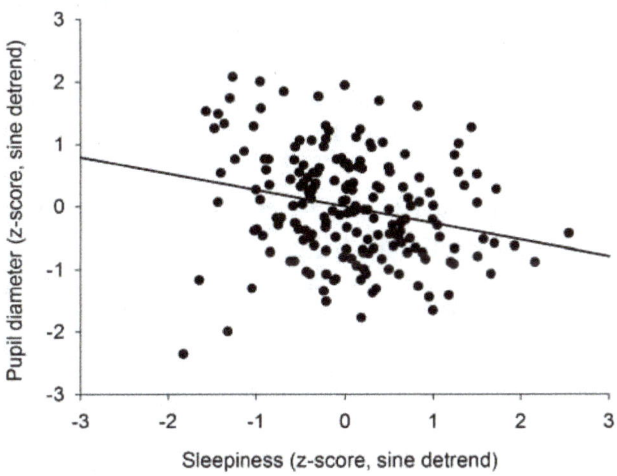

FIGURE 7 | Correlation between the homeostatic components of pupil diameter and subjective sleepiness ($R^2 = 0.06$; $p \leq 0.001$).

DISCUSSION

Our results show that the correlation between the size of the pupil and the subjective level of sleepiness is not systematic and that the pupil diameter cannot be a simple proxy for sleepiness. Sleepiness increases linearly as time spent awake increases and displays a circadian rhythm across the constant routine protocol. Pupil diameter shows a linear decrease with time spent awake, superimposed to a circadian 24-h rhythm. The separation of the two sleep regulatory processes (process S and process C) revealed that both homeostatic (S) processes correlate negatively. However, focusing the analysis on circadian (C) processes showed that the negative correlation between the two responses only appears at the beginning and the end of the biological day, but not in the afternoon or during the biological night.

Time-of-day Effect on Subjective Sleepiness

The subjective level of sleepiness increases as time spent awake and sleep pressure increases. This linear relationship between sleep pressure and subjective sleepiness (evaluated by the Stanford Sleepiness Scale or SSS) had already been identified in previous studies (23, 24). This homeostatic regulation of sleep (process S) could be explained by the accumulation of adenosine during wakefulness (17). A circadian variation of sleepiness (process C), modeled by a sinusoid regression, has also been identified, with a peak of sleepiness at 4:30. These data confirm previous results showing the existence of a 24-h rhythm of sleepiness (evaluated by the Karolinska Sleepiness Scale or KSS), and suggesting its control by the human endogenous circadian clock, located in the SCN (44, 45).

Time-of-day Effect on Baseline Pupil Diameter

We found that the size of the pupil showed a linear trend with time awake, suggesting that it is linked to the homeostatic increase in sleep pressure that occurs during the day. Therefore, the higher the sleep pressure, the smaller the pupil diameter. This result is in line with the study of Wilhelm et al., who showed a linear decreasing trend in pupil diameter in constant semi-darkness during a 30-h forced wakefulness protocol (23). Likewise, Ranzijn and collaborators showed that the pupil diameter is smaller after a 27-h constant routine protocol in constant ambient lighting (80 lux), than before the protocol (26). In our study, the constant routine protocol, conducted in highly controlled laboratory conditions, also allowed the identification of a circadian rhythm of the pupil size. This is the first evidence that the baseline pupil diameter in constant very dim-light conditions follows a 24-h rhythm in mammals (peak at 22:30) and that the origin of this rhythm is endogenous, and likely controlled by the SCN. One of the pioneer studies, in 1951, showed that the pupil diameter was not constant across the day with measures every 3 h (46). In 1998, Wilhelm

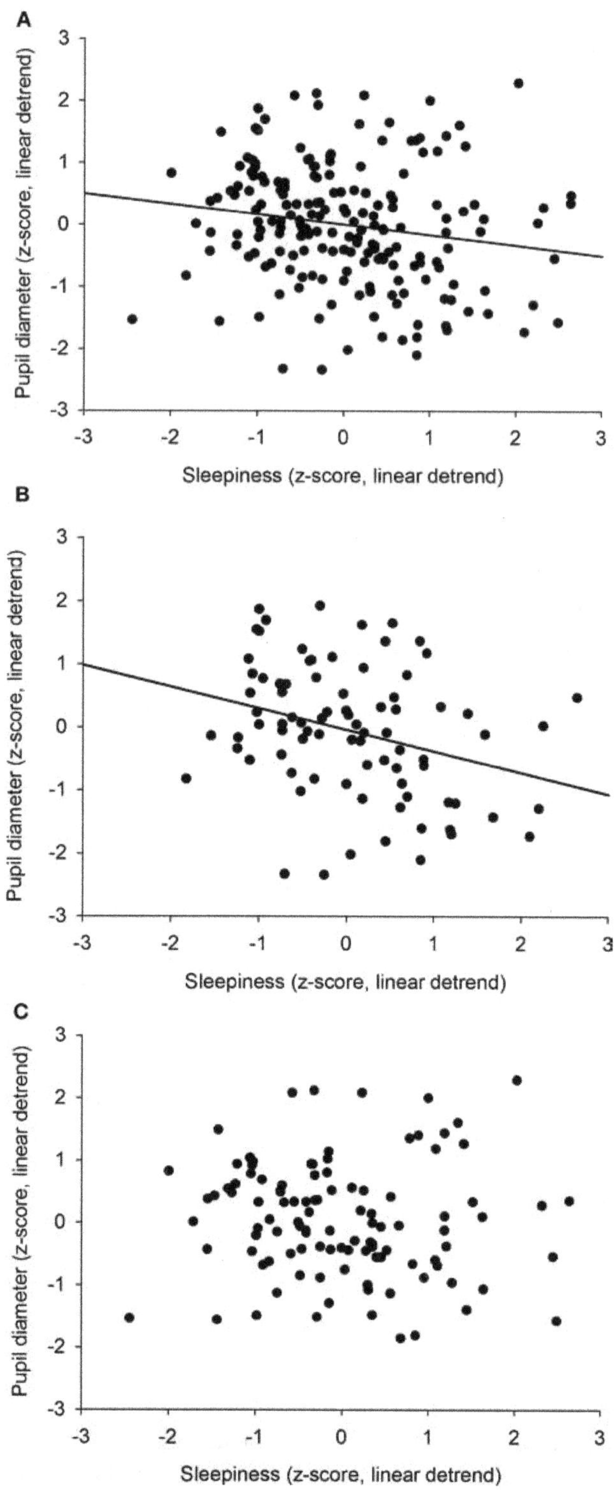

FIGURE 8 | Correlation between the circadian components of pupil diameter and subjective sleepiness. **(A)** all values across the 34-h constant routine segment ($R^2 = 0.03$; $p \leq 0.02$). **(B)** values when 2 curves vary in the same direction (between 4:30 and 10:30 and between 16:30 and 22:30; $R^2 = 0.09$; $p \leq 0.005$). **(C)** values when 2 curves vary in opposite directions (between 10:30 and 16:30 and between 22:30 and 4:30; $p = 0.57$).

and collaborators performed two pupil size measurements in constant darkness (82 s baseline) and found no time-of-day effect: no significant difference between the size of the pupil in the morning vs. afternoon (21). This lack of difference between morning and afternoon pupil diameter could be explained by the combination of a small sample size ($n = 7$) and of an insufficient sampling rate (only 2 measures). Zele et al. did not observe a significant variation of baseline pupil diameter with circadian time (10 s baseline), despite the hourly measures and the control of a number of environmental cues. The endogenous oscillation might have been masked by the lighting environment in 10 lux (compared to ~0.5 lux in our study) (47). On the opposite, a time-of-day effect of pupil size was shown by Kraemer et al. by measuring pupil diameter for 10 min every 2 h (after 2 min of dark adaptation) during a 16-h protocol (48). A few years later, Eggert et al. measured pupil size at two time points (once in the morning and once in the afternoon; 82 s baseline) on a large number of participants and they observed a smaller pupil diameter in the afternoon compared to the morning in constant darkness (12). Overall, the literature is not entirely consensual on the existence of a time-of-day effect on pupil diameter. This could be explained by the methodological differences in the protocols, such as ambient lighting ranging from darkness in some studies to relatively strong light (100 lux) in others, and/or the duration of the baseline pupil diameter measurement (values ranging from a few seconds to several minutes).

Correlation Between Subjective Sleepiness and Baseline Pupil Size

Sleepiness increased linearly whereas pupil diameter decreased linearly with time spent awake, revealing an overall negative correlation between the two responses. This correlation between pupil size and sleepiness was previously shown by a number of authors (20, 23, 25, 28, 29). Similarly, an association between pupil size and vigilance states (evaluated by measuring response times) has also been observed (27). However, other experiments with frequent pupillary measures did not find this association (24, 26, 30). The separation of the data according to the time of day (daytime = CR daytimes 2 & 3; nighttime = CR nighttime 2) revealed a correlation between the two responses during daytime only. This analysis allowed us to observe the changes in the relationship between pupil size and sleepiness, identifying for the first time that the pupil is a marker of sleepiness only at certain segments of the 24-h rhythm and therefore suggesting that their association is not solely linear.

Pupil Size as a Marker of Homeostatic (Process S) and Circadian (Process C) Sleepiness

The results of our study show that sleepiness and pupil size have opposite linear trends, and reveal that they also follow a 24-h rhythm. The linear trends suggest that the homeostatic component of pupil size could be a marker of homeostatic sleepiness and the 24-h rhythms suggest that circadian variation of pupil size could be a marker of circadian sleepiness. However, the peak of the circadian variation of sleepiness happens around

04:30, whereas the maximum pupil size is observed at 22:30, suggesting that the two circadian rhythms are phase-lagged by approximately 6 h. This large phase difference excludes a causal relationship between circadian sleepiness and circadian pupil size and suggests that they do not drive each other but that they are controlled by separate pathways, both depending on the circadian system. This phase-lag phenomenon between circadian rhythms is not unknown, and is in fact even classical. As an example, although body temperature and cortisol secretion are both driven by the circadian system, their rhythms are not in phase; while cortisol release peaks around habitual waketime, body temperature peaks 9 hours later (49).

The specific time epoch correlation analyses we have conducted according to circadian rhythmicity (signals varying in the same or in opposite directions) invalidate the use of pupil diameter as a reliable biomarker of sleepiness. Indeed, the fact that sleepiness and pupil size are not driven at the same circadian phase, makes pupil size a correlate of sleepiness only at certain times of the day (morning and evening, corresponding to 50% of the 24 hours,) and not at others. Along this line, a 24-h variation in the pupillary light reflex has been shown and interpreted as evidence that ipRGC activity is driven by the circadian system (47, 50). Given our results, the 24-h rhythm of pupil constriction should not be considered as a "pure" marker of circadian variation of ipRGC sensitivity to light.

Neurobiological Bases

Whereas the pupillary light reflex (PLR) depends on the activity of retinal photoreceptors (rods, cones and ipRGCs), the baseline pupil diameter in darkness is exclusively regulated by the autonomous nervous system (15, 22, 51). Wakefulness is associated with a large pupil size whereas during REM sleep small pupil sizes are observed (13). During anesthesia, a progressive dilation of the pupil indicates a greater loss of consciousness and a deepening of the anesthesia for certain anesthetics (18), however this has not been observed with other anesthetics, such as isoflurane (52). This result is in agreement with the literature and the results of our study, which show that overall as sleepiness increases, the pupil becomes smaller. Pupil dilation is known to originate from an activation of the sympathetic pathway or an inhibition of the parasympathetic circuitry (18). As it has been described by Samuels and collaborators (15, 53), an activation of the Locus Coeruleus (LC), conveyed to the VLPO, results in an increase in EEG signs of alertness, and a decrease in sleepiness. In parallel, an increased LC activity induces an increase in sympathetic activity and a decrease in parasympathetic activity, resulting in an increase in pupil diameter. This pupil dilation is mediated by the LC-Edinger-Westphal Nucleus (EW) pathway (15, 53). This dual circuitry shows that the LC influences both sleepiness and pupil diameter. This is in line with the results of Murphy and collaborators, who showed that there is a positive correlation between the pupil size and the BOLD signal in the LC (54). Therefore, we hypothesize that as sleepiness increases during the day, with the accumulation of homeostatic sleep pressure, the LC firing decreases, also inducing a decrease in pupil diameter. In this case the absence of stimulation of the fibers from the LC and the A1-A5 nuclei of the brainstem desinhibits the EW, which in turn activates the descending parasympathetic pathway, resulting in a pupil constriction (12, 15, 22). However, as we have seen previously, baseline pupil diameter and sleepiness do not simply vary linearly, as both of these responses also show a circadian rhythm, suggesting an interaction between the SCN and the LC. In this line, a circadian variation of the firing of the LC neurons has been observed in rats placed in constant darkness, with a faster firing rate during the active phase than during the inactive phase (55). Similarly, Takahashi et al. showed that in mice the noradrenergic neurons of the LC have a higher discharge rate during active wake compared to quiet wake, confirming that the LC is a wake-promoting structure (56). Here, we could hypothesize that the SCN regulates the LC activity, activating the LC neurons during the day and inactivating them during the night.

Limitations

This study exposes a few limitations. Firstly, the population examined in this study is only composed of men. However, we do not expect different results in women as no gender effect on pupillometry measures was observed by Eggert et al. on a large population (12). Similarly, although the amplitude of the circadian drive might be slightly more important in women vs. men, sleepiness has never been shown to be driven by different mechanisms (57). Secondly, the duration of the baseline pupil measurement was only 5 s, and one might think that a longer duration would be preferable. We do not think that our short segment is a problem, as the baseline measurements were very stable across and within subjects (mean $SD < 0.05$ mm), and ranged from (5.8 to 8.7 mm) which does not differ from those of previous studies (23, 25). Thirdly, even though we believe this is highly unlikely, we cannot exclude that exposure to very dim light intensity of ~0.5 lux may have had an effect on the pupil size subsequently measured in darkness. Fourthly, this protocol was conducted in an extremely controlled environment which does not reflect real life conditions, such as light exposure. Indeed, it is well known that light increases vigilance, decreases sleepiness and decreases pupil size (10, 58), suggesting that in real life conditions, the effect of light on the pupil could mask the effect of sleepiness that is hoped to be observed (59, 60).

CONCLUSION

Overall, our results show that even though baseline pupil diameter and sleepiness vary in opposite directions over the course of the day, their association is not that simple and is not solely the result of a homeostatic mechanism. The additional drive from the circadian timing system makes it more complex as it reveals an association only during half of the 24-h day, corresponding to 62% of the biological day and 25% of the biological night. These results demonstrate that due to the dual regulation of sleepiness by the homeostatic and circadian processes, baseline pupil diameter cannot be used as a reliable biomarker of sleepiness. Yet, finding an objective and convenient marker of sleepiness remains a priority as the subjective evaluation of sleepiness is not representative of performances or physiological sleepiness (20). Such a marker would be particularly useful to evaluate sleepiness in night workers, who are the highest at risk of making mistakes or injuring themselves (61, 62).

AUTHOR CONTRIBUTIONS

The experiment was conceived by CG and designed by CG and ID. Data collection was performed by ID and CG. Data analyses were conducted by ID. ID and CG interpreted the data and wrote the manuscript. DB provided edits. All authors agreed to be accountable for all aspects of the work.

FUNDING

This work was supported by a research award from the Societé Française de Recherche et Médecine du Sommeil (SFRMS) to ID and a grant from the French National Research Agency (ANR-12-TECS-0013-01) to CG. ID was funded by Ministère de l'Enseignement Supérieur et de la Recherche Français.

ACKNOWLEDGMENTS

We wish to thank all the volunteers who participated in this study. We also wish to thank the staff and students who helped with the measures and technical aspects of the protocol. A special thanks to Pauline Kirchhoff who was involved in collection and analysis of preliminary data.

REFERENCES

1. Roehrs T, Carskadon MA, Dement WC. Daytime sleepiness and alertness. In: Meir HK, Thomas R, William CD, editors. *Principles and Practice of Sleep Medicine*, Vol. 5. Elsevier Saunders (2011). pp. 42–53.
2. Strijkstra AM, Beersma DGM, Drayer B, Halbesma N, Daan S. Subjective sleepiness correlates negatively with global alpha (8–12 Hz) and positively with central frontal theta (4–8 Hz) frequencies in the human resting awake electroencephalogram. *Neurosci Lett.* (2003) 340:17–20. doi: 10.1016/S0304-3940(03)00033-8
3. Borbély AA, Daan S, Wirz-Justice A, Deboer T. The two-process model of sleep regulation: a reappraisal. *J Sleep Res.* (2016) 25:131–43. doi: 10.1111/jsr.12371
4. Dijk D-J, Czeisler CA. Paradoxical timing of the circadian rhythm of sleep propensity serves to consolidate sleep and wakefulness in humans. *Neurosci Lett.* (1994) 166:63–8.
5. Canisius S, Penzel T. Vigilance monitoring - review and practical aspects. *Biomed Tech Eng.* (2007) 52:77–82. doi: 10.1515/BMT.2007.015
6. Mitler MM, Miller JC. Methods of testing for sleepiness [corrected]. *Behav Med.* (1996) 21:171–83.
7. Lowenstein O, Loewenfeld IE. Types of central autonomic innervation and fatigue: pupillographic studies. *AMA Arch Neurol Psychiatry* (1951) 66:580–99. doi: 10.1001/archneurpsyc.1951.02320110045004
8. Lowenstein O. Pupillography; methods and diagnostic system. *AMA Arch Ophthalmol.* (1956) 55:565–71. doi: 10.1001/archopht.1956.00930030569015
9. Lowenstein O, Loewenfeld IE. Electronic pupillography: a new instrument and some clinical applications. *AMA Arch Ophthalmol.* (1958) 59:352–63. doi: 10.1001/archopht.1958.00940040058007
10. Wilhelm H. The pupil. *Curr Opin Neurol.* (2008) 21:36–42. doi: 10.1097/WCO.0b013e3282f39173
11. Chua EC-P, Yeo S-C, Lee IT-G, Tan L-C, Lau P, Tan SS, et al. Individual differences in physiologic measures are stable across repeated exposures to total sleep deprivation. *Physiol Rep.* (2014) 2:e12129. doi: 10.14814/phy2.12129
12. Eggert T, Sauter C, Popp R, Zeitlhofer J, Danker-Hopfe H, on behalf of the working group "Vigilance" of the German Society for Sleep Research and Sleep Medicine (DGSM). The pupillographic sleepiness test in adults: effect of age, gender, and time of day on pupillometric variables. *Am J Hum Biol.* (2012) 24:820–8. doi: 10.1002/ajhb.22326
13. Yüzgeç Ö, Prsa M, Zimmermann R, Huber D. Pupil size coupling to cortical states protects the stability of deep sleep via parasympathetic modulation. *Curr Biol.* (2018) 28:392–400.e3. doi: 10.1016/j.cub.2017.12.049
14. Iovino M, Messana T, De Pergola G, Iovino E, Guastamacchia E, Giagulli VA, et al. Vigilance states: central neural pathways, neurotransmitters and neurohormones. *Endocrine Metab Immune Dis Drug Targets* (2019) 19:26–37. doi: 10.2174/1871530318666180816115720
15. Samuels E, Szabadi E. Functional neuroanatomy of the noradrenergic Locus Coeruleus: its roles in the regulation of arousal and autonomic function part I: principles of functional organisation. *Curr Neuropharmacol.* (2008) 6:235–53. doi: 10.2174/157015908785777229
16. Markov D, Goldman M. Normal sleep and circadian rhythms: neurobiologic mechanisms underlying sleep and wakefulness. *Psychiatr Clin.* (2006) 29:841–53. doi: 10.1016/j.psc.2006.09.008
17. Landolt H-P. Sleep homeostasis: a role for adenosine in humans? *Biochem Pharmacol.* (2008) 75:2070–9. doi: 10.1016/j.bcp.2008.02.024
18. Larson MD, Behrends M. Portable infrared pupillometry: a review. *Anesth Analg.* (2015) 120:1242–53. doi: 10.1213/ANE.00000000000000314
19. Münch M, Kawasaki A. Intrinsically photosensitive retinal ganglion cells: classification, function and clinical implications. *Curr Opin Neurol.* (2013) 26:45–51. doi: 10.1097/WCO.0b013e32835c5e78
20. Danker-Hopfe H, Kraemer S, Dorn H, Schmidt A, Ehlert I, Herrmann WM. Time-of-day variations in different measures of sleepiness (MSLT, pupillography, and SSS) and their interrelations. *Psychophysiology* (2001) 38:828–35. doi: 10.1111/1469-8986.3850828
21. Wilhelm H, Lüdtke H, Wilhelm B. Pupillographic sleepiness testing in hypersomniacs and normals. *Graefes Arch Clin Exp Ophthalmol.* (1998) 236:725–9.
22. Wilhelm BJ, Widmann A, Durst W, Heine C, Otto G. Objective and quantitative analysis of daytime sleepiness in physicians after night duties. *Int J Psychophysiol.* (2009) 72:307–13. doi: 10.1016/j.ijpsycho.2009.01.008
23. Wilhelm B, Giedke H, Lüdtke H, Bittner E, Hofmann A, Wilhelm H. Daytime variations in central nervous system activation measured by a pupillographic sleepiness test. *J Sleep Res.* (2001) 10:1–7. doi: 10.1046/j.1365-2869.2001.00239.x
24. Wilhelm B, Wilhelm H, Lüdtke H, Streicher P, Adler M. Pupillographic assessment of sleepiness in sleep-deprived healthy subjects. *Sleep* (1998) 21:258–65.
25. Morad Y, Lemberg H, Yofe N, Dagan Y. Pupillography as an objective indicator of fatigue. *Curr Eye Res.* (2000) 21:535–42. doi: 10.1076/0271-3683(200007)2111-ZFT535
26. Ranzijn R, Lack L. The pupillary light reflex cannot be used to measure sleepiness. *Psychophysiology* (1997) 34:17–22. doi: 10.1111/j.1469-8986.1997.tb02411.x
27. Massar SAA, Lim J, Sasmita K, Chee MWL. Sleep deprivation increases the costs of attentional effort: performance, preference and pupil size. *Neuropsychologia* (2018). 123:169–77. doi: 10.1016/j.neuropsychologia.2018.03.032
28. Pressman MR, Spielman AJ, Korczyn AD, Rubenstein AE, Pollak CP, Weitzman ED. Patterns of daytime sleepiness in narcoleptics and normals: a pupillometric study. *Electroencephalogr Clin Neurophysiol.* (1984) 57:129–33. doi: 10.1016/0013-4694(84)90171-8
29. Yoss RE, Moyer NJ, Hollenhorst RW. Pupil size and spontaneous pupillary waves associated with alertness, drowsiness, and sleep. *Neurology* (1970) 20:545–54. doi: 10.1212/WNL.20.6.545
30. Lavie P. Ultradian rhythms in alertness - a pupillometric study. *Biol Psychol.* (1979) 9:49–62. doi: 10.1016/0301-0511(79)90022-X
31. Pressman MR, Fry JM. Relationship of autonomic nervous system activity to daytime sleepiness and prior sleep. *Sleep* (1989) 12:239–45. doi: 10.1093/sleep/12.3.239

32. Loving RT, Kripke DF, Glazner LK. Circadian rhythms in the human pupil and eyelid. *Am J Physiol-Regul Integr Comp Physiol.* (1996) 271:R320–4. doi: 10.1152/ajpregu.1996.271.2.R320
33. Beck AT, Ward CH, Mendelson M, Mock J, Erbaugh J. An inventory for measuring depression. *Arch Gen Psychiatry* (1961) 4:561–71. doi: 10.1001/archpsyc.1961.01710120031004
34. Buysse DJ, Reynolds CF, Monk TH, Berman SR, Kupfer DJ. The Pittsburgh sleep quality index: a new instrument for psychiatric practice and research. *Psychiatry Res.* (1989) 28:193–213. doi: 10.1016/0165-1781(89)90047-4
35. Horne JA, Ostberg O. A self-assessment questionnaire to determine morningness-eveningness in human circadian rhythms. *Int J Chronobiol.* (1976) 4:97–110.
36. Duffy JF, Dijk D-J. Getting through to circadian oscillators: why use constant routines? *J Biol Rhythms* (2002) 17:4–13. doi: 10.1177/0748730021290 02294
37. Mills JN, Minors DS, Waterhouse JM. Adaptation to abrupt time shifts of the oscillator (s) controlling human circadian rhythms. *J Physiol.* (1978) 285:455–70. doi: 10.1113/jphysiol.1978.sp012582
38. Mifflin MD, Jeor STS, Hill LA, Scott BJ, Daugherty SA, Koh YO. A new predictive equation for resting energy expenditure in healthy individuals. *Am J Clin Nutr.* (1990) 51:241–7. doi: 10.1093/ajcn/51.2.241
39. Jung CM, Melanson EL, Frydendall EJ, Perreault L, Eckel RH, Wright KP. Energy expenditure during sleep, sleep deprivation and sleep following sleep deprivation in adult humans. *J Physiol.* (2011) 589:235–44. doi: 10.1113/jphysiol.2010.197517
40. Jewett ME, Wyatt JK, Ritz-De Cecco A, Khalsa SB, Dijk DJ, Czeisler CA. Time course of sleep inertia dissipation in human performance and alertness. *J Sleep Res.* (1999) 8:1–8. doi: 10.1111/j.1365-2869.1999.00128.x
41. Burke TM, Scheer FAJL, Ronda JM, Czeisler CA, Wright KP. Sleep inertia, sleep homeostatic and circadian influences on higher-order cognitive functions. *J Sleep Res.* (2015) 24:364–71. doi: 10.1111/jsr. 12291
42. Gronfier C, Wright KP, Kronauer RE, Czeisler CA. Entrainment of the human circadian pacemaker to longer-than-24-h days. *Proc Natl Acad Sci USA.* (2007) 104:9081–6. doi: 10.1073/pnas.0702835104
43. Duffy JF, Cain SW, Chang A-M, Phillips AJK, Münch MY, Gronfier C, et al. Sex difference in the near-24-hour intrinsic period of the human circadian timing system. *Proc Natl Acad Sci USA.* (2011) 108(Suppl. 3):15602–8. doi: 10.1073/pnas.1010666108
44. Cajochen C, Khalsa SB, Wyatt JK, Czeisler CA, Dijk DJ. EEG and ocular correlates of circadian melatonin phase and human performance decrements during sleep loss. *Am J Physiol.* (1999) 277:R640–9. doi: 10.1152/ajpregu.1999.277.3.R640
45. Wyatt JK, Cecco AR-D, Czeisler CA, Dijk D-J. Circadian temperature and melatonin rhythms, sleep, and neurobehavioral function in humans living on a 20-H day. *Am J Physiol Regul Integr Comp Physiol.* (1999) 277:R1152–63. doi: 10.1152/ajpregu.1999.277.4.R1152
46. Döring GK, Schaefers E. Ueber die Tagesrhythmik der pupillenweite beim menschen. Pflügers Arch Gesamte Physiol. (1951) 252:337–41.
47. Zele AJ, Feigl B, Smith SS, Markwell EL. The circadian response of intrinsically photosensitive retinal ganglion cells. *PLoS ONE* (2011) 6:e17860. doi: 10.1371/journal.pone.0017860
48. Kraemer S, Danker-Hopfe H, Dorn H, Schmidt A, Ehlert I, Herrmann WM. Time-of-day variations of indicators of attention: performance, physiologic parameters, and self-assessment of sleepiness. *Biol Psychiatry* (2000) 48:1069–80. doi: 10.1016/S0006-3223(00)00908-2
49. Czeisler CA, Klerman EB. Circadian and sleep-dependent regulation of hormone release in humans. *Recent Prog Horm Res.* (1999) 54:97–130; discussion 130–132.
50. Münch M, Léon L, Crippa SV, Kawasaki A. Circadian and wake-dependent effects on the pupil light reflex in response to narrow-bandwidth light pulses. *Invest Ophthalmol Vis Sci.* (2012) 53:4546–55.
51. Lowenstein O, Loewenfeld IE. The sleep-waking cycle and pupillary activity. *Ann NY Acad Sci.* (1964) 117:142–56. doi: 10.1111/j.1749-6632.1964.tb48169.x
52. Cullen DJ, Eger EI 2nd, Stevens WC, Smith NT, Cromwell TH, Cullen BF, et al. *Clinical Signs of Anesthesia.* Anesthesiology, ASA Publications. Available online at: http://anesthesiology.pubs.asahq.org/article.aspx?articleid=1962908 (Accessed December 20, 2018).
53. Samuels E, Szabadi E. Functional neuroanatomy of the noradrenergic locus coeruleus: its roles in the regulation of arousal and autonomic function part II: physiological and pharmacological manipulations and pathological alterations of locus coeruleus activity in humans. *Curr Neuropharmacol.* (2008) 6:254–85. doi: 10.2174/157015908785777193
54. Murphy PR, O'Connell RG, O'Sullivan M, Robertson IH, Balsters JH. Pupil diameter covaries with BOLD activity in human locus coeruleus: pupil diameter and locus coeruleus activity. *Hum Brain Mapp.* (2014) 35:4140–54. doi: 10.1002/hbm.22466
55. Aston-Jones G, Chen S, Zhu Y, Oshinsky ML. A neural circuit for circadian regulation of arousal. *Nat Neurosci.* (2001) 4:732. doi: 10.1038/ 89522
56. Takahashi K, Kayama Y, Lin JS, Sakai K. Locus coeruleus neuronal activity during the sleep-waking cycle in mice. *Neuroscience* (2010) 169:1115–26. doi: 10.1016/j.neuroscience.2010.06.009
57. Santhi N, Lazar AS, McCabe PJ, Lo JC, Groeger JA, Dijk D-J. Sex differences in the circadian regulation of sleep and waking cognition in humans. *Proc Natl Acad Sci USA.* (2016) 113:E2730–9. doi: 10.1073/pnas.1521637113
58. Xu Q, Lang CP. Revisiting the alerting effect of light: a systematic review. *Sleep Med Rev.* (2018) 41:39–49. doi: 10.1016/j.smrv.2017.12.001
59. Mure LS, Cornut P-L, Rieux C, Drouyer E, Denis P, Gronfier C, Cooper HM. Melanopsin bistability: a fly's eye technology in the human retina. *PLoS ONE* (2009) 4:e5991. doi: 10.1371/journal.pone.0005991
60. Warga M, Lüdtke H, Wilhelm H, Wilhelm B. How do spontaneous pupillary oscillations in light relate to light intensity? *Vision Res.* (2009) 49:295–300. doi: 10.1016/j.visres.2008.09.019
61. Reinberg A, Smolensky MH, Riedel M, Touitou Y, Le Floc'h N, Clarisse R, et al. Chronobiologic perspectives of black time-accident risk is greatest at night: an opinion paper. *Chronobiol Int.* (2015) 32:1005–18. doi: 10.3109/07420528.2015.1053911
62. Landrigan CP, Rothschild JM, Cronin JW, Kaushal R, Burdick E, Katz JT, et al. Effect of reducing interns' work hours on serious medical errors in intensive care units. *N Engl J Med.* (2004) 351:1838–48. doi: 10.1056/NEJMoa041406

4

Standards in Pupillography

Carina Kelbsch[1*], *Torsten Strasser*[1], *Yanjun Chen*[2], *Beatrix Feigl*[3,4,5], *Paul D. Gamlin*[6], *Randy Kardon*[7], *Tobias Peters*[1], *Kathryn A. Roecklein*[8], *Stuart R. Steinhauer*[9,10], *Elemer Szabadi*[11], *Andrew J. Zele*[3,12], *Helmut Wilhelm*[1] *and Barbara J. Wilhelm*[1]

[1] Pupil Research Group, Centre for Ophthalmology, University Hospitals Tübingen, Tübingen, Germany, [2] Department of Ophthalmology and Visual Sciences, University of Wisconsin School of Medicine and Public Health, Madison, AL, United States, [3] Institute of Health and Biomedical Innovation, Queensland University of Technology, Brisbane, QLD, Australia, [4] School of Biomedical Sciences, Queensland University of Technology, Brisbane, QLD, Australia, [5] Queensland Eye Institute, Brisbane, QLD, Australia, [6] Department of Ophthalmology and Visual Sciences, University of Alabama at Birmingham, Birmingham, AL, United States, [7] Neuro-Ophthalmology Division, University of Iowa and Iowa City VA Healthcare System, Iowa City, LA, United States, [8] Department of Psychology, University of Pittsburgh, Pittsburgh, PA, United States, [9] VA Pittsburgh Healthcare System, VISN 4 MIRECC, University Drive C, Pittsburgh, PA, United States, [10] Department of Psychiatry, University of Pittsburgh School of Medicine, Pittsburgh, PA, United States, [11] Developmental Psychiatry, University of Nottingham, Nottingham, United Kingdom, [12] School of Optometry and Vision Science, Queensland University of Technology, Brisbane, QLD, Australia

Correspondence:
Carina Kelbsch
carina.kelbsch@med.uni-tuebingen.de

The number of research groups studying the pupil is increasing, as is the number of publications. Consequently, new standards in pupillography are needed to formalize the methodology including recording conditions, stimulus characteristics, as well as suitable parameters of evaluation. Since the description of intrinsically photosensitive retinal ganglion cells (ipRGCs) there has been an increased interest and broader application of pupillography in ophthalmology as well as other fields including psychology and chronobiology. Color pupillography plays an important role not only in research but also in clinical observational and therapy studies like gene therapy of hereditary retinal degenerations and psychopathology. Stimuli can vary in size, brightness, duration, and wavelength. Stimulus paradigms determine whether rhodopsin-driven rod responses, opsin-driven cone responses, or melanopsin-driven ipRGC responses are primarily elicited. Background illumination, adaptation state, and instruction for the participants will furthermore influence the results. This standard recommends a minimum set of variables to be used for pupillography and specified in the publication methodologies. Initiated at the 32nd International Pupil Colloquium 2017 in Morges, Switzerland, the aim of this manuscript is to outline standards in pupillography based on current knowledge and experience of pupil experts in order to achieve greater comparability of pupillographic studies. Such standards will particularly facilitate the proper application of pupillography by researchers new to the field. First we describe general standards, followed by specific suggestions concerning the demands of different targets of pupil research: the afferent and efferent reflex arc, pharmacology, psychology, sleepiness-related research and animal studies.

Keywords: clinical standards, pupillography, application of pupillography, stimulus characteristics, parameters of evaluation, analysis, pupillometry

INTRODUCTION

Otto Lowenstein and Irene Loewenfeld established a new era of pupil research with the development of infrared-video-pupillography (1). In the first instance, each single picture of the pupil was analyzed manually, before Lowenstein and Loewenfeld introduced the first on-line analysis with their newly constructed photoelectric pupillograph in 1947. It was not until the late seventies, when videotaping became possible, allowing recording of the pupil diameter continuously in darkness via infrared-videography with a combined computerized data analysis. Based on the knowledge of Irene Loewenfeld's outstanding life work (2), and particularly since the description of melanopsin expressing intrinsically photosensitive retinal ganglion cells (ipRGCs), there has been an increased interest and broader application of pupillography in ophthalmology as well as other fields including psychology and psychiatry.

IpRGCs, a subclass of retinal ganglion cells, are capable of detecting light directly via the photopigment melanopsin (3, 4), in addition to receiving input from the traditional extrinsic pathway via photoreceptors of the outer retina. Thus, the pupillary light reflex consists of rhodopsin-driven rod responses, opsin-driven cone responses and melanopsin-driven ipRGC responses (5–11). Depending on the stimulus paradigms, such as stimulus size, brightness, duration, and wavelength as well as background illumination and adaptation state of the retina, pupillary responses reflect these different response components.

Color pupillography currently plays an important role in different clinical and research areas. On the one hand, there is fundamental basic science being performed based on pupillographic animal studies with knockout models (12–14), but also on the cellular level (15, 16). On the other hand, there are pupillographic clinical studies in humans in order to better understand the pupil circuitry [e.g., (17, 18)] and the pathomechanism and remaining retinal functionality of certain diseases, e.g., glaucoma (19–23), Retinitis pigmentosa (9, 24–27), age-related macular degeneration (28–30), diabetes (31–33) or hereditary optic neuropathy (34). Furthermore, pupillography comes into use in clinical observational and therapy studies like gene therapy of hereditary retinal degenerations (35), studies on attention-modulation (36), in chronobiology [(37–39), for a review see (40)] and in psychopathology, psychiatric disorders and neurodegenerative conditions (41–45). Additionally, pupillography is indispensable in sleepiness-related research and the pupillographic sleepiness test (PST) has been developed into an objective measures of day time sleepiness (46, 47). In the last years, automated pupillography also found its way into the evaluation of patients in intensive care units, particularly using pupillary abnormalities in the management of severe traumatic brain injury as an indicator for an increased intracranial pressure (48) or in the management of analgesia (49, 50).

In all disciplines, one takes advantage of analyzing the pupil behavior and pupillary responses to specific stimuli: Pupil measurements are contactless, easily accessible, and objective, with only minor cooperation required from the examined participant.

The number of researchers studying the pupil is increasing, as are the number of publications, which increased almost exponentially over the past 50 years. In order to achieve a higher comparability of pupillographic studies worldwide and to increase the scientific weight of pupillography and pupil research, standards in pupillography regarding methodology including recording conditions, stimulus characteristics, as well as an agreement about parameters of evaluation are needed. Standards particularly facilitate the steps to perform a technically appropriate pupillographic procedure and to analyze and report the data properly, and pupillographic guidelines serve as a common basis for pupillography in scientific and clinical applications between different labs.

Visual electrophysiology, which allows for an objective evaluation of the visual pathway similar to pupillography, was confronted with similar requirements: Research groups started to develop sophisticated stimulus paradigms, leveraged by advances of technology and companies started to implement them into electrophysiological equipment. With the growing and widespread importance of visual electrophysiology for research and clinical routine, it became apparent that a common agreement of the principles of conducting visual electrophysiological tests was necessary in order to guarantee the comparability of results obtained in different labs, especially in clinical settings. The International Society for Clinical Electrophysiology of Vision (ISCEV)[1] recognized the need for standardization at its founding in 1961 (51, 52), but it took until 1989 until the first standard for electroretinography was published (53). These standards describe a set of basic stimuli that should be recorded in electrophysiological tests performed clinically. Marmor and Zrenner, two of the authors of the standards, state: "This ensures that electrophysiologic testing will always produce a core of data that is recognizable and comparable everywhere, whether for clinical or research purposes. This program of standardization has been highly successful. Today, most publications using visual electrophysiology refer to these standards and the major manufacturers of clinical electroretinographic equipment have incorporated them into their stimulus protocols." (54). Nowadays, standards are available for the different examination techniques in visual electrophysiology (55–59) which are accompanied by guidelines for calibration of stimulus and recording parameters (60) as well as a general guide to visual electrodiagnostic procedures (61). These standards and documents could serve as blueprints for analogous standards concerning stimulus and recording parameters of pupillography.

Initiated at the 32nd International Pupil Colloquium 2017 in Morges, Switzerland, the aim of this manuscript is to outline standards in pupillography based on current knowledge and experience of pupil experts in order to achieve greater comparability of pupillographic studies. It is divided into two major parts with general recommendations and specific application areas of pupillography:

[1]https://iscev.wildapricot.org/

I. Part: General standards for Pupillography

- Data collection and processing
- Reported/provided data

II. Part: Specific standards for Pupillography

1. The afferent pupillary pathway
   - 1.1 Rod and cone photoreceptor contribution to the pupil light reflex
   - 1.2 Melanopsin - The Post-Illumination Pupil Response (PIPR)
   - 1.3 Special clinical applications
2. The efferent pupillary pathway
3. Pharmacology
4. Psychology and Psychiatry
5. Sleepiness-Related Pupillary Oscillations
6. Animals

The first part is concerned with general standards for pupillography which should be reported in any pupillographic study. It contains basic information about the pupillographic device, the adaptation status of the retina, the stimulus characteristic as well as general information about the examined species. The second part provides specific standards regarding the specific demands of different areas of pupil research: the afferent pupillary pathway, the efferent pupillary pathway, pharmacology, psychology and psychiatry, sleepiness-related research and animal studies. It begins with a description of appropriate stimulus characteristics, followed by a presentation of appropriate response analysis parameters.

I. PART: GENERAL STANDARDS FOR PUPILLOGRAPHY

Data Collection and Processing

In addition to time series data, all pupillographic recordings should include data based on the Minimum Information about a Neuroscience Investigation (MINI), published by the CARMEN consortium (62). These data allow for the interpretation and the evaluation of the data by independent readers and can facilitate later computational access and analysis. **Table 1** gives an overview of these guidelines adapted for pupillography.

Reported/Provided Data

Information on the following topics is essential and recommended being addressed in any paper containing typical experiments performed with pupillography.

Pupillographic Device

The pupillographic device should be sufficiently explained to allow replication. That requires primarily whether a commercially available device (including name, city, and country of producer) or a self-built pupillograph has been used. The different components should be outlined together with the characteristics of the device including spatial and temporal resolution of the camera and the method of measurement (direct vs. consensual vs. binocular measurement of the pupils). Moreover, the method of stimulus presentation should be reported as stimuli might be either presented as a full-field (Ganzfeld bowl, mini-Ganzfeld bowl/tube, Maxwellian view/glasses) or focally on a hemisphere (perimetry) or a flat monitor (campimetry). The respective distance between the examined participant's cornea and the presented stimulus' location is required.

Demographic Data

Information on the examined species is crucial; this includes whether human subjects or animals were tested and should always be accompanied by a statement of keeping the conditions of ethical standards according to the Declaration of Helsinki and animal standards. The age range is likewise required as information of the sex and specific features like clinically verified diseases or known genotypes. When comparing participants with a certain disease and healthy controls, information on which tests have been performed to verify the diagnosis should be given. The number of participants included is influenced by the design of the experiment and the requirements of the post-experiment statistical analysis. A prior power analysis will help to determine whether the number of participants included is sufficient to avoid Type I error. The health status of the participants should be reported; it is customary to do this in the form of inclusion and exclusion criteria. In the case of healthy volunteers, medication with potential influence on the pupillary responses should be excluded. Many drugs of different classes can affect the pupil, however, there are some general patterns. The most common offenders are drugs that interact with the sympathetic and parasympathetic innervations of the iris, either peripherally or centrally (**Figure 4**), and drugs that influence the level of arousal (63) due to the coupling between arousal and autonomic activity (64–66). Many drugs in overdose can induce non-specific effects, such as general CNS depression, leading to coma, or CNS over-excitation, leading to seizures. CNS depression is usually accompanied by miosis, and over-excitation by mydriasis. **Table 2** gives an overview of selected topical and general medication potentially interfering with the pupillary responses. However, if patients are included, it may not be possible to exclude all these medication; in this case, all medication should be documented.

Adaptation State of the Retina

We recommend to report the background and room illuminance (Lux) during the measurements and, if applicable, the pre-dark or pre-light adaptation times to room illumination (light-adapted vs. dark-adapted vs. mesopic condition vs. no adaptation). With regard to dark adaptation times, Wang et al. showed a significantly increased transient and sustained contraction amplitude of the pupil light response during dark adaptation and consequently suggested a period of 20 min of dark adaptation for consistent pupil responses (67).

The first pupillary response in a series may be excluded from analysis, e.g., due to a larger response owing to the pre-stimulus state of relative dark adaptation. This has to be applied in a

TABLE 1 | Overview of the MINI recommendations of the CARMEN consortium (62) adapted for pupillography.

Context	• Recording date and time • (examiner)
Study subject	• Subject identifier • sex / age • ethnicity / race • clinical information, *if appropriate* • genetic characteristics, *if appropriate* • iris colour, *if appropriate*
Stimulus	• protocol name • stimulation equipment/device (including open loop/closed loop) • adaptation state • stimulus paradigm • calibration details
Recording	• protocol name • camera equipment/device • frame rate/temporal resolution • spatial resolution • type of recording (direct, consensual, binocular) • filtering, blink and artefact removal
Time series data	• data format • type (raw data, average)

consistent way for all recordings and has to be reported in the methods.

Stimulus Characteristics

Particular importance is ascribed to the stimulus characteristics themselves to make an experiment transparent and comparable to others. These include the method of stimulus presentation (full-field stimulation vs. local stimulation) and, in the case of a local stimulation, the exact stimulus size.

Furthermore, information regarding the stimulus intensity, duration, inter-stimulus time and wavelength (color) should be reported. These parameters determine whether rhodopsin-driven rod responses, opsin-driven cone responses, or melanopsin-driven ipRGC responses are primarily elicited.

Baseline Diameter

For a reliable interpretation of the data and to facilitate replication of findings, the absolute pupil baseline diameter before the stimulation should be reported. This metric varies widely across participants with a characteristic decreasing pupil size with age (2) and hints for smaller pupil sizes in specific retinal diseases, e.g., in CNGA3-linked Achromatopsia (35). Further analyses should usually be based on relative values as pupillary responses are dependent on the initial baseline diameter, which should be obtained during a sufficiently long recording period to ensure a steady and reliable estimate. Such normalizations limit the effect of fluctuations in diameter and control for individual differences in pupil diameter, including senile miosis. To normalize pupillary responses, the absolute pupil diameter at any given time is converted to a relative pupil constriction amplitude in percent from baseline, e.g., by the following formula:

relative pupil constriction amplitude at time x = [(baseline pupil diameter – absolute pupil diameter at time x)/baseline pupil diameter] × 100.

For specific research questions, particularly in psychological experiments with additional behavioral or performance context and pharmacological studies, it might also be reasonable to evaluate the actual change in diameter; we discuss this issue in the specific chapters.

II. PART: SPECIFIC STANDARDS FOR PUPILLOGRAPHY

Beside the above mentioned general standards that we strongly encourage researchers to consider in a publication, specific standards for the different research areas and applications of pupillography are important. In the following, the proposed specific standards and suggested investigation strategies regarding suitable stimulus characteristics as well as appropriate response analysis parameters are presented.

TABLE 2 | Effect of drug treatment on the pupil.

Drug	Mechanism	Pupil
TOPICAL		
Pilocarpine	cholinergic	miosis[a]
Carbachol	cholinergic	miosis[a]
Aceclidine	cholinergic	miosis[a]
Atropine	anticholinergic	mydriasis[b]
Scopolamine	anticholinergic	mydriasis[b]
Tropicamide	anticholinergic	mydriasis
Phenylephrine	α_1-adrenoceptor agonist	mydriasis
Methoxamine	α_1-adrenoceptor agonist	mydriasis
Apraclonidine	α_1-adrenoceptor agonist	mydriasis[c]
Dapiprazole	α_1-adrenoceptor antagonist	miosis
Brimonidine	α_2-adrenoceptor agonist	miosis[d]
Cocaine	noradrenaline uptake inhibitor	mydriasis
SYSTEMIC		
Antihistamines	H1 histamine receptor antagonists	miosis[e]
ANTIHYPERTENSIVES		
Prazosin	α_1-adrenoceptor antagonist	miosis[f]
Clonidine	α_2-adrenoceptor agonist	miosis[g]
ANTIARRYTHMICS		
Disopyramide	anticholinergic	mydriasis
DRUGS FOR PARKINSON'S DISEASE		
Anticholinergics	blockade of muscarinic receptors	mydriasis[h]
Dopaminergics	stimulation of D2 dopamine receptors	mydriasis[i]
ANTIDEPRESSANTS		
Tricyclic	mainly noradrenaline uptake blockade	mydriasis[j]
Reboxetine	noradrenaline uptake blockade	mydriasis
Venlafaxine	noradrenaline/serotonin uptake blockade	mydriasis
SSRIs	serotonin uptake blockade	no effect[k]
ANTIPSYCHOTICS		
Phenothiazines	α_1-adrenoceptor antagonist, sedation	miosis[l]
Haloperidol	α_1-adrenoceptor antagonist	miosis
SEDATIVES		
Benzodiazepines	GABA receptor agonist → sedation	no effect[m]
PSYCHOSTIMULANTS		
Amphetamine	noradrenaline releaser	mydriasis
Modafinil	dopamine uptake blocker	mydriasis[n]
ANALGESICS		
Opiates	stimulation of inhibitory μ receptors	miosis[o]
ANTIEMETICS		
Scopolamine	anticholinergic	mydriasis
ANTI-INCONTINENCE DRUGS		
	anticholinergic	mydriasis[p]

[a] *glaucoma treatment.*

[b] *myopia treatment.*

[c] *in Horner's syndrome (supersensitive α_1-adrenoceptors).*

[d] *drug reduces noradrenaline release (glaucoma treatment).*

[e] *first generation antihistamines (e.g., diphenhydramine, cyclizine) penetrate into the brain where they block H1 histamine receptors, leading to sedation.*

[f] *drug blocks α_1-adrenoceptors in vascular smooth muscle.*

[g] *drug stimulates inhibitory α_2-adrenoceptors on central noradrenergic neurones, leading to sedation and sympatholysis.*

[h] *include orphenadrine, procyclidine, trihexyphenidyl.*

[i] *D2 dopamine receptor agonists (e.g., pramipexole) stimulate inhibitory D2 receptors on wake-promoting central dopaminergic neurones, leading to sedation. This is expected to cause miosis, however, paradoxically, pramipexole causes mydriasis [see (65)].*

[j] *Tricyclic antidepressants block the uptake of noradrenaline, potentiating noradrenergic neurotransmission, and this would lead to mydriasis. However, they have some other effects: blockade of muscarinic cholinoceptors would lead to mydriasis and sedation, and blockade of α_1 adrenoceptors would cause miosis. The overall effect reflects the balance between these actions: mydriasis due to noradrenaline uptake blockade and cholinoceptor blockade is counteracted by miosis due to α_1-adrenoceptor blockade and sedation. This explains the variable effects of tricylic antidepresssants on the pupil: imipramine and desipramine dilate it, while amitriptyline has little effect on it.*

[k] *Selective serotonin reuptake inhibitors (SSRIs) block serotonin receptors in a complex network of serotonergic neurones associated with different excitatory/inhibitory receptors. The overall effect is little or no change in pupil diameter.*

[l] *These drugs (e.g., chlorpromazine, trifluoperazine) also have anticholinergic effects that would lead to mydriasis. However, α_1-adrenoceptor blockade and sedation predominate, leading to miosis.*

[m] *Paradoxically, although the benzodiazepine diazepam is highly sedative, it has no effect on pupil diameter [see (66)].*

[n] *Modafinil blocks dopamine uptake at exciatatory synapses on central noradrenergic neurones: this leads to increase in arousal and sympathetic activity.*

[o] *Stimulation of inhibitory μ receptors on central noradrenergic neurones leads to sedation and sympatholysis.*

[p] *These drugs (oxybutynin, festerodine) inhibit voiding of the urinary bladder by blocking cholinoceptors in the detrusor muscle.*

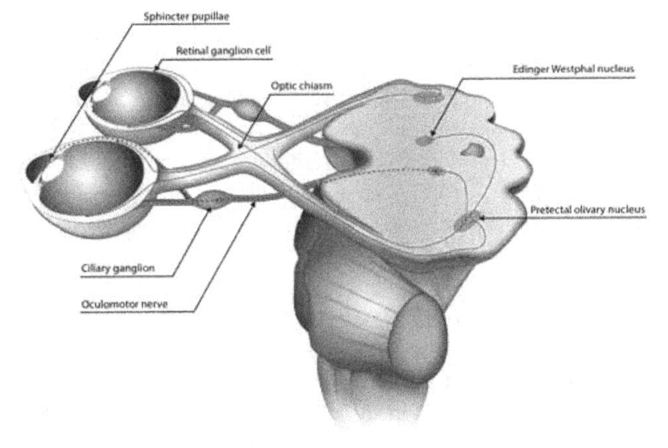

FIGURE 1 | The pupillary pathway. The afferent pupillary pathway comprises the retinal photoreceptors, the bipolar cells and the retinal ganglion cells whose axons form the optic nerve. Temporal fibers run ipsilaterally while the nasal fibers cross to the contralateral side in the optic chiasm. Afterwards, they form the optic tract and synapse at the olivary pretectal nucleus therefrom connecting to both Edinger Westphal nuclei (blue continuous line). The efferent pathway from the Edinger Westphal nucleus to the pupillary sphincter via the ciliary ganglion is depicted in dashed lines.

1. THE AFFERENT PUPILLARY PATHWAY Authors: Carina Kelbsch, Andrew J. Zele, Beatrix Feigl and Helmut Wilhelm

The afferent pupillary pathway consists of the retinal photoreceptors, the bipolar cells, the retinal ganglion cells, the optic nerve and optic tract, ends at the olivary pretectal nuclei which connect to the Edinger Westphal nuclei where the efferent pathway begins (see **Figure 1**).

The following variables influence the pupillary light response and should therefore be specified:

- Stimulus wavelength (nm; peak and bandwidth at half maximum)
- Stimulus irradiance (log photon.cm^{-2}.s^{-1}, W.m^{-2}), stimulus luminance (cd.m^{-2}) and/or stimulus illumination (Lux)
- Stimulus size (degrees visual angle) and shape (if not circular; e.g., quadrant)
- Stimulus localization/ fixation eccentricity (if not full-field)
- Stimulus duration (s) and frequency (Hz; for periodic temporal modulation)
- Background wavelength and irradiance (log photon.cm^{-2}.s^{-1}) or luminance (if not dark)
- Dark and light adaptation times (min)
- Inter-stimulus interval (s)
- Number of repetitions

To assess retinal function, specifically designed stimulation paradigms are required to stimulate the extrinsic pathway via rods and/or cones or the intrinsic pathway of melanopsin-expressing intrinsically photosensitive retinal ganglion cells (ipRGCs). In the following, we first provide recommendations for test stimulation protocols and analyses for objectively quantifying rod and cone photoreceptor inputs to the afferent pupillary pathway. These are based on an evaluation of modern approaches that we anticipate can provide a platform to facilitate the development of new protocols (Chapter 1.1). Then, we introduce a series of recommendations for the assessment of melanopsin inputs to the pupillary pathway (Chapter 1.2).

1.1 Rod and Cone Photoreceptor Contribution to the Pupil Light Reflex

Introduction

Human vision spans more than ~10 log of units of retinal illumination through the combined activity of rod and cone photoreceptors. In bright, photopic illumination, vision is initiated by the output of three different cone classes with overlapping absorption spectra and peak sensitivities at short wavelengths [S-cones: ~445 nm (corneal, 10° standard observer); ~420–430 nm (retinal)], medium wavelengths [M-cones: ~541 nm (corneal, 10° standard observer); ~530–534 nm (retinal)] and long wavelengths [L-cones: ~567 nm (corneal, 10° standard observer); ~561–563 nm (retinal)] (68–71). Rod photoreceptors [peak ~507 nm (corneal); ~491–498 nm (retinal)] initiate vision under dim, scotopic illumination and both the rods and cones are operational at intermediate, mesopic illuminations. In addition to their different spectral sensitivities, the rod and cone systems show different temporal, spatial and adaptation responses, and topographical retinal distributions. Taken together, their unique and combined contributions to vision (and the pupil light reflex) will vary with the spectral, temporal, spatial and adaptation characteristics of the stimulus conditions (72) and so differences in the stimulus conditions will be reflected in changes in the relative sensitivity of the two systems and their contributions to the pupil light reflex. Ultimately, spectral sensitivity measurements will be necessary to quantify the relative rod and cone contribution to the pupil light reflex for a particular set of stimulus conditions and analysis metrics as has been demonstrated for the pupil constriction during light stimulation (73) and the post-illumination pupil response, or PIPR (8, 74, 75).

Stimulus Characteristics

The separation and measurement of rod and/or cone contributions to the pupil has been assessed using techniques pioneered in visual psychophysics. A primary approach uses selective chromatic adaptation (76) with monochromatic test lights presented against monochromatic adapting background lights of different irradiances. The idea is that a background wavelength and irradiance can be chosen to desensitize (adapt) one or more photoreceptor classes, with the test wavelength chosen to bias the response to another photoreceptor class. The rod system has a higher luminous efficiency (V'λ) at shorter wavelengths than the cone pathway (Vλ), with this difference approaching zero at longer wavelengths (>650 nm) (77). Below cone threshold (~1 Troland), all stimulus wavelengths are mediated via rods (note that melanopsin contributions to vision and the pupil are still to be defined under scotopic illumination, but are believed to be negligible). In the mesopic and moderate photopic range (below rod saturation), no monochromatic light will isolate rods or cones, with the relative degree of separation dependent on the sensitivity of the two systems to the stimulus conditions. When possible, this should be estimated.

To favor detection to the rod system, Aguilar and Stiles (78) determined that a blue-green test stimulus (<490 nm) will provide a high ratio of rod to cone sensitivity; a red adapting background light (>610 nm) stimulates the cone system more than rods (a low ratio of rod to cone sensitivity) and reduces cone sensitivity. The stimulus light also entered the eye at the edge of the pupil to take advantage of the Stiles-Crawford (79) effect. To bias detection to the cone system, high irradiance adapting fields are required to saturate the rods, with the monochromatic test and field wavelengths reversed. When assessing the cone system, the stimulus properties, particularly the irradiance, size, duration and retinal eccentricity will influence the responsivity of the three primary post-receptoral pathways (80, 81). The success of selective chromatic adaptation is also limited by the assumption that the rod and cone systems are independent (the duplicity theory of vision), and this is not the case due to the rod and cone signals sharing the same post-receptoral neural pathways (72). For cone mediated pupillary responses, a high irradiance adapting field becomes problematic, as it drives the pupil into a relatively miotic state, reducing its dynamic range of movement to superimposed pedestal light stimuli. Therefore, there is usually a compromise between the background adapting field intensity and the level of rod suppression when attempting to isolate cone mediated pupillary responses.

Given that age-related changes in the optical media attenuate the stimulus corneal irradiance to modify pupillary responses, lens density should be estimated and controlled for in the study design [e.g., LOCS III; (82)]. However, an increase in lens density may also be partially compensated for by photoreceptor adaptation. The absorption of the stimulus light at the test wavelengths can be quantified (83, 84). It's necessary to highlight that when pupillary responses are measured with rods and cones in different states of sensitivity, this influences comparisons about the degree of rod and cone photoreceptor dysfunction detected in patients. Moreover, retinal and/or optic nerve disease can lead to a remodeling of the neural pathways (85) and so the level of photoreceptor separation may be dissimilar within and between patients and healthy control participants. Inferences about the relative degree of rod and cone dysfunction in disease are presumably possible when the two systems are measured under similar viewing conditions. Current research addresses this issue by using multiple-primary colorimetric techniques with the method of silent substitution (86–90). With this approach, specific photoreceptor classes (e.g., rods, cones, melanopsin) can be directly modulated to study the afferent pupillary response; it is evident that the pupillary responses from different photoreceptor classes vary in amplitude and phase depending on the photoreceptor input combination and so in the future these findings will be important for developing new approaches to isolate and separate rod, cone and melanopsin contribution to the pupillary response.

There are examples of chromatic pupillometry methodologies that provide initial efforts to separate rod and cone function through the careful control of the wavelength, irradiance, size and duration of the test stimuli; the degree of separation of rod and cone (and melanopsin) function that these conditions provide is still to be determined. At light levels below cone threshold, short wavelength lights are presented in the dark to bias the response to rods, with the PIPR amplitudes minimized under such conditions (9, 11, 35). To ensure maximal rod sensitivity, the pre-stimulus dark adaptation time should be at least 30 min (91); although this is not practical for all clinical protocols, shorter periods will influence the relative rod and cone sensitivity to the test stimuli. When using selective chromatic adaptation to bias pupil responses to the cone system, a red test stimulus (>610 nm) is presented against a blue background (<490 nm) to suppress rod function (11); a 467 nm, 0.78 log cd.m^{-2} background has a similar scotopic luminance to a 30 cd.m^{-2} white background as used in the standard ISCEV protocol (11, 92). Quantal matched long (and short) wavelength test stimuli can be included in each condition as a control. Because the pupil diameter returns to the dark-adapted baseline faster than after photopic test stimuli, the inter-stimulus interval is shorter for scotopic test conditions. As mentioned previously, a bright adapting light can present its own problem with reducing the dynamic range of pupil movement due to the relatively miotic state induced by a bright adapting background. Furthermore, in light-adapted condition, pupillary measurements become noisier as light-induced oscillations may occur during the exposure to the background light (2).

Analysis

During presentation of a light stimulus with low melanopsin excitation, the pupil light reflex is mainly driven by extrinsic cone and rod inputs to ipRGCs. For these conditions, analysis metrics include the transient response, latency to constriction and maximum pupil constriction amplitude. Both, absolute (in mm) or relative amplitudes (in %) relative to the baseline pupil diameter can be used, but the relative pupil constriction amplitude should always be provided (see Part I, general standards). Another parameter is the maximal constriction velocity which is proportional to the amplitude. Additional information may be gained by measuring the latency to constriction, inversely correlated to stimulus brightness and size and the time to maximal constriction. For an overview of typical pupillographic analysis metrics as well as more detailed information regarding stimulation characteristics, please refer to the following chapter (**Figure 2**; 1.2 Melanopsin-The Post-Illumination Pupil Response, PIPR).

Application

Chromatic pupillometry has been applied in various forms in clinical studies, including those with patients with rod and cone dystrophies such as Retinitis Pigmentosa (9, 24–27, 93, 94) and achromatopsia (35, 95), as well as in animals, including canine (96, 97) and mouse (98). These paradigms quantify the PLR metrics (see also **Figure 2**; 1.2 Melanopsin-The Post-Illumination Pupil Response, PIPR) after exposure to test stimuli specified according to their:

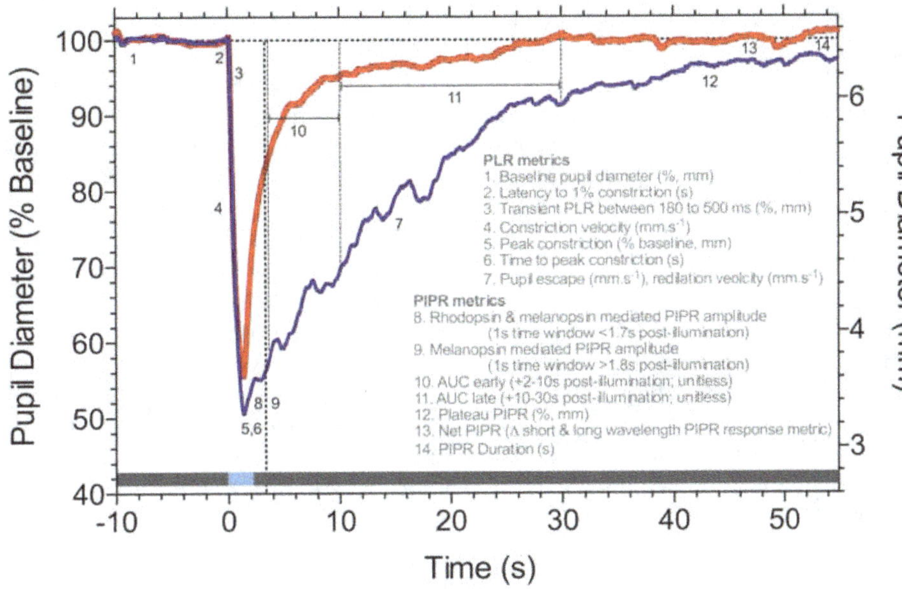

FIGURE 2 | Post-Illumination Pupil Response (PIPR) metrics. Consensual pupillary response to 1 s pulses (horizontal blue line at time 0; 465 nm blue, 637 nm red-the gray line represents the pre- and post-stimulus periods in the dark) measured in Maxwellian view (35.6° diameter stimulus; 15.1 log quanta.cm^{-2}.s^{-1}). Details of the pupil light response (PLR) and Post-Illumination Pupil Response (PIPR) metrics are described in the figure. Data are for a representative healthy observer (traces are the average of 3 repeats). Traces courtesy of Prakash Adhikari, Beatrix Feigl and Andrew J. Zele.

(a) stimulus wavelength (e.g., narrow band chromatic lights, broadband white lights), duration, area, fixation eccentricity and the dark- and light-adaptation levels (and pre-adaptation durations) that are optimized to stratify the rod-cone cut-offs under conditions of dark and light adaptation (11, 35, 99–103) that bias pupil responses to either rods or cones based on their characteristic spatial and temporal summation (104). A rod-favoring-condition may include a dim, short wavelength stimulus (e.g., 4 ms; 0.01 Lux corneal illumination) after prolonged dark adaptation and cone-favoring-condition with a brighter long wavelength stimulus (e.g., 1000 ms; 28 Lux) after a 10 min period of light adaptation (35);

(b) increment pulses increasing in a step-wise pattern from high mesopic to low photopic luminances (1, 10, 100 cd.m^{-2}; 45° diameter stimuli), which may be followed by a 30 s dark-period for additionally recording the Post-Illumination Pupil Response (95);

(c) a logarithmic increase in stimulus irradiance from 8.5 to ~14.5 log quanta (scotopic to photopic; full-field Ganzfeld stimuli) over a 2 min period, with 1 min pre- and post-stimulus periods of darkness (23);

(d) measurement of the peak-to-trough amplitude of the flicker (0.5 Hz) pupil response to blue test stimuli (with high melanopsin excitation) and red test stimuli (with low melanopsin excitation) (105), with the amplitude indicative of the level of interaction between the outer retina photoreceptors and inner retinal melanopsin, as calculated using the phase amplitude percentage (PAP) metric (28) that has application in disease detection (29, 44).

1.2 Melanopsin-The Post-illumination Pupil Response (PIPR)

Authors: Andrew J. Zele, Beatrix Feigl, Yanjun Chen, Paul D. Gamlin and Randy Kardon

Introduction

In human and non-human primate retina, melanopsin-expressing intrinsically photosensitive Retinal Ganglion Cells (ipRGCs) stratify the inner and outer regions of the inner plexiform layer, encircle the foveal pit, and increase in dendritic field diameter with increasing eccentricity, independent of their soma size (7, 16, 106). Signals originating in outer retinal rod and cone photoreceptors are transmitted extrinsically to ipRGCs via synaptic connections with DB6 diffuse bipolar cells and dopaminergic amacrine cells (16, 107–109). With a morphology and functionality distinct from conventional retinal ganglion cells (7), ipRGCs project 1) via the retinohypothalamic tract to multiple brain regions (110) for non-image forming functions including to the suprachiasmatic nucleus, the endogenous biological clock, to synchronize biological and physiological processes to the 24-hour light-dark cycle (5, 6, 111–115), 2) the pretectal olivary nucleus in the midbrain to regulate pupil diameter (8, 110), and 3) the lateral geniculate nucleus of the thalamus (7, 16, 110) for image forming visual functions (90, 116–118).

A signature biomarker of human melanopsin function is the Post-Illumination Pupil Response (PIPR), the sustained pupil constriction after light offset (**Figure 2**). This PIPR follows a characteristic irradiance-response relationship (8, 11, 74) with a half-maximal constriction for a retinal irradiance of ~13.5 log photons.cm^{-2}.s^{-1} (8); the largest sustained pupil constriction occurs at ~482 nm, the peak sensitivity of the melanopsin photopigment, as evidenced directly from spectral sensitivity measurements of the PIPR in humans (8, 28, 74) and non-human primates (8). Between light offset and ~1.7 s post-illumination, the peak sensitivity of the PIPR shifts to longer wavelengths to reflect major inputs from rhodopsin and melanopsin, with minor cone contributions (75).

Stimulus Characteristics

The following stimulus optimizations pertain to the measurement of the melanopsin-mediated PIPR measured in a darkened environment without immediate pre- or post-stimulus light adaptation. The optimal stimulus wavelength is nearer the melanopsin peak sensitivity (~482 nm), but any wavelength can produce PIPR amplitudes similar to the optimal wavelength by suitably scaling the irradiance according to the principle of univariance (119). Such alternate wavelength selections can be advantageous e.g., for limiting confounds from age-related lens attenuation. A long wavelength light (e.g., >635 nm) is typically included as a control to quantify non-specific autonomic factors, to measure extrinsic photoreceptor inputs to the pupil under conditions to which melanopsin has low sensitivity and to rule out the effect of lens attenuation.

Light output is ideally specified as the corneal or retinal irradiance using radiometric units (e.g., photon flux [log photons.cm^{-2}.s^{-1}] or irradiance [W.m^{-2}]). Stimuli of different wavelengths need to apply the same irradiance for comparability. Radiometric units are preferred because the photopic relative luminous efficiency (V) is defined exclusively in terms of additive L+M cone function (120). The quantification of the light in terms of its melanopsin excitation, that is the alpha-opic lux (121) or relative cone Trolands (122) will facilitate comparison between radiometric and photometric units.

Luminance (cd.m^{-2}) or corneal illumination (Lux), which are widely used in clinical applications, need to be combined with the stimulus wavelength.

Stimulus areas can be custom-selected to be full-field (e.g., Ganzfeld) or smaller focal-fields that localize responses to select visual field regions. The pupil pathway is presumed to integrate over larger retinal areas than image-forming vision (102, 123–126) and pupil measurements indicate that the PIPR follows a hill-of-vision with larger amplitudes in central than peripheral retina (127) which could be attributed to eccentricity related changes in ipRGC dendritic field density (7, 16, 106). Therefore, the select spatial stimulation of the PIPR will have advantages in the detection of early retinal dysfunction (21) due to the reduced number of ipRGCs [~3,000; (7)] compared to conventional ganglion cells [~1.5 million; (128)]. The PIPR has been assessed using stimulus durations ranging from 4 ms to 30 s (11, 74, 102), with 1 s test pulses (**Figure 2**) showing wide applicability due to their large, robust and repeatable PIPR amplitudes that are sustained for about 80 s with stimulus irradiances above 14 log photons.cm^{-2}.s^{-1} (74). The PIPR duration should be considered when determining the inter-stimulus interval, as well as the recovery from after-images of the stimulus light. The PIPR is typically measured using increment pulses. The flicker pupillary response to sinusoidal test stimuli has a low pass characteristic with a peak amplitude at ~0.5 Hz and high frequency cut-off near approaching 9 Hz (86, 105, 129, 130). With such sinusoidal temporal modulations the PIPR amplitude is presumed to be dependent on stimulus irradiance, and independent of temporal frequency in the range of 0.2–4 Hz (105).

A natural pupil is subject to fluctuations in diameter due to variation in autonomic nervous system tone, accommodation and vergence eye movements, environmental factors (ambient light, sounds, etc.) and interval (attention and alertness that reflects central nervous system adrenergic outputs) (131). A problem in closed-loop pupillographic paradigms is that the pupil of the test eye changes size during light presentation and subsequently alter the retinal irradiance (11, 132, 133). This could be overcome by mydriasis (in consensual pupil recordings) or using an open-loop Maxwellian view pupillometry system (with or without mydriasis) that focuses the stimulus image within the plane of the pupil (134). However, in clinical trials both methods may rarely be practicable because mydriasis interferes with other essential ophthalmological tests and not all laboratories have access to Maxwellian view systems.

Analysis

Post-illumination pupil response metrics quantified from 1.8 s post-stimulus onwards in time will provide a direct measure of human melanopsin function (**Figure 2**), with variability being the key determinant for the particular choice of metric (74); analyses are conducted with reference to the pre-stimulus baseline pupil diameter recorded prior to stimulus onset to achieve a stable and robust estimate in millimeters (mm, absolute pupil diameter) or percentage (%, relative pupil constriction amplitude). Under light adapted conditions, the pupil receives significant melanopsin input (88). Commonly implemented PIPR metrics include the plateau PIPR (8, 9); the PIPR amplitude [e.g., a 1s window at a pre-set time, such as 6 s post-illumination; (11, 74)] that is set for a participant cohort and specific stimulus conditions by determining the largest difference between the long wavelength (control) and short wavelength (test) PIPR amplitudes for the control group during a moving 1 s window (44); the PIPR average during pre-specified time epochs including the early and late Area Under Curve (AUC) [e.g., 2–10 s or 10–30 s post-illumination; (26, 135, 136)]; the net PIPR is the difference between the long wavelength (control) and short wavelength (test) PIPR amplitudes (19, 137); the redilation velocity (20) and the PIPR duration (74). Of these metrics, the PIPR amplitude and plateau PIPR show the lowest coefficient of variation which indicates these two metrics are the most reliable from one test to another in the same participant (78). During presentation of a light stimulus with low melanopsin excitation, the pupil light reflex is mainly driven by extrinsic cone and rod inputs to ipRGCs and metrics such as the transient response, latency to constriction and maximum pupil constriction amplitude are considered for analysis of outer retinal function (95). IpRGCs also act to keep the pupil constricted during light stimulation (73, 138, 139). The Phase Amplitude Percentage (PAP) can be used to study the interaction between inner and outer retinal inputs to the phasic pupil response during sinusoidal light stimulation (28).

Application

IpRGCs are presumed to be relatively robust to aging, with functional studies showing stable PIPR responses into the seventh decade (137, 140), and histological studies of human retina showing ipRGCs density is stable until this age, with a loss in density and dendritic arborization of human ipRGCs after the age 70 (141). The stability of PIPR amplitude across much of the lifespan (after controlling for age-related lens attenuation) makes it an objective reference marker of ophthalmic function for applications in clinical aging studies. No effect of refractive errors ranging between +3.00 and −9.25 D on the melanopsin mediated PIPR amplitude could be shown (140).

The melanopsin mediated PIPR can be applied in clinical cohorts to detect and monitor the progression of ipRGC dysfunction in disease. IpRGC dysfunction has been observed in a variety of retinal and optic nerve diseases, in particular at early stages, including in glaucoma (19–23), diabetic retinopathy (31, 32, 142), age-related macular degeneration (29, 30), and ischemic optic neuropathy (143). IpRGC function is largely preserved in mitochondrial optic neuropathy (135, 144) and in Retinitis Pigmentosa (9, 24–27). Altered melanopsin-dependent pupillary responses are also evident in neurologic and psychiatric conditions including seasonal affective disorder (41, 45), multiple sclerosis (145) and Parkinson's disease (44). As a direct measure of melanopsin function, the technique also has widespread application in the assessment of ipRGC function in chronobiology (37, 39).

1.3 Special Clinical Applications

Pupillographic Swinging Flashlight Test

Examination of the afferent pupillary pathway is a routine test in clinical and basic science investigations to determine the functionality of the retina and optic nerve signaling to the brain in the healthy eye or in specific disease. The comparison of the pupil light response between both eyes with the so-called swinging flashlight test is the standard for screening and diagnosing unilateral or asymmetric neuroretinal deficits by revealing a relative afferent pupillary defect (RAPD). The swinging flashlight test was first described by Levatin (146) and further developed by Thompson (147), and can be either assessed by an experienced clinician using a flashlight and neutral density filters, or by using pupillography that compares the pupil constriction amplitudes of both eyes quantitatively. With automated pupillography a stimulus response curve can quantify the difference between both eyes objectively (148) as opposed to the manual swinging flashlight test that is subjective and introduces examiner bias. The amplitude of the pupillary response is proportional to the logarithm of the intensity of the test light. Assessing the RAPD automatically might particularly help in precisely monitoring possible therapeutic effects in optic nerve diseases or serve as a screening method for defects of the afferent pathway. Pupillographic and swinging flashlight evaluation with neutral density filters of the RAPD have been performed e.g., in glaucoma (149–151) showing that the severity of RAPD correlates with the magnitude of field defects. However, diseases of the afferent visual system do not necessarily equally affect the results of perimetry or the RAPD (152).

The pupillographic swinging flashlight test should test the entire afferent pathway, and a white, full-field stimulus is recommended (151). The optimum stimulus brightness should constrict the pupil by approximately one third of its diameter. Stimulus length can be in accordance with the manual clinical swinging flashlight test that is usually between 1 and 3 s. The inter-stimulus interval should have at least the same length to allow the pupil's redilation, i.e., equal pupillary baseline conditions should be ensured for all stimuli. Fluctuations of pupil size or physiological anisocoria may influence the measurement. The best approach is therefore to measure both pupils simultaneously. Through this approach, the direct, bilateral pupil reactions to light, and the direct and consensual unilateral pupil reaction to light can be compared. At least four repeat measurements are recommended using pupillography as it is with the manual swinging flashlight test. This eliminates the problem of short term fluctuations of pupil size. Using a Maxwellian view condition (see also Chapter 1.2. Melanopsin) overcomes the fluctuating pupil size and hence irregular retinal irradiance. However, Maxwellian view is not always available in a clinical practice and does not eliminate fluctuations within the sympathetic system causing variations of the constriction speed and amplitude. It is therefore inevitable to repeat stimulus presentation several times to assess the afferent visual system. Adaptation before testing has to be considered: dark adaptation enhances the pupil light response while light adaptation will attenuate it. It is therefore mandatory to provide equal background illumination and equal stimulation length and brightness for both eyes but also an equal inter-stimulus interval.

Full-Field Pupillography, Pupil Perimetry/Campimetry

Pupillography is not only useful for the determination of an intact afferent limb of the pupillary pathway but can be performed to determine retinal functionality in certain retinal diseases. There are two strategies, either full-field pupillography to assess the entire neuroretinal function [e.g., in Retinitis pigmentosa: (24–26), or CNGA3-linked Achromatopsia: (35)], or pupil perimetry (stimulus presentation on a hemisphere) / campimetry (stimulus presentation on a flat monitor) to assess focal neuroretinal defects (94, 153–155).

When using focal stimuli, pupil visual field maps can be derived (156). Stimulus size may vary between large hemifields to small 1° stimuli to map visual fields objectively. Stimuli are classically presented one after another or using a multifocal pattern strategy (33, 157, 158). Ideally, a stimulus has to be large or bright enough to elicit a reliable pupil response but should avoid causing stray light. A challenge in pupil perimetry can be unstable fixation. Therefore, stimulus length is usually shorter (around 200 ms) in pupil perimetry/campimetry than the stimulus length used in pupillographic swinging flashlight testing (1–3 s) to avoid the patients wandering eyes during stimulus presentation. Nevertheless, fixation is essential in perimetric strategies for an accurate stimulus presentation on the retina, thus a gaze-controlled strategy (e.g., via eye-tracking) is recommended, as it allows for a retinotopic stimulation regardless of fixation problems (153). As pupil measurements are objective, pupil perimetry/campimetry also helps in distinguishing real visual field defects from functional visual field loss and malingering (153–155).

Each laboratory using pupil perimetry/campimetry needs to establish normative values or use a commercially available device with an existing database of normative (age corrected) values. This is not only important in a clinical setting but also for basic science evaluations of the pupil.

2. THE EFFERENT PUPILLARY PATHWAY Author: Helmut Wilhelm

Introduction

The efferent pupillary pathways comprise the cholinergic pathway to the sphincter muscle and the adrenergic pathway to the dilator muscle of the iris. The cholinergic pathway begins in the dorsal region of the oculomotor nucleus complex (159). It runs with the third nerve through the cavernous sinus via the ciliary ganglion where the second order neurons, named short ciliary nerves, begin. Those reach the sphincter muscle through the subchoroidal space. Nerve fibers supplying the ciliary muscle underlying accommodation run together with the pupillomotor fibers. The sympathetic pathway begins in the hypothalamus, projects down the brainstem to the centrum ciliospinale at the level of Th1–Th3, follows the sympathetic chain to the superior cervical ganglion where the terminal neurons innervating the dilator muscle start (160). Their axons run without synapse through the ciliary ganglion and are called long ciliary nerves.

Stimulus Characteristics and Analysis in Clinical Applications

Pupillographic examinations of the efferent pupillary system have mainly the purpose to detect pathologies like oculosympathetic paresis (Horner syndrome), oculomotor nerve palsy, and tonic pupil (damage of the ciliary ganglion). Those diagnoses are usually based on clinical observation and pharmacological testing (cocaine or apraclonidine in Horner syndrome (161–165) or dilute pilocarpine in tonic pupil (166). Pupillography is not necessary to establish a reliable diagnosis. However, it may be helpful to distinguish Horner syndrome from simple anisocoria or other causes of anisocoria in so far that it can help to decide whether pharmacological testing is necessary or not (167).

Horner-Syndrome

In Horner syndrome, pupil dilation is slowed down. Because this condition is, with very few exceptions, unilateral, comparison of the dilation behavior of both pupils is the best approach. Clinical studies establishing cut-off values are not available. A video study revealed the amount of anisocoria 4 s after switching off the light as the best parameter to diagnose Horner syndrome (168). It is recommended to use a bright stimulus to achieve a maximal possible pupillary constriction and then abruptly switch off the light and record the pupil behavior (169). A suitable parameter describing dilation is the ¾-redilation time in comparison between both eyes (169). This is the time between maximal constriction and the time point when ¾ of the constriction amplitude has been lost by redilation. The constriction amplitude is defined as the difference between baseline and pupil size with maximal constriction. Another possibility is to measure constriction speed or post-illumination response as described in the chapter about intrinsic photosensitive ganglion cells (Chapter 1.2). Which approach would best distinguish Horner syndrome from physiologic anisocoria has not yet been studied. Using dilation lag based on the measurement of the ¾ redilation time, a sensitivity of 70% and a specificity of 95% for diagnosing Horner syndrome by pupillography is possible (169). **Figure 3** shows the typical dilation behavior of a Horner pupil.

Independent from the parameters chosen, at least 3 tests per eye are necessary because pupil responses may vary and dilation lag might sometimes be detectable and sometimes not (170). Because a sympathetically denervated pupil dilates very slowly, it is recommended to extend the recording by at least 10 s or better 15 s after maximal constriction. Cocaine or apraclonidine testing (in children <1 year only cocaine) decides finally if Horner syndrome can be diagnosed.

Oculomotor Nerve Palsy and Neurological Emergency

In oculomotor nerve palsy, the accompanying outer eye muscle palsies determine the diagnosis. Oculomotor palsy limited to the pupil is extremely rare (171) and pupillography cannot contribute to the diagnosis. However, in the setting of raised intracranial pressure or uncal herniation or any other neurological emergency, pupillary light response is used to monitor the patients. There have been attempts to use pupillography instead of simple clinical observation to detect a light response (172). Indices based on pupillography have been used, but it is not yet clear if pupillography adds information additional to simple observation. By means of pupillography it may be easier to recognize a residual pupillary constriction in an emergency setting. By looking at the pupillogram it may be easier to decide whether a pupil has reacted to light or a random movement has been observed. The use of maximally bright light and at least 10 recordings per eye are recommended. Binocular recording has the advantage that afferent and efferent defects may be distinguished.

Tonic Pupil

The diagnosis of a tonic pupil is based on its clinical picture, reduced or absent response to light, preserved but slow near response and slow redilation. If the pupil is examined under magnification, small spontaneous segmental constrictions of the sphincter become visible (173). Also during near reaction, it may be observed that different parts of the sphincter react with different speed. The pupil is mostly not absolutely round but elliptically distorted. 0.1% pilocarpine constricts a tonic pupil and has less effect on a normal pupil.

It is possible to record both light and near response pupillographically (174). Constriction speed and amplitude are

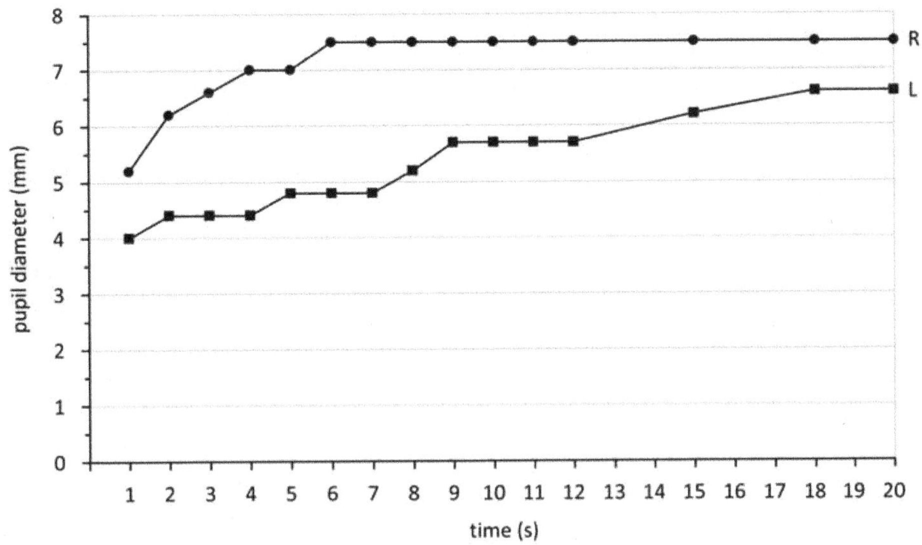

FIGURE 3 | Pupil diameter (mm) measured in darkness after switching off a light stimulus over a time period of 20 s. The right eye (R) shows the typical quick redilation behavior of a healthy pupil while the left eye (L) reveals a dilation lag, typical for Horner syndrome. Data are taken from a patient with Horner syndrome in the left eye collected during standard care.

relevant parameters. By comparing to normal subjects, criteria for the diagnosis of a tonic pupil may be defined. This is especially helpful when diagnosing a bilateral condition (174). It can of course be used for precise measurement of pupillary diameter before and after pharmacological testing.

Diabetic Autonomic Neuropathy

Pupillary abnormalities in patients with diabetes have been found indicating sympathetic and parasympathetic dysfunction in comparison to healthy controls. While Dütsch et al. (175) could not reveal a difference between diabetes patients with and without cardiac autonomic neuropathies or peripheral neuropathies, Lerner et al. (176) found hints for reduced baseline pupil diameters and constriction amplitudes in patients with diabetes-related cardiac autonomic neuropathy compared to those without cardiac autonomic neuropathies. Consequently, when examining pupillary responses from a diabetes patient cohort, it is important to consider that they are not consequences of an underlying efferent neuropathy.

Although the diagnosis of efferent pupillary defects is a domain of clinical observation and pharmacological testing, pupillography might be a valuable supplement. It is important to be aware that any defects in the efferent pupillary pathway may change pupil movements and thus confound the interpretation of the pupil-based test in the assessment of the afferent pupillary pathway. For example, the pupil constriction in a pseudophakic eye may show a slower direct response (due to perturbation of the iris mechanics from the cataract surgery) thus leading to a misperception reduced pupillary response to light. Using consensual pupillary responses may provide a more precise measurement of the integrity of the afferent pathway if the efferent pupillary defect is a concern in the studied eye.

3. PHARMACOLOGY

Author: Elemer Szabadi

Introduction

The anatomical and physiological features of the pupil make it eminently suitable for pharmacological studies. Its size (measured as diameter, or occasionally as area) is determined by the balance between two opposing smooth muscles in the iris that receive opposing sympathetic and parasympathetic innervations (**Figure 4**).

The two serially connected pre- and postganglionic neurons are under the influence of a network of premotor autonomic neurons in the brainstem and diencephalon which channel all physiological and psychological stimuli, including the effect of light, to the pupil. Changes in pupil diameter brought about by these stimuli, including drugs modulating them, are directly available to visual and instrumental inspection, recording, measurement and quantitative analysis. Furthermore, the iris is accessible to topically applied drugs creating, together with the concomitant recording of pupillary changes, a unique *in situ/in vivo* pharmacological test system.

Not surprisingly, pharmacological studies of the pupil are abundant, both in humans and non-human animal species. The use of drugs can help in unraveling the central neuronal network controlling the pupil, and can also provide valuable information about the drugs themselves by establishing their effects in a well-defined physiological/pharmacological system. Reports on the effect of drugs on the pupil require documentation of parameters of light stimulation and method of recording, like in any other field of pupillography, together with information on the pharmacological aspects of the study (characteristics of the participants and drug(s) used, design, measurement of drug effects, data analysis). It is important that all methodological

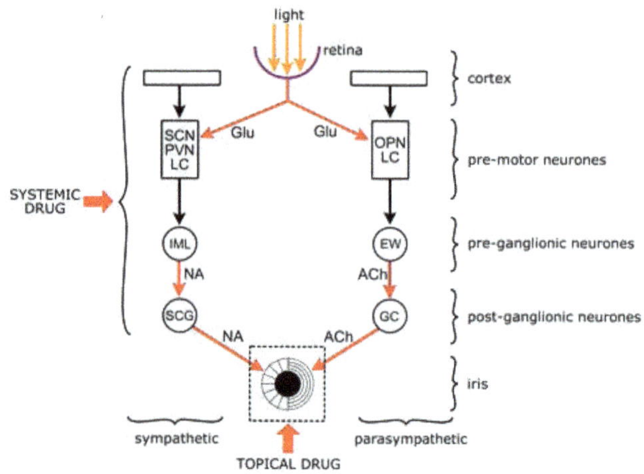

FIGURE 4 | Targets of drugs in the neuronal network controlling the pupil. The pupil is an aperture in a diaphragm, the iris. The size of the pupil reflects the interaction between the circular sphincter muscle and the radial dilator muscle. The sphincter receives a parasympathetic and the dilator a sympathetic output. Both autonomic outputs consist of serially linked preganglionic and postganglionic neurones that are under the influence of premotor autonomic neurones. The premotor neurones channel the influence of other brain structures (e.g., cortex) and light to the preganglionic neurones. Premotor neurones: SCN: suprachiasmatic nucleus (hypothalamus); PVN: paraventricular nucleus (hypothalamus); LC: locus coeruleus (brainstem: pons); OPN: olivary pretectal nucleus (pretectum). Preganglionic neurones: IML: intermediate lateral column (spinal cord); EWN: Edinger-Westphal nucleus (brainstem: midbrain). Postganglionic neurones: SCG: superior cervical ganglion; GC: ciliary ganglion. Arrows are neuronal connections, red arrows are excitatory connections with identified neurotransmitters (Glu, glutamate; NA, noradrenaline; Ach, acetylcholine). Drugs can be applied topically to the surface of the cornea to affect the iris and the noradrenergic and cholinergic neuro-effector junctions, or systemically when they can affect any part of the central neuronal network. It should be noted that topically applied drugs may get into the systemic circulation leading to systemic effects, and systemically applied drugs may also affect the iris directly.

detail is provided not only to help the reader to evaluate the study but also to help further investigators to replicate the study.

In this chapter, we propose some guidelines that should be adhered to when publishing the effects of drugs on the pupil. It is hoped that adherence to these guidelines would help the reader to better evaluate the study and facilitate replication. These guidelines relate to the study of human participants. However, many of them are also applicable to the study of non-human subjects.

Specification and Stimulus Characteristics

Participants

If the study involves topical drug application, in addition to general information as number, age and sex, the color of the iris should be specified since pigment in the iris binds the applied drug leading to a reduction in the response (177).

Drugs

Topical application

A major issue in case of topical application is bioavailability of the drug that is largely determined by penetration through the cornea (178). Drugs can be applied to the surface of the eye in different forms (179). For pharmacological studies, drugs are used in aqueous or oily solutions. The formulation of the drug should be specified: it should be made clear whether the drug is used as a base or a salt. The vehicle should be specified: penetration through the cornea is usually better from oily solutions (180). Although the possibility of applying drugs to the surface of the eye as a continuous superfusion has been explored (181), the "blob" application in the form of eye drops has remained the common form. A calibrated micropipette should be used to apply a standard volume of solution (e.g., 10 μl) into the conjunctival sac. The molar concentration of the drug should be specified, together with the pH of the solution. It should be made clear whether any "penetration enhancer" [e.g., a local anesthetic; see (182)] has been used. Although topical application assumes that the effect of the drug is restricted to the eye to which the drug was applied, occasionally systemic effects can occur, affecting the fellow eye, and /or other parts of the body (183).

Systemic application

Drugs are usually administered orally, however, occasionally parenteral administration (e.g., infusion) is used (184). The formulation (base vs. salt) should be specified. Dosage per single oral dose, or concentration in infusion fluid and rate of infusion, should be specified. In single dose experiments pharmacokinetic evidence is needed to make sure that measurements coincide with the peak blood concentration of the drug.

Design

The design can vary according to the questions to be answered. It should aim at eliminating bias and contamination by procedural factors (e.g., practice effects). Therefore, it is common practice to use a double-blind design, and to allocate participants to sessions and treatments according to a balanced cross-over design. The index treatment should be compared with positive (i.e., a known treatment with the expected effect) and negative (placebo) **controls.** In the case of topical application, the fellow eye should receive treatment with artificial tear (i.e., placebo). However, if the measurements are taken in light, the response to the topical drug cannot be taken as the size of the drug-induced anisocoria, due to the operation of a consensual interaction between the pupils (185). Therefore, measurements should either be taken in darkness, or the response should be measured from the pre-treatment baseline in the index eye.

Apart from using positive and negative control treatments, it is also necessary to include a number of **collateral measurements** with expected effects in the relevant area. For example, if the potential sedative effect of a drug on the pupil is studied, non-pupillary effects of sedation can be included in the design [e.g., battery of visual analog scales, critical flicker fusion frequency; see (66)], or when potential sympatholytic or sympathomimetic effects on the pupil are investigated, non-pupillary sympathetic effects can be incorporated [e.g., changes in blood pressure and heart rate: see (186)]. The collateral evidence is important in corroborating the genuineness of the pupillary findings.

Recording of Pupillary Effects of Drugs

Recording in Darkness

Infrared technology allows recording pupil diameter changes in darkness. Although some limited information may be obtained by studying the effects of drugs on **resting pupil diameter** in the dark, more comprehensive information can be gained by investigating their effects on light-evoked pupillary function (see below). Spontaneous **pupillary fluctuations** in the dark are recorded using the Pupillographic Sleepiness Test (PST). The PST and the specific standards for its use are discussed later in this paper (see Chapter 5). This test is amenable for the detection of the sedative and alerting effects of drugs, and its two quantitative indices (Pupillary Unrest Index and total power of fluctuations) correlate well with non-pupillary measures of the level of arousal (66).

Recording in Presence of Light Stimulation

For pharmacological studies both static (resting pupil diameter) and dynamic (pupillary reflexes) pupillometry can be used. The methodological requirements for light stimulation are the same as for other pupillographic investigations and are described in detail in the general standards section.

For pharmacological studies, it is desirable to study the effects of drugs on **resting pupil diameter** at a number of luminance levels, for several reasons. Firstly, in this way we obtain a much larger data set that would yield greater statistical power. Secondly, light can set the baseline at different levels that in turn would be reflected in the size of the responses, a lower baseline favoring dilator responses and a higher baseline constrictor responses (187). It should be noted, however, that apart from its mechanistic effect of setting the baseline, light also has a more specific effect in the case of sympathetic drugs, potentiating sympatholytic and antagonizing sympathomimetic effects (188).

The pupillary light reflex is evoked by a brief light pulse and the darkness reflex by sudden withdrawal of illumination. For pharmacological studies, the **light reflex response** is divided into two parts, latency and amplitude reflecting parasympathetic activation, and recovery time sympathetic activation (189). The parameters of the **darkness reflex response** (initial velocity, amplitude) are indices of sympathetic activation (66). For the light reflex response, it is recommended to use a range of stimulus intensities: this would enable the construction of light intensity/amplitude, light intensity/latency and light intensity/75% recovery time curves. The large dataset obtained in this way yields enhanced statistical robustness.

Analysis

Baseline pupillary measures (resting pupil diameter, parameters of pupil reflexes) should be presented in absolute units. It may be appropriate to use percentage changes in responses (e.g., after the application of an antagonist) only if the absolute sizes of the unaffected responses are available. Full details of the statistical analysis should be provided (e.g., for analysis of variance, F ratios and degrees of freedom, and not only levels of significance).

4. PSYCHOLOGY AND PSYCHIATRY

Authors: Stuart R. Steinhauer and Kathryn A. Roecklein

Introduction

Since the late 1950's, assessment of dynamic changes in the pupil (pupillography or pupillometry) have become a primary measure of increased cognitive and emotional activity (190–193). Both sympathetic and parasympathetic systems contribute to these pupillary modulations. The light reaction, which is primarily under parasympathetic control, can be reduced by emotional and cognitive activity. Suppression of the light reaction has been associated with fear and pain (194). Light can drive pupil constriction directly through the pupil light reflex, but also indirectly through retinal input to the suprachiasmatic nucleus and its pathways recruiting the dorsomedial hypothalamus and locus coeruleus, underlying wakefulness (193). Dilation in response to cognitive, effortful or emotional stimulation is mediated by both direct activation of the sympathetic system on dilator muscles of the iris, and by inhibition of the parasympathetic pathway leading to relaxation of the sphincter muscles (195–197). As in pure physiological experiments, the interaction of these systems may involve considerable reciprocal inhibition: the stimulation of one pathway is accompanied by decreased activity in the complementary pathway. The PIPR, described in Chapter 1, is a third type of pupil response potentially affected by psychological processes and is the dilation after illumination offset that persists as a function of melanopsin cell responses (8, 9).

Stimulus Characteristics

The characteristics of stimuli that elicit pupillary dilation, or that modify parameters of the light reaction, are related to virtually all sensory modalities, and are sensitive to different contextual states. Thus, in relation to psychology and psychophysiology, there are three essential domains that need to be considered [after Sutton (198)]: (1) the physiological response (in this case, modulation of the pupil), (2) stimulus characteristics, and (3) the contingencies for behavioral response and task demand. In contrast to absolute stimulation and analysis approaches employed in clinical ophthalmological work, psychological and neuropsychiatric research employing pupillary assessment does not involve any standardized paradigms and is more often related to the parameters of complex instructions and varying complexity in stimuli. Reporting characteristics discussed and adopted at the 1999 meeting of the International Colloquium on the Pupil (ICP99) are provided below and serve as standards for reporting.

Stimuli

In most non-psychological research, the varying stimulus element is light. For psychological studies, there are also changes in auditory and even more rarely, tactile or olfactory stimuli (the latter not discussed further). Light stimuli have their most direct effect in producing constriction of the pupil, but in psychological studies, complex visual stimuli are often used to convey different meanings. Thus, the classical digit span task involves presenting a series of auditory stimuli which are later repeated, but the same effect psychologically could be produced by presenting brief visual digits. Specific experiments may provide a visual background after which target stimuli are presented. When the difference between background and stimulus is significant, a light reaction may be produced, which confounds the accurate assessment of dilation to the task demands in several potential ways: the light reaction may be magnitudes of order greater than the dilation, or baseline from which the dilation is measured may be shifted. At the very least, the luminance of the display should be specified in candelas/square meter ($cd.m^{-2}$; ICP99). For single discrete stimuli, it is often possible to report the wavelength in nanometers. This is more difficult when using complex pictures, which vary in brightness across the visual field. One approach to minimizing hue effects (and stimulation of different photoreceptors) is to transform pictures into gray scales (199). For example, when presenting words, numbers, or small figures, use of black stimuli on a gray background minimizes contrast effects, and using pre- and post-stimulus masks (a row of X's, then the target, then X's again) also tends to minimize contrast effects (200). In such cases, the size of the stimuli needs to be provided in degrees of visual angle (which can be calculated using actual size and distance from the display). Distance of the visual stimulus from the eye is a consideration, as very close stimuli will result in constriction of the pupil related to vergence and accommodation effects.

Similarly, auditory stimuli need to be specified in loudness and duration. For pure tones, frequency should be specified, though this is not practical for spoken words or other complex sounds. Except for abrupt transients (that can elicit orienting reflexes), rise and fall times for auditory stimuli are not so critical in pupillary studies as in electrophysiology.

Finally, there are interactions related to the illumination of the testing situation. Pupillary oscillations are always greater in the presence of increasing ambient light, which decreases signal-to-noise ratio. Thus, recording in darkness minimizes oscillations, though provides more emphasis on sympathetic activation than parasympathetic inhibition. In darkness, there may be a ceiling effect on maximum pupillary dilation.

Behavior

This aspect is related to the task demands in psychological experiments. The participant may be asked just to sit passively, but most studies involve an interaction based on instructions. There may be cues that instruct subjects to have different expectancies (which increases pre-stimulus diameter), or to remember and modulate responses to stimuli (remember and repeat; calculate; sort numbers; categorize). The parameters of procedures and instructions to subjects are critical to communicate to readers. It is not unusual to ascribe a complex psychological context to a task manipulation, but without knowing exactly what the subject is being asked, it is difficult to know whether the proposed construct has actually been implemented.

Minor instructional differences can have significant effects. For example, asking a subject to make a simple button press every time a tone occurs seems overtly simple, and results in a dilation beginning around 500 ms and peaking around 1,200–1,400 ms. If instead the subject is asked just to make a voluntary press every few seconds, the early portion of the response is seen, but with a smaller dilation that ends before 1,000 ms. Even the presence of an experimenter near the participant can influence pupillary findings (201).

Analysis

Initial Pupillary Recording and Data Reduction

Most current pupil and eye tracking devices have a minimum temporal resolution of 50 or 60 Hz, though some handheld devices use a slower sampling rate. As maximum frequency response of the pupil is <9 Hz, even a 20 Hz sampling rate is enough to capture critical aspects of pupillary oscillations. The pupil has a relatively large signal-to-noise ratio so that for most processing tasks, use of repeated conditions and averaging of the same condition provides a waveform that eliminates artifacts due to other factors, though only 5–10 repetitions of a condition may be necessary compared to the larger number of repetitions needed for event-related potentials and other physiological measures. In many studies, there may be up to 40 repetitions of a condition contributing to an average for an individual. Electrical noise, accuracy of edge detection of the pupil, and resolution of the recording device all may add some noise to the signal. The resolution of the recording system in mm should be specified—is it accurate to the nearest 0.02 or 0.05 mm or better? Some instruments provide a number that is confusing—the data file may give pupil diameter to the nearest 0.0001 mm, but this is not meaningful, it is a rounding error of the manufacturer. Most of the more accurate systems either provide direct measurement or a means for calibrating measurements to a known standard.

Preprocessing of the data to eliminate blinks or other artifacts is mandatory; short-duration artifacts can be corrected by linear interpolation between valid points (except at peaks and troughs of the signal). It is reasonable to filter pupillary data that have a high sampling rate (this can be easily performed by averaging of points around each original point, though peaks and troughs will be slightly attenuated). Filtering can be performed either before or after signal averaging. However, filtering and averaging can make determination of abrupt latency changes (time of light reaction or dark reaction onset) less precise.

The Parameters of the Light Reaction and PIPR

The parameters of the light reaction and PIPR are more clearly detailed in Chapter 1. For most psychological studies, the key measures will be prestimulus diameter (which can also be determined from onset of the light stimulus until the beginning of the light reaction), latency of the light reaction, and amplitude and latency of the light reaction. Other measures may include times to reach greatest constriction velocity, and times at which 50 or 75% of redilation are reached. Note that for very brief stimuli, there may be an incomplete light reaction (2), and for prolonged light stimuli, the pupil will begin to enlarge (pupillary escape) after the initial constriction.

Measures Related to Pupillary Dilation

Measures related to pupillary dilation are more complex and variable across studies as appropriate. The pupil may show a slowly increasing tonic change as working memory load is gradually increased, or phasic changes during the 1–2 s after presentation of more discrete stimuli. From the average response, it is somewhat standard to use a pre-stimulus average of 500–1,000 ms as a baseline diameter. Where a simple peak is observed, either amplitude of the peak (or simple average of a few points around the peak within a pre-specified range) may be calculated after subtracting the baseline diameter. In some experiments, the difference between baseline diameters by condition may be of interest. In experiments in which there is differential processing complexity, the peak may be delayed, as seen when sorting increasing numbers of digits (202) so that either amplitude or latency to peak may be of interest. In some experiments, including complex processing of emotional stimuli, there may be a prolonged dilation with no clear peak, resulting in a need for an average measurement over a prolonged interval rather than a specific peak. Measurement of dilation may be complicated by the occurrence of multiple peaks in the pupillary dilation waveform. When recordings are obtained in relatively bright conditions, there may be both an early dilation related to parasympathetic inhibition, as well as a later peak related to both parasympathetic inhibition and sympathetic activation.

Diameter/Change in mm vs. per Cent Change

The ICP99 standard was that pupil diameter in mm should be reported, rather than area or radius. There is also a question as to whether absolute measures of diameter or change in diameter should be reported, as compared to % change in baseline. Per cent change is often used in ophthalmologic practice to evaluate change across treatment conditions (e.g., % reduction of the light reaction due to pharmacological instillation). However, in psychological experiments, it is important to evaluate the actual change in diameter, since this may vary across conditions, as well as different baselines across conditions. Even where a rationale for using % change is presented, some reference to absolute pupil diameter and pupil change is necessary in order to replicate findings. Note that similar real changes in diameter will be underestimated for participants with larger initial diameter compared to smaller pupil diameter, a major problem in utilizing per cent change (203).

Statistical Analyses

Several alternative statistical approaches have been used. When comparing groups or variables within a group, *t*-tests or ANOVA models to evaluate differences in maximum constriction, peak dilation, or latency are most often appropriate. Often, there is interest in evaluating prolonged periods of pupillary activity rather than peak measures. A Principal Components Analysis (PCA) can be used to isolate orthogonally independent factors, which describe for each component how it is related to variation over the time of the waveform; factor scores may be derived which can then be subject to separate analyses (204). Another approach based on the Guthrie-Buchwald (205) procedure provides a minimum number of successive points that must all be significantly different across conditions (by *t*-test or ANOVA) to define *post-hoc* regions of significant effects (200). There has recently been increased interest in utilizing Bayesian statistics to define regions of significant differences.

Abbreviations

There is often much confusion in the pupillary literature associated with unique or uninformative abbreviations. Acceptable and readily recognized abbreviations include PLR (pupillary light reaction) or PIPR (post-illumination pupil response). All other abbreviations are recommended to be mnemonic as appropriate to a paper: for example PkDil or AvgDil communicates peak or average dilation (which still needs to be defined as the absolute value or difference from baseline). Beatty (206) had earlier introduced TEPR (task evoked pupillary response), but this is a confusing terminology as it referred to dilations, but could as easily be misinterpreted as a constriction response. Even PDR for pupillary dilation response is confusing and probably should be avoided.

Application

Loewenfeld documented the two millennia history of pupillary movements in her dissertation (207) and epic tome on the pupil (2). The more sustained interest in psychological constructs was initiated after 1960 with studies of dilation in response to emotional stimuli (208) working memory tasks (209), orienting stimuli (210), and processing load (206), among others. Responses to orienting or novelty, emotionally salient, and simple feedback stimuli tend to peak at slightly after one second (193, 211–213). Mental effort or arousal responses which require greater processing time occur with greater peak latencies related to the complexity of the task, such as performing arithmetic (214), memorizing digits using working memory (202, 209), both positive and negatively salient arousal (199), reward processing (215), as well as numerous other types of cognitive or emotional processes (193). Convergent validity for pupillographic measures of arousal comes from correlation with psychophysiological measures of arousal such as skin conductance [e.g., (199)], and associations with pupillary and electrocortical activity [e.g., (211)]. Change in pupil diameter with alertness and sleepiness, including decreased diameter and increasing pupillary oscillations, are discussed in Chapter 5. Thus, pupillary assessment continues to be employed as a significant window on complex psychological processes (193). The pupil has been a strong investigative tool in psychopathology for over 70 years (particular schizophrenia and depression studies), with well documented decreased processing-related dilations in schizophrenia (204, 216, 217) and enhanced dilations to negatively valenced stimuli in depressed patients (200, 218, 219).

More recently, the PIPR has been evaluated among individuals with seasonal affective disorder (SAD), and is highlighted here in somewhat more detail. Initially, Roecklein et al. (41) found a reduced PIPR in SAD participants compared to nondepressed, nonseasonal participants. Laurenzo et al. (220) subsequently reported an attenuation of the PIPR in those with nonseasonal Major Depressive Disorder (MDD) compared to nondepressed controls, but only when using low intensity red and blue stimuli, and not under higher intensity chromatic stimuli. A seasonal variation was identified such that high intensity blue light responses in the post-illumination period were more pronounced during longer photoperiods (220). This is in contrast to the findings of Roecklein et al. (under review) presented in this issue. In a study of Age-Related Macular Degeneration (AMD) and healthy controls, AMD was associated with depression, but the PIPR was not correlated with depression (30). Depression was measured with a short self-report questionnaire and mean scores for both groups were below the cutoff of 16 indicating that the AMD group was, on average, not reporting symptoms of clinical depression. All individuals in this study were below self-report threshold on a screening implement for seasonal affective disorder. Münch et al. (221) reported a larger PIPR in winter in individuals without cataracts, and low levels of depression which is consistent with the seasonal variation found by Roecklein et al. (under review) in the present issue. Discrepancies, while few, in the emerging literature attempting to evaluate melanopsin cell responses to light in seasonal and nonseasonal depression have largely motivated the above review of melanopsin oriented pupillometry methods. Because light can impact both mood and learning and memory processes through melanopsin pathways (222), future work may employ the PIPR in studies on learning and memory as well as depression.

5. SLEEPINESS-RELATED PUPILLARY OSCILLATIONS

Authors: Barbara J. Wilhelm, Kathryn A. Roecklein and Tobias Peters

Introduction

Oscillations of pupil diameter in darkness related to sleepiness of a subject were first described by Lowenstein et al. (223) and called "fatigue waves" at that time. Today, there is a differentiation between sleepiness (related to either quantity or quality of sleep) and fatigue (not necessarily related to sleep, but also evocable by physical or psychological exhaustion) in sleep research and sleep medicine. Therefore, the terms "sleepiness waves" and "sleepiness-related oscillations" are preferable because fatigue does not result in oscillations in pupil diameter. Lowenstein et al. (223) confirmed the central nervous system origin of sleepiness-related oscillations of pupil diameter in darkness using pharmacological experiments. Subsequently, Yoss et al. used the Lowenstein device clinically in the diagnosis and treatment of patients with narcolepsy and developed a classification of pupillary oscillations related to eye lid movements and EEG signs of increased sleepiness (224, 225). In the following two decades few clinical applications emerged due to complicated apparatuses and a lack of automation (226, 227). The pupillographic sleepiness test (PST) developed by Lüdtke et al. (228) utilized modern technical possibilities regarding recording, image analysis, artifact elimination and automated analysis. Classical test quality criteria of the PST have been evaluated and are adequate (229–231). The PST is now established and widely used in sleep research and sleep medicine as well as in psychology (232–234).

Experimental Conditions for the Pupillographic Sleepiness Test

Darkness

Light is the major contributing factor of the pupil diameter. To capture measures of autonomic arousal, all light sources need to be excluded (235). Therefore, infrared goggles are used for the recording of sleepiness-related pupillary oscillations. Depending on individual face shape such goggles may not be completely light-tight and for this reason the examination room should be as dark as possible (in the mesopic range, i.e., below 3 $cd.m^{-2}$) and the illumination level needs to be quantified. Infrared indicators can be used for orientation.

Silence

It is important to protect the subject from acoustic influences in a silent room with sound dampening or by the use of noise canceling headphones. During the recording period communication with the participant is prohibited and the examiner is meant to be silent during examination.

Temperature

Room temperature needs to be comfortable because cold temperatures stimulate the sympathetic nervous system and may have an alerting effect. In addition, high temperatures may result in higher pupillary unrest index (PUI) due to reduced alertness. Stable room temperature between 68 and 72°F (20–23°C) is ideal.

Time of Day

Normative values for the PST have been collected during the first half of the day [8 a.m. to 1 p.m.; (231)]. Patients with obstructive sleep apnea show their highest sleepiness values during this timeframe. For hospital use, this time frame is recommended to allow for comparison with the reference values.

Medication

Topical medication (eye drops) with effects on pupil size should be avoided prior to testing. In addition, systemic medications with psychoactive or alerting effects or influence on the sympathetic/parasympathetic nervous system should be avoided if feasible or documented. The PST can also be used to quantify improvement in sleepiness due to a therapeutic regimen when measured pre-treatment and post-treatment.

Caffeine and Nicotine Consumption

Participants should be reminded to abstain from caffeine for 8–10 h prior to testing (236). However, this recommendation may be relaxed in field studies to avoid withdrawal effects or poor compliance. Nicotine has a minimal impact on the PUI and performing the PST 1 h after the last use of tobacco or nicotine products is sufficient (237).

Preparation and Standardized Instruction of the Participant

Reference values have been collected previously only after a 10 min period of sedentary rest to minimize any impact of physical activity on the PST (238). The following verbal instructions have been provided in past studies, including those reporting normative PUI values, and are provided here to be used broadly in future studies as a standardized set of instructions prior to recording the PST.

"The measurement will last 11 min. During the recording it will be dark and quiet in the room. We will not talk to you before the recording is completed. Please look in the direction of the red fixation light; you do not need to focus on it.

You may want to avoid thinking about problems or plans for your day, or about difficult issues in your life. Just look straight ahead and relax. We will now adjust the camera and we will inform you when the recording is about to start."

Preliminary Pupil Examination

Before the pupillographic sleepiness test is started, a basic pupil examination (160) should be performed with a flashlight or other light source to make sure that the recorded pupil shows normal and unrestricted mobility.

Test Duration and Interval of Consecutive Measurements

The standard test duration, which also has been used when collecting normative values, is 11 min of recording (230, 233). In the case of series of recordings an interval of 2 h is recommended to avoid possible sequence effects.

Data Surveillance During the Recording

Because participants may fall asleep, or the camera may need to be adjusted if data loss occurs, experimenters should monitor data acquisition continuously either in the same room or from outside of the testing room via monitor to ensure the quality of the recording.

Falling Asleep

If a participant falls asleep during testing, we recommend that the experimenter provides a brief acoustic signal if the participant does not awaken in 20 s. A louder or longer signal should be used if the first is unsuccessful, and a verbal request to open the eyes may be delivered by the examiner, if ultimately necessary. We recommend that all such sleep events should be documented, and that a test with multiple sleep events should be considered as pathological and/or as excessive sleepiness.

Subjective Rating of Sleepiness

The Stanford Sleepiness Scale or the Karolinska Sleepiness Scale assess self-reported sleepiness and can be included to determine the degree of awareness or insight into the degree of sleepiness retrospectively after recording in the clinical setting.

The Suggested Experimental Order of Procedures Is:

1. 10 min of physical rest
2. Preliminary pupil examination
3. Assessment of medication, caffeine, and nicotine use; entry into database
4. PST recording for 11 min
5. Subjective sleepiness scale.

Analysis

Before analysis of a recording, high frequency noise (e.g., due to blinks) is excluded and, for missing values, a linear interpolation is applied which is standard in pupillographic recordings in general (239). Parameters of evaluation may be gained by Fast Fourier Transformation (FFT) or calculation of the Pupillary Unrest Index (PUI). FFT normally is characterized by the amplitude spectrum (or "power") in the frequency range $\leq$0.8 Hz (228). The PUI is the sum of the absolute changes in pupil diameter over the time of recording and is given in mm/min (230). For statistical analysis the natural logarithm of the PUI is recommended due to its normal distribution in larger samples (231).

Data Reporting Recommendations

a) Participants

Besides general aspects as age and sex (see general standards Part I), the time lag to the consumption of nicotine and caffeine should be provided.

In addition: sleep habits, method of assessing sleep behavior during the days before the recording (e.g., diary, actigraphy), use of alerting or sedative medication.

b) Technical information on test system, camera (video frequency in hertz), sampling rate, image analysis.

c) Method of artifact management. Specify methods for blink removal.

d) General conditions of the pupillographic sleepiness

Information on all conditions listed above should be provided. Deviations from these standard conditions should be described and substantiated.

e) Pupil parameters (averages of the recording period): pupil size (absolute), Pupillary Unrest Index (PUI, absolute and ln) and interpolation rate should be given for the investigated sample.

f) Classification of test result in normal, suspicious or pathological, according to the "green ($\pm$1 SD), yellow (between 1 and 2 SD) or red (above 2 SD)" flag in relation to normative sample (231).

g) Number of recordings with sleep events, if occurred. Such recordings should be classified as pathological, regardless of PUI value.

6. ANIMALS

Author: Paul D. Gamlin

Introduction

Pupillary responses in animals, as in humans, are driven by the parasympathetic and sympathetic components of the autonomic nervous system (131), and are studied for a number of reasons. First, animals serve as potential models for humans for understanding the retinal and central processing of pupillary control signals, both those driven by light and those modulated by eye movements, attention, or cognition. Second, pupillary responses can be used to assess animal models of retinal degeneration. Third, pupillary responses can be used to assess autonomic function. Fourth, the discovery of intrinsically photosensitive retinal ganglion cells (ipRGCs) and their contribution to a non-image forming visual system that drives pupillary responses, entrains circadian rhythms, and can affect sleep and mood has resulted in the pupil being studied as a surrogate for, or to complement, studies of these other systems. Indeed, all mammals studied to date show pupillary responses consistent with rod, cone, and melanopsin driven responses [e.g., (6, 8, 13, 96, 97, 240)].

In this chapter, we propose some standards that should be followed when studying pupillary responses in animals.

Stimulus Characteristics

In studies of light-evoked pupillary responses, it is important to fully characterize the visual stimulus. Authors should specify: (1) the spectral content or the light source, and provide either the corneal or estimated retinal irradiance (121); (2) the spatial extent and retinal locus of the stimulus; (3) the duration of the stimulus; (4) the duration of recording–ensuring that a period of time prior to the stimulus is recorded for baseline purposes; (5) whether the stimulus is binocular or monocular; (6)whether either pupil is dilated pharmacologically; (7) whether pupil responses are measured monocularly or binocularly; (8) whether direct or consensual pupil responses were measured.

Restraint

In many cases, animals will be restrained by either physical or chemical means. Each approach presents a challenge to reliable measurements of the pupil. In the case of physical restraint, whether it consists of body and head restraint, or just head restraint, animals must undergo significant acclimation, usually with positive reward, such that their stress responses are minimal when pupillary measurements are taken. Failure to do so will result in increased sympathetic tone, and unreliable measurement of resting state pupil diameters and light-evoked responses. In case of chemical restraint, the challenges are greater, and the ability to compare results between laboratories will rely heavily on the use of the same chemical restraint protocol. Further, the results obtained under chemical restraint are unlikely to match those that would be obtained from a physically restrained, but relaxed animal.

Species Specific Recommendations

Monkeys

Sedated Protocol

In some cases, pupillary responses can be studied in sedated monkeys. Animals in such studies will not require the surgically implanted head holder that is generally used for studies in alert monkeys. For this procedure, one acceptable protocol is as follows: animals are lightly anesthetized (heart rate maintained at awake levels) using intramuscular injections of a low dose of anesthetic (<10 mg/kg ketamine and 0.1 mg/kg acepromazine) with supplementation as needed to maintain anesthesia. If the heart rate is seen to decrease, this is a sign that the level of anesthesia is too deep and will result in suppressed pupillary responses. The head of the animal is stabilized by a bite bar and head holder.

Alert Protocol

In almost all cases, monkeys will be chair-trained, will receive a surgically implanted head holder, and will be extensively acclimated to head fixation for periods of up to a few hours while viewing visual targets for liquid or food reward. Such procedures have been used in studies of the pupillary light reflex in macaques [e.g., (8)] and cognition [reviewed by Binda and Gamlin (241)].

For open-loop studies of the pupillary light reflex, either the stimuli should be presented to one eye in which the pupil has been dilated, or the stimulus duration should be brief enough to ensure that it is extinguished prior to pupil constriction. For closed-loop experiments, in which pupil constriction alters retinal irradiance, no such limitations are necessary. In general, pupil diameters should be measured in both eyes under infrared illumination using video cameras. For open-loop experiments, the pupil of one eye will be dilated with 1.0% tropicamide and 2.5% phenylephrine. Therefore, pupillary responses elicited by stimuli presented to this eye are measured by evaluating the consensual pupil response of the fellow eye. Animals fixate with the fellow eye on a target presented on a computer monitor. Pupil diameter in the fellow eye is monitored continuously. After a period of fixation, a stimulus is presented to the eye with the dilated pupil. The duration, extent, intensity, and spectral content of the stimulus will be appropriately varied for the planned experiment. The stimulus is then extinguished, and the participant maintains fixation for up to 30 s (8).

For studies of cognitively-related pupil responses, very similar procedures to the above are followed. The animal is head-fixed performing a behavioral task for water or food. In general, pupil diameters are measured by the eye movement systems used in these experiments. If the pupil is to be measured at anything other than primary position, then the investigator should try to calibrate pupil measurements throughout the range of expected eye movements, and should not rely solely on the cosine correction factors that are often used by these systems.

For these alert monkey protocols to yield reliable data, it is essential that the animal is fully acclimated to both the required head fixation and the task, and be actively engaged in the required task. Pupillary hippus and signs of sleepiness should be monitored since, as in humans, these will affect resting pupil diameter and light-evoked pupillary responses.

Dogs

While it is feasible to measure resting pupil diameter in conscious dogs (96), studies of light-evoked pupillary responses generally use chemical restraint. In an early study, dogs were mildly sedated with medetomidine administered intramuscularly in a dose of 5 micrograms/kg body weight (240). In later studies, this level of sedation was found to be unsuitable for more extensive pupil light reflex testing. Whiting and colleagues (96) evaluated five different chemical restraint protocols for measurement of the pupillary light reflex in purpose-bred long-haired miniature Dachshunds. They found that 5 μg/kg dexmedetomidine provided them with insufficient restraint to place a speculum, while higher doses of dexmedetomidine alone (35 μg/kg) or dexmedetomidine/ketamine (18 μg/kg/3.5 mg/kg) or dexmedetomidine/butorphanol (5 μg/kg/0.17 mg/kg) resulted in large spontaneous fluctuations in pupil size. Therefore, they recommended the following protocol: Dexmedetomidine (20–25 lg/kg IM) is given 30 min before induction of anesthesia with propofol (intravenous [IV] to effect, 1.49 ± 0.59 mg/kg [mean ± SD]). Dogs are intubated with a cuffed endotracheal tube and restraint maintained with 1.5% isoflurane in oxygen. This protocol is similar to that used recently by Yeh and colleagues in both wild type dogs, and dogs with retinal and optic nerve disease (97). In this study, animals were first premedicated using acepromazine, at an intravenous dose of 0.02 mg/kg and induced with propofol given intravenously to effect (starting dose, 4 mg/kg). The dogs were then intubated, and general anesthesia was maintained with 2–3% isoflurane in oxygen. The differences between the two studies in the propofol and isoflurane doses used may result from the different breeds of dog used in these studies.

Mice

PLR testing can be conducted in completely awake mice without the use of general anesthetic or sedation. The mice are initially habituated to extensive handling with food rewards, in order for them to remain calm during recording [e.g., (242)]. Acclimated animals can be lightly held by the scruff of the neck to ensure they are correctly positioned during pupil measurements without increased stress (S. Hattar, Personal communication). In most studies, the steady state pupil diameter (~30 s light) is measured. Prior to stimulation, animals are usually dark adapted for 1 h. For ease of measurement, one eye is usually exposed to the stimulus while the consensual pupil response is measured. Animals can also be acclimated to head fixation [e.g., (243, 244)], and similar procedures followed for measurement of the pupillary light reflex.

FINAL REMARKS

The authors understand these standards in pupillography as a "living" standard; new insights in retinal and pupillary circuitries as well as in stimulation and response analysis parameters of future projects will consequently be amended.

AUTHOR CONTRIBUTIONS

The introduction and I. Part were written by CK and TS; II. Part: 1. CK, AZ, BF, HW, YC, PG, RK; 2. HW; 3. ES; 4. SS, KR; 5. BW, KR, TP; 6. PG. Additional details are included within the manuscript sub-parts. All authors critically reviewed the manuscript.

FUNDING

This project was supported in part by an unrestricted research grant from Research to Prevent Blindness, Inc. to the Department of Ophthalmology and Visual Sciences at the University of Wisconsin (YC). Australian Research Council Discovery Projects ARC-DP170100274 (AZ and BF); Australian Research Council Future Fellowship ARC-FT180100458 (AZ). Department of Veterans Affairs Rehabilitation Research and Development Division, Department of Defense (Chronic Effects of Neurotrauma Consortium, CENC) and National Eye Institute (RK). United States Public Health Service Grant MH55762 and Dept. of Veterans Affairs (SS). This project was also supported by Egon Schumacher-Stiftung, Barnstorf, Germany, a private foundation without commercial interest (CK, TS, TP, BW, and HW). The views expressed in this article are those of the authors and do not necessarily reflect the position or policy of the Department of Veterans Affairs or the United States government.

ACKNOWLEDGMENTS

We thank the Organizing Committee of the 32nd International Pupil Colloquium 2017 in Morges, Switzerland, where the foundation of this joint project was laid.

We thank Dipl. Ing. Irena Stingl for her graphical support with the **Figures 1, 3**.

We are grateful to Mr. R.W. Langley for drawing **Figure 4**.

REFERENCES

1. Lowenstein O, Loewenfeld IE. Electronic pupillography; a new instrument and some clinical applications. *AMA Arch Ophthalmol.* (1958) 59:352–63 doi: 10.1001/archopht.1958.00940040058007
2. Loewenfeld I.E. *The Pupil: Anatomy, Physiology, and Clinical Applications.* Detroit, MI: Wayne State University Press (1993).
3. Provencio I, Rodriguez IR, Jiang G, Hayes WP, Moreira EF, Rollaq MD. A novel human opsin in the inner retina. *J Neurosci.* (2000) 20:600–5. doi: 10.1523/JNEUROSCI.20-02-00600.2000
4. Qiu X, Kumbalasiri T, Carlson SM, Wong KY, Krishna V, Provencio I, et al. Induction of photosensitivity by heterologous expression of melanopsin. *Nature* (2005) 433:745–9. doi: 10.1038/nature03345
5. Berson DM, Dunn FA, Takao M. Phototransduction by retinal ganglion cells that set the circadian clock. *Science* (2002) 295:1070–3. doi: 10.1126/science.1067262
6. Hattar S, Lucas RJ, Mrosovsky N, Thompson S, Douglas RH, Hankins MW, et al. Melanopsin and rod-cone photoreceptive systems account for all major accessory visual functions in mice. *Nature* (2003) 424:76–81. doi: 10.1038/nature01761
7. Dacey DM, Liao HW, Peterson BB, Robinson FR, Smith VC, Pokorny J, et al. Melanopsin expressing ganglion cells in primate retina signal colour and irradiance and project to the LGN. *Nature* (2005) 433:749–54. doi: 10.1038/nature03387
8. Gamlin PD, McDougal DH, Pokorny J, Smith VC, Yau KW, Dacey DM. Human and macaque pupil responses driven by melanopsin-containing retinal ganglion cells. *Vis Res.* (2007) 47:946–54. doi: 10.1016/j.visres.2006.12.015
9. Markwell EL, Feigl B, Zele AJ. Intrinsically photosensitive melanopsin retinal ganglion cell contributions to the pupillary light reflex and circadian rhythm. *Clin Exp Optom.* (2010) 93:137–49. doi: 10.1111/j.1444-0938.2010.00479.x
10. Schmidt TM, Do MTH, Dacey D, Lucas R, Hattar S, Matynia A. Melanopsinpositive intrinsically photosensitive retinal ganglion cells:from form to function. *J Neurosci.* (2011) 31:16094–101. doi: 10.1523/JNEUROSCI.4132-11.2011
11. Park JC, Moura AL, Raza AS, Rhee DW, Kardon RH, Hood DC. Toward a clinical protocol for assessing rod, cone, and melanopsin contributions to the human pupil response. *Invest Ophthalmol Vis Sci.* (2011) 52:6624–35. doi: 10.1167/iovs.11-7586

12. Lucas RJ, Douglas RH, Foster RG. Characterization of an ocular photopigment capable of driving pupillary constriction in mice. *Nat Neurosci.* (2001) 4:621–6. doi: 10.1038/88443
13. Lucas RJ, Hattar S, Takao M, Berson DM, Foster RG, Yau KW. Diminished pupillary light reflex at high irradiances in melanopsin-knockout mice. *Science* (2003) 299:245–7. doi: 10.1126/science.1077293
14. Lall GS, Revell VL, Momiji H, Al Enezi J, Altimus CM, Güler AD, et al. Distinct contributions of rod, cone, and melanopsin photoreceptors to encoding irradiance. *Neuron* (2010) 66:417–28. doi: 10.1016/j.neuron.2010.04.037
15. Graham DM, Wong KY, Shapiro P, Frederick C, Pattabiraman K, Berson DM. Melanopsin ganglion cells use a membrane-associated rhabdomeric phototransduction cascade. *J Neurophysiol.* (2008) 99:2522–32. doi: 10.1152/jn.01066.2007
16. Liao HW, Ren X, Peterson BB, Marshak DW, Yau KW, Gamlin PD, et al. Melanopsin-expressing ganglion cells on macaque and human retinas form two morphologically distinct populations. *J Comp Neurol.* (2016) 524:2845–72. doi: 10.1002/cne.23995
17. Kelbsch CB, Maeda F, Strasser T, Peters TM, Wilhelm BJC, Wilhelm HM. Color pupillography in dorsal midbrain syndrome. *J Neuroophthalmol.* (2017) 37:247–52. doi: 10.1097/WNO.0000000000000527
18. Maeda F, Kelbsch C, Straßer T, Skorkovská K, Peters T, Wilhelm B, et al. Chromatic pupillography in hemianopia patients with homonymous visual field defects. *Graefes Arch Clin Exp Ophthalmol.* (2017) 255:1837–42. doi: 10.1007/s00417-017-3721-y
19. Kankipati L, Girkin CA, Gamlin PD. The post-illumination pupil response is reduced in glaucoma patients. *Invest Ophthalmol Vis Sci.* (2011) 52:2287–92. doi: 10.1167/iovs.10-6023
20. Feigl B, Mattes D, Thomas R, Zele AJ. Intrinsically photosensitive (melanopsin) retinal ganglion cell function in glaucoma. *Invest Ophthalmol Vis Sci.* (2011) 52:4362–7. doi: 10.1167/iovs.10-7069
21. Adhikari P, Zele AJ, Thomas R, Feigl B. Quadrant field pupillometry detects melanopsin dysfunction in glaucoma suspects and early glaucoma. *Sci Rep.* (2016) 6:33373. doi: 10.1038/srep33373
22. Kelbsch C, Maeda F, Strasser T, Blumenstock G, Wilhelm B, Wilhelm H, et al. Pupillary responses driven by ipRGCs and classical photoreceptors are impaired in glaucoma. *Graefes Arch Clin Exp Ophthalmol.* (2016) 254:1361–70. doi: 10.1007/s00417-016-3351-9
23. Najjar RP, Sharma S, Atalay E, Rukmini AV, Sun C, Lock JZ, et al. Pupillary responses to full-field chromatic stimuli are reduced in patients with early-stage primary open-angle glaucoma. *Ophthalmology* (2018) 125:1362–71. doi: 10.1016/j.ophtha.2018.02.024
24. Kardon R, Anderson SC, Damarjian TG, Grace EM, Stone E, Kawasaki A. Chromatic pupillometry in patients with retinitis pigmentosa. *Ophthalmology* (2011) 118:376–81. doi: 10.1016/j.ophtha.2010.06.033
25. Lorenz B, Strohmayr E, Zahn S, Friedburg C, Kramer M, Preising M, et al. Chromatic pupillometry dissects function of the three different light-sensitive retinal cell populations in RPE65 deficiency. *Invest Ophthalmol Vis Sci.* (2012) 53:5641–52. doi: 10.1167/iovs.12-9974
26. Kelbsch C, Maeda F, Lisowska J, Lisowski L, Strasser T, Stingl K, et al. Analysis of retinal function using chromatic pupillography in retinitis pigmentosa and the relationship to electrically evoked phosphene thresholds. *Acta Ophthalmol.* (2017) 95:e261–9. doi: 10.1111/aos.13259
27. Kawasaki A, Crippa SV, Kardon R, Leon L, Hamel C. Characterization of pupil responses to blue and red light stimuli in autosomal dominant retinitis pigmentosa due to NR2E3 mutation. *Invest Ophthalmol Vis Sci.* (2012) 53:5562–9. doi: 10.1167/iovs.12-10230
28. Feigl B, Zele AJ. Melanopsin-expressing intrinsically photosensitive retinal ganglion cells in retinal disease. *Optom Vis Sci.* (2014) 91:894–903. doi: 10.1097/OPX.0000000000000284
29. Maynard ML, Zele AJ, Feigl B. Melanopsin-mediated post-illumination pupil response in early age-related macular degeneration. *Invest Ophthalmol Vis Sci.* (2015) 56:6906–13. doi: 10.1167/iovs.15-17357
30. Maynard ML, Zele AJ, Kwan AS, Feigl B. Intrinsically photosensitive retinal ganglion cell function, sleep efficiency and depression in advanced age-related macular degeneration. *Invest Ophthalmol Vis Sci.* (2017) 58:990–6. doi: 10.1167/iovs.16-20659
31. Feigl B, Zele AJ, Fader SM, Howes AN, Hughes CE, Jones KA, et al. The post-illumination pupil response of melanopsin-expressing intrinsically photosensitive retinal ganglion cells in diabetes. *Acta Ophthalmol.* (2012) 90:e230–4. doi: 10.1111/j.1755-3768.2011.02226.x
32. Park JC, Chen YF, Blair NP, Chau FY, Lim JI, Leiderman YI, et al. Pupillary responses in non-proliferative diabetic retinopathy. *Sci Rep.* (2017) 7:44987. doi: 10.1038/srep44987
33. Sabeti F, Nolan CJ, James AC, Jenkins A, Maddess T. Multifocal pupillography identifies changes in visual sensitivity according to severity of diabetic retinopathy in Type 2 Diabetes. *Invest Ophthalmol Vis Sci.* (2015) 56:4504–13. doi: 10.1167/iovs.15-16712
34. Kawasaki A, Collomb S, Léon L, Münch M. Pupil responses derived from outer and inner retinal photoreception are normal in patients with hereditary optic neuropathy. *Exp Eye Res.* (2014) 120:161–6. doi: 10.1016/j.exer.2013.11.005
35. Lisowska J, Lisowski L, Kelbsch C, Maeda F, Richter P, Kohl S, et al. Development of a chromatic pupillography protocol for the first gene therapy trial in patients with CNGA3-linked achromatopsia. *Invest Ophthalmol Vis Sci.* (2017) 58:1274–82. doi: 10.1167/iovs.16-20505
36. Binda P, Straßer T, Stingl K, Richter P, Peters T, Wilhelm H, et al. Pupil response components:attention-light interaction in patients with Parinaud's syndrome. *Sci Rep.* (2017) 7:10283. doi: 10.1038/s41598-017-10816-x
37. Münch M, Léon L, Crippa SV, Kawasaki A. Circadian and wake-dependent effects on the pupil light reflex in response to narrow-bandwidth light pulses. *Invest Ophthalmol Vis Sci.* (2012) 53:4546–55. doi: 10.1167/iovs.12-9494
38. Münch M, Léon L, Collomb S, Kawasaki A. Comparison of acute non-visual bright light responses in patients with optic nerve disease, glaucoma and healthy controls. *Sci Rep.* (2015) 5:15185. doi: 10.1038/srep15185
39. Zele AJ, Feigl B, Smith SS, Markwell EL. The circadian response of intrinsically photosensitive retinal ganglion cells. *PLoS ONE* (2011) 6:e17860. doi: 10.1371/journal.pone.0017860
40. Lazzerini Ospri L, Prusky G, Hattar S. Mood, the circadian system, and melanopsin retinal ganglion cells. *Annu Rev Neurosci.* (2017) 40:539–56. doi: 10.1146/annurev-neuro-072116-031324
41. Roecklein K, Wong P, Ernecoff N, Miller M, Donofry S, Kamarck M, et al. The post illumination pupil response is reduced in seasonal affective disorder. *Psychiatry Res.* (2013) 210:150–8. doi: 10.1016/j.psychres.2013.05.023
42. Münch M, Kourti P, Brouzas D, Kawasaki A. Variation in the pupil light reflex between winter and summer seasons. *Acta Ophthalmol.* (2016) 94:e244–6. doi: 10.1111/aos.12966
43. Granholm EL, Panizzon MS, Elman JA, Jak AJ, Hauger RL, Bondi MW, et al. Pupillary Responses as a biomarker of early risk for Alzheimer's disease. *J Alzheimers Dis.* (2017) 56:1419–28. doi: 10.3233/JAD-161078
44. Joyce DS, Feigl B, Kerr G, Roeder L, Zele AJ. Melanopsin-mediated pupil function is impaired in Parkinson's disease. *Sci Rep.* (2018) 8:7796. doi: 10.1038/s41598-018-26078-0
45. Feigl B, Ohja G, Hides L, Zele AJ. Melanopsin function and light exposure in non-seasonal, major depressive disorder. *Front. Neurol.* (2018) 9:764. doi: 10.3389/fneur.2018.00764
46. Wilhelm H, Lüdtke H, Wilhelm B. Pupillographic sleepiness testing in hypersomniacs and normals. *Graefes Arch Clin Exp Ophthalmol.* (1998) 236:725–9.
47. Wilhelm B, Bittner E, Hofmann A, Koerner A, Peters T, Lüdtke H, Wilhelm H. Short- term reproducibility and variability of the pupillographic sleepiness test. *Am J Hum Biol.* (2015) 27:862–6. doi: 10.1002/ajhb.22726
48. Chen JW, Gombart ZJ, Rogers S, Gardiner SK, Cecil S, Bullock RM. Pupillary reactivity as an early indicator of increased intracranial pressure:the introduction of the Neurological Pupil index. *Surg Neurol Int.* (2011) 2:82. doi: 10.4103/2152-7806.82248
49. Paulus J, Roquilly A, Beloeil H, Théraud J, Asehnoune K, Lejus C. Pupillary reflex measurement predicts insufficient analgesia before endotracheal suctioning in critically ill patients. *Crit Care* (2013) 17:R161. doi: 10.1186/cc12840
50. Lukaszewicz AC, Dereu D, Gayat E, Payen D. The relevance of pupillometry for evaluation of analgesia before noxious procedures in the intensive care unit. *Anesth Analg* (2015) 120:1297–300. doi: 10.1213/ANE.0000000000000609

51. Wouters K. INTERNATIONAL SOCIETY FOR CLINICAL ELECTRORETINOGRAPHY (ISCERG). *Acta Ophthalmol Suppl.* (1962) 40:264–8. doi: 10.1111/j.1755-3768.1962.tb00330.x
52. Tweel LH. Some proposals for standardization of ERG equipment. *Acta Ophthalmol Suppl.* (1962) 40:87–96.
53. Marmor MF, Arden GB, Nilsson SEG, et al. Zrenner E. Standard for clinical electroretinography. *Arch Ophthalmol.* (1989) 107:816–9.
54. Heckenlively JR, Arden GB, editors. *Principles and Practice of Clinical Electrophysiology of Vision.* 2nd ed. Cambridge:MIT Press (2006). p. 1016.
55. McCulloch DL, Marmor MF, Brigell MG, Hamilton R, Holder GE, Tzekov R, et al. ISCEV Standard for full-field clinical electroretinography (2015 update). *Doc Ophthalmol.* (2015) 130:1–12. doi: 10.1007/s10633-014-9473-7
56. Hood DC, Bach M, Brigell M, Keating D, Kondo M, Lyons JS, et al. ISCEV standard for clinical multifocal electroretinography (mfERG) (2011 edition). *Doc Ophthalmol.* (2012) 124:1–13. doi: 10.1007/s10633-011-9296-8
57. Bach M, Brigell MG, Hawlina M, Holder GE, Johnson M a, McCulloch DL, et al. ISCEV standard for clinical pattern electroretinography (PERG):2012 update. *Doc Ophthalmol.* (2013) 126:1–7. doi: 10.1007/s10633-012-9353-y
58. Odom JV, Bach M, Brigell M, Holder GE, McCulloch DL, Mizota A, et al. ISCEV standard for clinical visual evoked potentials:(2016 update). *Doc Ophthalmol.* (2016) 133:1–9. doi: 10.1007/s10633-016-9553-y
59. Constable PA, Bach M, Frishman LJ, Jeffrey BG, Robson AG. ISCEV Standard for clinical electro-oculography (2017 update). *Doc Ophthalmol.* (2017) 134:1–9. doi: 10.1007/s10633-017-9573-2
60. Brigell M, Bach M, Barber C, Kawasaki K, Kooijman A. Guidelines for calibration of stimulus and recording parameters used in clinical electrophysiology of vision. Calibration Standard Committee of the International Society for Clinical Electrophysiology of Vision (ISCEV). *Doc Ophthalmol.* (1998) 95:1–14. doi: 10.1023/A:1001724411607
61. Robson AG, Nilsson J, Li S, Jalali S, Fulton AB, Tormene AP, et al. ISCEV guide to visual electrodiagnostic procedures. *Doc Ophthalmol.* (2018) 136:1–26. doi: 10.1007/s10633-017-9621-y
62. Gibson F, Overton P, Smulders T, Schultz S, Eglen S, Ingram C, et al. *Minimum Information About A Neuroscience Investigation (MINI): Electrophysiology* (2009). Aailable online at: http://precedings.nature.com/documents/1720/version/2/files/npre20091720-2.pdf
63. Szabadi E. Neuronal networks regulating sleep and arousal:effect of drugs. In: Guglietta A, editor. *Drug Treatment of Sleep Disorders* (Cham: Springer), p. 25–70.
64. Szabadi E. The integrated control of arousal and pupil function:role of the noradrenergic locus coeruleus. *Neuro-opthalmol Jpn.* (2008) 25:176–89.
65. Samuels ER, Hou RH, Langley RW, Szabadi E, Bradshaw CM. Comparison of pramipexole and modafinil on arousal, autonomic, and endocrine functions in healthy volunteers. *J Psychopharmacol.* (2006) 20:756–70. doi: 10.1177/0269881106060770
66. Hou RH, Samuels ER, Langley RW, Szabadi E, Bradshaw CM. Arousal and the pupil:why diazepam-induced sedation is not accompanied by miosis. *Psychopharmacology* (2007) 195:41–50. doi: 10.1007/s00213-007-0884-y
67. Wang B, Shen C, Zhang L, Qi L, Yao L, Chen J, et al. Dark adaptation-induced changes in rod, cone and intrinsically photosensitive retinal ganglion cell (ipRGC) sensitivity differentially affect the pupil light response (PLR). *Graefes Arch Clin Exp Ophthalmol.* (2015) 253:1997–2005. doi: 10.1007/s00417-015-3137-5
68. Smith VC, Pokorny J. Spectral sensitivity of the foveal cone photopigments between 400 and 500 nm.*Visi Res.* (1975) 15:161–71. doi: 10.1016/0042-6989(75)90203-5
69. CIE 170-1:2006. *Fundamental Chromaticity Diagram With Physiological Axes–Part 1.* (2006). ISBN:978 3 901906 46 6.
70. Schnapf JL, Kraft TW, Nunn BJ, Baylor DA. Spectral sensitivity of primate photoreceptors. *Vis Neurosci.* (1988) 1:255–61. doi: 10.1017/S0952523800001917
71. Bowmaker JK, Dartnall HJ. Visual pigments of rods and cones in a human retina. *J Physiol.* (1980) 298:501–11 doi: 10.1113/jphysiol.1980.sp013097
72. Zele AJ, Cao D. Vision under mesopic and scotopic illumination. *Front Psychol.* (2015) 5:1594. doi: 10.3389/fpsyg.2014.01594
73. McDougal DH, Gamlin PD. The influence of intrinsically-photosensitive retinal ganglion cells on the spectral sensitivity and response dynamics of the human pupillary light reflex. *Vis Res.* (2010) 50:72–87. doi: 10.1016/j.visres.2009.10.012
74. Adhikari P, Zele AJ, Feigl B. The post-illumination pupil response (PIPR). *Invest Ophthalmol Vis Sci.* (2015) 56:3838–49. doi: 10.1167/iovs.14-16233
75. Adhikari P, Feigl B, Zele AJ. Rhodopsin and melanopsin contributions to the early redilation phase of the post-illumination pupil response (PIPR). *PLoS ONE* (2016) 11:e0161175. doi: 10.1371/journal.pone.0161175
76. Stiles WS. Color vision:the approach through increment threshold sensitivity. *Proc Natl Acad Sci USA.* (1959) 45:100–14. doi: 10.1073/pnas.45.1.100
77. Roufs JAJ. *Light As a True Visual Quantity :Principles of Measurement*, Vol. 41. Paris: Commission Internationale de l'Éclairage (1978).
78. Aguilar M, Stiles WS. Saturation of the rod mechanism of the retina at high levels of stimulation. *Optica Acta* (1954) 1:59–65. doi: 10.1080/713818657
79. Stiles WS, Crawford BH. The luminous efficiency of rays entering the eye pupil at different points. *Proc R Soc Lond B* (1933) 112:428–50. doi: 10.1098/rspb.1933.0020
80. King-Smith PE, Carden D. Luminance and opponent-color contributions to visual detection and adaptation and to temporal and spatial integration. *J Opt Soc Am.* (1976) 66:709–17. doi: 10.1364/JOSA.66.000709
81. Sperling HG, Harwerth RS. Red-green cone interactions in the increment-threshold spectral sensitivity of primates. *Science* (1971) 172:180–4. doi: 10.1126/science.172.3979.180
82. Chylack LT Jr, Wolfe JK, Singer DM, Leske MC, Bullimore MA, Bailey IL, et al. The lens opacities classification system III. The longitudinal study of cataract study group. *Arch Ophthalmol.* (1993) 111:831–6. doi: 10.1001/archopht.1993.01090060119035
83. Pokorny J, Smith VC. How much light reaches the retina? In: Cavonius editor. *Colour Vision Deficiencies XIII.* 59:491–511. Dordrecht: Kluwer Academic Publishers. (1997).
84. van de Kraats J, van Norren D. Optical density of the aging human ocular media in the visible and the UV. *J Opt Soc Am A Opt Image Sci Vis.* (2007) 24:1842–57. doi: 10.1364/JOSAA.24.001842
85. Jones BW, Kondo M, Terasaki H, Lin Y, McCall M, Marc RE. Retinal remodeling. *Jpn J Ophthalmol.* (2012) 56:289–306. doi: 10.1007/s10384-012-0147-2
86. Barrionuevo PA, Nicandro N, McAnany JJ, Zele AJ, Gamlin P, Cao D. Assessing rod, cone, and melanopsin contributions to human pupil flicker responses. *Invest Ophthalmol Vis Sci.* (2014) 4;55:719–27. doi: 10.1167/iovs.13-13252
87. Barrionuevo PA, Cao D. Luminance and chromatic signals interact differently with melanopsin activation to control the pupil light response. *J Vis.* (2016) 16:29. doi: 10.1167/16.11.29
88. Tsujimura S, Ukai K, Ohama D, Nuruki A, Yunokuchi K.Contribution of human melanopsin retinal ganglion cells to steady-state pupil responses. *Proc Biol Sci.* (2010) 277:2485–92. doi: 10.1098/rspb.2010.0330
89. Tsujimura S, Tokuda Y.Delayed response of human melanopsin retinal ganglion cells on the pupillary light reflex. *Ophthalmic Physiol Opt.* (2011) 31:469–79. doi: 10.1111/j.1475-1313.2011.00846.x
90. Zele AJ, Feigl B, Adhikari P, Maynard ML, Cao D. Melanopsin photoreception contributes to human visual detection, temporal and colour processing. *Sci Rep.* (2018) 8:3842. doi: 10.1038/s41598-018-22197-w
91. Hecht S, Haig C, Wald G. THE DARK ADAPTATION OF RETINAL FIELDS OF DIFFERENT SIZE AND LOCATION. *J Gen Physiol.* (1935) 19:321–37. doi: 10.1085/jgp.19.2.321
92. Marmor MF, Fulton AB, Holder GE, Miyake Y, Brigell M, Bach M. International society for clinical electrophysiology of vision. ISCEV Standard for full-field clinical electroretinography (2008 update). *Doc Ophthalmol.* (2009) 118:69–77. doi: 10.1007/s10633-008-9155-4
93. Birch EE, Birch DG. Pupillometric measures of retinal sensitivity in infants and adults with retinitis pigmentosa. *Vis Res.* (1987) 27:499–505. doi: 10.1016/0042-6989(87)90034-4
94. Chibel R, Sher I, Ben Ner D, Mhajna MO, Achiron A, Hajyahia S, et al. Chromatic multifocal pupillometer for objective perimetry and diagnosis of patients with retinitis pigmentosa. *Ophthalmology* (2016) 123:1898–911. doi: 10.1016/j.ophtha.2016.05.038
95. Kardon R, Anderson SC, Damarjian TG, Grace EM, Stone E, Kawasaki A. Chromatic pupil responses:preferential activation

of the melanopsin-mediated versus outer photoreceptor-mediated pupil light reflex. *Ophthalmology* (2009) 116:1564–73. doi: 10.1016/j.ophtha.2009.02.007
96. Whiting RE, Yao G, Narfström K, Pearce JW, Coates JR, Dodam JR, et al. Quantitative assessment of the canine pupillary light reflex. *Invest Ophthalmol Vis Sci.* (2013) 54:5432–40. doi: 10.1167/iovs.13-12012
97. Yeh CY, Koehl KL, Harman CD, Iwabe S, Guzman JM, Petersen-Jones SM, et al. Assessment of rod, cone, and intrinsically photosensitive retinal ganglion cell contributions to the canine chromatic pupillary response. *Invest Ophthalmol Vis Sci.* (2017) 58:65–78. doi: 10.1167/iovs.16-19865
98. Kostic C, Crippa SV, Martin C, Kardon RH, Biel M, Arsenijevic Y, et al. Determination of rod and cone influence to the early and late dynamic of the pupillary light response. *Invest Ophthalmol Vis Sci.* (2016) 57:2501–8. doi: 10.1167/iovs.16-19150
99. Berman SM, Fein G, Jewett DL, Saika G, Ashford E. Spectral determinants of steady-state pupil size with full field of view. *J Illum Eng Soc.* (1992) 21:3–13. doi: 10.1080/00994480.1992.10747995
100. Crawford BH. The dependence of pupil size upon external light stimulus under static and variable conditions. *Proc Roy Soc B.* (1936) 121:376–95 doi: 10.1098/rspb.1936.0072
101. De Groot SG, Gebhard JW. Pupil size as determined by adapting luminance. *J Opt Soc Am.* (1952) 42:492–5. doi: 10.1364/JOSA.42.000492
102. Lei S, Goltz HC, Chandrakumar M, Wong AM. Test-retest reliability of hemifield, central-field, and full-field chromatic pupillometry for assessing the function of melanopsin-containing retinal ganglion cells. *Invest Ophthalmol Vis Sci.* (2015) 56:1267–73. doi: 10.1167/iovs.14-15945
103. Winn B, Whitaker D, Elliott DB, Phillips NJ. Factors affecting light-adapted pupil size in normal human subjects. *Invest Ophthalmol Vis Sci.* (1994) 35:1132–7.
104. Barlow HB.Temporal and spatial summation in human vision at different background intensities. *J Physiol.* (1958) 141:337–50.
105. Joyce DS, Feigl B, Cao D, Zele AJ. Temporal characteristics of melanopsin inputs to the human pupil light Reflex. *Vision Res.* (2015)107:58–66. doi: 10.1016/j.visres.2014.12.001
106. Nasir-Ahmad S, Lee SC, Martin PR, Grünert U. Melanopsin-expressing ganglion cells in human retina:Morphology, distribution, and synaptic connections. *J Comp Neurol.* (2017) 527:312–27. doi: 10.1002/cne.24176
107. Jusuf PR, Lee SC, Hannibal J, Grünert U. Characterization and synaptic connectivity of melanopsin-containing ganglion cells in the primate retina. *Eur J Neurosci.* (2007) 26:2906–21. doi: 10.1111/j.1460-9568.2007.05924.x
108. Grünert U, Jusuf PR, Lee SC, Nguyen DT. Bipolar input to melanopsin containing ganglion cells in primate retina. *Vis Neurosci.* (2011) 28:39–50. doi: 10.1017/S095252381000026X
109. Joo HR, Peterson BB, Dacey DM, Hattar S, Chen SK. Recurrent axon collaterals of intrinsically photosensitive retinal ganglion cells. *Vis Neurosci.* (2013) 30:175–82. doi: 10.1017/S0952523813000199
110. Hannibal J, Kankipati L, Strang CE, Peterson BB, Dacey D, Gamlin PD. Central projections of intrinsically photosensitive retinal ganglion cells in the macaque monkey. *J Comp Neurol.* (2014) 522:2231–48. doi: 10.1002/cne.23555
111. Brainard GC, Hanifin JP, Greeson JM, Byrne B, Glickman G, Gerner E, Rollag MD. Action spectrum for melatonin regulation in humans:evidence for a novel circadian photoreceptor. *J Neurosci.* (2001) 21:6405–12. doi: 10.1523/JNEUROSCI.21-16-06405.2001
112. Gooley JJ, Lu J, Chou TC, Scammell TE, Saper CB. Melanopsin in cells of origin of the retinohypothalamic tract. *Nat Neurosci.* (2001) 4:1165. doi: 10.1038/nn768
113. Lucas RJ, Freedman MS, Muñoz M, Garcia-Fernández JM, Foster RG. Regulation of the mammalian pineal by non-rod, non-cone, ocular photoreceptors. *Science* (1999) 284:505–7.
114. Hannibal J, Hindersson P, Ostergaard J, Georg B, Heegaard S, Larsen PJ, et al. Melanopsin is expressed in PACAP-containing retinal ganglion cells of the human retinohypothalamic tract. *Invest Ophthalmol Vis Sci.* (2004) 45:4202–9. doi: 10.1167/iovs.04-0313
115. Panda S, Provencio I, Tu DC, Pires SS, Rollag MD, Castrucci AM, et al. Melanopsin is required for non-image-forming photic responses in blind mice. *Science* (2003) 301:525–7. doi: 10.1126/science.1086179
116. Brown TM, Tsujimura S, Allen AE, Wynne J, Bedford R, Vickery G, et al. Melanopsin-based brightness discrimination in mice and humans. *Curr Biol.* (2012) 22:1134–41. doi: 10.1016/j.cub.2012.04.039
117. Spitschan M, Bock AS, Ryan J, Frazzetta G, Brainard DH, Aguirre GK. The human visual cortex response to melanopsin-directed stimulation is accompanied by a distinct perceptual experience. *Proc Natl Acad Sci USA.* (2017) 114:12291–6. doi: 10.1073/pnas.1711522114
118. Zele AJ, Adhikari P, Feigl B, Cao D. Cone and melanopsin contributions to human brightness estimation. *J Opt Soc Am A Opt Image Sci Vis.* (2018) 35:B19–25. doi: 10.1364/JOSAA.35.001783
119. Rushton WAH. Review lecture. Pigments and signals in colour vision. *J Physiol.* (1972) 220:1–31.
120. Lennie P, Pokorny J, Smith VC. Luminance. *J Opt Soc Am A.* (1993) 10:1283–93. doi: 10.1364/JOSAA.10.001283
121. Lucas RJ, Peirson SN, Berson DM, Brown TM, Cooper HM, Czeisler CA, et al. Measuring and using light in the melanopsin age. *Trends Neurosci.* (2014) 37:1–9. doi: 10.1016/j.tins.2013.10.004
122. Cao D, Nicandro N, Barrionuevo PA. A five-primary photostimulator suitable for studying intrinsically photosensitive retinal ganglion cell functions in humans. *J Vis.* (2015) 15:15.1.27. doi: 10.1167/15.1.27
123. Ferree CE, Rand G, Harris ET. Intensity of light and area of illuminated field as interacting factors in size of pupil. *J Exp Psychol.* (1933) 16:408–422. doi: 10.1037/h0072100
124. Stanley PA, Davies AK. The effect of field of view size on steady-state pupil diameter. *Ophthalmic Physiol Opt.* (1995) 15:601–3. doi: 10.1016/0275-5408(94)00019-V
125. Atchison DA, Girgenti CC, Campbell GM, Dodds JP, Byrnes TM, Zele AJ. Influence of field size on pupil diameter under photopic and mesopic light levels. *Clin Exp Optom.* (2011) 94:545–8. doi: 10.1111/j.1444-0938.2011.00636.x
126. Park JC, McAnany JJ. Effect of stimulus size and luminance on the rod-, cone-, and melanopsin-mediated pupillary light reflex. *J Vis.* (2015) 15:13. doi: 10.1167/15.3.13
127. Joyce DS, Feigl B, Zele AJ. Melanopsin-mediated post-illumination pupil response in the peripheral retina. *J Vis.* (2016) 16:5. doi: 10.1167/16.8.5
128. Curcio CA, Allen KA. Topography of ganglion cells in human retina. *J Comp Neurol.* (1990) 300:5–25. doi: 10.1002/cne.903000103
129. Stark L. Biological rhythms, noise, and asymmetry in the pupil-retinal control system. *Ann N Y Acad Sci.* (1962) 98:1096–108 doi: 10.1111/j.1749-6632.1962.tb30621.x
130. Clarke RJ, Zhang H, Gamlin PD. Characteristics of the pupillary light reflex in the alert rhesus monkey. *J Neurophysiol.* (2003) 89:3179–89. doi: 10.1152/jn.01131.2002
131. McDougal DH, Gamlin PD. Autonomic control of the eye. *Comp Physiol.* (2015) 5:439–73. doi: 10.1002/cphy.c140014
132. Miller SD, Thompson HS. Edge-light pupil cycle time. *Br J Ophthalmol.* (1978) 62:495–500. doi: 10.1136/bjo.62.7.495
133. Troland LT. On the measurement of visual sensation intensities. *J Exp Psychol.* (1917). 2:1–34. doi: 10.1037/h0071652
134. Westheimer G. The Maxwellian view. *Vis Res.* (1966) 6:669–82. doi: 10.1016/0042-6989(66)90078-2
135. Kawasaki A, Herbst K, Sander B, Milea D. Selective wavelength pupillometry in Leber hereditary optic neuropathy. *Clin Exp Ophthalmol.* (2010) 38:322–4. doi: 10.1111/j.1442-9071.2010.02212.x
136. Herbst K, Sander B, Milea D, Lund-Andersen H, Kawasaki A. Test-retest repeatability of the pupil light response to blue and red light stimuli in normal human eyes using a novel pupillometer. *Front Neurol.* (2011) 2:10. doi: 10.3389/fneur.2011.00010
137. Kankipati L, Girkin CA, Gamlin PD. Post-illumination pupil response in subjects without ocular disease. *Invest Ophthalmol Vis Sci.* (2010) 51:2764–9. doi: 10.1167/iovs.09-4717
138. Gooley JJ, Ho Mien I, St Hilaire MA, Yeo SC, Chua EC, van Reen E, et al. Melanopsin and rod-cone photoreceptors play different roles in mediating pupillary light responses during exposure to continuous light in humans. *J Neurosci.* (2012) 32:14242–53. doi: 10.1523/JNEUROSCI.1321-12.2012
139. Zele AJ, Feigl B, Adhikari P, Cao D. *IOVS e-abstract 5036-A0232* (2018).

140. Adhikari P, Pearson CA, Anderson AM, Zele AJ, Feigl B. Effect of age and refractive error on the melanopsin mediated post-illumination pupil response (PIPR). *Sci Rep.* (2015) 5:17610. doi: 10.1038/srep17610
141. Esquiva G, Lax P, Pérez-Santonja JJ, García-Fernández JM, Cuenca N. Loss of melanopsin-expressing ganglion cell subtypes and dendritic degeneration in the aging human retina. *Front Aging Neurosci.* (2017) 9:79. doi: 10.3389/fnagi.2017.00079
142. Obara EA, Hannibal J, Heegaard S, Fahrenkrug J. Loss of melanopsin-expressing retinal ganglion cells in patients with diabetic retinopathy. *Invest Ophthalmol Vis Sci.* (2017) 58:2187–92. doi: 10.1167/iovs.16-21168
143. Herbst K, Sander B, Lund-Andersen H, Wegener M, Hannibal J, Milea D. Unilateral anterior ischemic optic neuropathy:chromatic pupillometry in affected, fellow non-affected and healthy control eyes. *Front Neurol.* (2013) 4:52. doi: 10.3389/fneur.2013.00052
144. Ba-Ali S, Lund-Andersen H. Pupillometric evaluation of the melanopsin containing retinal ganglion cells in mitochondrial and non-mitochondrial optic neuropathies. *Mitochondrion* (2017) 36:124–9. doi: 10.1016/j.mito.2017.07.003
145. Meltzer E, Sguigna PV, Subei A, Beh S, Kildebeck E, Conger D, et al. Retinal architecture and melanopsin-mediated pupillary response characteristics: a putative pathophysiologic signature for the retino-hypothalamic tract in multiple sclerosis. *JAMA Neurol.* (2017) 74:574–82. doi: 10.1001/jamaneurol.2016.5131
146. Levatin P. Pupillary escape in disease of the retina or optic nerve. *Arch Ophthalmol.* (1959) 62:768–79. doi: 10.1001/archopht.1959.04220050030005
147. Thompson HS. Afferent pupillary defects. Pupillary findings associated with defects of the afferent arm of the pupillary light reflex arc. *Am J Ophthalmol.* (1966) 62:860–73.
148. Wilhelm B, Lüdtke H, Peters T, Schmid R, Wilhelm H, Zrenner E. [Automated swinging flashlight test in patients with optic nerve diseases] German. *Klin Monbl Augenheilkd.* (2001) 218:21–5. doi: 10.1055/s-2001-11256
149. Jonas JB, Zach FM, Naumann GO. Quantitative pupillometry of relative afferent defects in glaucoma. *Arch Ophthalmol.* (1990)108:479–80. doi: 10.1001/archopht.1990.01070060025009
150. Schiefer U, Dietzsch J, Dietz K, Wilhelm B, Bruckmann A, Wilhelm H, et al. Associating the magnitude of relative afferent pupillary defect (RAPD) with visual field indices in glaucoma patients. *Br J Ophthalmol.* (2012) 96:629–33. doi: 10.1136/bjophthalmol-2011-300776
151. Ozeki N, Yuki K, Shiba D, Tsubota K.Pupillographic evaluation of relative afferent pupillary defect in glaucoma patients. *Br J Ophthalmol.* (2013) 97:1538–42. doi: 10.1136/bjophthalmol-2013-303825
152. Kardon RH, Haupert CL, Thompson HS. The relationship between static perimetry and the relative afferent pupillary defect. *Am J Ophthalmol.* (1993) 115:351–6. doi: 10.1016/S0002-9394(14)73587-1
153. Stingl K, Peters T, Strasser T, Kelbsch C, Richter P, Wilhelm H, et al. Pupillographic campimetry:an objective method to measure the visual field. *Biomed Tech (Berl).* (2018) 63:729–34. doi: 10.1515/bmt-2017-0029
154. Skorkovská K, Wilhelm H, Lüdtke H, Wilhelm B. How sensitive is pupil campimetry in hemifield loss? *Graefes Arch Clin ExpOphthalmol.* (2009) 247:947–53. doi: 10.1007/s00417-009-1040-7
155. Schmid R, Luedtke H, Wilhelm BJ, Wilhelm H. Pupil campimetry in patients with visual field loss. *Eur J Neurol.* (2005) 12:602–8. doi: 10.1111/j.1468-1331.2005.01048.x
156. Naber M, Roelofzen C, Fracasso A, Bergsma DP, van Genderen M, Porro GL, et al. Gaze-contingent flicker pupil perimetry detects scotomas in patients with cerebral visual impairments or glaucoma. *Front Neurol.* (2018) 9:558. doi: 10.3389/fneur.2018.00558
157. Maddess T, Bedford SM, Goh XL, James AC. Multifocal pupillographic visual field testing in glaucoma. *Clin Exp Ophthalmol.* (2009) 37:678–86. doi: 10.1111/j.1442-9071.2009.02107.x
158. Sabeti F, Maddess T, Essex RW, Saikal A, James AC, Carle CF. Multifocal pupillography in early age-related macular degeneration. *Optom Vis Sci.* (2014) 91:904–15. doi: 10.1097/OPX.0000000000000319
159. Horn AK, Eberhorn A, Hartig W, Ardeleanu P, Messoudi A, Buttner-Ennever JA. Perioculomotor cell groups in monkey and man defined by their histochemical and functional properties:reappraisal of the Edinger-Westphal nucleus. *J Comp Neurol.* (2008) 507:1317–35. doi: 10.1002/cne.21598
160. Wilhelm H. Disorders of the pupil. *Handb Clin Neurol.* (2011) 102:427–66. doi: 10.1016/B978-0-444-52903-9.00022-4
161. Brown SM. The utility of 0.5% apraclonidine in the diagnosis of horner syndrome. *Arch Ophthalmol.* (2005) 123:578; author reply. doi: 10.1001/archopht.123.4.578-a
162. Chen PL, Hsiao CH, Chen JT, Lu DW, Chen WY. Efficacy of apraclonidine 0.5% in the diagnosis of Horner syndrome in pediatric patients under low or high illumination. *Am J Ophthalmol.* (2006) 142:469–74. doi: 10.1016/j.ajo.2006.04.052
163. Martin GC, Aymard PA, Denier C, Seghir C, Abitbol M, Boddaert N, et al. Usefulness of cocaine drops in investigating infant anisocoria. *Eur J Paediatr Neurol.* (2017) 21:852–7. doi: 10.1016/j.ejpn.2017.07.020
164. Morales J, Brown SM, Abdul-Rahim AS, Crosson CE. Ocular effects of apraclonidine in Horner syndrome. *Arch Ophthalmol.* (2000) 118:951–4. doi: 10.1001/pubs.Ophthalmol.-ISSN-0003-9950-118-7-ecs90240
165. Kardon RH, Denison CE, Brown CK, Thompson HS. Critical evaluation of the cocaine test in the diagnosis of Horner's syndrome. *Arch Ophthalmol.* (1990) 108:384–7. doi: 10.1001/archopht.1990.01070050082036
166. Thompson HS. Adie's syndrome:some new observations. *Trans Am Ophthalmol Soc.* (1977) 75:587–626.
167. Bremner F, Smith S. Pupillographic findings in 39 consecutive cases of harlequin syndrome. *J Neuroophthalmol.* (2008) 28:171–7. doi: 10.1097/WNO.0b013e318183c885
168. Krzizok T, Gräf M, Klaus S. Foto- und videographische Messungen des Dilatationsdefizits zur Differentialdiagnose beim Horner-Syndrom. *Ophthalmologe* (1995) 92:125–31.
169. Smith SA, Smith SE. Bilateral Horner's syndrome:detection and occurrence. *J Neurol Neurosurg Psychiatry* (1999) 66:48–51. doi: 10.1136/jnnp.66.1.48
170. Crippa SV, Borruat FX, Kawasaki A. Pupillary dilation lag is intermittently present in patients with a stable oculosympathetic defect (Horner syndrome). *Am J Ophthalmol.* (2007) 143:712–5. doi: 10.1016/j.ajo.2006.10.049
171. Wilhelm H, Klier R, Wilhelm B, Tóth B. Isolated internal ophthalmoplegia as sign of a third nerve palsy. *Neuroophthalmology* (1995) 15:211–5.
172. Papangelou A, Zink EK, Chang WW, Frattalone A, Gergen D, Gottschalk A, et al. Automated pupillometry and detection of clinical transtentorial brain herniation: a case series. *Mil Med.* (2018) 183:e113–21. doi: 10.1093/milmed/usx018
173. Thompson HS. Segmental palsy of the iris sphincter in Adie's syndrome. *Arch Ophthalmol.* (1978) 96:1615–20. doi: 10.1001/archopht.1978.03910060249012
174. Bremner FD, Smith SE. Bilateral tonic pupils: holmes adie syndrome or generalised neuropathy? *Br J Ophthalmol.* (2007) 91:1620–3. doi: 10.1136/bjo.2007.118968
175. Dütsch M, Marthol H, Michelson G, Neundörfer B, Hilz MJ. Pupillography refines the diagnosis of diabetic autonomic neuropathy. *J Neurol Sci.* (2004) 222:75–81. doi: 10.1016/j.jns.2004.04.008
176. Lerner AG, Bernabé-Ortiz A, Ticse R, Hernandez A, Huaylinos Y, Pinto ME, et al. CRONICAS Cohort Study Group. Type 2 diabetes and cardiac autonomic neuropathy screening using dynamic pupillometry. *Diabet Med.* (2015) 32:1470–8. doi: 10.1111/dme.12752
177. Anderson HA, Bertrand KC, Many RE, Hu Y-S, Fern KD. A comparison of two drug combinations for dilating dark irides. *Optom. Vis. Sci.* (2010) 87, 120–4. doi: 10.1097/OPX.0b013e3181cc8da3
178. Mishima, S. Clinical pharmacokinetics of the eye. Invest. *Ophthalmol Vis Sci.* (1981) 21:504–41.
179. Baranowski P, Karolewicz B, Gada M, Pluta, J. Ophthalmic drug dosage forms:characterisation and research methods. *ScientificWorldJournal* (2014) 2014:861904. doi: 10.1155/2014/861904
180. Smith SA, Smith SE, Lazare, R. An increased effect of pilocarpine on the pupil by application of the drug in oil. *Br. J. Ophthalmol.* (1978) 62:314–17. doi: 10.1136/bjo.62.5.314
181. Birmingham AT, Galloway NR, Spencer SA. A comparison of the pupilloconstrictor effect of pilocarpine solution administered to the conjunctival sac as a single drop or as a continuous infusion in normal subjects. *Br. J. Ophthalmol.* (1976) 60:568–72. doi: 10.1136/bjo.60.8.568
182. Ghose S, Garodia VK, Sachdev MS, Kumar H, Biswas NR, Pandey RM. Evaluation of potentiating effect of a drop of lignocaine on tropicamide-induced mydriasis. *Invest Ophthalmol Vis Sci.* (2001) 42, 1581–1585.

183. Farkouh A, Frigo P, Czejka, M. Systemic side effects of eye drops:a pharmacokinetic perspective. *Clin Opthalmol.* (2016) 10:2433–41. doi: 10.2147/OPTH.S118409
184. Tavernor SJ, Abduljawad KAJ, Langley RW, Bradshaw CM, Szabadi E. Effects of pentagastrin and the cold pressor test on the acoustic startle response and pupillary function in man. *J Psychopharmacol.* (2000) 14:387–94. doi: 10.1177/026988110001400407
185. Theofilopoulos N, Longmore J, Kerr FA, Szabadi E, Bradshaw CM. Consensual pupillary responses to mydriatic and miotic drugs. *Br J Clin Pharm.* (1988) 26:697–702.
186. Hou RH, Freeman C, Langley RW, Szabadi E, Bradshaw CM. Does modafinil activate the locus coeruleus in man? Comparison of modafinil and clonidine on arousal and autonomic functions in human volunteers. *Psychopharmacology (Berl)* (2005) 181:537–49. doi: 10.1007/s00213-005-0013-8
187. Szabadi E. The influence of the baseline on the size of pharmacological responses:a theoretical model. *Br J Clin Pharmacol.* (1977) 61, 492–3.
188. Phillips MA, Szabadi E, Bradshaw CM. Comparison of the effects of clonidine and yohimbine on pupillary diameter at different illumination levels. *Br J Clin Pharmacol.* (2000) 50:65–8. doi: 10.1046/j.1365-2125.2000.00225.x
189. Bitsios P, Szabadi E, Bradshaw CM. Comparison of the effects of venlafaxine, paroxetine and desipramine on the pupillary light reflex in man. *Psychopharmacology (Berl)* (1999) 143:286–92.
190. Beatty J, Lucero-Wagoner B. The pupillary system. In: Cacioppo JT, Tassinary LG, Berntson GG editors. Vol. 2, *Handbook of Psychophysiology.* New York, NY: Cambridge University Press (2000). p. 142–62.
191. Janisse M-P. editor. *Pupillary Dynamics and Behavior.* New York, NY: Plenum Press (1974).
192. Janisse M-P. *Pupillometry: The Psychology of the Pupillary Response.* Washington, DC: Hemisphere Publishing (1977).
193. Mathôt S. Pupillometry: psychology, physiology, and function. *J Cogn.* (2018) 1:16. doi: 10.5334/joc.18
194. Szabadi, E. Modulation of physiological reflexes by pain:role of the locus coeruleus. *Front Integr Neurosci.* (2012) 6:94. doi: 10.3389/fnint.2012.00094
195. Löwenstein, O. Pupillary reflex shapes and topical clinical diagnosis. *Neurology* (1955) 5:631–44.
196. Steinhauer SR, Hakerem G. The pupillary response in cognitive psychophysiology and schizophrenia. *Ann N Y Acad Sci.* (1992) 658:182–204. doi: 10.1111/j.1749-6632.1992.tb22845.x
197. Steinhauer SR, Siegle GJ, Condray R, Pless, M. Sympathetic and parasympathetic innervation of pupillary dilation during sustained processing. *Int J Psychophysiol.* (2004) 52:77–86. doi: 10.1016/j.ipsycho.2003.12.005
198. Sutton S. The specification of psychological variables in an average evoked potential experiment. In: Donchin E, Lindsley DB editors. *Average Evoked Potentials:Methods, Results and Evaluations.* Washington, DC: U.S. Government Printing Office (1969). pp. 237–62.
199. Bradley MM, Miccoli L, Escrig MA, Lang PJ. The pupil as a measure of emotional arousal and autonomic activation. *Psychophysiology* (2008) 45:602–7. doi: 10.1111/j.1469-8986.2008.00654.x
200. Siegle GJ, Steinhauer SR, Thase ME. Pupillary assessment and computational modeling of the Stroop task in depression. *Int J Psychophysiol.* (2004) 52:63–76. doi: 10.1016/j.ijpsycho.2003.12.010
201. Hess EH, Seltzer AL, Shlien JM. Pupil response of hetero-and homosexual males to pictures of men and women: a pilot study. *J Abnorm Psychol.* (1965) 70:165–8. doi: 10.1037/h0021978
202. Siegle GJ, Steinhauer SR, Stenger V, Konecky R, Carter CS. Use of concurrent pupil dilation assessment to inform interpretation and analysis of fMRI data. *Neuroimage* (2003) 20:114–24. doi: 10.1016/S1053-8119(03)00298-2
203. Mathôt S, Fabius J, Van Heusden E, Van der Stigchel S. Safe and sensible preprocessing and baseline correction of pupil-size data. *Behav Res Methods* (2018) 50:94–106. doi: 10.3758/s13428-017-1007-2
204. Granholm E, Verney SP. Pupillary responses and attentional allocation problems on the backward masking task in schizophrenia. *Int J Psychophysiol.* (2004) 52:37–51. doi: 10.1016/j.ijpsycho.2003.12.004
205. Guthrie D, Buchwald JS. Significance testing of difference potentials. *Psychophysiology* (1991) 28:240–44. doi: 10.1111/j.1469-8986.1991.tb00417.x
206. Beatty J. Task-evoked pupillary responses, processing load, and the structure of processing resources. *Psychol Bull.* (1982) 91:276–92. doi: 10.1037/0033-2909.91.2.276
207. Loewenfeld IE. Mechanisms of reflex dilatation of the pupil. *Doc Ophthalmol.* (1958) 12:185–448. doi: 10.1007/BF00913471
208. Hess EH, Polt JM. Pupil size as related to interest value of visual stimuli. *Science* (1960) 132:349–50. doi: 10.1126/science.132.3423.349
209. Kahneman D, Beatty J. Pupil diameter and load on memory. *Science* (1966) 154:1583–5. doi: 10.1126/science.154.3756.1583
210. Sokolov YN. *Perception and the Conditioned Reflex.* Translated by S.W. Waydenfeld. Oxford: Pergamon Press (1963).
211. Friedman D, Hakerem G, Sutton S, Fleiss JL. Effect of stimulus uncertainty on the pupillary dilation response and the vertex evoked potential. *Electroencephal Clin Neurophysiol.* (1973) 34:475–84. doi: 10.1016/0013-4694(73)90065-5
212. Wang C, Boehnke SE, Itti L, Munoz DP. Transient pupil response is modulated by contrast-based saliency. *J Neurosci.* (2014) 34:408–17. doi: 10.1523/JNEUROSCI.3550-13.2014
213. Wang C, Munoz DP. Modulation of stimulus contrast on the human pupil orienting response. *Eur J Neurosci.* (2014) 40:2822–32. doi: 10.1111/ejn.12641
214. Hess EH, Polt JM. Pupil size in relation to mental activity during simple problem-solving. *Science* (1964) 143:1190–2. doi: 10.1126/science.143.3611.1190
215. Aston-Jones G, Cohen JD. An integrative theory of locus coeruleus-norepinephrine function:adaptive gain and optimal performance. *Ann Rev Neurosci.* (2005) 28:403–50. doi: 10.1146/annurev.neuro.28.061604.135709
216. Steinhauer SR, Hakerem G, Spring BJ. The pupillary response as a potential indicator of vulnerability to schizophrenia. *Psychopharmacol Bull.* (1979) 15:44–45.
217. Granholm E, Morris SK, Sarkin AJ, Asarnow RF, Jeste DV. Pupillary responses index overload of working memory resources in schizophrenia. *J Abnorm Psychol.* (1997) 106:458–67. doi: 10.1037/0021-843X.106.3.458
218. Siegle GJ, Granholm E, Ingram RE, Matt GE. Pupillary response and reaction time measures of sustained processing of negative information in depression. *Biol Psychiatry* (2001) 49:624–36. doi: 10.1016/S0006-3223(00)01024-6
219. Siegle GJ, Steinhauer SR, Carter CS, Ramel W, Thase ME. Do the seconds turn into hours? Relationships between sustained pupil dilation in response to emotional information and self reported rumination. *Cogn Therapy Res.* (2003) 27:365–83. doi: 10.1023/A:1023974602357
220. Laurenzo SA, Kardon R, Ledolter J, Poolman P, Schumacher AM, Potash JB, et al. Pupillary response abnormalities in depressive disorders. *Psychiatry Res.* (2016) 246:492–9. doi: 10.1016/j.psychres.2016.10.039
221. Münch M, Ladaique M, Roemer S, Hashemi K, Kawasaki A. Melanopsin-mediated acute light responses measured in winter and in summer:seasonal variations in adults with and without cataracts. *Front Neurol.* (2017) 8:464. doi: 10.3389/fneur.2017.00464
222. LeGates TA, Altimus CM, Wang H, Lee HK, Yang S, Zhao H, et al. Aberrant light directly impairs mood and learning through melanopsin-expressing neurons. *Nature* (2012) 491:594–8. doi: 10.1038/nature11673
223. Lowenstein O, Feinberg R, Loewenfeld IE. Pupillary movements during acute and chronic fatigue. *Invest Ophthalmol Vis Sci.* (1963) 2:138–57.
224. Yoss RE, Moyer NJ, Ogle KN. The pupillogram and narcolepsy. A method to measure decreased levels of wakefulness. *Neurology* (1969) 19:921–28. doi: 10.1212/WNL.19.10.921
225. Yoss RE, Moyer NJ, Hollenhorst RW. Pupil size and spontaneous pupillary waves associated with alertness, drowsiness, and sleep. *Neurology* (1970) 20:545–54. doi: 10.1212/WNL.20.6.545
226. Schmidt HS, Jackson EI, Knopp W. Electronic pupillography (EPG): objective assessment of sleepiness and differentiation of disorders of excessive somnolence. *Sleep Res.* (1981) 10:48.
227. Merritt SL, Keegan AP, Mercer PW. Artifact management in pupillometry. *Nurs Res.* (1994) 43:56–9. doi: 10.1097/00006199-199401000-00012
228. Lüdtke H, Wilhelm B, Adler M, Schaeffel F, Wilhelm H. Mathematical procedures in data recording and processing of pupillary fatigue waves. *Vis Res.* (1998) 38:2889–96.
229. Weeß H-G, Sauter C, Geisler P, Böhning W, Wilhelm B, Rotte M, et al. Vigilanz, Einschlafneigung, Daueraufmerksamkeit, Müdigkeit,

Schläfrigkeit-Diagnostische Instrumentarien zur Messung müdigkeits- und schläfrigkeitsbezogener Prozesse und deren Gütekriterien. *Somnologie* (2000) 4:20–38. doi: 10.1046/j.1439-054x.2000.00116.x

230. Wilhelm B, Wilhelm H, Lüdtke H, Streicher P, Adler M. Pupillographic assessment of sleepiness in sleep-deprived healthy subjects. *Sleep* (1998) 21:258–65.
231. Wilhelm B, Körner A, Heldmaier K, Moll K, Wilhelm H, Lüdtke H. Normwerte des pupillographischen Schläfrigkeitstests für Frauen und Männer zwischen 20 und 60 Jahren. *Somnologie* (2001) 5:115–20. doi: 10.1046/j.1439-054X.2001.01156.x
232. Regen F, Dorn H, Danker-Hopfe H. Association between pupillary unrest index and waking electroencephalogram activity in sleep-deprived healthy adults. *Sleep Med.* (2013) 14:902–12. doi: 10.1016/j.sleep.2013.02.003
233. Wilhelm B, Neugebauer P, Lüdtke H, Hohenstein E, Ederle K, Wilhelm H. Pupillographischer Schläfrigkeitstest zur Therapiekontrolle beim Schlafapnoe-Syndrom nach drei Monaten nächtlicher Beatmung. *Somnologie* (1999) 3:53–56.
234. Urschitz MS, Heine K, Brockmann PE, Peters T, Durst W, Poets CF, et al. Subjective and objective daytime sleepiness in schoolchildren and adolescents:results of a community-based study. *Sleep Med.* (2013) 14:1005–12. doi: 10.1016/j.sleep.2013.05.014
235. Warga M, Lüdtke H, Wilhelm H, Wilhelm B. How do spontaneous pupillary oscillations in light relate to light intensity? *Vis Res.* (2009) 49:295–300. doi: 10.1016/j.visres.2008.09.019
236. Wilhelm B, Stuiber G, Lüdtke H, Wilhelm H. The effect of caffeine on spontaneous pupillary oscillations. *Ophthalmic Physiol Opt.* (2014) 34:73–81. doi: 10.1111/opo.12094
237. Heneka C, Lüdtke H, Wilhelm B. Effects of nicotine on the results of the pupillographic sleepiness test (PST) in normal healthy subjects. *Somnologie* (2003) 7(Suppl. 1):69. doi: 10.1002/ajhb.22326
238. Möller M, Schläfke ME, Schäfer T. On the influence of pretest conditions on the reproducibility of the pupillographic sleepiness test. *Somnologie* (2002) 6:75–8. doi: 10.1046/j.1439-054X.2002.02179.x
239. Steinhauer SR, Condray R, Kasparek A. Cognitive modulation of midbrain function:task-induced reduction of the pupillary light reflex. *Int J Psychophysiol.* (2000) 39:21–30. doi: 10.1016/S0167-8760(00)00119-7
240. Grozdanic SD, Matic M, Sakaguchi DS, Kardon RH. Evaluation of retinal status using chromatic pupil light reflex activity in healthy and diseased canine eyes. *Invest Ophthalmol Vis Sci.* (2007) 48:5178–83. doi: 10.1167/iovs.07-0249
241. Binda P, Gamlin PD. Renewed attention on the pupil light reflex. *Trends Neurosci.* (2017) 40:455–7. doi: 10.1016/j.tins.2017.06.007
242. Mohan K, Harper MM, Kecova H, Ye EA, Lazic T, Sakaguchi DS, et al. Characterization of structure and function of the mouse retina using pattern electroretinography, pupil light reflex, and optical coherence tomography. *Vet Ophthalmol.* (2012) 15(Suppl. 2):94–104. doi: 10.1111/j.1463-5224.2012.01034.x
243. Cahill H, Nathans J. The optokinetic reflex as a tool for quantitative analyses of nervous system function in mice:application to genetic and drug-induced variation. *PLoS ONE* (2008) 3:e2055. doi: 10.1371/journal.pone.0002055
244. Somasundaram P, Wyrick GR, Fernandez DC, Ghahari A, Pinhal CM, Simmonds Richardson M, et al. C-terminal phosphorylation regulates the kinetics of a subset of melanopsin-mediated behaviors in mice. *Proc Natl Acad Sci USA.* (2017) 114:2741–6. doi: 10.1073/pnas.1611893114

5

Buzzing Sympathetic Nerves: A New Test to Enhance Anisocoria in Horner's Syndrome

Rawan Omary[1], Christopher J. Bockisch[1,2,3], Klara Landau[1], Randy H. Kardon[4] and Konrad P. Weber[1,2]*

[1] Department of Ophthalmology, University Hospital Zurich, University of Zurich, Zurich, Switzerland, [2] Department of Neurology, University Hospital Zurich, University of Zurich, Zurich, Switzerland, [3] Department of ENT, University Hospital Zurich, University of Zurich, Zurich, Switzerland, [4] Department of Ophthalmology, University of Iowa and Veterans Medical Center, Iowa City, IA, United States

***Correspondence:**
Konrad P. Weber
konrad.weber@usz.ch

Introduction: Patients with suspected Horner's syndrome having equivocal pupil dilation lag and pharmacologic testing may undergo unnecessary MR imaging and work up in the case of false positive pupil test results. Our goal was to increase the diagnostic accuracy of pupillometry by accentuating the inter-ocular asymmetry of sympathetic innervation to the iris dilator with surface electrical stimulation of the median nerve using a standard electromyography machine. We hypothesized that an accentuated difference in sympathetic response between the two eyes would facilitate the diagnosis of Horner's syndrome.

Methods: Eighteen patients with pharmacologically proven Horner's syndrome were compared to ten healthy volunteers tested before and after monocular instillation of 0.2% brimonidine tartrate ophthalmic solution to induce pharmacological Horner's syndrome. Pupillary responses were measured with binocular pupillometry in response to sympathetic activation by electrical stimulation of the median nerve in darkness and at various times after extinction of a light stimulus. Sudomotor sympathetic responses from the palm of the stimulated arm were recorded simultaneously.

Results: In subjects with Horner's syndrome and pharmacologically induced unilateral sympathetic deficit, electrical stimulation in combination with the extinction of light greatly enhanced the anisocoria during the evoked pupil dilation, while there was no significant increase in anisocoria in healthy subjects. The asymmetry of the sympathetic response was greatest when the electrical stimulus was given 2 s after termination of the light or under constant low light conditions. When given 2 s after termination of light, the electrical stimulation increased the mean anisocoria from 1.0 to 1.2 mm in Horner's syndrome ($p = 0.01$) compared to 0.22–0.26 mm in healthy subjects ($p = 0.1$). In all subjects, the maximal anisocoria induced by the electrical stimulation appeared within a 2 s interval after the stimulus. Correspondingly, the largest change in anisocoria between light and dark without electrical stimulation was seen between 3 and 4 s after light-off. While stronger triple stimulation further enhanced the anisocoria, it was less well tolerated.

Conclusions: Electrical stimulation 2 s after light-off greatly enhances the sensitivity of pupillometry for diagnosing Horner's syndrome. This new method may help to rule in or rule out a questionable Horner's syndrome, especially if the results of topical pharmacological testing are inconclusive.

Keywords: Horner's syndrome, pupillometry, sympathetic activation, electrical stimulation, anisocoria, brimonidine

INTRODUCTION

The clinical diagnosis of Horner's syndrome (HS) relies on the classical triad of ipsilateral pupillary miosis, blepharoptosis, and facial anhidrosis, which result from an interruption of the sympathetic innervation to the eye and ocular adnexa. Pupillary dilation lag, which is considered to be the most specific feature of Horner's syndrome, is not routinely used for diagnosis due to the difficulty in detecting it with clinical certainty, leaving pharmacologic testing with cocaine or apraclonidine as the gold standard despite their own limitations of availability, added time to a clinic visit, and correct interpretation. The resulting diagnostic uncertainty in borderline cases often leads to patient anxiety, unnecessary neuroimaging and workup.

Previous attempts to use automated pupillometry for the diagnosis of HS through the detection of pupillary dilation lag have shown very high specificity yet the sensitivity was low (1).

Knowing that unilateral Horner's syndrome occurs due to a sympathetic innervation defect in one eye, we suggest that by delivering a generalized sympathetic stimulation to both eyes, we can cause enhancement of the anisocoria in patients with HS but not in healthy subjects.

General sympathetic activation can be achieved through a painful stimulus (2, 3), such as that caused by an electrical surface stimulation to the median nerve at the wrist using a standard electromyography (EMG) machine. Using automated pupillometry, we look for an increase in the anisocoria and difference in pupil dilation velocity in reaction to the enhanced sympathetic activation, to more sensitively detect a unilateral sympathetic innervation deficit.

Patients with HS can have different degrees of ocular sympathetic deficit, depending on the underlying site of nerve damage or the duration of HS. In order to control for those variables, we treated one eye of healthy subjects with 0.2% brimonidine tartrate ophthalmic solution, which is known to induce a sympathetic block in the eye owing to the alpha-2 adrenergic agonist effect (4, 5), blocking the release of norepinephrine, resulting in a complete pharmacological HS.

With this new method, our goal is to enhance the diagnostic accuracy of pupillometry for the diagnosis of Horner's syndrome with electrically induced sympathetic activation.

MATERIALS AND METHODS

Protocol Approval, Registrations, and Patient Consents

Written informed consent was obtained from all participants, and the protocol was approved by the Zurich cantonal ethics committee, Switzerland (BASEC-Nr. 2016-02151), in accordance with the Helsinki Declaration.

Participants

Participants were tested at the University Hospital of Zurich between October 2017 and August 2018. Eighteen patients (8 female) with proven Horner's syndrome (HS) (age mean 59 years, range 38–83 years) and 10 healthy volunteers (4 female, age mean 39 years, range 25–52 years) took part in the study. Etiologies for HS included: long-standing and new onset HS of unknown etiology, surgically induced HS, cervical lesions, and internal carotid artery dissection. Inclusion criteria for the patients' group were: older than 18 years, unilateral HS previously confirmed using cocaine eye drops test (6), no past ocular surgery or trauma with residual iris sphincter damage, and no topical or systemic medications that could affect pupillary responses. Healthy subjects' inclusion criteria: older than 18 years, no past pupillary disorders, no past ocular surgery or trauma, no chronic topical or systemic medications use. Exclusion criteria for both groups: the presence of a cardiac pacemaker or defibrillator.

Study Design

Case-control study.

Experimental Procedure

A binocular pupillometer (DP-2000, Neuroptics, Irvine, CA, USA) was used to produce light stimuli and record the pupils of all subjects. Electrical stimulation was provided using a standard electromyography (EMG) machine (Nicolet Viking Quest, Natus Medical Incorporated, Pleasanton, CA, USA).

With the participant sitting and looking into the eyepieces of the pupilometer, binocular pupillary recording (frame rate 30 Hz) was done for each test paradigm (**Figure 1**). In a dark and quiet examination room, the participants were asked to look straight ahead into the video cameras for about 1–1.5 min depending on the test paradigm, during which they were asked to close

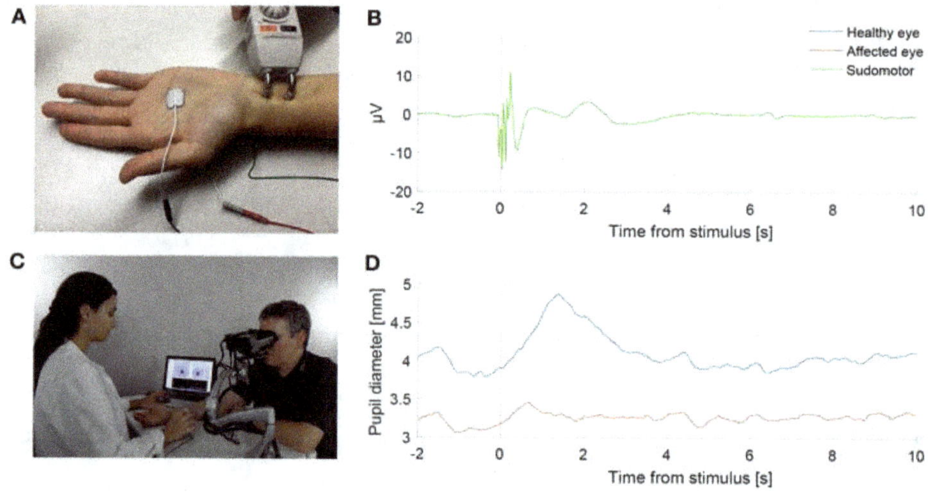

FIGURE 1 | Pupillometry with a "buzz". **(A)** Electrical sympathetic stimulation ("a buzz") is delivered to the median nerve using a standard electromyography (EMG) stimulator. Red and black electrodes record sympathetic skin response (SSR). Green electrode is ground. **(B)** Normal SSR recording in a patient with Horner's syndrome. **(C)** Pupil dynamics are recorded simultaneously using automated binocular pupillometry. **(D)** Pupil size over time in a patient with Horner's syndrome as measured with pupillometry, showing the timely synchronized appearance of the increase in anisocoria with the SSR in response to the electrical stimulation. (Photograph in C is published after obtaining a written informed consent from the appearing persons).

their eyes for 4 s at the end of each repetition to prevent ocular irritation and blinking at critical recording times. An electrical stimulus was delivered using the stimulator of the EMG machine to the median nerve at the wrist (**Figure 1A**), similar to that used in the sympathetic skin response test (SSR) (7). Conducting gel [Ten20, Weaver and Company, Aurora, USA] for the tip of the stimulator, as well as a grounding sticker electrode [Neuroline Ground, Ambu, Copenhagen, Denmark] at the back of the hand, were used, as in the standard SSR test. The electric current of a single electrical stimulus was chosen to be 55 mA during 0.2 ms, and a triple stimulus was defined as three consecutive single stimuli (12 Hz). The devices were synchronized so that the pupillometer triggered the EMG machine to deliver an electrical stimulus at specified times as programmed for each test paradigm.

The SSR was recorded from electrodes at both sides of the hand (**Figure 1A**) in 2 patients and 2 healthy volunteers as a reference. SSR represents the potential generated in skin sweat glands in response to sympathetic stimulation. SSR in response to median nerve stimulation was recorded simultaneously to the pupil reaction to compare the timing of the pupillary reflex dilation to the SSR.

Patients with HS received the stimulation to the ipsilateral median nerve (same side as the HS), and healthy volunteers were assigned randomly to receive the electrical stimulation to the right or left median nerve. The purpose of the electric stimulus was to induce a general sympathetic activation through the associated pain, rather than a direct activation of the median nerve (2, 3).

After completing the initial tests, healthy volunteers were treated with 0.2% brimonidine tartrate ophthalmic solution to one eye only, assigned randomly, and the tests were all repeated 45 min after the drop instillation. Brimonidine is an alpha-2 adrenergic agonist, which causes inhibition of norepinephrine secretion, resulting in a sympathetic block to the iris dilator (4, 5), resembling the pupil's state in a complete HS.

Test Paradigms

Pupil responses were recorded in response to cycles of light and dark, to electrical stimulation during constant low (0.1 log-lux) and high (2.5 log-lux) illumination, and to electrical stimulation at different time points during the cycles of light and dark. Examples of test paradigms are shown in **Supplementary Videos 1–5.**

Each subject first underwent baseline binocular pupil recordings, without electrical stimulation. The main paradigm consisted of cycles with 4 s of white light-on (3 log-lux) followed by 20 s of darkness, and was repeated at least four times. Pupil responses were also recorded for 17 s of constant light stimulation with levels of 0.1 and 2.5 log lux. Next, the paradigms were repeated with the addition of electrical stimulation. For the cyclic paradigm, the stimulation occurred at different time points (at 0.5 s before, simultaneously with, and 2 s after the termination of light). Only one stimulation was presented per light/dark cycle, and four repetitions of each stimulation time point were included. In the constant light paradigms, the electrical stimulation occurred after 4 s of constant light stimulation.

To avoid an "order bias" which can be caused by response habituation after repeated nerve stimulation (8), the test paradigms with electrical stimulation were performed in a randomized order for each subject, and a 5–10 min break with turning the room light on and engaging the subject in a conversation were taken half way through the experiment.

In order to assess the pupils' reaction to different levels of electrical stimulation, three of the aforementioned test paradigms, namely the electrical stimulus given at 0.5 s before and 2 s after light-off, and the electrical stimulation alone paradigm with 0.1 log-lux light intensity, were repeated with a triple stimulus, performed last in each testing session.

Data Analysis and Statistics

Videos recorded by the pupillometer were analyzed with custom programs written in MATLAB and the Image Processing and Statistics toolboxes 2016b (The MathWorks Inc., Natick, Massachusetts, United States). Pupils were found by thresholding the image, the pupil edge identified with the MATLAB function "bwboundaries.m," and an ellipse was fitted to the edge (9). The vertical diameter of the fitted ellipse was used as a measure of pupil size, since this will not change with horizontal eye movements, which seemed more common than vertical

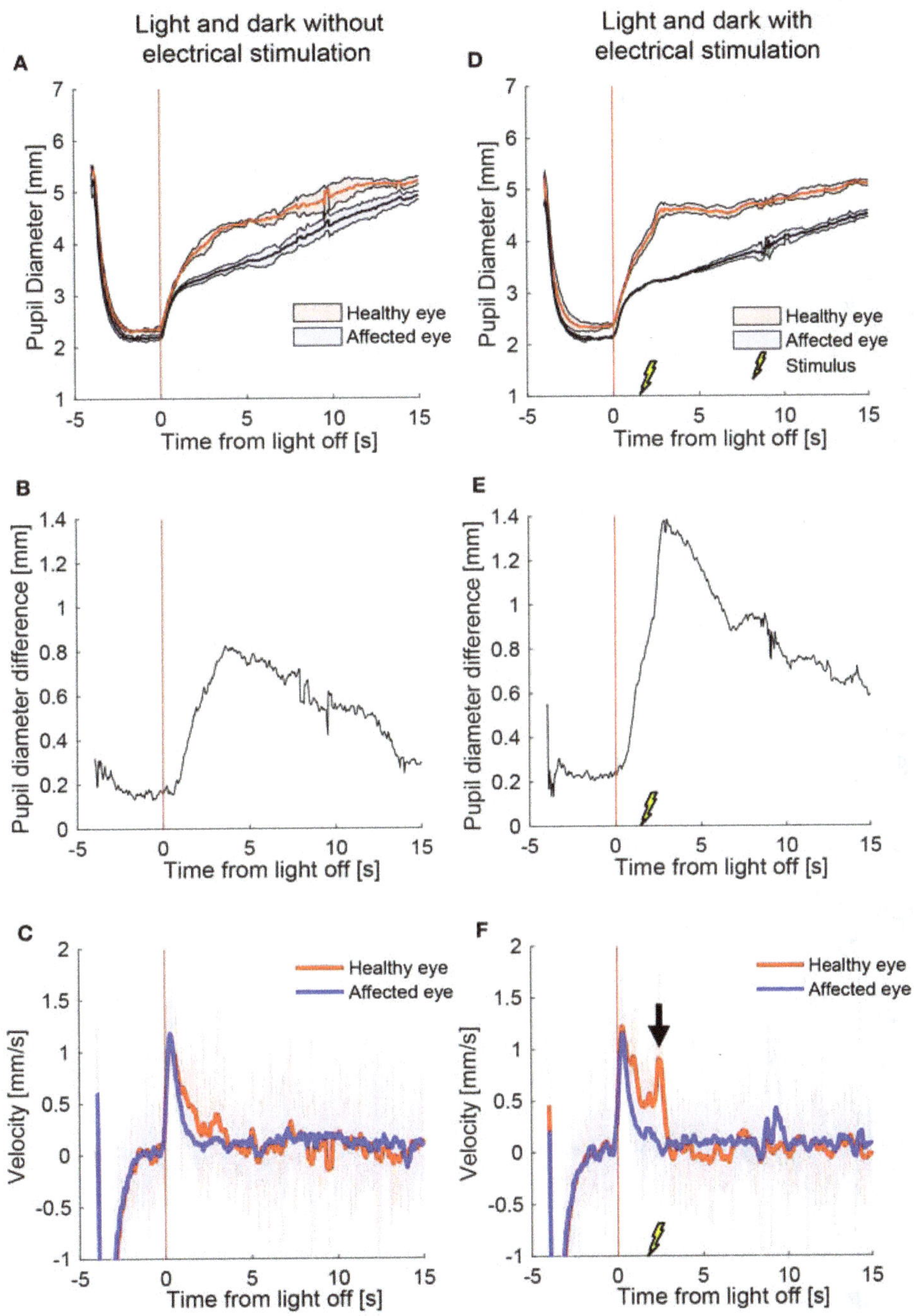

FIGURE 2 | The effect of electrical stimulation ("buzzing") in a patient with Horner's syndrome. The left column shows the pupil response to a cycle of light and dark alone, and the right column shows the response with the addition of electrical stimulation delivered 2 s after light-off **(A)** Pupils size over time in a patient with HS, as seen on pupillometry with light/dark alone. The dark lines are the means of 5 trials, and the shaded region represents ± 1 standard deviation. Time zero indicates extinction of the light, after which the difference between the pupils starts to increase. **(B)** The difference in mean pupil size, showing a maximal difference of about 0.8 mm, 4 s after the light is turned off **(C)** Pupil dilation velocity over time for the same test: a difference is noted in the early dilation phase between the healthy and affected pupils. **(D–F)** When an electrical stimulation is introduced at 2 s after light-off, a clear increase in anisocoria **(D,E)** and second dilation velocity peak (arrow) of the healthy eye **(F)** appear.

eye movements in our paradigms (a fixation target was not present during recording, and subjects were reminded to try and maintain straight-ahead gaze as necessary). Recordings of artificial pupils were used to calibrate the pupilometer and to convert pupil diameter from pixels to millimeters. The measured values were removed (usually owing to full or partial blinks or large eye movements) if the fitted ellipse deviated too far from a circle (ratio of major to minor axes >1.3), if the pupil diameter was <1.25 or >8 mm, if pupil constriction/dilation velocity exceeded 10 mm/s, or the duration of the eyes being open was <0.5 s. Entire trials were rejected if more than one third of the data of either eye was lost.

Pupillary dilation lag was defined as the change in anisocoria (difference in pupil diameter) between 5 and 15 s after the light stimulus was removed (1). For patients, we always measured anisocoria as the healthy pupil size minus the affected pupil size; for healthy subjects we took the absolute value of the difference in pupil size. Pilot experiments showed that the effect of electrical stimulation was limited to the 2 s period following stimulation, so we defined the electrically-induced anisocoria as the maximum anisocoria during this period. To determine the effect of electrical stimulation during trials where there was a changing light stimulus, compared to a baseline measure of ansiocoria, we also calculated the maximum anisocoria during the 2 s interval on

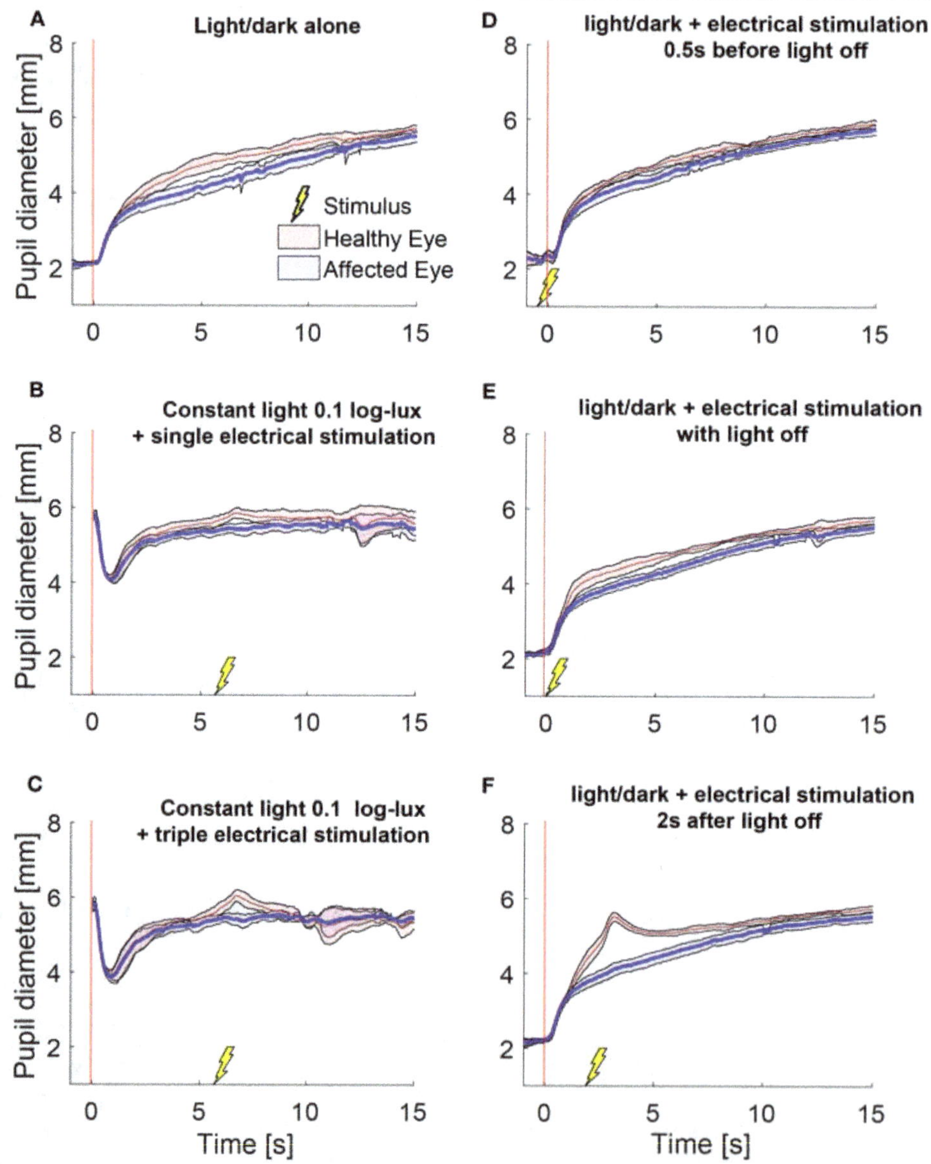

FIGURE 3 | Pupillary responses to light/dark alone, electrical stimulation alone, and the combination of the two in a patient with HS. All traces are the means (thick lines) ±1 standard deviation (shaded areas). **(A)** Pupillometry with light and dark alone (no electrical stimulation). **(B)** Electrical stimulation alone during constant low light with single stimulus and **(C)** with triple stimulus. After the initial constriction in response to the low light, pupils are allowed to reach a steady state for 5 s before the electrical stimulation is given at 6 s. **(D–F)** Combined test paradigms: electrical stimulation during cycle of light/dark at minus 0.5 s **(D)**, 0 s **(E)**, and 2 s **(F)** from-light-off.

the equivalent trials without electrical stimulation. For constant light-on trials, we used the anisocoria just prior to electrical stimulation as the baseline.

To determine the optimal time point for measuring anisocoria that differentiates patients from healthy subjects without electrical stimulation, we calculated the relative change in anisocoria between light and dark over 1 s for each second after light-off. The relative change in anisocoria was defined as the median anisocoria during that time interval minus the anisocoria at the end of the light-on period. The area under the receiver operating characteristic curve (AUC) was then calculated at each time interval.

To evaluate the effect of electrical stimulation, we performed paired *t*-tests with Holm's correction for multiple comparisons within each subject group. In order to evaluate which electrical stimulation condition produced the most consistent differences from non-electrical stimulation conditions, we calculated the mean differences to z-scores (mean difference/standard deviation of the pair differences). Larger z-scores thus indicated that electrical stimulation produced a larger consistent effect, and could be produced either by a larger mean difference, or by smaller variability.

RESULTS

We measured 18 patients with Horner's syndrome (HS) and 10 healthy volunteers before and after monocular instillation of brimonidine drops. Using automated pupillometry, we compared the anisocoria and difference in pupillary dilation velocity with and without electrical stimulation.

Figure 2 shows a representative example of the pupil light responses of a patient with left HS without (left column) and with (right column) electrical stimulation delivered 2 s after the extinction of light. The healthy right pupil (red) of this patient dilated normally in the dark, expanding from a little more than 2 mm in diameter in the light to about 5 mm after 15 s (**Figure 2A**). The affected left pupil (blue), however, dilated similarly in the first second, but then dilation slowed, with a maximum anisocoria of about 0.8 mm appearing about 4 s after light off (**Figure 2B**). In **Figure 2C** the dilation velocity graph for each pupil shows that the right healthy pupil (red) has a larger dilation velocity in the first 3 s after light off. Electrical stimulation 2 s after light off increased the dilation in the healthy right pupil, but had no discernable effect in the affected left pupil (**Figure 2D**), resulting in an increase in maximum anisocoria to about 1.4 mm (**Figure 2E**) as well as an increase in the difference in pupillary dilation velocity between the healthy and affected pupil (**Figure 2F**, arrow).

We also tested the effect of electrical stimulation at different times relative to light-off. **Figure 3** shows the average responses of one patient during different test paradigms. A single electrical stimulus in low light (0.1 log-lux) (**Figure 3B**) produced a small change in anisocoria, whereas the triple stimulus during similar light conditions produced a noticeable dilation response in the healthy eye (**Figure 3C**) causing a larger increase in anisocoria. When electrical stimulation occurred 0.5 s before (**Figure 3D**) or with (**Figure 3E**) the light extinction, the effect of the stimulus was smaller and no discernable increase in anisocoria was noticed. Electrical stimulation at 2 s after light off (**Figure 3F**) produced the largest increase in anisocoria as compared to the other test paradigms.

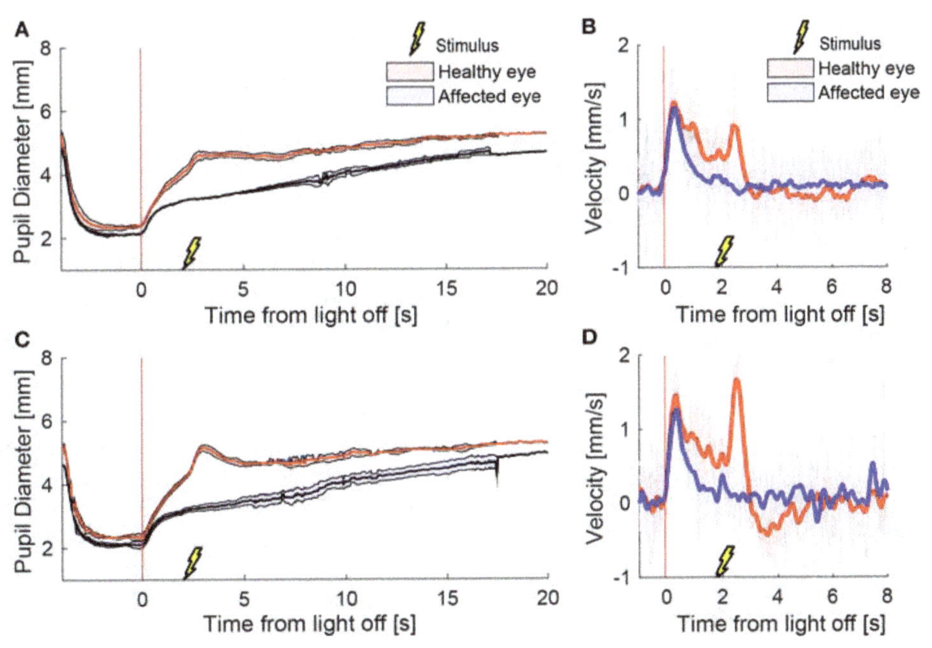

FIGURE 4 | Different stimulation intensities. In a patient with HS, a single electrical stimulus (55 mA, 0.2 ms) causes an increase in difference between the pupils in size **(A)** and dilation velocity **(B)**. A triple stimulus (3x single stimulus, 12 Hz) causes a larger difference between the pupils **(C,D)** compared to the single stimulus.

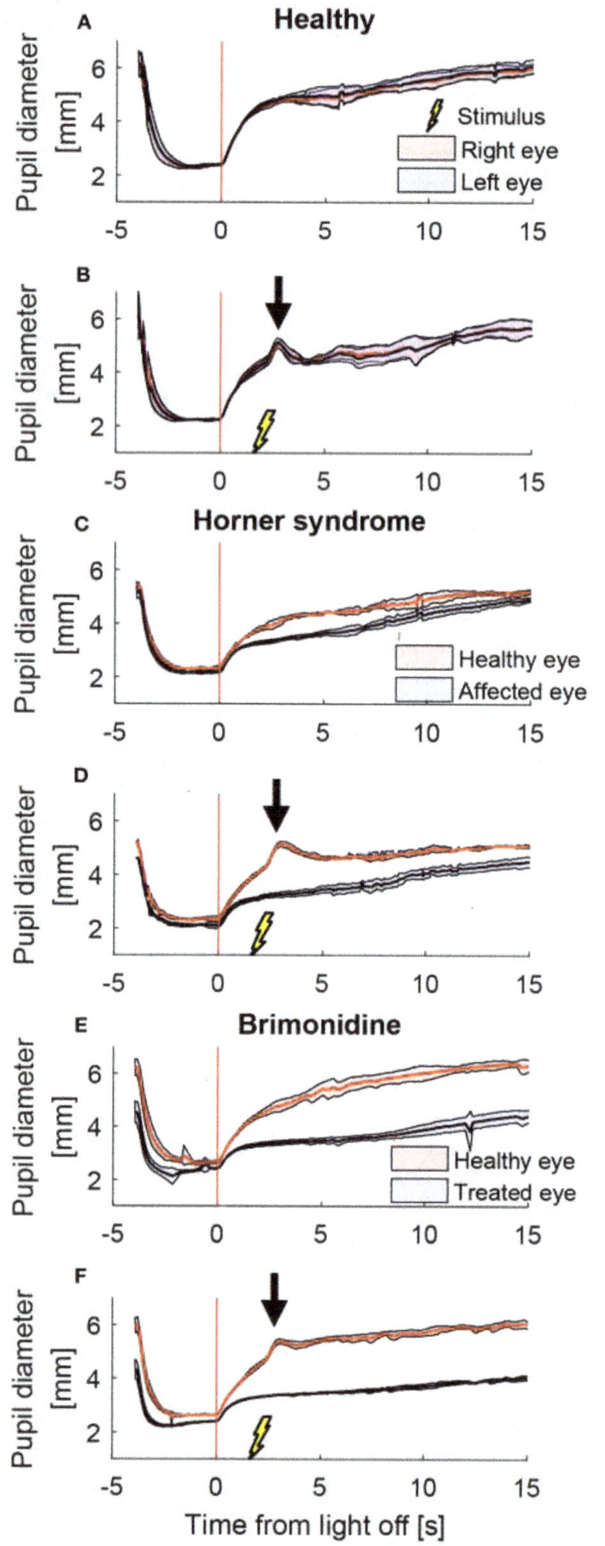

FIGURE 5 | Comparison of pupillary response with and without electrical stimulus. All traces are the means (thick lines) ±1 standard deviation (shaded areas) of 4–5 trials (trials could be lost due to blinks) **(A)** a cycle of light and dark alone in a healthy subject, shows no anisocoria. **(B)** Adding an electrical *(Continued)*

FIGURE 5 | stimulus 2 s after light-off in a light and dark cycle results in a second dilation peak (arrow) yet does not provoke a difference between the pupils as compared to light and dark alone. In a patient with Horner's syndrome **(C,D)** as well as in a healthy subject treated with brimonidine **(E,F)**, electrical stimulation results in an increase in the anisocoria as compared to a similar test paradigm of light and dark alone (arrows).

To test the effect of stimulus intensity, we applied three electrical stimuli in quick succession at 12 Hz (triple stimulus). **Figure 4** shows an example of mean pupil responses in a patient with HS to the triple stimulation compared to the single stimulation during a cycle of light and dark. The increase in both the anisocoria (**Figure 4A**) and difference in pupil dilation velocity (**Figure 4B**) produced by the single stimulus were further increased in the same patient when a triple stimulus was given (**Figures 4C,D**).

A representative example of mean pupil responses to electrical stimulation (triple stimulus condition) compared to the condition without electrical stimulation is shown in **Figure 5** in a healthy subject (**Figures 5A,B**), a patient with HS (**Figures 5C,D**), and a healthy subject treated with brimonidine (**Figures 5E,F**). The triple-stimulus produced a prominent increase in anisocoria in the HS patient and the subject with brimonidine for a couple of seconds, whereas no increase or induction of anisocoria was seen in the healthy subject as a result of the stimulation.

Average anisocoria traces for each of the groups are shown in **Figure 6** (**Figures 6A–C** during light and dark cycles, **Figures 6D–F** in constant light-on conditions). As expected, there was little measured anisocoria in healthy subjects, whereas substantial increases in anisocoria were noted in HS patients and healthy subjects with brimonidine in response to electrical stimulation as compared to without. Note that in our patients during cycles of light and dark without electrical stimulation, the average anisocoria was largely constant in the period from 5 s after light off (1.0 mm) to the end of the trial (0.9 mm) (**Figure 6A**).

We observed that the effect of electrical stimulation was generally confined to 2 s after the stimulus. Therefore, we assessed the effect of the electrical stimulation by measuring the maximum anisocoria within 2 s after electrical stimulation, and compared it to the anisocoria during the same time interval in the conditions without electrical stimulation. **Figure 7** shows the measured anisocoria in each condition after electrical stimulation (color bars), along with the associated condition without electrical stimulation for each test paradigm (yellow bars) for comparison. **Figure 7** also shows a measurement of dilation lag as it was previously defined in literature (1, 10) as the change in anisocoria from 5 to 15 s after light off. Of note is that none of our HS patients or brimonidine subjects had an average dilation lag of 0.4 mm or larger with these parameters. In subjects treated with brimonidine the anisocoria slightly increased over time after light off, giving a negative result when calculating the dilation lag using this method.

For HS patients, electrical stimulation produced a significant increase in anisocoria in all test paradigms except for the

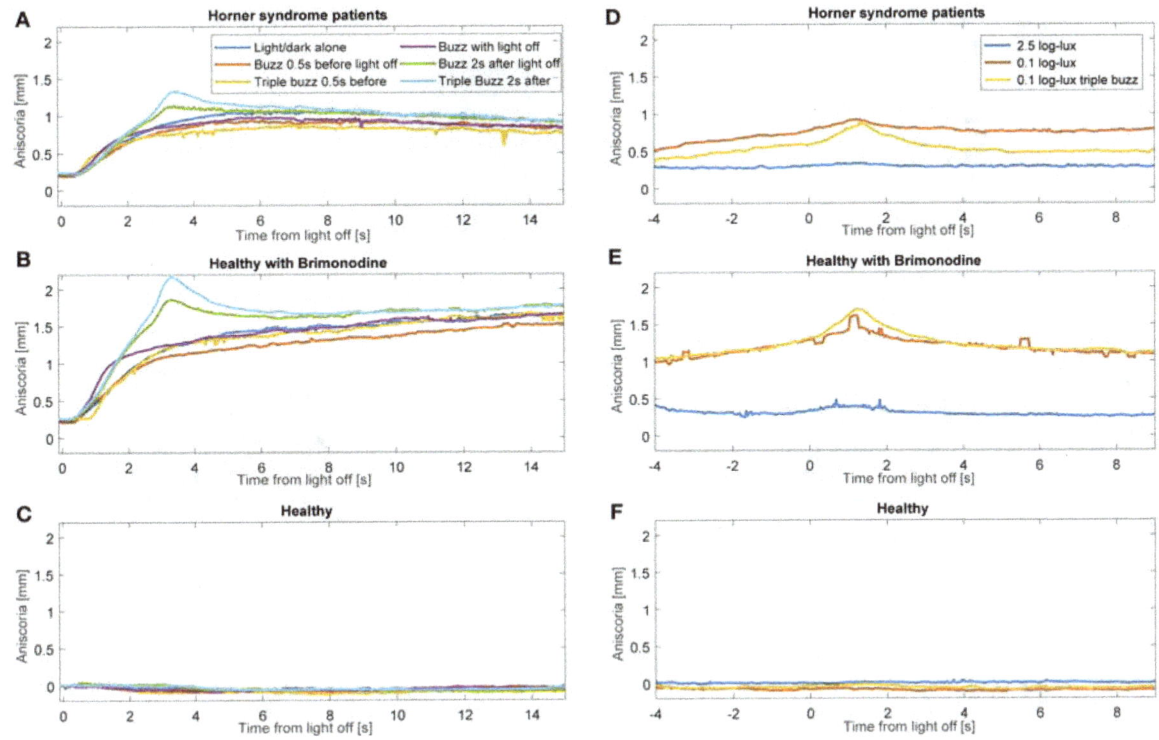

FIGURE 6 | Average anisocoria traces for each group. Graphs **(A–C)** show the average anisocoria resulting from different conditions during cycles of light and dark. In the patient group **(A)** and the brimonidine group **(B)** we notice a larger transient increase in anisocoria in response to single and triple electrical stimulation at 2 s after light goes off as compared to the test paradigm without electrical stimulation. Electrical stimulation at the other times did not produce as discernable increase. **(C)** In the healthy group, no anisocoria was measured or induced during all the test paradigms. Graphs **(D–F)** show the average anisocoria resulting from different conditions during constant light-on conditions. Single electrical stimulation during constant light on of 0.1 log-lux intensity produced an increase in anisocoria in both the patients group **(A)** and brimonidine group **(B)** but not in the healthy group **(C)**. Triple stimulation during similar light conditions produced a larger increase in anisocoria for the patient **(A)** and brimonidine **(B)** groups. Stimulation during constant light on of 2.5 log-lux intensity did not increase the anisocoria in any of the 3 groups.

single electrical stimulus given 0.5 s before light off during a cycle of light and dark (**Figure 7A**). The largest increase in anisocoria was found when electrical stimulation occurred 2 s after light off (mean = 1.3 mm, standard deviation (*SD*) = 0.4, $p < 0.01$ for difference from baseline *t*-test) for triple stimulus, and 1.2 mm for single stimulus ($SD = 0.4$, $p < 0.0001$) as compared to 1 mm ($SD = 0.41$, $p < 0.0001$) without stimulus. Electrical stimulation also significantly increased the anisocoria in the constant light condition, particularly with the lower light intensity of 0.1 log-lux. Subjects treated with brimonidine showed the same pattern of results as the HS, though the amount of anisocoria was higher. Healthy subjects did not, in general, show an increase in anisocoria with electrical stimulation (because we took the absolute difference in pupil size for healthy subjects, any change in anisocoria was likely just an increase in variability). Overall, the increase in anisocoria for the healthy group in response to a single and triple electrical stimuli given 2 s after light of was similar and equal to 0.04 ($p > 0.1$). Within the healthy group, three subjects had some physiological anisocoria (mean 0.3 mm). The mean increase in anisocoria for those subjects in response to a single and triple electrical stimuli 2 s after light-off was 0.07 and 0.09 mm, respectively, and for subjects without physiological anisocoria was 0.03 and 0.015 mm, respectively ($p = 0.5$ and 0.42).

We also determined the best time point after light off at which the change in anisocoria, relative to light on, best differentiated HS from healthy subjects based on pupillometry without electrical stimulation. The time interval after light termination which gave the greatest area under the receiver operating characteristic curve (AUC) and the best discrimination between patients with HS and healthy subjects, was 3–4 s after light-off, with an AUC of 0.98 (**Figure 8**). For this time interval, the best discriminating criterion (cut-off value for relative change in anisocoria) was 0.4 mm. Note, however, that AUC was >0.97 for all time intervals between 3 and 8 s, and was above 0.9 for all time intervals except the first second after light off. The AUC for pupillary dilation lag (change in anisocoria from 5 to 15 s after light-off) was only 0.5, and the AUC for all test paradigms with electrical stimulation was more than 0.97.

To determine which of the electrical stimulation conditions gave the largest consistent change in anisocoria, thus taking within-subject variability into account, we converted the differences (electrical stimulation minus no stimulation) into standardized z-scores. The largest z-score was given by the single electrical stimulus under 0.1 log-lux constant light condition (*z*

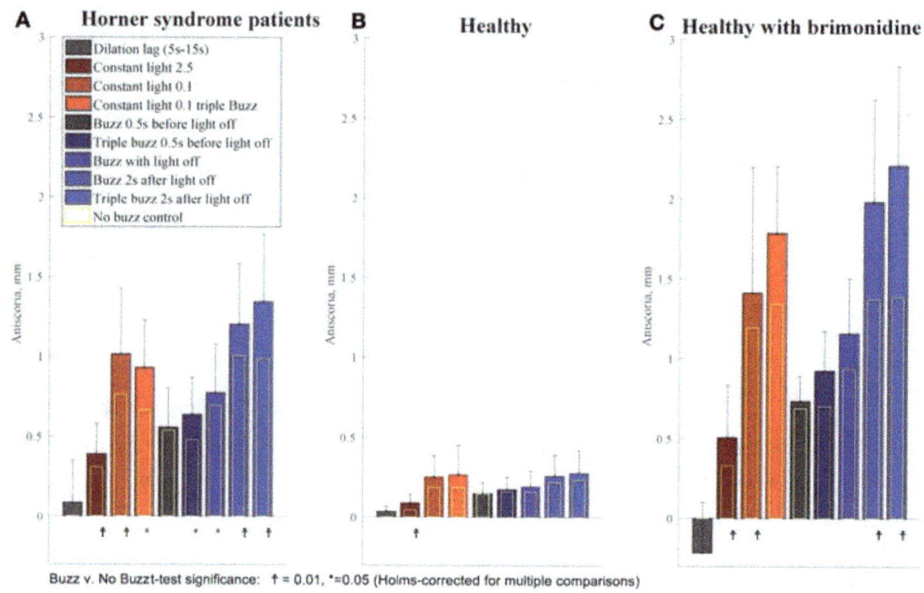

FIGURE 7 | Summary of buzzing effect. Each bar shows the measured anisocoria in response to electrical stimulation compared to the baseline anisocoria (yellow bars) for each matched condition with no electrical stimulation. **(A)** In Horner's syndrome patients, electrical stimulation produced a significant increase in aniscoria in all conditions except for the single stimulus given 0.5 s before light off. **(B)** Except for the constant bright light condition (2.5 log-lux), healthy subjects did not show any significant increase in anisocoria in the test paradigms as compared to parallel no electrical stimulation paradigms. **(C)** Subjects treated with brimonidine showed similar reaction patterns to electrical stimulation as seen in HS group, yet with larger increases in anisocoria.

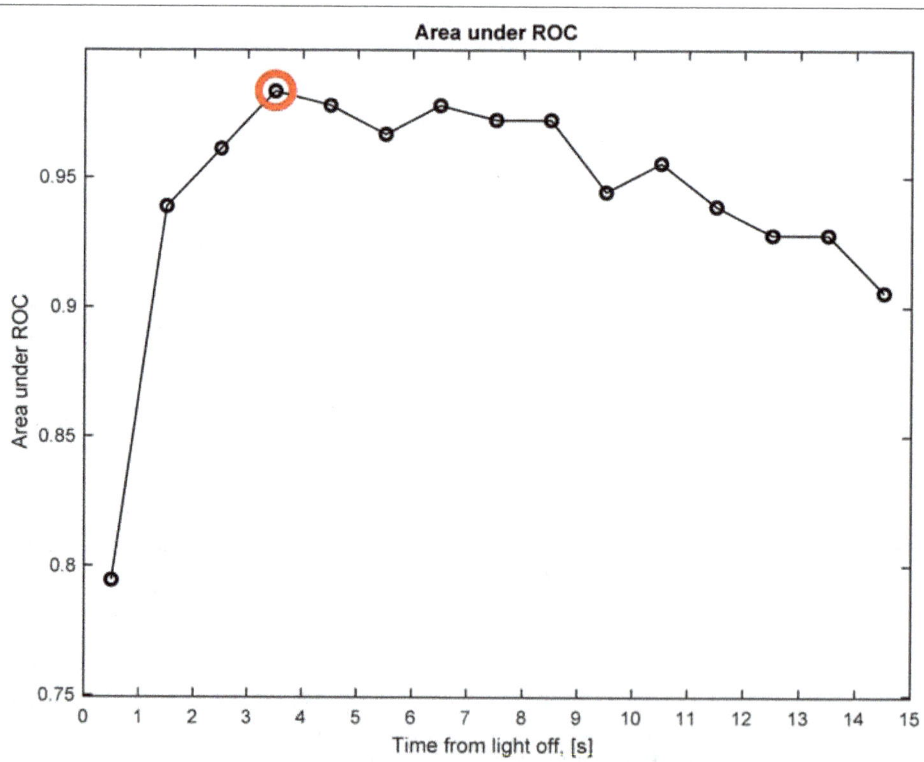

FIGURE 8 | Anisocoria in Horner's syndrome without electrical stimulation. This graph shows the area under the receiver operating characteristic (ROC) curve (AUC) for the anisocoria at each time interval of 1 s after light-off relative to the anisocoria at the end of the light-on period, presented at the matching time interval, e.g., a circle at 0.5 represents the time interval of 0–1 s. The largest AUC occurs at the 3–4 s interval (red circle), indicating that the largest relative change in anisocoria that helps differentiating Horner's syndrome patients from healthy subjects occurs at the 3–4 s interval after light-off.

= 2.6). For the light and dark cycles, the triple stimulus given 2 s after light off condition ($z = 1.1$) was best, though just slightly larger than the single stimulus 2 s after light off condition.

DISCUSSION

Summary of Results

We found that electrical stimulation increases the anisocoria and difference in dilation velocity between the pupils of subjects with unilateral ocular sympathetic deficit both in Horner's syndrome (HS) and a pharmacologically induced sympathetic block. In contrast, no significant anisocoria was induced in healthy volunteers in response to the electrical stimulation including those with slight physiological anisocoria. The combination of electrical stimulation with cycles of light and dark produced the largest and most consistent enhancement in anisocoria, as compared to either one alone. Pupillary dilation lag with its previous definition is not helpful as a diagnostic measure for HS. Electrical stimulation 2 s after light off and stimulation during constant low light of 0.1 log-lux produced the largest increase in anisocoria compared to the other test paradigms. Electrical stimulation alone caused a larger increase in low light conditions (0.1 log-lux) than in high light condition (2 log-lux). Higher electrical stimulation intensities (triple stimulus) produced a larger increase in anisocoria in HS and pharmacological HS groups as compared to a single stimulus, yet was less well tolerated.

Previous and Current Tests

The current gold standard for the diagnosis of HS using pharmacologic eye drops testing with either cocaine or apraclonidine, carries several disadvantages, including limited availability of cocaine, longer test duration, and possible false-positive and false negative results (6, 11–14).

Pupillary dilation in response to sympathetic stimulation in the form of auditory stimulus in healthy subjects as well as an increase in anisocoria in subjects with unilateral pharmacological ocular sympathetic block (15), and in patients with HS (16) has been described. In neither study, however, were those stimuli clinically implemented.

The detection of a pupillary dilation lag using pupillometry in patients with HS has been defined as the difference in anisocoria between 5 and 15 s after extinction of the light, and regarded positive when the value is equal to or more than 0.4 mm (1). By this definition, dilation lag had very high specificity for HS yet relatively low sensitivity (48%). In addition, dilation lag was found to be only intermittently present and not consistent from one test to the next in patients with HS, making it unreliable as a clinical diagnostic test (10). In our HS patient group, a positive dilation lag according to this definition was also found in some patients in single cycles of light and dark, yet when averaging the 4–5 test repeats performed for each subject, this value was <0.4 mm for all subjects, thus considered negative. Therefore, our results are in agreement with the previous findings about the intermittent nature of dilation lag in this patient group. This encouraged us to improve the diagnostic accuracy for HS with new pupillometry paradigms and better measurement algorithms.

The Procedure

Automated binocular pupillometry is a short and easy test to perform, and patient cooperation required is minimal. Electrical nerve stimulation is routinely used in neurology in the sympathetic skin response test (SSR) test among others, and its safety has been long established (17). The synchronization of the EMG machine to the pupillometer facilitates the precise timing of the electrical stimulation during cycles of light and dark. Both the pupillometer and the EMG machines are portable, making it possible to test immobile patients at the bedside.

Pupillometry With a "Buzz"

All HS patients exhibited anisocoria on pupillometry with cycles of light and dark alone, which significantly increased with the addition of an electrical stimulation. Electrical stimulation before the termination of light (0.5 s before light off) as well as simultaneously with light off produced a smaller enhancement of anisocoria when compared to stimulation at 2 s after light off. This smaller response is likely due to the parasympathetic tone induced by the light stimulus (18), which is no longer present 2 s after the light goes off. At 2 s after light off the pupils are close to the secondary dilation phase which is in the larger part due to sympathetic activity (18) resulting from the termination of light. The addition of the electrical stimulation during this phase seemed to produce the best synergistic sympathetic response between the termination of light and electrical stimulation, resulting in a significant increase in anisocoria. Similarly, electrical stimulation alone (during constant light) produced a larger increase in anisocoria with low background illumination than with higher illumination, which can as well be correlated with the higher parasympathetic tone induced by brighter light.

The triple electrical stimulation resulted in a larger increase in anisocoria compared to similar test paradigms with a single stimulus. The higher the intensity of the stimulus, the larger the increase in anisocoria both in patients and in the brimonidine group. Similar effects of stimulus intensity were demonstrated by Hirano et al. (15) where they showed that louder auditory stimuli produced larger pupillary dilation in healthy pupils.

Using pupillometry without electrical stimulation, we found that the biggest difference in relative anisocoria between patients with HS and healthy subjects occurred when comparing the anisocoria at 3–4 s after light off to that at the end of the light-on period. Using those time points, a 0.4 mm cut-off was found to be the upper limit of relative anisocoria in our normal subjects. This finding is also important since it confirms that the optimal test paradigm for electrical stimulation was where the stimulus was given 2 s after light off, compared to the best measurement of HS found on pupillometry without electrical stimulation.

Patients showed good tolerance to the single electrical stimulation, but tolerance to the triple stimulus was variable. Seven out of eighteen patients declined trying the triple stimulus simply due to the idea of a stronger stimulus, in spite of reporting no pain and minimal discomfort with the single electrical stimulus. Of the 11 patients who agreed to the triple stimulus, 2 patients found it intolerable and stopped, the other 9 completed the experiment and reported it to be "less pleasant" than the lower (single) stimulation, yet still tolerable. Of note, during the experiment the subjects underwent multiple stimulations during all the different test paradigms, which may have influenced the tolerance of patients and increased the discomfort. In a clinical setting, however, only few repetitions would be needed for making the diagnosis of HS, which might lead to less discomfort and higher tolerance for the electrical stimulation. In addition, of the healthy subjects group, all 10 subjects completed the experiment with the triple stimulus twice (before and after brimonidine drops), with only one subject reporting considerable discomfort.

SUMMARY

In a clinical setting, physicians are facing the challenge of ruling out HS in borderline cases, especially when pharmacological test results are equivocal. We found that compared to pupillometry alone, pupillometry with electrical stimulation 2 s after light off results in an increase of anisocoria in subjects with ocular sympathetic deficit, but not in healthy subjects, which may help distinguish healthy from HS patients.

We found that all patients with HS as well as subjects with brimonidine demonstrated an increase in anisocoria in response to electrical sympathetic stimulation as compared to similar test paradigms without stimulation. The increase in anisocoria in the brimonidine group was larger and more consistent than in HS group, which can be attributed to the complete nature of the sympathetic block induced by brimonidine, compared to the possibly partial sympathetic deficit in patients with HS. This could be due to the different degrees of nerve damage in different HS patients depending on the mechanism and duration of the nerve injury. Healthy subjects demonstrated no significant increase of anisocoria in response to electrical stimulation in contrast to HS patients or brimonidine treated subject on similar test paradigms.

LIMITATIONS

Due to the relatively small number of subjects in this study, it was not possible to assess the effect of different HS etiologies and durations on the responses to electrical stimulation. The reduced tolerability of patients to the triple stimulus resulted in fewer subjects undergoing such test paradigms. In the current study, we only had three patients with some physiological anisocoria, a topic that we plan to address in a follow-up study.

CONCLUSIONS

In this "proof of concept" study, we showed that patients with HS as well as pharmacological ocular sympathetic block demonstrate a significant increase in anisocoria in response to electrical stimulation as measured with binocular pupillometry, while healthy subjects demonstrated no significant anisocoria, reflecting that electrical stimulation may help increase the diagnostic accuracy of pupillometry for HS in a clinical setting.

AUTHOR CONTRIBUTIONS

RO: study design, data collection, data analysis, and paper writing; CB: data analysis, statistical analysis, and paper writing; KL: paper revision; RK: study design, paper revision; KW: study design, data analysis, and paper writing.

FUNDING

This study was supported by The Frieda Magdalena Cattaruzza Foundation and the Albert Bruppacher foundation, Switzerland (RO), The Swiss National Science Foundation [320030_166346] and the Uniscientia Stiftung, Vaduz, Liechtenstein (KW), The Department of Veterans Affairs USA C9251-C, Rehabilitation Research & Development (RR&D), VA-ORD and the Lavern and Audrey Busse Foundation (RK).

ACKNOWLEDGMENTS

Marco Penner for the technical support.

SUPPLEMENTARY MATERIAL

Supplementary Video 1 | Pupillometry without electrical stimulation in a patient with left Horner's syndrome. 5 cycles of light and dark alone without electrical stimulation.

Supplementary Video 2 | Pupillometry with electrical stimulation in a patient with left Horner's syndrome. A single electrical stimulation is delivered during constant low light-on (0.1 log-lux).

Supplementary Video 3 | Pupillometry with electrical stimulation in a patient with left Horner's syndrome. A triple electrical stimulation is delivered during constant low light-on (0.1 log-lux).

Supplementary Video 4 | Pupillometry with electrical stimulation in a patient with left Horner's syndrome. A single electrical stimulation is delivered during each cycle of light and dark, 2 seconds after the termination of light.

Supplementary Video 5 | Pupillometry with electrical stimulation in a patient with left Horner's syndrome. A triple electrical stimulation is delivered during each cycle of light and dark, 2 seconds after the termination of light.

REFERENCES

1. Kawasaki A, Kardon RH. Evaluation of a simple photographic technique to detect pupillary dilation lag due to Horner's syndrome. *Neuro-Ophthalmol.* (2004) 28:215–9. doi: 10.1080/01658100490887913
2. Szabadi E. Modulation of physiological reflexes by pain: role of the locus coeruleus. *Front Integr Neurosci.* (2012) 6:94. doi: 10.3389/fnint.2012.00094
3. Jänig W. The sympathetic nervous system in pain. *Eur J Anaesthesiol Suppl.* (1995) 10:53–60.
4. McDonald JE, El-Moatassem Kotb AM, Decker BB. Effect of brimonidine tartrate ophthalmic solution 0.2% on pupil size in normal eyes under different luminance conditions. *J Cataract Refract Surg.* (2001) 27:560–4. doi: 10.1016/S0886-3350(01)00769-6

5. Gerente VM, Biondi AC, Barbosa CP, Lottenberg CL, Paranhos A. Effect of brimonidine tartrate 0.15% on scotopic pupil: controlled trial. *J Ocul Pharmacol Ther Off J Assoc Ocul Pharmacol Ther.* (2007) 23:476–80. doi: 10.1089/jop.2007.0017.R1
6. Wilhelm H. The pupil. *Curr Opin Neurol.* (2008) 21:36–42. doi: 10.1097/WCO.0b013e3282f39173
7. Buchmann SJ, Penzlin AI, Kubasch ML, Illigens BM-W, Siepmann T. Assessment of sudomotor function. *Clin Auton Res.* (2019) 29:41–53. doi: 10.1007/s10286-018-0530-2
8. Donadio V, Lenzi P, Montagna P, Falzone F, Baruzzi A, Liguori R. Habituation of sympathetic sudomotor and vasomotor skin responses: neural and non-neural components in healthy subjects. *Clin. Neurophysiol. Off. J. Int. Fed. Clin. Neurophysiol.* (2005) 116:2542–9. doi: 10.1016/j.clinph.2005.07.009
9. Fitzgibbon A, Pilu M, Fisher RB. Direct least square fitting of ellipses. *IEEE Trans Pattern Anal Mach Intell.* (1999) 21:476–80.
10. Crippa SV, Borruat F-X, Kawasaki A. Pupillary dilation lag is intermittently present in patients with a stable oculosympathetic defect (Horner syndrome). *Am J Ophthalmol.* (2007) 143:712–5. doi: 10.1016/j.ajo.2006.10.049
11. Freedman KA, Brown SM. Topical apraclonidine in the diagnosis of suspected Horner syndrome. *J Neuroophthalmol.* (2005) 25:83–5. doi: 10.1016/j.ajo.2005.08.011
12. Martin TJ. Horner syndrome: a clinical review. *ACS Chem Neurosci.* (2018) 9:177–86. doi: 10.1021/acschemneuro.7b00405
13. Dewan MA, Harrison AR, Lee MS. False-negative apraclonidine testing in acute Horner syndrome. *Can J Ophthalmol J Can Ophtalmol.* (2009) 44:109–10. doi: 10.3129/i08-162
14. Kawasaki A, Borruat F-X. False negative apraclonidine test in two patients with Horner syndrome. *Klin Monatsbl Augenheilkd.* (2008) 225:520–2. doi: 10.1055/s-2008-1027349
15. Hirano T, Inoue H, Uemura T, Matsunaga K. Pupillary responses in normal subjects following auditory stimulation. *Eur Arch Otorhinolaryngol.* (1994) 251(Suppl. 1):S3–6.
16. Pilley SF, Thompson HS. Pupillary 'dilatation lag' in Horner's syndrome. *Br. J. Ophthalmol.* (1975) 59:731–5.
17. Al-Shekhlee A, Shapiro BE, Preston DC. Iatrogenic complications and risks of nerve conduction studies and needle electromyography. *Muscle Nerve* (2003) 27:517–26. doi: 10.1002/mus.10315
18. Heller PH, Perry F, Jewett DL, Levine JD. Autonomic components of the human pupillary light reflex. *Invest Ophthalmol Vis Sci.* (1990) 31:156–62.

6

Chromatic Pupillometry in Children

*Sylvain V. Crippa[1,2], Fatima Pedrosa Domellöf[3] and Aki Kawasaki[1]**

[1] Neuro-Ophthalmology Unit, Jules-Gonin Eye Hospital, University of Lausanne, Lausanne, Switzerland, [2] Group for Retinal Disorder Research, Jules-Gonin Eye Hospital, University of Lausanne, Lausanne, Switzerland, [3] Ophthalmology, Department of Clinical Science, Umeå University, Umeå, Sweden

***Correspondence:**
Aki Kawasaki
aki.kawasaki@fa2.ch

Chromatic pupillometry is a technique that is increasingly used to assess retinal disorders. As age may be one of the various factors which can influence the pupillary light reaction, this study aimed to evaluate the pupil responses to colored light stimuli in the pediatric population. Fifty-three children with normal vision and without any history of ocular disorders were tested with a portable pupillometer. Four test sequences were used: five dim blue (470 nm) stimuli presented in half log steps ranging from −3.15 to −1.15 log cd/m^2 after 3 min of dark adaptation, five red (622 nm) stimuli of −1.15, −0.7, −0.15, 0.3, and 0.85 log cd/m^2 after 1 min light adaptation, one bright blue stimulus of 2.2 log cd/m^2 and one bright red of 2 log cd/m^2. The results were grouped by age: a younger group included 27 children aged from 3 to 10 years old and an older group included 26 from 10 and 1 month to 18 years old. The younger group had a smaller pupil diameter after dark adaptation compared with the older group. A linear regression defining the photopic threshold showed that younger subjects had a higher threshold, e.g., needed a brighter red stimulus to evoke a threshold pupil response comparable that of subjects. Age thus seems to influence outer retinal sensitivity at least as evaluated by the pupillary photopic threshold intensity. The post-illumination pupillary reaction was used as a marker of intrinsic melanopsin activity and did not show any difference between the two age groups.

Keywords: pupil, chromatic pupillometry, children, pupillary light reaction, growth

INTRODUCTION

The use of colored light stimuli under conditions of dark and light adaptation facilitates rod versus cone mediation of retinal light signaling. More than 3 decades ago, Drs Lowenstein and Loewenfeld were recording the pupil response to focal green light flashes presented parafoveally at sub-photopic intensities to define the response curve of rods (1). In 1987, Birch and Birch (2) described a method using the steady-state pupil diameter after dark adaptation to determine the pupillometric threshold of rods, both in normal eyes and in eyes with retinal degeneration. The threshold was the retinal illumination necessary to evoke a criterion pupil response (defined as a decrease in pupil size by 1.0 mm). Adults with retinitis pigmentosa with reduced scotopic amplitude on electroretinography had elevated pupillometric rod threshold (mean 2.23 log units). Patients with nondetectable responses on electroretinography had pupil thresholds 3.27 log units higher than controls.

These early pioneering works which measured the pupil response to colored light stimuli under conditions of dark- and light-adaptation were the basis for quantifying rod and cone activity from the pupil light reflex. The discovery of the photopigment melanopsin and the identification of a non-rod, non-cone retinal photoreceptor have renewed interest in the pupil as a biomarker and have demonstrated that examination of the post-stimulus pupillary dynamics provides additional information about retinal light sensitivity.

In the 1960s, Bouma described that the steady-state pupil size that was largely determined by the scotopic spectral sensitivity using a large test field (3). Notably, he defined the pupil size against the intensity for different wavelengths and extracted the static pupillary sensitivity curve showing a peak at 490 nm. This is remarkably similar to the spectral sensitivity curve of melanopsin.

In terms of afferent pupillary signaling from the retina, melanopsin appears to be the predominant contribution for steady state pupil size and for sustained pupillary constriction following light stimulus offset. Various methods have been described to quantify this post-illumination pupil response (PIPR) which has a spectral sensitivity matching that of melanopsin (4–7).

Pupillometry using colored light stimulation has technologically advanced since the early experiments of the 60s and 70s. Chromatic pupillometry is now available as a small desktop or portable model (8–10). The simplicity of the technique broadens the patient population to be tested and is thus well-suited for use in patients with limited mobility. However, testing protocols still tend to be longer than most typical clinical tests and the dark adaptation needed to improve rod sensitivity could be difficult in patients with limited comprehension or attention span, such as patients with cognitive decline and young children. Yet it is the pediatric population in whom chromatic pupillometry may be a potentially important tool to evaluate outer and inner retinal activity in a variety of retinal and neurologic disorders (11).

Portable chromatic pupillometry for children may be an alternative to electroretinography for assessing photoreceptor function. The distinct advantage of pupillometry is that electrodes are not necessary. One foreseeable application is the school vision screening test. The ease of portable pupillometry permits on-site testing of children who fail the screening test. Chromatic pupillometry may also be used to monitor children with retinal degenerative disorders. In patients with endstage photoreceptor degeneration, chromatic pupillometry has been shown to be more sensitive than full-field electroretinography in detecting residual levels of cone function (12). Conversely chromatic pupillometry has promise as a tool to detect recovery of photoreceptor function in children who undergo gene therapy who are still too young to provide reliable responses to subjective tests of vision.

Thus, this pilot study was undertaken to evaluate chromatic pupillometry in children using a portable pupillometer.

SUBJECTS AND METHOD

The study was conducted according to the tenets of the Declaration of Helsinki and received authorization from the Regional Ethical Review Board for human research. Because study participants were under-age minors, one parent of each subject provided oral and written informed consent for participation in the study. Healthy children from families and acquaintances of the staff of the eye clinic of the University Hospital of Umeå (NUS) in Umeå were invited to participate in the study. Premature birth, a history of ocular trauma or diagnosis, use of ophthalmic or systemic medications were exclusionary criteria. Visual acuity, a Donders confrontation test, microscopic examination of anterior segment and examination of the macula and optic nerve head with 90D lens was performed and were normal for all children included in the study. No child was wearing glasses for refractive error at the time of the study. Refraction with cyclopentolate was not performed. Fifty-three children aged 3–18 years old were included. Because the axial length of the eye reaches its adult size at 10 years of age (13), the children were divided into two groups: those aged 10 years or less, here forth called the younger group and those over age 10 years called the older group. Detailed information was provided to the child and the accompanying parent prior to the recordings. The smaller children were given the opportunity to explore the environment and to "test" the different steps of the procedure before starting.

Pupil recordings were made using the IDMed Neurolight (Marseille, France) portable device. The light source is composed of three trichromatic light emitting diodes with a 6 log unit range of intensity placed in a kurbisfeld. For this study, only the blue (470 nm) and red (622 nm) lights were used. In this kurbisfeld, an infrared camera records the pupil continuously at 67 Hz with telecentric optics. A touchscreen graphical user interface is situated on the back of the stimulation chamber. It allows the examiner to enter the name of the subject and to select the pre-programmed stimulus sequence. This touchscreen offers a window where the pupil image is shown continuously during the recording. An occlusive rubber ocular is placed over the eye to be tested and the subject is instructed to look straight ahead. The examiner may stabilize head movement by placing a hand gently on the subject's forehead. In this study, the right eye was the tested eye.

We developed four test sequences (**Supplemental Figure 1**), modified from a previously-described stimulus protocol which was used to evaluate photoreceptor function in patients with rod-cone degeneration due to NR2E3 mutation (14). The relatively short times for dark and light adaptation in this study were selected from pre-study trial-and-error experiences noting child comfort and cooperation as well as the practicality of pupil testing in a clinical outpatient setting. We have retained the naming of the stimulus light sequence as "scotopic" and "photopic" for those following dark and light adaptation respectively. For this study, we use these light sequences with shortened adaptation times to grossly assess outer photoreceptor function: the scotopic sequence with blue lights biased toward rod function and the photopic sequence with red lights biased to cone function. We acknowledge that the shortened adaptation times used in this study are, however, not standard and not validated for true measuring of rod and cone function.

The first test sequence is performed after dark adaptation. For dark adaptation in this study, both eyes of the child are covered with sticky patches and the child sits quietly, accompanied by a parent if needed, in a dark, windowless room (0 cd/m2) for 3 min. The testing is performed in darkness as the pupilometer is placed over the right eye and the left (non-tested) eye remains under occlusion with a sticky patch. The pupil recording is started and the scotopic test sequence begins with 5 s of darkness (0 log cd/m2) followed by a series of five stimulations from a dim blue light having an intensity from −3.15 to −1.15 log cd/m^2, in increasing half log steps. Each stimulation is 1 s in duration. The inter-stimulus interval is 3 s as this had been previously determined to be sufficient time to permit the pupil to return to baseline size before the arrival of the next light stimulus. The pupillometer is then removed from the right eye, the occlusive patch is removed from the left eye and the room light is turned on (900 lux) to start light adaptation for 1 min before the second test sequence. The second test sequence (photopic sequence) also begins with pupil recording during 5 s of darkness (0 log cd/m2) which is followed by a series of 5 stimulations from a red light having an intensity starting at −1.15 followed by −0.7, −0.15, 0.3, and 0.85 log cd/m^2. Each stimulation is 1 s in duration and the inter-stimulus interval is 3 s. The eyes are again light adapted for 1 min before the third and before the fourth pupil tests sequences, each of which consists of a single light stimulation (1 s) having a high intensity and recording the pupillary response during the light stimulus and for 20 s in darkness after the light stimulus. The prolonged post-light recording of the pupil allows determination of the post-illumination pupil response (see PIPR calculation below). For the third test sequence, the stimulus is a blue light 160 cd/m^2 and for the fourth test sequence, a red light stimulus 102 cd/m^2, respectively 2.2 and 2 log cd/m2. In sum, the full protocol of this study consists of 12 stimuli divided into four test sequences; two with 5 stimuli and two with a single stimulus.

The pupil recordings were qualitatively assessed for validity of recording after each of the 4 testing sequences. For the first and second test sequences, pupil recordings having artifacts other than rapid blinks which occurred during 2 s of light stimulus onset were considered invalid responses and were removed from further analysis.

Scotopic and photopic test sequences having less than 4 valid responses out of five stimuli were considered invalid recordings. In cases where the first recording was deemed invalid, a second recording of the same test sequence was performed on the same eye (data not shown).

The pupil data were exported and analyzed in a spreadsheet (Microsoft Excel 2010; Microsoft, Redmond, WA). Blink artifacts were removed from the raw pupil tracings with a customized semi-automated filter function. The baseline pupil size (diameter) was determined from the first test sequence following dark-adaption and defined as the mean diameter during 250 ms just before the first light stimulus. This baseline pupil size was used to determine the pupil contraction amplitude. The maximal contraction amplitude is reported in this study as the maximal decrease in pupil size (in %) within 2 s of the light stimulus onset and calculated by the following formula: % maximal contraction amplitude at time x = ([baseline pupil diameter minus pupil diameter at time x]/[baseline pupil diameter]) × 100. A criterion level of 5% contraction amplitude was applied to distinguish evoked pupil responses from random noise.

The post illumination pupil response (PIPR) (7, 15) was calculated for the two last test sequences (single stimulus sequences having either a blue light or a red light). The PIPR (in %) was calculated as following: 100 – ([mean pupil diameter between 5.75 and 6.25 s after termination of the light stimulus/baseline pupil diameter] × 100) (6). The PIPR is a clinical marker of the melanopsin contribution to the pupil light response and is generally greater following a blue light stimulus compared to a red light stimulus as melanopsin has relatively poor sensitivity to long wavelength light (7).

Outcome parameters were compared using student *t*-test for normalized data. The significance threshold was defined as ≤0.05.

RESULTS

In the younger group (<10 years old) there were 9 boys and 18 girls and in the older group (>10 and <18 years old), 13 girls and 13 boys. The ages of children in the younger group ranged from 3 years and 4 months old to 10 years old (mean ± SD: 80 ± 23 months; the oldest of this group had her recording during her 10th anniversary month) and the older group were aged from 10 years and 1 month old to 17 years old and 10 months (153 ± 26 months).

The first test sequence was valid in every subject except two; one in the younger group and one in the older. For the second photopic test sequence, three children in the younger group had an invalid recording. For the two last test sequences, the older group had no difficulties, but four in the younger group had invalid recording due to prolonged eye closure: one with the bright blue stimulus of the third test sequence and three with both bright red and blue sequences.

All subjects had at least two valid sequences for analysis except one 9 year old subject who only had the 1st sequence deemed valid. Forty-five subjects could complete the full protocol (four test sequences); these were 21 of 27 (78%) in the younger group and 25 of 26 (96%) in the older group.

Pupil Size

The younger group showed a significantly smaller baseline pupil size, 7.2 ± 0.8 mm compared to the older group of 7.6 ± 0.8 mm ($p = 0.03$).

Contraction Amplitude

In the scotopic test sequence, the pupil contraction amplitude increased with increasing stimulus intensity for both subject groups (**Figure 1**). This relationship appeared to be linear with a mean individual coefficient of determination of $r^2 = 0.92 \pm 0.07$ (0.92 ± 0.07 for the younger group and 0.93 ± 0.07 for the older group; $p = 0.59$). The slopes were compared and considered as equal ($p = 0.61$).

For the photopic test sequence, the contraction amplitude increased with increasing stimulus intensity for both groups. This relationship appeared to be linear with a mean individual coefficient of determination of $r^2 = 0.88 \pm 0.10$ (0.86 ± 0.11 for

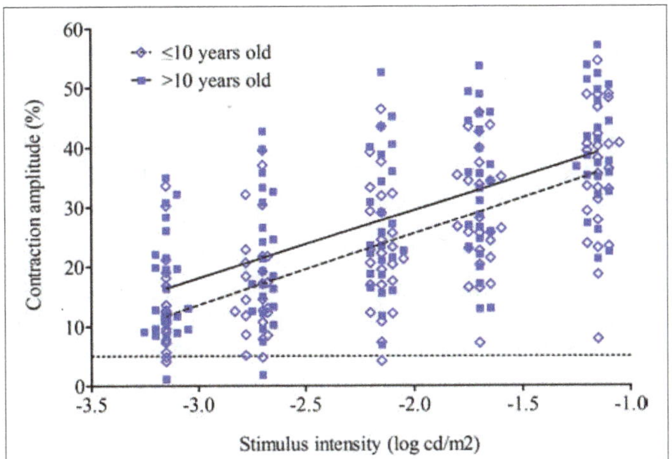

FIGURE 1 | Maximal contraction amplitude to dim blue lights (scotopic test sequence) for 52 subjects (26 in younger group and 26 in older group). The mean contraction amplitude for younger (open diamonds) and older (closed squares) groups is plotted as a regression line across a range of intensities. The dashed line is the younger group; the solid line is the older group. The dotted line represents the threshold (5%) for defining an evoked pupil response.

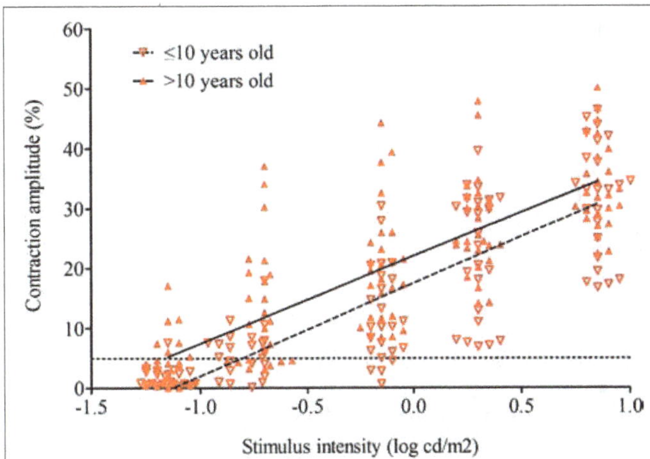

FIGURE 2 | Maximal contraction amplitude to dim red lights (photopic test sequence) for 50 subjects (24 in younger group and 26 in older group). The mean contraction amplitude for younger (open triangles) and older (closed triangles) groups is plotted as a regression line across a range of intensities. The dashed line is the younger group; the solid line is the older group. The dotted line represents the threshold (5%) for defining an evoked pupil response.

the younger group and 0.90 ± 0.10 for the older group; $p = 0.23$); the slopes were compared and considered as equal ($p = 0.91$; **Figure 2**). Only one subject aged 6 years in the younger group had an observable pupil reaction (defined as >5% decrease in pupil diameter) to the dimmest red stimulus having intensity of −1.15 log cd/m^2 whereas seven older subjects clearly show an evoked response at this dimmest red light stimulus. This and the generally lower pupil responses in the younger group suggest that threshold intensity for a pupil contraction to red light stimulation under conditions of light adaptation is slightly higher for younger children and overall retinal light sensitivity is lower.

Threshold

From the regression lines determined for the scotopic and photopic test sequences, the threshold intensity could be extrapolated to the intercept at y = 5 which is the dimmest stimulus that produces a 5% pupil contraction. Only subjects with at least on 4 out of 5 valid stimuli were considered for this analysis. Twenty-six of 27 the younger group were included for the scotopic test sequence and 24 of 27 for the photopic test sequence. For the older group, these were 25 of 26 and 26 of 26 for the scotopic and photopic test sequences, respectively.

The mean threshold intensity for the scotopic test sequence is −3.75 ± 0.96 log cd/m^2 for the younger group and −4.14 ± 1.03.log cd/m^2 for the older group ($p = 0.17$) and for the photopic test sequence, the mean threshold is −0.77 ± 0.25 log cd/m^2 for the younger group and −1.17 ± 0.48 log cd/m^2 for the older group ($p = <0.01$; **Figure 3**).

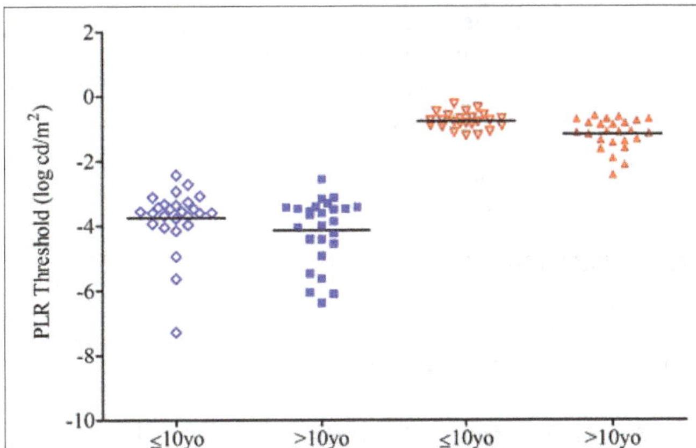

FIGURE 3 | Dot plot of the threshold for 26 subjects of the younger group and 26 from the older one. Threshold intensity is the light intensity needed to produce a 5% contraction amplitude using a regression line. See **Figures 1**, **2**. Horizontal bars represent the mean for younger (open symbols) and older (closed symbols) groups.

PIPR

The post-illumination pupil response for the third test sequence (single blue light stimulus) was larger (10.47 ± 7.04%), i.e., pupil size remained smaller after light offset, compared to that for the fourth test sequence having a single red light stimulus (2.45 ± 4.52%). This difference was statistically significant ($p = <0.01$). The older group showed a larger blue light PIPR in response (11.09 ± 7.92%) compared to younger group (9.75 ± 5.92%) but the difference was not statistically significant ($p = 0.51$). For the PIPR to bright red light, the older group showed a larger PIPR (2.97 ± 3.98%) compared to the younger group: 1.91 ± 5.05%; but again, the difference was not significant ($p = 0.42$; **Figure 4**).

The PIPR in response to the last red light test sequence for all children was expectedly very small (mean 2.45 ± 4.52%), and this is consistent with results from other studies made with primates and adult humans (6, 15, 16) The bright red light test sequence

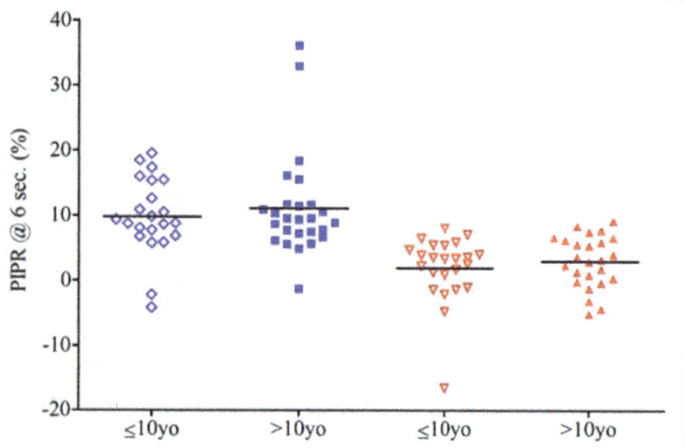

FIGURE 4 | PIPR to blue light for 23 subjects in younger group and 26 subjects in older group and PIPR to red light for 24 in younger group and 26 in older group. Horizontal bars show the mean. Subjects in the younger group are shown in open diamond for the blue stimulation and open triangle for the red one. Those in the older group are respectively shown as closed squares and closed triangles.

PIPR generally serves as a control stimulus in which melanopsin stimulation is presumed to be null-to-minimal. In order to relate the melanopsin contribution from the blue light stimulus to the control response, we also evaluated difference in between the blue light PIPR and the red light PIPR (difference PIPR). There is no difference in the difference PIPR between the younger groups (7.59 ± 8.81%) and the older group (8.21 ± 8.01%; $p = 0.80$).

DISCUSSION

This study used a portable, hand-held device to record the pupil response to a range of chromatic light stimuli in children. The ages of the children ranged from 3 years and 4 months to 17 years and 10 months old. The dark and light adaptation times were reduced in order to enhance subject cooperation. The two light-adapted test sequences using a single bright stimulus, one blue and one red, showed the most artifacts in the younger group. Three children for whom a valid recording was not possible in these two test sequence were aged of 6 years and 11 months, 8 years and 9 months, and 9 years and 8 months; showing that nonetheless the youngest of the participants (aged 3 years and 4 months) could cooperate enough to complete tests sequences with bright lights and a long post stimulus dark period.

The mean scotopic baseline pupil diameter was larger in the older group compared to the younger group; respectively a pupillary diameter of 7.2 ± 0.8 mm for the younger and 7.6 ± 0.8 mm for the older group ($p = 0.03$). This finding is consistent with the published literature (1, 17, 18).

From linear regression analysis, the intensity for a threshold pupil response (threshold intensity) was determined. We found the scotopic threshold showed a tendency to be higher in the younger group compared to the older group (−3.75 ± 0.96 log cd/m^2 vs. −4.14 ± 1.03 log cd/m2, respectively, $p = 0.17$). The range of scotopic threshold values of the older group of children in this study were similar to those of adults (−4.7 ± 0.4 log cd/m2) who were tested with a ganzfeld stimulator and more rigorous protocol of light and dark adaptation (14).

The similarity in threshold intensity between children tested with the portable pupillometer and previously reported values in adults suggest that the abbreviated testing protocol of this study may be sufficient to assess rod-weighted pupil responses. For the threshold intensity of the photopic test sequence, we found a higher threshold in the younger group (−0.79 ± 0.28 log cd/m^2) compared to the older group (−1.17 ± 0.48 log cd/m^2) and this difference was significant ($p = <0.01$). Our finding that younger children have a higher scotopic and photopic threshold intensity may have importance when interpreting results of chromatic pupillometry for clinical purposes in children.

While it is beyond the scope of this study to examine the reason behind this age-related difference in threshold values, we may postulate on several possibilities for why the younger group requires a greater light intensity to evoke a minimum 5% pupillary contraction. These include: decreased neural signal from the retina to the olivary pretectal nucleus, greater supranuclear inhibition of the afferent pupillomotor signal at the level of the olivary pretectal nucleus, lesser neural signal from the Edinger-Westphal nucleus or greater mechanical resistance to pupillary movement at the level of the iris. We favor the first emitted hypothesis that decreased retinal light sensitivity related to ongoing postnatal retinal development is the basis for the higher thresholds seen in younger children. Anatomic and functional studies provide some support data (19–21).

From a histopathologic study, cone density at the fovea is 108,400/mm^2 at age 3.8 years which is still far under the density of 208,200/mm^2 in adults (19, 20). However, cone packing is completed before age 10 years after which the fovea attains its adult characteristics. From an electrophysiologic study, it has been shown that the rod and cone response (b-wave amplitude) increases between age 1 and 20 years with peak values occurring between age 10 and 20 years (21). Specifically, the rod b-wave median amplitude was 45% higher in children aged 10–20 years compared to those aged 1–10 years. Similarly the cone b-wave median amplitude and the cone a-wave median amplitude by electroretinography were larger in the older group by 21 and 26%, respectively. These anatomic and functional studies suggest that the outer retina in children under age 10 is still developing and is yet less light sensitive than a fully mature one.

In all four test sequences the older group had a larger pupillary contraction compared to the younger group. In the scotopic test sequence, the pupil contraction amplitude increased with increasing stimulus intensity for younger and older groups (**Figure 1**). This relationship appeared to be linear for both groups (younger group: slope 14.73 ± 5.19, $r^2 = 0.92 \pm 0.07$; older group: slope 14.87 ± 3.0, $r^2 = 0.93 \pm 0.07$). There was no difference in the slope or the variance between the two groups ($p = 0.61$ and $p = 0.59$, respectively).

For the photopic test sequence, the contraction amplitude increased with increasing stimulus intensity for younger and older groups (**Figure 2**). This relationship appeared to be linear for both groups (younger group: slope 12.11 ± 3.68, $r^2 = 0.86 \pm 0.11$; older group: slope 11.66 ± 2.35, $r^2 = 0.90 \pm 0.10$).

There was no difference in the slope or the variance between the two groups, $p = 0.91$ and $p = 0.23$, respectively. Only one subject aged 6 years in the younger group had an observable pupil reaction (defined as >5% decrease in pupil diameter) to the dimmest red stimulus having intensity of -1.15 log cd/m^2 whereas seven older subjects clearly show an evoked response at this dimmest red light stimulus. This and the generally lower pupil responses in the younger group suggest that threshold intensity for a pupil contraction to red light stimulation under conditions of light adaptation is slightly higher for younger children and overall retinal light sensitivity is lower.

The blue light PIPR in this study was relatively small, suggesting suboptimal stimulation of melanopsin. We selected the intensities for these two test sequences in part from a widely shared methodology (6) and in part from consideration for light tolerance in children. There were no differences between the two age groups in the PIPR determined from the single stimulus sequences. This is contrary to the age-related differences observed with the scotopic and photopic sequences. We can postulate that the absence of an age effect on PIPR indicates that melanopsin-mediated phototransduction matures early in human development. It is also possible that the PIPR determined by this methodology is not sensitive enough to detect developmental changes in melanopsin light sensitivity (22). For purposes of using PIPR as a clinical biomarker of melanopsin activity, we suggest that a larger population of children be tested so that trends in PIPR as a function of age can be verified as absent or present.

Overall, we found that portable pupillometry using four short test sequences permits, in children as young as age 3 years, a valid recording of pupil responses to light stimuli biased to favor one photoreceptive element: rods or cones or melanopsin. Ocular development, estimated by age, seems to influence outer retinal sensitivity at least as evaluated by the pupillary and in general, supports lower threshold intensity (greater light sensitivity of the outer retina) in children after age 10 years. The melanopsin sensitivity estimated from the blue light PIPR was not influenced by age.

AUTHOR CONTRIBUTIONS

AK and FP conceived, designed, and supervised the project. FP performed the experiments. All authors participated in the analysis and interpretation of the experiments. SC and AK wrote the manuscript. All authors critically revised and approved the final manuscript version.

SUPPLEMENTARY MATERIAL

Supplemental Figure 1 | Graphical presentation of the full pupil protocol consisting of four test sequences. Each numbered line represents one of the four test sequences. The 1st test sequence starts after 3 min of dark adaptation (DA; 0 lux) whereas the following 3 sequences start after 1 min of light adaptation (LA; 900 lux). The pupil recording is represented by the x axis; the scale bar equals 1 s. Each pupil recording starts with 5 s of darkness before the first light stimulus is presented. The vertical bars represent the light stimuli; the intensity is given above each stimulus and each stimulus is 1 s in duration. The inter-stimulus interval for sequences 1 and 2 is 3 s. Recording during non-stimulus segments occurs in darkness (0 lux).

REFERENCES

1. Loewenfeld IE, Lowenstein O. *The Pupil: Anatomy, Physiology, and Clinical Application.* Ames, IA; Detroit, MI: Iowa State University Press; Wayne State University Press (1993).
2. Birch EE, Birch DG. Pupillometric measures of retinal sensitivity in infants and adults with retinitis pigmentosa. *Vision Res.* (1987) 27:499–505. doi: 10.1016/0042-6989(87)90034-4
3. Bouma H. Size of the static pupil as a function of wave-length and luminosity of the light incident on the human eye. *Nature* (1962) 193:690–1. doi: 10.1038/193690a0
4. Kardon RH, Anderson SC, Damarjian TG, Grace EM, Stone E, Kawasaki A. Chromatic pupillometry in patients with retinitis pigmentosa. *Ophthalmology* (2011)118:376–81. doi: 10.1016/j.ophtha.2010.06.033
5. Kankipati L, Girkin CA, Gamlin PD. The post-illumination pupil response is reduced in glaucoma patients. *Invest Ophthalmol Vis Sci.* (2011) 52:2287–92. doi: 10.1167/iovs.10-6023
6. Park JC, Moura AL, Raza AS, Rhee DW, Kardon RH, Hood DC. Toward a clinical protocol for assessing rod, cone, and melanopsin contributions to the human pupil response. *Invest Ophthalmol Vis Sci.* (2011) 52:6624–35. doi: 10.1167/iovs.11-7586
7. Adhikari P, Zele AJ, Feigl B. The Post-Illumination Pupil Response (PIPR). *Invest Ophthalmol Vis Sci.* (2015) 56:3838–49. doi: 10.1167/iovs.14-16233
8. Narita A, Shirai K, Kubota N, Takayama R, Takahashi Y, Onuki T, et al. Abnormal pupillary light reflex with chromatic pupillometry in Gaucher disease. *Ann Clin Transl Neurol.* (2014) 1:135–40. doi: 10.1002/acn3.33
9. Tsika C, Crippa SV, Kawasaki A. Differential monocular vs. binocular pupil responses from melanopsin-based photoreception in patients with anterior ischemic optic neuropathy. *Sci Rep.* (2015) 5:10780. doi: 10.1038/srep 10780
10. Münch M, Kourti P, Brouzas P, Kawasaki A. Variation in the pupil light reflex between winter and summer seasons. *Acta Ophthalmol.* (2016) 94:244–6. doi: 10.1111/aos.12966
11. Ikeda T, Ishikawa H, Shimizu K, Asakawa A, Goseki T. Pupillary size and light reflex in premature infants. *Neuroophthalmology* (2015) 39:175–8. doi: 10.3109/01658107.2015.1055363
12. Kawasaki A, Munier FL, Leon L, Kardon RH. Pupillometric quantification of residual rod and cone activity in Leber congenital amaurosis. *Arch Ophthalmol.* (2012) 130:798–800. doi: 10.1001/archophthalmol.2011.1756
13. Gordon RA, Donzis PB. Refractive development of the human eye. *Arch Ophthalmol.* (1985) 103:785–9. doi: 10.1001/archopht.1985.010500600 45020
14. Kawasaki A, Crippa SV, Kardon R, Leon L, Hamel C. Characterization of pupil responses to blue and red light stimuli in autosomal dominant retinitis pigmentosa due to NR2E3 mutation. *Invest Ophthalmol Vis Sci.* (2012) 53:5562–9. doi: 10.1167/iovs.12-10230
15. Gamlin PD, McDougal DH, Pokorny J, Smith VC, Yau KW, Dacey DM. Human and macaque pupil responses driven by melanopsin-containing retinal ganglion Cells. *Vision Res.* (2007) 47:946–54. doi: 10.1016/j.visres.2006.12.015

16. Kardon R, Anderson SC, Damarjian TG, Grace EM, Stone E, Kawasaki A. Chromatic pupil responses: preferential activation of the melanopsin-mediated versus outer photoreceptor-mediated pupil light reflex. *Ophthalmology* (2009) 116:1564–73. doi: 10.1016/j.ophtha.2009.02.007
17. Kohnen EM, Zubcov AA, Kohnen T. Scotopic pupil size in a normal pediatric population using infrared pupillometry. *Graefes Arch Clin Exp Ophthalmol.* (2004) 242:18–23. doi: 10.1007/s00417-003-0735-4
18. Suh SH, Suh DW, Benson C. The degree of anisocoria in pediatric patients with Horner syndrome when compared to children without disease. *J Pediatr Ophthalmol Strabismus* (2016) 53:186–9. doi: 10.3928/01913913-20160405-07
19. Hendrickson A, Possin D, Vajzovic L, Toth C. Histological development of the human fovea from midgestation to maturity. *Am J Ophthalmol.* (2012) 154:767–78. doi: 10.1016/j.ajo.2012.05.007
20. Yuodelis C, Hendrickson A. A qualitative and quantitative analysis of the human fovea during development. *Vision Res.* (1986) 26:847–55. doi: 10.1016/0042-6989(86)90143-4
21. Fulton AB, Hansen RM, Westall CA. Development of ERG responses: the ISCEV rod, maximal and cone responses in normal subjects. *Doc Ophthalmol.* (2003) 107:235–41. doi: 10.1023/B:DOOP.0000005332.88367.b8
22. Schmidt TM, Taniguci K, Kofuji P. Intrinsic and extrinsic light responses in melanopsin-expressing ganglion cells during mouse development. *J Neurophysiol.* (2008) 100:371–84. doi: 10.1152/jn.00062.2008

7

Maturation of the Pupil Light Reflex Occurs Until Adulthood in Mice

Noémie Kircher[1], Sylvain V. Crippa[1,2], Catherine Martin[1], Aki Kawasaki[2] and Corinne Kostic[1]*

[1] Group for Retinal Disorder Research, Department of Ophthalmology, Hôpital Ophtalmique Jules Gonin, University of Lausanne, Lausanne, Switzerland, [2] Neuro-Ophtalmology, Department of Ophthalmology, Hôpital Ophtalmique Jules Gonin, University of Lausanne, Lausanne, Switzerland

***Correspondence:**
Corinne Kostic
corinne.kostic@fa2.ch

With respect to photoreceptor function, it is well known that electroretinogram (ERG) amplitudes decrease with age, but to our knowledge, studies describing age-related changes in the pupil light response (PLR) of mice are lacking. This study recorded the PLR and ERG in C57BL/6 and Sv129S6 wild-type mice at three different ages during early adulthood. Dark- and light-adapted PLR and ERG measurements were performed at 1, 2, and 4 months of age. For PLR measurements, we used either a red (622 nm) or blue (463 nm) light stimulus (500 ms) to stimulate one eye. We selected various light intensities ranging across almost 4 log units and subsequently classified them as low, medium, or high intensity. From the recorded PLR, we selected parameters to quantify the early and late phases of the response such as the baseline pupil size, the maximal constriction amplitude, the maximal velocity, the early partial dilation (area under the curve of the positive peak of the first derivative of PLR tracing), and the sustained constriction amplitude. For ERG measurements, both scotopic and photopic responses were recorded following stimulation with green light (520 nm) at preselected intensities. The amplitudes and latencies of the a-wave and the b-wave were also analyzed. In both strains, 1-month-old animals presented with a smaller baseline pupil diameter compared to that in 2- and 4-month-old mice. They also exhibited greater maximal constriction amplitude in response to red stimuli of medium intensity. Further, 1-month-old Sv129S6 mice responded with greater constriction amplitude to all other red and blue stimuli. One-month-old C57BL/6 mice also demonstrated faster early partial dilation and smaller sustained response to low blue stimuli. The ERG of 1-month-old C57BL/6 mice showed a greater scotopic a-wave amplitude compared to that of 2-month-old mice, whereas no significant differences were found in Sv129S6 mice. These results suggest that the functional maturation of the neuronal pathway that mediates the PLR continues after 1 month of age. In studies that measure PLR to determine retinal integrity in adult mice, it is thus important to determine normative values in animals of 2 months of age.

Keywords: pupil light response, electroretinography, C57BL6, Sv129S6, age-related changes, retina, maturation

INTRODUCTION

The electroretinogram is a standardized test to described outer photoreceptor function, and normative values for rod and cone activity have been established in adult humans (1, 2). This technique has the advantage of recording the electrical activity of photoreceptors and interneurons, eliminating potential post-retinal effects. However, when vision is severely affected and reaches the level of light perception, the full-field electroretinogram (ERG) response becomes undetectable, as observed in patients affected by retinitis pigmentosa (3–7).

Alternatively, the pupillary light response (PLR) can provide a functional evaluation of outer and inner photoreceptors (7, 8). By modifying the wavelength, intensity, and background conditions of the light stimulus, the specific contribution of different photoreceptors to the PLR can be altered to favor rods, cones, or intrinsically photosensitive retinal ganglion cells (ipRGCs) (6, 9–12). However, a standardized protocol and normative values to assess the PLR in adult humans has not been defined.

In a previous study, we developed a PLR protocol for mice to characterize changes in the pupil response that are related to rod and cone degenerative diseases. When *Rho*$^{-/-}$ (rodless) mice were exposed to blue- and red-light stimuli, the initial maximal constriction amplitude was decreased, whereas the response after light termination (sustained constriction amplitude) was increased compared to that in wild-type mice. These findings implied that rod photoreceptors are a major contributor to both initial and post-illumination pupil constriction. Furthermore, low- or medium-intensity red light was not able to elicit any pupil response in *Cnga3*$^{-/-}$; *Rho*$^{-/-}$ (coneless and rodless) mice demonstrating that both rods and cones are required to promote pupil responses under these particular conditions (13). Many other studies, each using different methodologies, have examined the origin of the photosensitive input with respect to the murine PLR. In addition to rods and cones, a small subset of retinal ganglion cells expressing the melanopsin protein, termed ipRGCs, was found to contribute to the mouse PLR (14–18). The general model is that rods are required for PLR sensitivity to lower intensity stimuli, whereas cones and melanopsin cells induce responses to more intense levels of light (16, 17). Moreover, rods and cones are mainly involved in the rapid and transient pupil response, whereas ipRGCs are the predominant players in the sustained pupillary response (17, 18).

ERG recordings change with age in young rodents. Specifically, the response amplitudes recorded from photoreceptors and second-order neurons increase gradually from eye-opening (postnatal day 12, P12) until adulthood, which is approximately P30 in mice (19). In rats, oscillatory potential (OP) amplitude and the implicit time also change with age. The amplitudes of OP2, OP3, and OP4 are larger at P31 than at P18 and P67, suggesting the functional refinement of the inner retina (20). Moreover, between 1 and 2 months of age, the mixed rod–cone response and the photopic cone response decrease (21). These observations suggest that the development of retinal processing continues after the first 2 postnatal weeks.

The development of the mouse retina starts at the embryonic stage and continues after birth. Retinal ganglion cells (RGCs) differentiate first followed by amacrine, cone, and horizontal cells. However, the neurogenesis of rods and bipolar cells continues for 1–2 weeks after birth (22). The process that converts bistratified ON-OFF responsive RGCs to monostratified ON or OFF responsive RGCs occurs 2–3 weeks after eye-opening (P12) and depends on light exposure (23). The synaptic strength, measured as the frequency of spontaneous synaptic inputs, also continues to mature after P12, and RGC spontaneous activities peak at P25, finally decreasing to reach adult levels at P60 (23). OFF-type bipolar cells, for example, those responsive to decreases in light, retain the ability to form new synapses in the intact adult retina and continue to increase synapse numbers and the complexity of dendritic arborization to at least 6 months of age, well after the mouse retina is considered mature (24). It has been shown that the presence of abnormal synaptic ribbons (synaptic ribbons floating in the cytoplasm without post-synaptic processes) correlates with abnormal ERG responses (reduction in the amplitude and increase in the implicit time of the b-wave) (25). Although impaired synaptogenesis has an effect on ERG measurements, the influence of normally developing synaptogenesis on the ERG remains unclear.

Five subtypes of ipRGCs (1–3% of the RGC population) were described in rodents based on the stratification of their dendrites (26). McNeil et al. (27) showed that ipRGC neurogenesis begins from embryonic day (ED) 11 to ED14, similar to that observed for other RGCs, but continues after ED15 when other types of RGC neurogenesis stop. At ED15, ipRGCs are not present in the peripheral retina and reach the ciliary margin at birth (P0). IpRGCs begin innervating the suprachiasmatic nucleus at P3 and P4 until the second postnatal week, whereas most RGCs innervate their image-forming targets during embryogenesis. Moreover, the appearance of ipRGC axons in the olivary pretectal nucleus coincides precisely with the onset of the PLR at P7 (27). However, the consequence of retina circuitry refinement, observed after eye opening on visual function is still not well understood.

In this study, we examined the effect of continued retinal maturation after 1 month of age, based on functional tests of the retina, in mice. Specifically, we aimed to better characterize how age affects the mouse PLR and ERG response under non-pathological conditions. Two wild-type mouse strains, C57BL/6 and Sv129S6, were examined because many retinal dystrophy mouse models are based on these genetic backgrounds. Additionally, a difference in the course of degeneration was observed when comparing *Rho*$^{-/-}$ mice between C57BL/6 and Sv129S6 backgrounds (28). The development of such normative values will help to differentiate pathological responses from non-relevant variations, when assessing functional retinal integrity.

MATERIALS AND METHODS

Animals

Animals were handled in accordance with the statement of the "Animals in Research Committee" of the Association for Research in Vision and Ophthalmology, and protocols were approved by the local institutional committee (VD1367). The mice were maintained at 22°C with a 12-h light/12-h dark cycle with light on at 7:00 a.m. and were feed *ad libitum*. C57BL/6 wild-type (males, $n = 15$; females, $n = 12$) and Sv129S6 wild-type (males, $n = 7$; females, $n = 11$) mice were tested at 1, 2, and 4 months. Dark- and light-adapted PLR and ERG examination were always performed on separate days and during the morning, specifically during the first 6 h of the light cycle, at week 4 (1 month), week 8 (2 months), and week 16 (4 months). ERG examinations were always performed after the light and dark-adapted PLR to avoid the effects of the anesthesia on the PLR.

Light Stimuli and Pupil Response Recording

Mice were dark-adapted overnight and tested under mesopic (<5 lux) red light. Pupillary recordings were performed as previously described (13). Animals were not anesthetized to avoid the effects of medication, but were manually restrained in front of the camera. Pupils were maintained at a constant distance from the camera of the A2000 pupillometer (Neuroptics Inc., Irvine, CA). This apparatus presents a light stimulus to one eye while continuously recording the pupil diameter at 31 Hz in the same eye. For this study, the light stimulus had a duration of 500 ms and was either red (622 nm) or blue (463 nm), both with a half-maximum bandwidth of 8 nm, with a range of intensities covering almost 4 log units. Light is emitted through a diffusing screen (approximately 50° × 35° of the visual angle). Based on a previous study, we used pre-selected light intensities that were considered "low," "medium," and "high" [(13); **Table 1**]. Low light intensities are sufficient to generate more than 10% constriction. The maximum red intensity was determined based on the limit of the pupillometer apparatus, whereas the maximum blue intensity was limited to restrict the response to less than 50% of the constriction amplitude in an effort to minimize mouse discomfort. We used the following light stimulus sequence to test all animals under scotopic or photopic conditions: low red, low blue, medium red, medium blue, high red, high blue (**Table 1**). We recorded the pupil response once after administering each stimulus in this sequence for any given animal of a particular age.

The pupil recording started 500 ms before administering the light stimulus and continued 29 s after the blue light stimulus offset or 17 s after the red-light stimulus offset. The interval between stimuli was at least 49 s after blue-light stimulations or 37 s after red-light stimulations; this provided the opportunity for the mouse to freely move for at least 20 s after recording each stimulus to calm the animals before the next stimulus.

The PLR recordings under photopic conditions were taken in an independent session 1 day before or after the dark-adapted recordings. Mice were exposed to room light (fluorescent tube white light emitting 200 ± 50 lux at the level of the mice) for 30 min before the test and both eyes were constantly exposed to the same ambient light during pupil response recordings for the stimulated eye.

TABLE 1 | Light stimulus intensities converted to different units and the order of stimuli applied during the protocol of this study.

Stimuli name	Intensity		
	(log cds/m^2)	(log W/m^2)	(W/m^2)
Low red	1.2	−1.2	0.065
Low blue	0.6	−1.1	0.074
Medium red	2	−0.4	0.408
Medium blue	1.2	−0.5	0.3
High red	4.5	2.1	129.018
High blue	2	0.3	1.893

PLR Analysis

The raw data were exported to a worksheet and all pupil diameters were converted to a percentage of the baseline diameter. The following parameters were determined from the data.

The baseline pupil diameter was set as the mean pupil diameter during the 500 ms before light onset; thereafter, all pupil sizes were converted to a relative size that was a function of the baseline value.

The pupil response was then divided into the constriction phase (defined as the time from the light onset to 2 s after light onset) and the recovery phase (defined as the time from the maximal constriction amplitude to the end of the recording at 29 or 17 s after blue or red stimuli offset, respectively). To evaluate the constriction phase, we determined the maximal constriction amplitude and the maximal velocity (see below). The recovery phase was analyzed at two different stages as follows: at an early phase, to determine the early partial dilation, until 2.5 s after light onset (first derivative, as follows) and at a later time point 9.5 s after light offset (sustained constriction amplitude and ratio, as follows). These features are more precisely described in the following text and in the formula listed in **Table 2**.

The maximal constriction amplitude was the percent change from the baseline value to the minimal diameter reached after application of the light stimuli during the first 2 s following stimulus onset. For the photopic protocol, instead of using the maximal constriction amplitude, we used the minimal diameter reached during the first 1.8 s following stimulus onset, which is the absolute value of the diameter (mm) at the maximal constriction point.

To characterize the early response dynamics by determining the maximal velocity (constriction phase) and the early partial dilation (early recovery phase), the first derivative curve was created using GraphPad Prism 5.01 software (GraphPad Software, Inc., San Diego, CA, USA) comprising the first 3 s of the protocol (2.5 s from light onset). When the pupil was in a steady state, for example before the stimulus onset, the derivative values were essentially zero. A change resulting in a smaller pupil size was indicated by negative values, and the rate of change was indicated by the magnitude of these negative values. The peak negative value thus represented the maximum velocity of constriction, which becomes slower as constriction continues toward the maximum amplitude. When constriction stabilized briefly at the minimum pupil size, the derivative value returned to zero. Thereafter, if the derivative values became positive, this indicated a change resulting in an increase in pupil size, which corresponds to a dilation movement. When these positive

TABLE 2 | Formulas related to pupil light response (PLR) parameters used for quantification.

Baseline pupil diameter	Sum of the pupil diameters (mm) during 500 ms before the light stimulus/total number of pupil diameter values during 500 ms before the light stimulus.
Maximal constriction amplitude	Baseline pupil diameter—minimal pupil diameter expressed in percentage.
Area under the curve	The first derivative of individual pupil tracing was created using GraphPad Prism 5.01 software (GraphPad Software, Inc., San Diego, CA, USA). Individual curves were then exported into excel for identification of positif peak by the formula: = SI(ET(Cn>0;Cn+1>0);($An-$An-1)*(Cn+Cn+1)/2;"") where C is the column of data for one individual, A is the colunm for time values, n is the row number. The AUC of each individual is then determined by the sum of these values.
Sustained response	Percentage of constriction amplitude at 9.5 s following stimulus offset.
Ratio of the sustained response	Percentage of constriction amplitude at 9.5 s following stimulus offset above the maximal constriction amplitude.

values increased rapidly, a peak was distinguishable, indicating a rapid and early dilation for which the maximal velocity (the positive peak) was reached within the first 3 s of the recording. Alternatively, if the derivative was maintained at approximately zero, without reaching a peak positive value, this indicated the absence of a rapid dilation within this 3 s period. To quantify this early partial dilation, we calculated the area under the curve (AUC) below this peak, when the first derivative was positive.

The sustained constriction amplitude was the percent change from the baseline value to the diameter reached at 9.5 s following stimulus offset. In the recovery phase, this time point was previously demonstrated to reveal the most significant difference between the different photoreceptor cell input conditions (13).

To evaluate the relative recovery from the maximal constriction, we calculated the ratio of the sustained constriction amplitude to the maximal constriction amplitude.

Electroretinography

Mice were dark-adapted overnight for another session of ERG measurements 1 or 2 days after pupillometry. They were anesthetized with a mixture of ketamine (20 mg/kg, Streuli, Uznach, CH) and xylazine (20 mg/kg, Bayler, Lyssach, CH) and both pupils were dilated with a single eye drop of 0.5% tropicamide (Théa, Schaffausen, CH) and 5% phenylephrine hydrochloride (Bausch and Lomb, London, UK). As mice are temperature-sensitive, animals were maintained on a heating pad connected to a temperature control unit to maintain temperature at 37–38°C throughout the experiment. Responses to standard single light flashes [520 nm; half-bandwidth, 35 nm; at 0.0001 cds/m^2 (2.2×10^{-7} W/sr/m^2), 0.001 cds/m^2 (2.2×10^{-6} W/sr/m^2), 0.01 cds/m^2 (2.2×10^{-5} W/sr/m^2), 0.03 (6.6×10^{-5} W/sr/m^2), 0.1 cds/m^2 (2.2×10^{-4} W/sr/m^2), 0.3 cds/m^2 (6.6×10^{-4} W/sr/m^2), 1 cds/m^2 (2.2×10^{-3} W/sr/m^2), 3 cds/m^2 (6.6×10^{-3} W/sr/m^2), 10 cds/m^2 (1.9×10^{-2} W/sr/m^2), and 30 cds/m^2 (5.9×10^{-2} W/sr/m^2) for scotopic ERG and 1 cds/m^2 (2.2×10^{-3} W/sr/m^2), 3 cds/m^2 (6.6×10^{-3} W/sr/m^2), 10 cds/m^2 (1.9×10^{-2} W/sr/m^2), and 30 cds/m^2 (5.9×10^{-2} W/sr/m^2) for photopic ERG] generated by a stroboscope (Ganzfeld stimulator, Espion E3 apparatus; Diagnosys LLC, Lowell, MA, USA) were recorded binocularly with corneal electrodes. The a-wave (photoreceptor-driven first negative wave) amplitude was measured from baseline to the bottom of the a-wave trough and the b-wave (second order neuron-driven, first positive wave) amplitude was measured from the bottom of the a-wave trough to the b-wave peak.

Immunohistochemistry

Three eyes from three different C57BL/6 mice, 1 and 2 months of age, were prepared for immunohistochemistry. A cauterization mark was made in the inner corner of the eye as a marker for orientation. After enucleation, eyes were incubated at room temperature (RT) in 4% paraformaldehyde for 1.25 h, washed twice with PBS, and incubated sequentially for 2 h each in 10% and 20% sucrose and finally overnight in 30% sucrose. Eyes were embedded in yazzulla (30% egg albumin and 3% gelatin in water) and cut with a cryostat to generate 14-µm-thick sections.

For all staining procedures, blocking was performed at RT for 1–1.5 h, and the primary antibody was incubated with the samples at 4°C overnight, whereas the secondary antibody was added to the section for 1 h at RT. For protein kinase C-alpha (PKC) and bassoon double staining, sections were blocked with 5% normal goat serum with 0.2% triton X-100, and anti-PKC-alpha (sc-10800, Santa Cruz, Dallas, USA) and anti-Bassoon (VAM-PS003, Stressgen, Lausen, Switzerland) were diluted to 1:200 and 1:400, respectively. For calbindin and cholinergic amacrine cell (ChAT) double staining, blocking was performed with 10% NDS with 0.2% triton X-100 before incubation with anti-Calbindin (1:5000, SWANT CB 38, Swant Inc., Marly, Switzerland) and anti-ChAT (1:2500, kind gift from Prof. J.P Hornung, UNIL, Lausanne, Switzerland) antibodies. The blocking solution for transducin Gαt1 rods (GNAT1) was 10% NGS with 0.3% triton X-100 in PBS and anti-GNAT1 antibody was diluted to 1:1000 (Sc-389 Santa Cruz, Dallas, USA). S-opsin/MWL-opsin double staining was performed by first blocking with 5% normal donkey serum with 0.2% triton X-100 and anti-S-opsin (sc-14363, Santa Cruz, Dallas) and anti-MWL-Opsin (AB5405, Chemicon, Temecula, CA, USA) were diluted to 1:1000. Secondary antibodies including Alexa Fluor 488, 633, or 594 goat anti-rabbit, goat anti-mouse, donkey anti-goat, or donkey anti-rabbit antibodies (depending on the primary antibody) were diluted to 1:2000 in PBS and counterstaining was finally performed with DAPI. Sections were mounted in Mowiol® 4-88 reagent (Sigma, Buchs, Switzerland), a poly(vinyl)alcohol medium used to preserved stained sections.

Immunohistochemistry Analysis

Images of the different labeled samples were obtained in 3D using LAST X software driving a DM6 Leica microscope and were merged to obtain a composite picture. Noise was removed by performing deconvolution using Huygens Essential software (Scientific Volume Imaging B.V. Hilversum, The Netherlands).

TABLE 3 | Pupil light response (PLR) analysis of C57BL/6 mice at 1, 2, and 4 months of age.

	1 month			2 months			4 months		
	Mean	**SEM**	***n***	**Mean**	**SEM**	***n***	**Mean**	**SEM**	***n***
BASELINE PUPIL DIAMETER (mm)									
	1.11	0.07	16	1.74*	0.08	15	1.93*	0.05	12
MAXIMUM CONSTRICTION AMPLITUDE (%)									
Low blue	36.27	1.02	23	36.38	1.34	13	35.09	1.58	13
Medium blue	43.86	1.32	23	45.43	2.45	14	45.07	1.49	10
High blue	52.41	1.87	16	53.10	1.82	16	49.84	3.54	8
Low red	20.19	1.26	22	15.35	1.14	17	18.19	2.14	14
Medium red	32.61	1.32	24	27.15#	0.86	16	25.29†	1.36	11
High red	44.96	1.80	20	43.79	1.74	16	41.22	2.21	12
MAXIMAL CONSTRICTION VELOCITY (mm/s)									
Low blue	−0.71	0.04	17	−0.87	0.06	13	−0.98†	0.04	13
Medium blue	−0.76	0.04	24	−0.95#	0.05	14	−1.05*	0.04	10
High blue	−0.84	0.06	16	−1.15*	0.09	15	−0.95	0.06	8
Low red	−0.46	0.05	22	−0.51	0.05	17	−0.59	0.06	14
Medium red	−0.73	0.05	24	−0.79	0.04	17	−0.79	0.05	12
High red	−0.82	0.05	20	−1.03†	0.06	16	−1.05#	0.06	12
AREA UNDER THE CURVE OF THE POSITIVE PEAK OF THE 1ST DERIVATIVE									
Low blue	9.63	1.11	24	5.78†	0.93	13	6.28#	1.35	13
Medium blue	2.91	0.89	24	1.34	0.49	14	1.27	1.06	10
High blue	0.39	0.28	17	0.13	0.086	15	0.11	0.08	8
Low red	8.67	1.02	21	6.13	0.62	16	7.46	0.67	14
Medium red	10.07	0.98	25	8.37	0.74	16	8.98	1.04	12
High red	2.79	0.55	27	2.28	0.44	15	1.64	0.49	12
SUSTAINED CONSTRICTION AMPLITUDE (%)									
Low blue	14.08	1.80	23	17.49	2.23	13	13.09	1.35	13
Medium blue	19.92	2.41	23	28.22#	1.84	14	25.63	1.83	10
High blue	32.25	2.98	17	45.51*	3.55	16	31.72	4.00	8
Low red	11.95	4.38	22	6.57	1.32	17	4.12	0.82	14
Medium red	9.16	1.73	24	16.81	5.33	17	9.24	1.17	12
High red	22.36	1.73	20	25.94	2.36	16	19.35	2.00	12
RATIO									
Low blue	0.38	0.04	23	0.48	0.06	13	0.38	0.04	13
Medium blue	0.46	0.05	25	0.64#	0.05	14	0.57	0.04	10
High blue	0.65	0.05	16	0.84#	0.06	15	0.64	0.07	8
Low red	0.46	0.08	21	0.41	0.08	17	0.27	0.06	14
Medium red	0.29	0.05	23	0.45	0.05	16	0.37	0.06	12
High red	0.50	0.03	20	0.59	0.04	16	0.47	0.04	12

*Quantification of the baseline pupil diameter (mm), the relative maximal constriction amplitude (%), the maximal constriction velocity (mm/s), the area under the curve of the positive peak of the first derivative (arbitrary unit), the relative sustained constriction amplitude (%), and the ratio of sustained to maximal constriction amplitude. *Significantly different compared to 1-month-old mice, $p < 0.001$; †significantly different compared to 1-month-old animals, $p < 0.01$; #significantly different compared to 1-month-old mice, $p < 0.05$.*

Quantification of the number of labeled cells was performed in the central section bisecting the optic nerve along the vertical axis, which represents the most sagittal region of the retina. The number of positive cells, based on different markers, was determined for the inferior and the superior hemispheres through manual counting during visualization using a microscope. Both inferior and superior counts were added together to obtain the final number of labeled cells in the entire section. Three eyes from three different mice were analyzed for each age group.

Statistical Analysis

All statistical analyses were performed using GraphPad Prism software (San Diego, CA, USA). For the statistical analysis, each PLR characteristic obtained for each age group was analyzed by performing a two-way ANOVA with Bonferroni tests to compare males and females. As no sex-based difference was noted, males and females were then grouped as a single experimental group for each age tested. Two-way ANOVA and Bonferroni tests were then performed for each feature to compare the three C57BL/6 age groups or the two Sv129S6 age groups.

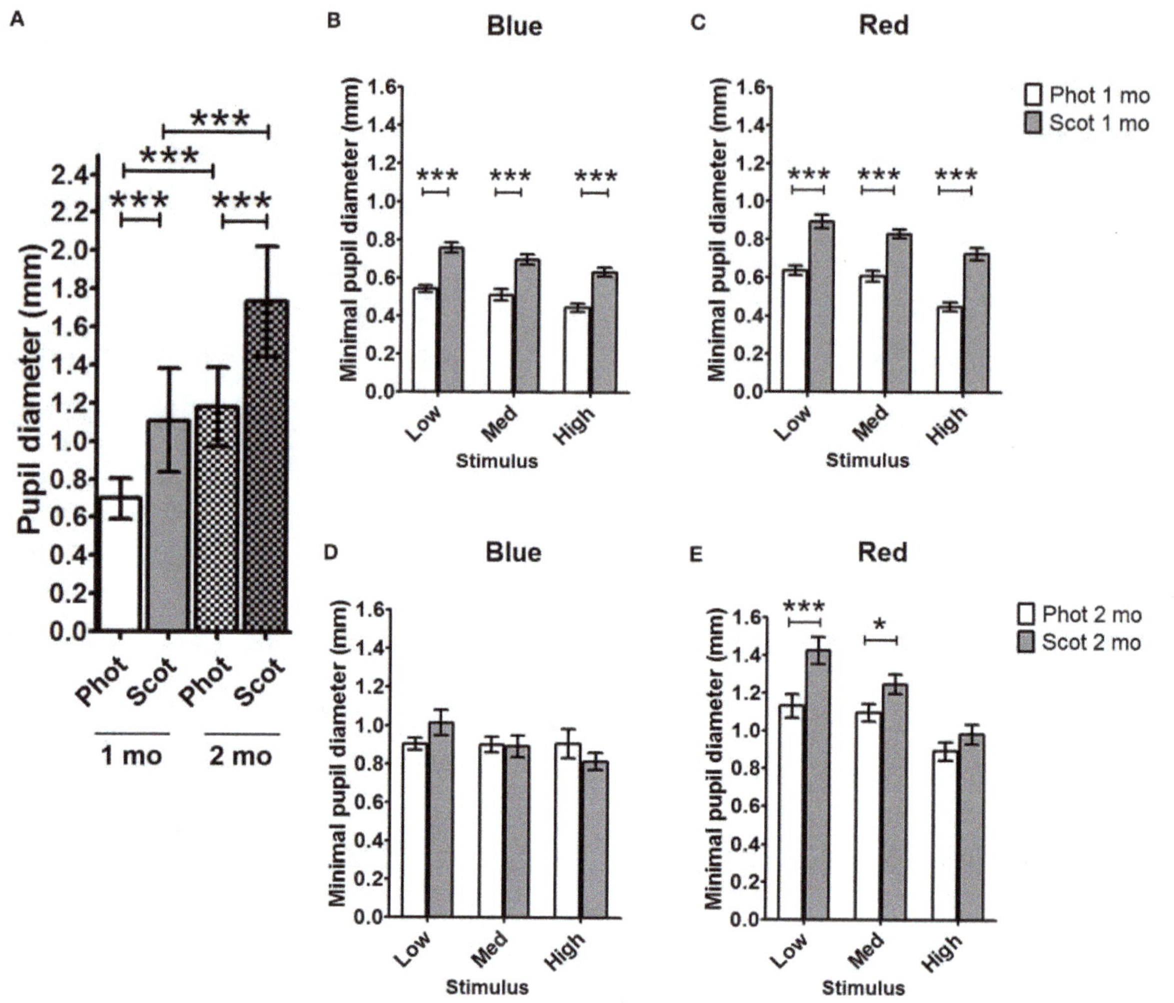

FIGURE 1 | Comparison of C57BL/6 pupil diameters under photopic and scotopic conditions for 1- and 2-month-old animals. **(A)** Baseline pupil diameters for photopic and scotopic conditions in 1- and 2-month-old animals were compared. The minimal pupil diameter for 1-month- **(B,C)** and 2-month- **(D,E)** old mice under scotopic and photopic conditions in response to blue light stimuli **(B,D)** and red-light stimuli **(C,E)** were compared. Phot, photopic conditions; Scot, scotopic conditions; mo, months; Med, medium; $^*p < 0.05$; $^{***}p < 0.001$.

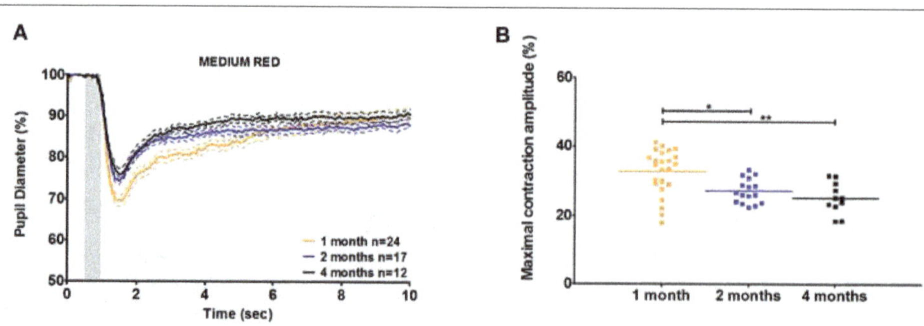

FIGURE 2 | C57BL/6 pupil responses to medium red light in 1-, 2-, and 4-month-old mice. **(A)** Mean pupil diameter (in %) of 1-, 2-, and 4-month-old mice in response to medium red stimulus. The plain lines represent the mean responses of 1-, 2-, and 4-month-old mice and the dotted lines represent the SEM of these means with the same color code. **(B)** Dot plot of the maximal constriction amplitude of 1-, 2-, and 4-month-old mice in response to medium red stimulus. Horizontal lines represent the mean of the different age groups. $^*p < 0.05$; $^{**}p < 0.01$.

TABLE 4 | Pupil light response (PLR) analysis of Sv129S6 mice at 1 and 2 months of age.

	1 month			2 months		
	Mean	**SEM**	***n***	**Mean**	**SEM**	***n***
BASELINE PUPIL DIAMETER (mm)						
	1.30	0.04	17	1.58*	0.04	25
MAXIMAL CONSTRICTION AMPLITUDE (%)						
Low blue	42.87	1.007	24	36.74#	1.09	24
Medium blue	46.99	1.67	21	41.63#	1.34	24
High blue	50.91	1.68	22	43.75†	2.28	23
Low red	32.51	1.70	22	24.32*	1.29	25
Medium red	42.95	1.45	21	33.84*	0.97	25
High red	48.29	1.50	20	41.60†	1.49	26
AREA UNDER THE CURVE OF THE POSITIVE PEAK OF THE 1ST DERIVATIVE						
Low blue	15.71	1.17	24	14.07	0.71	24
Medium blue	7.94	1.11	20	6.99	0.82	27
High blue	2.27	0.77	20	1.94	0.61	25
Low red	17.19	1.13	21	12.67†	0.82	28
Medium red	20.56	1.23	24	15.95†	0.66	29
High red	9.60	1.00	20	9.19	0.92	32
SUSTAINED CONSTRICTION AMPLITUDE (%)						
Low blue	8.38	1.33	24	9.50	1.32	24
Medium blue	13.74	1.58	21	15.51	2.19	24
High blue	23.77	2.07	21	18.82	1.84	23
Low red	9.71	4.42	22	6.48	0.66	25
Medium red	7.03	1.09	22	8.11	1.09	25
High red	10.39	1.32	20	17.04	3.47	26
RATIO						
Low blue	0.17	0.03	24	0.22	0.03	24
Medium blue	0.26	0.04	21	0.30	0.03	24
High blue	0.41	0.03	21	0.38	0.03	23
Low red	0.34	0.22	22	0.21	0.03	25
Medium red	0.13	0.02	22	0.20	0.03	25
High red	0.18	0.02	20	0.37	0.07	26

*Quantification of the baseline pupil diameter (mm), the relative maximal constriction amplitude (%), the area under the curve of the positive peak of the first derivative (arbitrary unit), the relative sustained constriction amplitude (%), and the ratio of sustained to maximal constriction amplitude. *Significantly different compared to 1-month-old mice, $p < 0.001$; †significantly different compared to 1-month-old animals, $p < 0.01$; #significantly different compared to 1-month-old mice, $p < 0.05$.*

For immunochemistry, *t*-tests were performed for each marker to compare counts between 1 and 2 months of age. A value was considered significant if $p < 0.05$.

RESULTS

Age-Related Changes in Baseline Pupil Diameter

Under scotopic conditions, the pupil baseline diameter increased significantly with age in both C57BL/6 (**Table 3**; 55% increase at 2 months and 74% increase at 4 months compared to that at 1 month; $p < 0.001$ for 1 vs. 2 and 4 months) and Sv126S6 strains (**Table 4**; 22% increase at 2 months compared to that at 1 month; $p < 0.001$). We also observed significantly larger pupil diameters in 2-month-old mice compared to those in 1-month-old C57BL/6 mice under photopic conditions (**Figure 1A**). Four-month-old C57BL/6 mice and Sv129S6 mice were not tested under photopic conditions. The smaller pupil diameter of 1-month-old mice consequently resulted in a reduction in the pupil area through which the light stimuli can enter. For the C57BL/6 strain, in dark-adapted conditions, a 60% reduction in pupil area was estimated compared to that in 2-month-old mice and a 77% reduction was calculated compared to that in 4-month-old animals. In the dark-adapted Sv126S6 strain, 1-month-old mice presented with a 33% reduced pupil area compared to that in 2-month-old animals. Since in the following experiments, the stimulus light intensities were kept constant, the amount of light entering the eye would proportionally decrease in 1-month-old mice.

Age-Related Changes During the Constriction Phase of the Pupil Response

To determine whether age affects the initial pupil constriction in response to light, we compared the maximal constriction amplitude of 1-, 2-, and 4-month-old animals. Except in reaction to medium red stimulus, there were no significant differences in the maximal constriction amplitude between ages. However, 1-month-old C57BL/6 mice showed a greater maximal constriction amplitude in response to medium red stimulus compared to that in 2- and 4-month-old animals (20 and 30% increases, respectively; $p < 0.01$; **Figure 2**, **Table 3**, **Supplementary Figures 1**, **2**). This greater constriction amplitude seemed to contrast the smaller pupil diameter of the 1-month-old mice and we subsequently repeated the measurements in another wild-type strain, namely Sv129S6. Similar to that observed with the C57BL/6 strain, 1-month-old Sv129S6 mice showed greater maximal constriction amplitude in response to medium red stimulus. However, unlike the C57BL/6 strain, Sv129S6 mice also showed greater maximal constriction amplitude in response to all other red and all blue stimuli compared to that in 2-month-old mice (**Table 4**, **Supplementary Figures 3**, **4**).

To better understand the differential pupil response between 1 and 2 months of age, we recorded the PLR in C57BL/6 mice using the same protocol but under photopic conditions. As expected, the baseline pupil diameter was smaller under photopic conditions than under scotopic conditions for both 1- and 2-month-old C57BL/6 animals (**Figure 1A**, **Table 5**; 37 and 32% decreases in diameter at 1 and 2 months, respectively; $p < 0.001$). The maximal constriction amplitude was also decreased under photopic conditions compared to that under scotopic conditions at both ages for all stimuli (**Table 5**; $p < 0.001$). However, age influenced the effect of light conditions on the minimal diameter (at maximal constriction). Whereas for 1-month-old animals the minimal diameter in response to all stimuli was 28–34% smaller under photopic conditions compared to that with scotopic conditions (**Figure 1**, **Table 5**; $p < 0.001$), for 2-month-old animals, the minimal diameters in response to high red and all blue stimuli were

TABLE 5 | Comparison of pupil light response (PLR) under photopic and scotopic conditions in C57BL/6 mice at 1 and 2 months of age.

	1 month			2 months		
	Mean	**SEM**	***n***	**Mean**	**SEM**	***n***
PHOTOPIC BASELINE PUPIL DIAMETER (mm)						
	0.70[1]	0.02	19	1.18*[1]	0.06	13
SCOTOPIC BASELINE PUPIL DIAMETER (mm)						
	1.11	0.07	16	1.74*	0.08	15
PHOTOPIC MAXIMAL CONSTRICTION AMPLITUDE (%)						
Low blue	20.74[1]	0.99	21	19.77[1]	1.53	13
Medium blue	25.63[1]	1.80	20	26.46[1]	1.40	12
High blue	33.16[1]	1.93	20	29.80[1]	3.11	9
Low red	8.82[1]	1.06	19	4.54[1]	0.873	13
Medium red	14.01[1]	1.49	19	10.51[1]	0.80	15
High red	30.64[1]	1.45	21	28.47[1]	1.69	15
SCOTOPIC MAXIMAL CONSTRICTION AMPLITUDE (%)						
Low blue	36.27	1.02	23	36.38	1.34	13
Medium blue	43.86	1.32	23	45.43	2.45	14
High blue	52.42	1.87	16	53.10	1.82	16
Low red	20.19	1.26	22	15.35	1.14	17
Medium red	32.61	1.32	24	27.15#	0.86	16
High red	44.96	1.80	20	43.79	1.74	16
PHOTOPIC MINIMAL DIAMETER (mm)						
Low blue	0.54[1]	0.02	21	0.90*	0.03	13
Medium blue	0.51[1]	0.03	20	0.90*	0.03	12
High blue	0.45[1]	0.02	20	0.91*	0.08	9
Low red	0.64[1]	0.03	19	1.13*[1]	0.06	13
Medium red	0.61[1]	0.03	19	1.10*[2]	0.05	15
High red	0.45[1]	0.02	21	0.89*	0.05	14
SCOTOPIC MINIMAL DIAMETER (mm)						
Low blue	0.76	0.03	23	1.01*	0.07	13
Medium blue	0.70	0.03	23	0.89*	0.06	14
High blue	0.65	0.03	16	0.81†	0.05	15
Low red	0.88	0.04	21	1.43*	0.07	17
Medium red	0.84	0.03	25	1.25*	0.05	17
High red	0.68	0.03	25	0.98*	0.05	16

*Quantifications of the baseline pupil diameter (mm) and the relative maximal constriction amplitude (%) are reported. *Significantly different compared to 1-month-old mice under the same conditions, $p < 0.001$; †significantly different compared to 1-month-old animals under the same conditions, $p < 0.01$; #significantly different compared to 1-month-old mice under the same conditions, $p < 0.05$. [1]significantly different compared to scotopic conditions based on mice of the same age, $p < 0.001$; [2]significantly different compared to scotopic conditions based on mice of the same age, $p < 0.05$.*

not significantly different between the two conditions. At 2 months of age, the only significant decrease in minimal diameter under photopic conditions (compared to that under scotopic conditions) occurred in response to low and medium red stimuli (**Figure 1**, **Table 5**; 29 and 12% decreases in diameter; $p < 0.001$ and $p < 0.05$, respectively). These results showed that the response of 1-month-old mouse pupils is highly affected by the light conditions (scotopic or photopic), whereas in 2-month-old mice, only responses to low and medium red are modified by photopic conditions.

The maximal peak velocity in response to low and medium red stimuli was not significantly different among C57BL/6 mice aged 1, 2, and 4 months. However, in response to high red and low and medium blue, 1-month-old animals exhibited significantly smaller maximal velocity compared to that in 4-month-old animals (**Figure 3**). Measures for 2-month-old animals followed a trend regarding the age-dependent effect on maximal velocity, but significant differences compared to those in 1-month-old mice were only observed in response to high red and medium blue stimuli. In response to high blue, the 1-month-old maximal velocity was smaller than the 2-month-old maximal velocity but not that of 4-month-old animals. Thus, we showed that during the constriction phase, age can affect both the maximal constriction amplitude and maximal velocity of the pupil response to particular stimuli based on our protocol.

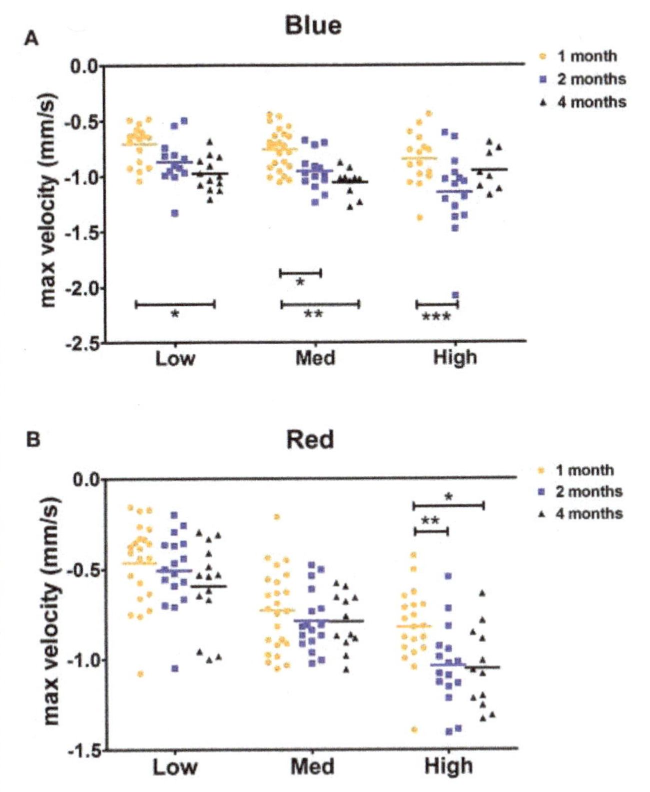

FIGURE 3 | C57BL/6 maximal constriction velocity for 1-, 2-, and 4-month-old animals. Dot plot of the maximal velocity of constriction in response to blue **(A)** and red **(B)** light stimuli is shown. Horizontal lines represent the means of different age groups. $^*p < 0.05$; $^{**}p < 0.01$; $^{***}p < 0.001$.

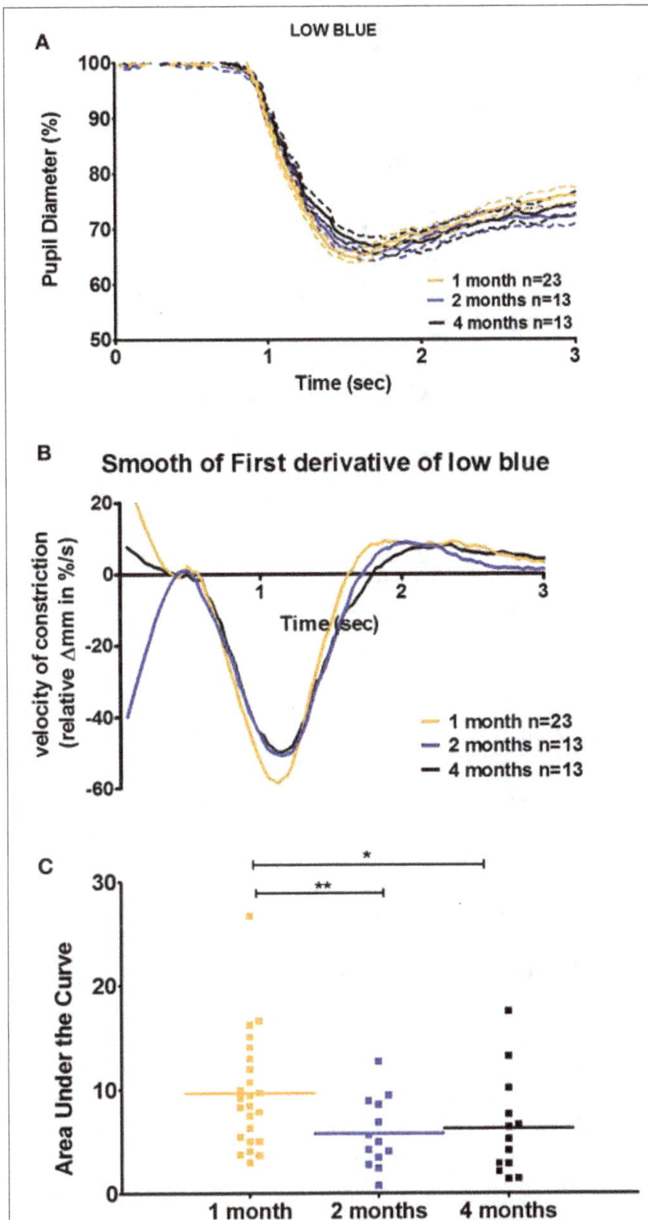

FIGURE 4 | Quantification of the positive peak of the first derivative of the response to low blue stimuli in C57BL/6 mice. **(A)** Magnification of the mean pupil response to low blue stimuli during the first 3 s of the protocol. The plain lines represent the mean responses and dotted lines represent the respective SEMs of these means. **(B)** The smooth first derivative of the pupil response is shown in **(A)**. **(C)** Dot plot of the area under the curve of the positive peak observed after light offset, based on the graph **(B)**. Horizontal lines represent the means of the different age groups. $^*p < 0.05$; $^{**}p < 0.01$.

Age-Related Changes During the Recovery Phase of the Pupil Response

For C57BL/6 mice, except in response to low blue stimulus, there was no significant difference between ages with respect to the early partial dilation of the recovery phase in response to all other stimuli. The AUC of the first derivative of the response to low blue was significantly greater in 1-month-old mice compared to that in 2- and 4-month-old mice (66 and 53% increase at 1 month compared to that at 2 and 4 months, $p < 0.01$ and $p < 0.05$, respectively; **Figure 4**, **Table 3**). For Sv129S6 mice, significantly larger AUC values were noted for both low and medium red responses at 1 month compared to those at 2 months (**Table 4**).

To analyze the later phase of recovery, we compared relative pupil diameters 9.5 s after stimuli offset (sustained constriction). The only significant difference between age groups was in response to medium and high blue stimuli. Specifically, 1-month-old C57BL/6 mice a had decreased sustained constriction amplitude in response to these stimuli compared to that in 2-month-old, but not 4-month-old, mice (**Figure 5**, **Table 3**, 30% decreased amplitude at 1 month compared to that in 2 months, in response to medium and high blue stimuli, $p < 0.05$ and $p < 0.001$ respectively). A significant decrease was even observed in 4-month-old animals in response to high blue light compared to that in 2-month-old mice (**Table 3**, $p < 0.01$). Assessing the ratio of sustained constriction amplitude to maximal constriction amplitude gave similar results. No significant differences between ages were observed in terms of the relative recovery in response to all stimuli, except in response to medium blue and high blue

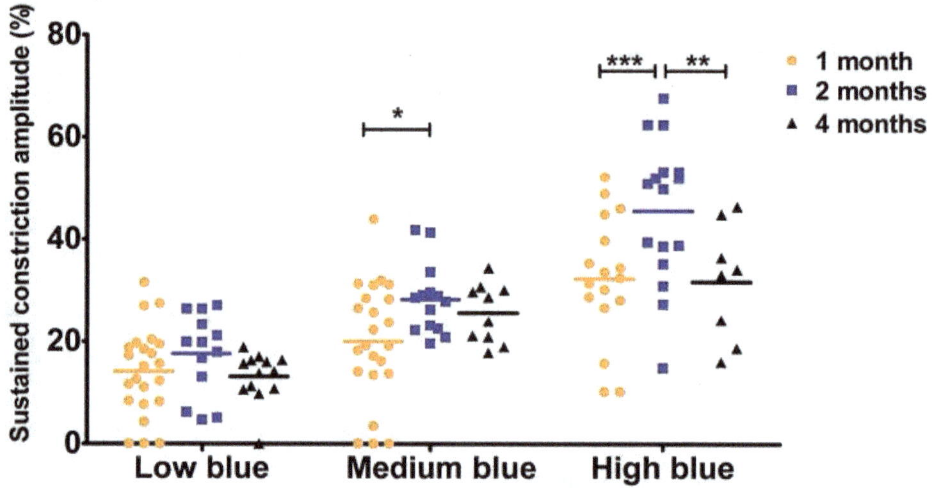

FIGURE 5 | Sustained constriction amplitude for 1-, 2-, and 4-month-old C57BL/6 mice in response to blue stimuli. Dot plot of sustained response after 9.5 s of light offset for 1-, 2-, and 4-month-old mice. One-month old mice exhibited significantly smaller sustained constriction in response to medium and high blue light compared to that in 2-month-old animals. Horizontal lines represent the mean of the different age groups. *$p < 0.05$; **$p < 0.01$; ***$p < 0.001$.

light (**Table 3**, $p > 0.05$). In response to these stimuli, 1-month-old mice exhibited a significantly smaller ratio than 2-month-old, but not 4-month-old, mice. For Sv129S6 mice, no significant differences were found in terms of the sustained response or the ratio of response to all stimuli (**Table 4**, $p > 0.05$). These results revealed the limited modification of the recovery phase in response to medium and high blue light at 2 months of age in C57BL/6, but not Sv129S6, mice.

Age-Related Changes in Retinal Activity

In parallel to PLR recordings, retinal activity was measured by ERG. For C57BL/6 mice, we observed significant increase in the scotopic a-wave amplitude of 1-month-old mice compared to that of 2-month-old animals only in response to the highest stimulus intensity; however, with an intermediate value, the amplitude in 4-month-old mice was not significantly different from that in either 1- or 2-month-old mice (1 month = -138.1 ± 10.27 μV, 2 months = -96.84 ± 9.84 μV, and 4 months = -112.01 ± 10.06; 1 month vs. 2 month, $p < 0.001$; **Figure 6A**). No other significant differences were found in terms of the ERG parameters among the three age groups in this strain (**Figure 6B**). Further, no significant age-specific effects on any ERG parameters examined were noted in Sv129S6 mice (**Supplementary Figure 5**).

Comparison of Retina Structure Between Mice of 1 and 2 Months of Age

The origin of the modified pupil response between 1 and 2 months of age was unknown, but one possibility was suggested to be changes in retinal structure, particularly in the outer layer. We thus evaluated the histopathology of the retina in these two age groups. Specifically, we labeled cones, rods, bipolar cells, horizontal cells, and amacrine cells with different antibodies and analyzed the central section bisecting the optic nerve of each eye ($n = 3$ for each group; **Figure 7**).

Cone photoreceptors were labeled with anti-S-opsin and anti-MWL-opsin antibodies; no significant difference in the number of positive cells was observed. In the central section, an average of 573 ± 91.25 S-opsin-positive cells were counted for 1-month-old animals, whereas 472 ± 21 positive cells were observed for 2-month-old mice ($p > 0.05$). For MWL-opsin, 822 ± 133 and 710 ± 14 positive cells were counted for 1- and 2-month-old animals, respectively ($p > 0.05$). To study rod photoreceptors, we labeled the outer segment with an antibody directed against the rod transducing GNAT1 protein. No differences in labeling intensity in the outer segments were found between 1- and 2-month-old mice. The thickness of the photoreceptor layers was also similar between both age groups. Rod bipolar cells were then analyzed using the marker PKC-alpha. No differences in the number of PKC-alpha-positive cells were observed (638 ± 50 at 1 month and 650 ± 26 at 2 months of age; $p > 0.05$). For the presynaptic nerve terminals labeled with an anti-bassoon antibody, no obvious changes in intensity or amount of staining were noted between 1- and 2-month-old animals.

Next, we used an anti-calbindin antibody to quantify horizontal cells and amacrine cells in the inner nuclear layer and displaced amacrine cells in the ganglion cell layer, in addition to ganglion cells. No difference was observed in terms of horizontal cells (96 ± 25 at 1 month and 94 ± 3.2 at 2 months of age), amacrine cells (373 ± 44 at 1 month and 268 ± 21 at 2 months of age), or displaced amacrine cells and ganglion cells (163 ± 18.5 at 1 month and 141 ± 9.8 at 2 months of age).

Finally, an anti-ChAT antibody was used to label cholinergic amacrine cells. No differences in the number of positive cells were noted (140 ± 0 vs. 100 ± 81 at 1 and 2 months of age, respectively).

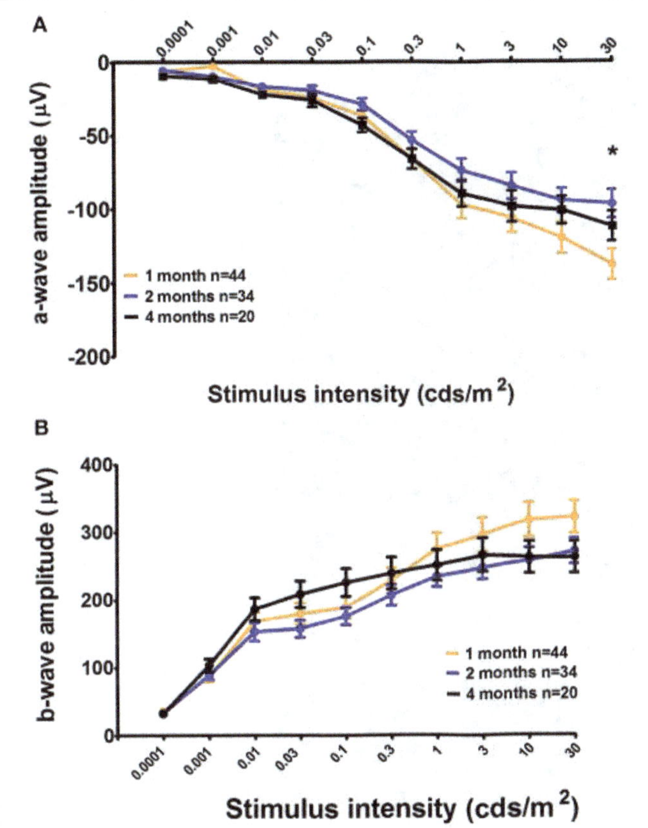

FIGURE 6 | Retinal activity in 1-, 2-, and 4-month-old C57BL/6 mice. The mean a-wave and b-wave amplitudes, with SEM error bars, measured under scotopic conditions, are represented as a function of the stimulus intensities for graph **(A)** and **(B)**, respectively. One-month-old C57BL/6 mice (light gray) displayed a larger maximal retinal response for the a-wave under scotopic conditions as measured by an electroretinogram (ERG) compared to that in 2-month-old mice (medium gray). The 4-month-old animal responses were not significantly different from those at 1 and 2 months. $^{*}p < 0.05$.

DISCUSSION

The comparison of PLR and ERG measurements at different ages revealed alterations in pupil and retinal responses that occurred with age. Specifically, 1-month-old animals clearly showed different features compared to older animals. Currently, we cannot identify the mechanisms underlying these age-related changes, but several explanations can be proposed, such as morphological differences, the maturation of the iris sphincter, changes in retinal sensitivity, or refined central control of the pupil. These hypotheses will be considered in relation to the significant results discussed as follows.

The smaller baseline diameters (in scotopic and photopic conditions) of 1-month-old animals (36% decrease compared to that in 2-month-old C57BL/6 mice) cannot be entirely explained by morphological size differences between 1- and 2-month-old groups because the eye cup diameter was found to only be decreased by 4% in 1-month-old animals (personal unpublished data). Furthermore, morphological differences would not explain the increase in maximal constriction amplitude in response to particular photoreceptor stimuli at 1 month of age because the relative quantification of baseline parameters took into account the starting diameter.

Another explanation for these age-related differences could be the maturation of the iris sphincter. The smaller baseline pupil diameter and increased maximal constriction amplitudes could result from an immature and stronger iris at 1 month of age. However, the slower maximal velocity and faster recovery suggest decreased iris sphincter efficacy at this age. Additionally, variations in these PLR features were observed only following specific stimuli, which is not consistent with general iris immaturity that would affect all responses similarly. For these reasons, maturation of the iris sphincter is probably not the origin of PLR variations observed with age.

Several of the PLR metrics analyzed in our study suggest higher retinal sensitivity at 1 month of age compared to that in older mice. First, the baseline diameter after dark adaptation was smaller at 1 month of age for both strains. The same difference was noticed under photopic conditions for 1-month-old C57BL/6 mice. Second, the maximal constriction amplitudes in response to medium (C57BL/6) or low and medium (Sv129S6) red stimuli were larger at 1 month of age. Considering that these stimuli were previously shown to be rod- and cone-driven in mice (13), these results suggest an increase in rod and cone input in 1-month-old mice. Likewise, in C57BL/6 mice, the ERG response to scotopic conditions was associated with a larger maximal mixed cone–rod response at this age, demonstrating that 1-month-old animals exhibit heightened response to light. Of note, in Sv129S6 mice, we could not confirm the increased maximal cone–rod response. Moreover, in this genetic background, the maximal constriction amplitude was greater in response to all other stimuli at 1 month of age. This latter result suggests that in this strain, a major change in the PLR process occurs between 1 and 2 months of age, which might not be directly linked to rods and cones, but rather to variation in pathways that control the entire pupil. At this stage of the study, we cannot distinguish between changes in peripheral or central pathways. Natural variances exist between wild-type mouse strains, which could explain the differences between C57BL/6 and Sv129S6 mice observed in our study. Previously, different neurochemical profiles have been highlighted, which could account for different behavioral responses between strains (29). For example, basal levels of ionotropic glutamate receptor subunit vary according to mouse strain (30). Such diversity might also be present in the neural retina and could induce small deviations in terms of retinal visual processing among non-pathological mouse strains. A variation in the course of retinal degeneration was noted between C57BL/6 and Sv129S6 mice when examining the effect of rhodopsin knockouts on the retina (28). Genetic modifiers were proposed to modulate the survival of photoreceptors in these models and could also affect neural development processes, which might account for the dissimilarity of pupillary and ERG responses observed between these strains.

An additional hypothesis for the mechanism responsible for age-related changes in the PLR is that the pupil circuitry, associated with all three types of photosensitive cells, is adjusted after 1 month. Since melanopsin cells were previously shown

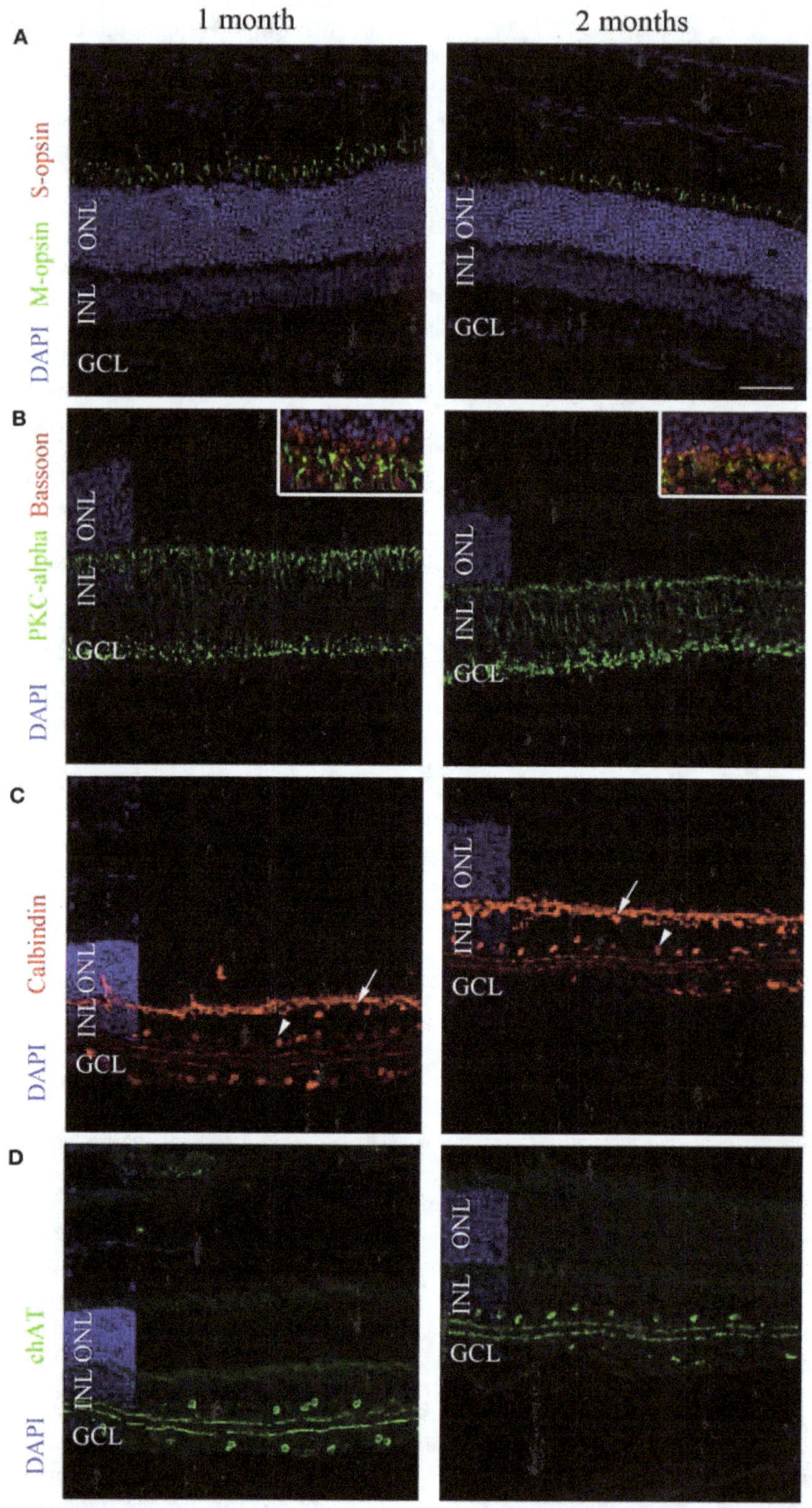

FIGURE 7 | Representative immunolabeling of the retinas of 1- and 2-month-old C57BL/6 mice. **(A)** A region in the superior hemisphere of 1- and 2-month-old retinas showed a similar number of M-cones (green) and S-cones (red) labeled by anti-MWL-opsin and anti-S-opsin antibodies, respectively. **(B)** Bipolar cells labeled with anti-PKCalpha (green) were similar between 1- and 2-month-old retinas. The inset shows 2-fold magnification of B at the photoreceptor termini with co-labeling for Bassoon (red). **(C)** The calbindin labeling of horizontal (arrows), amacrine (arrowheads), displaced amacrine, and ganglion cells was similar at 1 and 2 months. **(D)** The labeling of cholinergic amacrine cells using an anti-ChAT antibody was similar at 1 and 2 months. DAPI (blue) was used as a counterstain for panels **(A–D)**. The horizontal line in **(A)** represents 50 μm for all panels and 25 μm for the inset of **(B)**. ONL, outer nuclear layer; INL, inner nuclear layer; GCL; ganglion cell layer.

to mediate the steady state of the pupil, these cells could be implicated in the reduced baseline pupil size observed at 1 month. Recording the PLR under photopic conditions allows for the examination of potential changes in retina circuitry that have been implicated in adaptation between 1 and 2 months of age (16, 17). As expected, because of the adaptation to background light and the subsequent smaller baseline diameter, the maximal constriction amplitude (in %) in C57BL/6 mice was reduced under photopic conditions compared to that under scotopic conditions. More importantly, age was found to influence the effect of photopic conditions on the minimal diameter (in mm). Whereas at 1 month of age, in response to all stimuli, the minimal diameter was smaller under photopic conditions, at 2 months of age, this only occurred in response to low and medium red light (rod and cone-driven stimuli). Thus, in response to the specific rod- and cone-driven stimuli, photopic conditions induce a decrease in the minimal diameter independent of age. However, in response to all other stimuli (also directly implicating melanopsin cells), photopic conditions promoted a decrease in the minimal diameter only in 1-month-old animals. In this case, the smaller diameter could indicate improper integration of background light, which would result in some type of additive process comprising rod and cone input and melanopsin input. This experiment revealed the immature control of the PLR under photopic conditions at 1 month of age in C57BL/6 mice; however, we did not perform similar photopic examinations using Sv129S6 mice to confirm this result. Replicating such experiments in this strain could determine if this change in photopic sensitivity between 1 and 2 months is common to both wild-type strains.

In the early phase of recovery, the more pronounced early partial dilation observed in younger animals is a precise characteristic of rod and cone inputs (13). The setup of early recovery control thus also occurs between 1-month-old and older-aged mice. How the rod and cone inputs, which are transient and linked to light onset, play a role in the recovery phase is not well understood. In 1-month-old C57BL/6 mice, faster recovery was also observed when measuring the sustained amplitude at 9.5 s in response to medium and high blue light, two stimuli expected to be biased toward melanopsin input (13, 16). In humans, Adhikari et al. (12) reported the contribution of rhodopsin and melanopsin to the early recovery phase when subjects were pre-adapted to light. They showed that during the 1.7 s after stimulus offset, both rods and melanopsin were implicated in the early phase of recovery, whereas after 1.7 s post-stimulus offset, dilation was mainly controlled by melanopsin. The faster early and late recovery described in this study at 1 month of age is in accordance with the incomplete maturation of rod- and melanopsin-driven circuitry.

The changes in the pupil response at 1 month of age could reveal the functional refinement of photoreceptor (rod, cone, and/or melanopsin cells) input between 1 and 2 months of age. This hypothesis is consistent with the ERG results obtained from C57BL/6 mice and with the literature wherein most studies showed that ERG measures of retinal response differ between young animals after eye opening and adult mice, and increases until 1 month of age (19, 31). More importantly, in rats, Chaychi et al. (21) showed that the ERG response decreases with age between 1 and 2 months of age (21), consistently with results described in this study. In C57BL/6 mice, Vistamehr and Tian (32) observed the same decrease in a- and b-wave amplitudes from P30 to P60, but this effect did not reach significance (32). Nevertheless, in this study, oscillatory potential amplitudes were significantly reduced from P30 to P60 and to P90. Since oscillatory potential reflects the interaction between bipolar, amacrine cells and retinal ganglion cells, this finding could also reflect the refinement of the retinal circuitry for the PLR.

Whereas our results suggest modifications of the PLR circuitry that occur with age, our histological data did not reveal obvious changes in retinal composition between 1- and 2-month-old mice for classical rod, cone, amacrine, horizontal, and ganglion cells. However, we cannot exclude subtle changes in connections between cells at the outer or inner plexiform layer, as well as in the afferent and efferent pathways involved in the PLR. Further work using whole-mount techniques and electron microscopy is essential to reveal cellular morphological changes and are needed to define the biological basis of PLR refinement between 1 and 2 months of age. Nevertheless, this report shows that in mice, age affects both transient and steady-state mouse pupil diameters. Our results suggest that functional maturation of the retina still takes place after 1 month of age, indicating that studies on adult mouse retinal function should be performed on animals 2 months of age or older. This work also emphasizes the need for the use of adequate control animals of the same background age when PLR is used to explore retinal dystrophy models.

AUTHOR CONTRIBUTIONS

CK and NK conceived, designed, and supervised the project. NK, CM, and SC performed the experiments. NK, SC, AK, and CK participated in the analysis and interpretation of the data. NK and CK wrote the manuscript. All authors critically revised and approved the final version of the manuscript.

ACKNOWLEDGMENTS

We thank Nathalie Terrier for her technical support and Dana Wanner for editing. We would like to thank Editage (www.editage.com) for English language editing. This work was supported by the Foundation Gelbert, the Fondation Kattenburg (project RETPUP), and the Fondation Asile des Aveugles.

REFERENCES

1. McCulloch DL, Marmor MF, Brigell MG, Hamilton R, Holder GE, Tzekov R, et al. ISCEV Standard for full-field clinical electroretinography (2015 update). *Doc Ophthalmol.* (2015) 130:1–12. doi: 10.1007/s10633-014-9473-7
2. Robson AG, Nilsson J, Li S, Jalali S, Fulton AB, Tormene AP, et al. ISCEV guide to visual electrodiagnostic procedures. *Doc Ophthalmol.* (2018) 136:1–26. doi: 10.1007/s10633-017-9621-y
3. Kremmer S, Eckstein A, Gal A, Apfelstedt-Sylla E, Wedemann H, Ruther K, et al. Ocular findings in patients with autosomal dominant retinitis pigmentosa and Cys110Phe, Arg135Gly, and Gln344stop mutations of rhodopsin. *Graefes Arch Clin Exp Ophthalmol.* (1997) 235:575–83. doi: 10.1007/BF00947087
4. Hanein S, Perrault I, Gerber S, Tanguy G, Barbet F, Ducroq D, et al. Leber congenital amaurosis: comprehensive survey of the genetic heterogeneity, refinement of the clinical definition, and genotype-phenotype correlations as a strategy for molecular diagnosis. *HumMutat.* (2004) 23:306–17. doi: 10.1002/humu.20010
5. Dai H, Zhang X, Zhao X, Deng T, Dong B, Wang J, et al. Identification of five novel mutations in the long isoform of the USH2A gene in Chinese families with Usher syndrome type II. *Mol Vis.* (2008) 14:2067–75.
6. Park JC, Moura AL, Raza AS, Rhee DW, Kardon RH, Hood DC. Toward a clinical protocol for assessing rod, cone, and melanopsin contributions to the human pupil response. *Invest Ophthalmol Vis Sci.* (2011) 52:6624–35. doi: 10.1167/iovs.11-7586
7. Kawasaki A, Munier FL, Leon L, Kardon RH. Pupillometric quantification of residual rod and cone activity in leber congenital amaurosis. *Arch Ophthalmol.* (2012) 130:798–800. doi: 10.1001/archophthalmol.2011.1756
8. Kawasaki A, Crippa SV, Kardon R, Leon L, Hamel C. Characterization of pupil responses to blue and red light stimuli in autosomal dominant retinitis pigmentosa due to NR2E3 mutation. *Invest Ophthalmol Vis Sci.* (2012) 53:5562–9. doi: 10.1167/iovs.12-10230
9. Kardon R, Anderson SC, Damarjian TG, Grace EM, Stone E, Kawasaki A. Chromatic pupil responses: preferential activation of the melanopsin-mediated versus outer photoreceptor-mediated pupil light reflex. *Ophthalmology* (2009) 116:1564–73. doi: 10.1016/j.ophtha.2009.02.007
10. Adhikari P, Zele AJ, Feigl B. The Post-Illumination Pupil Response (PIPR). *Invest Ophthalmol Vis Sci.* (2015) 56:3838–49. doi: 10.1167/iovs.14-16233
11. Joyce DS, Feigl B, Cao D, Zele AJ. Temporal characteristics of melanopsin inputs to the human pupil light reflex. *Vision Res.* (2015) 107:58–66. doi: 10.1016/j.visres.2014.12.001
12. Adhikari P, Feigl B, Zele AJ. Rhodopsin and melanopsin contributions to the early redilation phase of the Post-Illumination Pupil Response (PIPR). *PLoS ONE* (2016) 11:e0161175. doi: 10.1371/journal.pone.0161175
13. Kostic C, Crippa SV, Martin C, Kardon RH, Biel M, Arsenijevic Y, et al. Determination of rod and cone influence to the early and late dynamic of the pupillary light response. *Invest Ophthalmol Vis Sci.* (2016) 57:2501–8. doi: 10.1167/iovs.16-19150
14. Lucas RJ, Douglas RH, Foster RG. Characterization of an ocular photopigment capable of driving pupillary constriction in mice. *Nat Neurosci.* (2001) 4:621–6. doi: 10.1038/88443
15. Hattar S, Lucas RJ, Mrosovsky N, Thompson S, Douglas RH, Hankins MW, et al. Melanopsin and rod-cone photoreceptive systems account for all major accessory visual functions in mice. *Nature* (2003) 424:75–81. doi: 10.1038/nature01761
16. Lall GS, Revell VL, Momiji H, Al Enezi J, Altimus CM, Guler AD, et al. Distinct contributions of rod, cone, and melanopsin photoreceptors to encoding irradiance. *Neuron* (2010) 66:417–28. doi: 10.1016/j.neuron.2010.04.037
17. Keenan WT, Rupp AC, Ross RA, Somasundaram P, Hiriyanna S, Wu Z, et al. A visual circuit uses complementary mechanisms to support transient and sustained pupil constriction. *Elife* (2016) 5:e15392. doi: 10.7554/eLife.15392
18. Hayter EA, Brown TM. Additive contributions of melanopsin and both cone types provide broadband sensitivity to mouse pupil control. *BMC Biol.* (2018) 16:83. doi: 10.1186/s12915-018-0552-1
19. Gibson R, Fletcher EL, Vingrys AJ, Zhu Y, Vessey KA, Kalloniatis M. Functional and neurochemical development in the normal and degenerating mouse retina. *J Comp Neurol.* (2013) 521:1251–67. doi: 10.1002/cne.23284
20. Liu K, Akula JD, Hansen RM, Moskowitz A, Kleinman MS, Fulton AB. Development of the electroretinographic oscillatory potentials in normal and ROP rats. *Invest Ophthalmol Vis Sci.* (2006) 47:5447–52. doi: 10.1167/iovs.06-0702
21. Chaychi S, Polosa A, Lachapelle P. Differences in retinal structure and function between aging male and female sprague-dawley rats are strongly influenced by the estrus cycle. *PLoS ONE* (2015) 10:e0136056. doi: 10.1371/journal.pone.0136056
22. Young RW. Cell differentiation in the retina of the mouse. *Anat Rec.* (1985) 212:199–205. doi: 10.1002/ar.1092120215
23. Tian N. Visual experience and maturation of retinal synaptic pathways. *Vision Res.* (2004) 44:3307–16. doi: 10.1016/j.visres.2004.07.041
24. Simmons AB, Bloomsburg SJ, Sukeena JM, Miller CJ, Ortega-Burgos Y, Borghuis BG, et al. DSCAM-mediated control of dendritic and axonal arbor outgrowth enforces tiling and inhibits synaptic plasticity. *Proc Natl Acad Sci USA.* (2017) 114:E10224–33. doi: 10.1073/pnas.171354 8114
25. Allwardt BA, Lall AB, Brockerhoff SE, Dowling JE. Synapse formation is arrested in retinal photoreceptors of the zebrafish nrc mutant. *J Neurosci.* (2001) 21:2330–42. doi: 10.1523/JNEUROSCI.21-07-02330.2001
26. Zhao X, Stafford BK, Godin AL, King WM, Wong KY. Photoresponse diversity among the five types of intrinsically photosensitive retinal ganglion cells. *J Physiol.* (2014) 592:1619–36. doi: 10.1113/jphysiol.2013.262782
27. McNeill DS, Sheely CJ, Ecker JL, Badea TC, Morhardt D, Guido W, et al. Development of melanopsin-based irradiance detecting circuitry. *Neural Dev.* (2011) 6:8. doi: 10.1186/1749-8104-6-8
28. Humphries MM, Kiang S, McNally N, Donovan MA, Sieving PA, Bush RA, et al. Comparative structural and functional analysis of photoreceptor neurons of Rho-/- mice reveal increased survival on C57BL/6J in comparison to 129Sv genetic background. *Vis Neurosci.* (2001) 18:437–43. doi: 10.1017/S0952523801183100
29. Yilmazer-Hanke DM. Morphological correlates of emotional and cognitive behaviour: insights from studies on inbred and outbred rodent strains and their crosses. *Behav Pharmacol.* (2008) 19:403–34. doi: 10.1097/FBP.0b013e32830dc0de
30. Dobo E, Torok I, Mihaly A, Karoly N, Krisztin-Peva B. Interstrain differences of ionotropic glutamate receptor subunits in the hippocampus and induction of hippocampal sclerosis with pilocarpine in mice. *J Chem Neuroanat.* 64–65, 1–11. doi: 10.1016/j.jchemneu.2015.02.002
31. Fisher LJ. Development of synaptic arrays in the inner plexiform layer of neonatal mouse retina. *J Comp Neurol.* (1979) 187:359–72. doi: 10.1002/cne.901870207
32. Vistamehr S, Tian N. Light deprivation suppresses the light response of inner retina in both young and adult mouse. *Vis Neurosci.* (2004) 21:23–37. doi: 10.1017/S0952523804041033

8

Pupil Size as a Gateway into Conscious Interpretation of Brightness

Irene Sperandio [1*], *Nikki Bond* [1] *and Paola Binda* [2,3*]

[1] The School of Psychology, University of East Anglia, Norwich, United Kingdom, [2] Department of Translational Research and New Technologies in Medicine and Surgery, University of Pisa, Pisa, Italy, [3] Institute of Neuroscience, Consiglio Nazionale delle Ricerche (CNR), Pisa, Italy

***Correspondence:**
Irene Sperandio
i.sperandio@uea.ac.uk
Paola Binda
paola1binda@gmail.com

Although retinal illumination is the main determinant of pupil size, evidence indicates that extra-retinal factors, including attention and contextual information, also modulate the pupillary response. For example, stimuli that evoke the idea of brightness (e.g., pictures of the sun) induce pupillary constriction compared to control stimuli of matched luminance. Is conscious appraisal of these stimuli necessary for the pupillary constriction to occur? Participants' pupil diameter was recorded while sun pictures and their phase-scrambled versions were shown to the left eye. A stream of Mondrian patterns was displayed to the right eye to produce continuous flash suppression, which rendered the left-eye stimuli invisible on some trials. Results revealed that when participants were aware of the sun pictures their pupils constricted relative to the control stimuli. This was not the case when the pictures were successfully suppressed from awareness, demonstrating that pupil size is highly sensitive to the contents of consciousness.

Keywords: pupillometry, pupillary constriction, high-level visual processing, visual awareness, brightness

INTRODUCTION

Increments or decrements of light are associated with pupillary constrictions or dilations, respectively. This is known as the pupillary light reflex, and has been traditionally considered as a low-level mechanism that simply regulates the amount of light that enters the eye to optimize vision. However, since pupillometry—i.e., the measurement of the diameter and rate of reactivity of the pupil—was introduced more than 50 years ago, it soon became evident that pupillary responses can be used to index cognitive operations, such as thinking and emotional processing [(1, 2) for a review see (3)]. More recently, it has been argued that high-level visual processing, including attention, mental imagery, and contextual modulation, can also influence pupillary responses under conditions of constant retinal illumination, demonstrating that the pupil diameter is not solely determined by physiological factors [for reviews, see (4, 5)]. For example, it has been shown that covert shifts of attention to brighter surfaces cause pupillary constrictions (6–8) and that similar changes in pupil diameter can be induced even in the absence of visual stimulation by asking participants to mentally visualize a bright scene (9). By the same token, the pupil constricts in response to visual illusions of brightness (10) and stimuli that evoke the idea of bright objects, like pictures of the sun (11, 12) or words conveying brightness (13). Another line of experiments showing pupil changes in conditions of constant retinal stimulation examined the phenomenon of binocular rivalry between stimuli of different luminance. The typical finding is that pupil size follows the dominant percept, with a relative constriction when the brighter stimulus dominates conscious perception (14–16), and an attenuation of pupillary responses to light flashes when these were presented to the suppressed eye (14, 17–19). There is also a line of experiments demonstrating the importance of cortical signals, and specifically signals from the occipital visual cortex, for modulating the pupillary response to light. For example, pupil perimetry (measurement of the pupillary response to light stimuli located at different loci across the visual field) has provided clear evidence of reduced or absent pupillary light reflex in the blind visual area of patients with lesions to the occipital lobe [e.g., (20–23)].

Taken together, these findings provide compelling evidence in support of the view that the pupillary light reflex is sensitive to top-down modulation. This suggests that pupil light responses may be used as a read-out of the idiosyncrasies of visual perception—a simple, non-invasive, objective, and quantitative measure of our attentional biases, our illusion susceptibility, our ability to use contextual information etc., and an initial success of this strategy has recently been reported (24). However, before these exciting avenues can be explored, it is necessary to demonstrate that top-down effects on pupil response do in fact reflect the contents of visual awareness. One possibility to address this issue is to look for correlations between perceptual (e.g., brightness) judgments and pupillary responses (9, 25). Here we took a more radical approach and tested whether one such top-down effect requires visual awareness of the stimuli—and whether it is absent when stimuli are not consciously perceived.

The perceptual visibility of the stimuli, specifically pictures of the sun (11), was manipulated by means of continuous flash suppression [CFS; (26)], a widely used technique that enables to reliably erase stimuli from visual awareness for extended periods of time [for reviews, see (27, 28)]. During CFS, a static image presented to one eye is rendered invisible by ever-changing Mondrian patterns displayed to the other eye. This interocular suppression technique seems to be particularly effective at disrupting high-level visual processing completely [for a review, see (28)]. A particularly clear case can be made from adaptation studies. Aftereffects specific to complex motion [e.g., (29)], facial expression of emotions [(30); but see (31)], and subordinate information about faces, such as gender or race (32), all of which require higher order visual processing, were abolished when adapters were suppressed from awareness by CFS. In contrast, aftereffects specific to low-level stimulus attributes, such as orientation [e.g., (33)] and contrast [e.g., (34)], were only attenuated by CFS. Evidence from other paradigms, such as priming and braking-CFS, is more mixed. A suppressed stimulus is more likely to break CFS and come back to awareness when it is familiar and provided with emotional values [e.g., (35, 36)], suggesting that at least some form of high-level information may be processed even when the stimulus is suppressed from awareness [for a review, see (37)]. Similarly, a subliminal form of priming by stimuli made invisible by CFS, may in some cases be observed for numerosity [e.g., (38)], object category [e.g., (39)] and emotional content [e.g., (40)]; however, in other cases, priming effects for complex stimulus features, such as word stimuli (41), emotional faces (42), and threatening animal stimuli (43), vanish completely when the prime is rendered invisible by CFS. Thus, the literature on the effects of CFS on low- and high-level visual processing is mixed, suggesting that processing of many stimulus features can take place outside of conscious awareness. Nevertheless, high-level visual properties are likely to succumb suppression [e.g., (28, 44)], at least more than low-level simple visual features, which continue to adapt and shape perceptual processes quite irrespectively of awareness.

With the support of this literature, here we aimed to study how CFS would affect the pupillary response to sun image (vs. their phase scrambled versions). If—as argued before—the relative pupillary constriction evoked by the sun images depends on high-level visual processing, we predict that it should be abolished, or at least diminished, under CFS.

METHODS

Participants

Twenty-four participants (16 females, all right handed) ranging in age from 18 to 27 years ($M = 20.48$, $SD = 2.24$) with normal or corrected-to-normal vision, took part in the experiment. This sample size was deemed to be appropriate to attain a moderate effect size with $\alpha = 0.05$ and power $= 0.80$, according to calculations performed in G*Power (45). Two participants were excluded due to technical issues and an additional participant was excluded due to poor stereoacuity, as assessed using the Frisby stereotest (Clement Clarke International Ltd, Essex, UK). This resulted in a final sample size of 21 participants (13 females) with an age range of 18–27 years ($M = 20.42$, $SD = 2.03$). Participants received either 2 study credits or £5 for their time. Written consent was obtained prior to testing. All procedures were approved by the School of Psychology Research Ethics Committee of the University of East Anglia and were carried out in accordance with the Declaration of Helsinki.

Apparatus and Stimuli

The experiment was programmed in E-Prime 2.0 (Psychology Software Tools, Pittsburg, PA, USA) on a Viglen DQ77MK, running Windows 7. Stimuli were presented on a 16-inch Dell monitor with a resolution of 1,280 × 1,024 pixels and a refresh rate of 60 Hz. Participants were seated in front of the computer monitor in a dark room with their head fixed on a chin rest at a distance of 57 cm and viewed the stimuli through a mirror stereoscope. A divider (i.e., a sheet of cardboard) was placed between the stereoscope's midline and the center of the monitor to ensure that images displayed on each half of the monitor would be seen by each eye separately (46). Participants wore SMI™ (SensoMotoric Instruments) eye tracking glasses to measure their pupil diameter (see "Eye Tracking" for details).

Stimuli consisted of 13 different pictures of the sun and their phase-scrambled counterparts of matched luminance, as developed by Binda et al. (11) (available at: http://faculty.washington.edu/somurray/PupilSun/). The Supplementary material reports an analysis of the luminance profile of all images as a function of distance from image center (i.e., eccentricity, since fixation was maintained at image center). Across all images, there was a tendency for the sun images to have higher luminance than their phase scrambled versions near the center (although luminance was always lower than that of the pre-stimulus white screen), but this was not always the case (it is possible to select a subsample of pictures with matched luminance profiles, where additional analyses of the pupillary responses can be performed, see **Figures S2, S3**).

The stimulus was presented on the left half of the monitor. The rival stimulus consisted of a series of high-contrast Mondrian patterns with a flicker rate of 10 Hz, which were displayed to the right half of the monitor (26). The series of Mondrian patterns consisted of five distinct images cycling in a sequential order with individual frames refreshing every 100 ms (mean luminance = 70.84 cd/m^2). Both static and flickering stimuli were preceded and followed by a plain white background of maximum luminance, i.e., 196.30 cd/m^2, and subtended 7° × 7° of visual angle. A 1°-thick frame of various grayscale squares was placed around the stimuli to assist binocular alignment and a white small fixation cross was centered in each eye's stimulus to aid stable fixation (**Figure 1**). Participants' response was recorded by means of a keyboard.

Procedure

Prior to the beginning of the experiment, two frames with a fixation cross in each were presented dichoptically to the eyes and participants were instructed to adjust the stereoscope's mirrors until the left and right stimuli were correctly aligned and fused. In addition, to ensure that binocular fusion was maintained throughout the experiment, the same calibration stimuli were presented at the beginning of each trial and participants were asked to initiate the trial by pressing the spacebar on the keyboard only after they perceived a single frame and fixation cross.

To manipulate the perceptual visibility of the stimuli, participants were tested both in CFS and no_CFS conditions. In the CFS condition, the right eye was presented with a continuous stream of Mondrian images while static pictures of the sun or their scrambled versions were displayed to the left eye. Under this condition, the CFS mask typically renders perceptually invisible the static images for prolonged periods of time (26). In the no_CFS condition, the Mondrians were replaced by a blank background. The removal of the CFS mask should make the left-eye stimulus easily visible to the participants [e.g., (47)].

Each trial lasted for 6 s, which consisted of: (a) 2-s blank *pre-stimulus interval* where participants' eyes were exposed to the maximum luminance of the monitor; (b) 2-s *stimulus interval* where a static picture (sun or scrambled version) was displayed to the left-eye while flickering Mondrians (CFS) or a blank background (no_CFS) were displayed to the right-eye; (c) 2-s *post-stimulus interval* where the monitor returned to the maximum luminance (11). Participants were discouraged from blinking or making saccades over the entire duration of the trial but they were allowed to do so in between trials.

To ensure that stimuli were truly suppressed from conscious perception under the CFS condition, participants were asked at the end of each trial to report whether or not they saw an image besides the CFS mask (i.e., failure of suppression) by pressing designated keys on the keyboard. These unsuccessful trials were labeled as "failed CFS." In order to compare pupil traces in failed and successful CFS trials (characterized by identical stimulation but different conscious percept), we aimed to collect a significant amount of "failed CFS" trials, ideally as many as the successful ones. To this end, we chose to flash the sun/scrambled image abruptly, rather than gradually ramping it in, since flashing the stimulus is known to encourage CFS-breaking [e.g., (48)].

The experiment consisted of 52 trials in total, namely 2 suppression conditions × 2 image types × 13 repetitions. The suppression conditions (i.e., CFS vs. no_CFS) were tested in two separate blocks. The order of these two blocks was counterbalanced across participants. Within each block, trials were presented in a random fashion.

Eye Tracking

SMI^{TM} eye tracking glasses registered pupil diameter binocularly at a sampling rate of 60 Hz. A 3-point calibration was performed at the beginning of each block. Time points with impossible pupil size (i.e., exceeding the range 2–8 mm) were considered as signal losses and removed from the analysis. To measure the change in pupil diameter evoked by the static pictures, individual data were baseline-corrected against a 500-ms window preceding the stimulus presentation. The time course of the pupillary response was determined by averaging baseline-corrected data in 250-ms bins (25 data points). To allow comparisons across conditions, an average of the baseline-corrected data during the last second of stimulus presentation was also calculated (this window was selected based on previous data, as the interval where the difference across image types is expected to be the largest, see 11).

Data Analysis

A two-way repeated measures analysis of variance (ANOVA) was carried out on average baseline-corrected pupil diameter during the last second of stimulus presentation, to evaluate the main effects of Condition (no CFS vs. CFS) and Image Type (sun vs. phase-scrambled), and their interaction. To establish if changes in pupil diameter could predict individual differences in visual awareness of the pictures, we further analyzed the effect of Image Type separately in CFS trials where pictures were successfully suppressed or where they could still be seen by the participant. For this analysis, we relied on a Linear Mixed Model approach, motivated by the considerable sample size variability across subjects (due to the variability of the CFS success). In this approach, individual trials from all subjects are compared with a model comprising both the effect of experimental variables ("fixed effects") and the variability across participants ("random effects"). Fixed effects were coded as categorical variables Image type (sun vs. phase-scrambled) and Visibility Condition (no-CFS, failed-CFS and successful CFS). Random effects were coded by allowing subject-by-subject variations of both the slope and intercept for each of the fixed effects. An additional analysis reported in the Supplementary material combines the two approaches described above and directly compares pupil responses when the sun or scrambled images were seen (no-CFS and failed-CFS trials) or unseen (successful CFS trials), either considering all images or a subset of sun/scrambled images with matching luminance profiles.

For all analyses, we used standard MATLAB functions provided with the Statistics and Machine Learning Toolbox

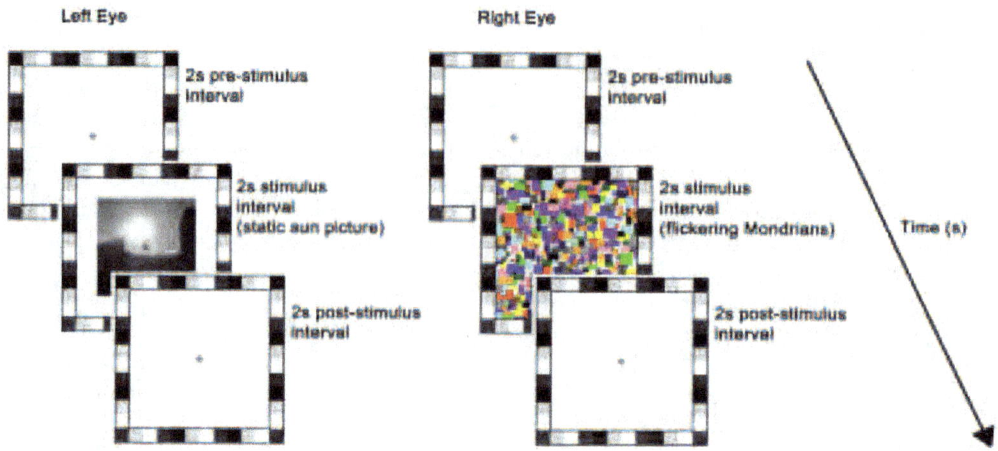

FIGURE 1 | Trial sequence and timing. At the beginning of each trial, a white background of maximum luminance was presented for 2 s (i.e., pre-stimulus interval). This was followed by a 2 s stimulus interval where a static picture (sun or scrambled version) was displayed to the left-eye while flickering Mondrians (CFS; as depicted here) or a blank background (No_CFS) were displayed to the right-eye. Finally, a blank screen was presented for 2 s during the post-stimulus interval. The flickering Mondrians successfully suppressed the static image in ~50% of trials on average, whereas images were always seen when accompanied by the blank.

(R2015b, The MathWorks). Specifically, the function "fitlme (data, model)" fit the linear-mixed model to the data, yielding an object "lme" with associated method "anova" that returns *F* statistics and *P*-values for each of the fixed effect terms. The function "fitrm (data, model)" fit the ANOVA for repeated measures, returning *F* statistics, degrees of freedom and associated *P*-values. Standard *t*-test functions were complemented with Bayes Factors estimations, using the "Bayes Factors" toolbox for Matlab available online at https://figshare.com/articles/Bayes_Factors_Matlab_functions/1357917. All reported *p*-values were based on two-tailed criteria.

RESULTS

We tracked changes in pupil diameter induced by the presentation of pictures of the sun and their scrambled version (11) and manipulated the perceptual visibility of the stimuli by means of CFS. The CFS mask successfully suppressed the unchanging image in 58.29% (s.e.m. 7.17%) of trials, while images were constantly visible under the no_CFS condition. The average baseline pupil size (during blanks, when screen luminance was maximum) was 3.66 mm (s.e.m = 0.11 mm); pupil baseline values were tightly distributed around this value, and never exceeded the 2.5–6.5 mm range, ensuring that our measurements were clear of the physiological limits of pupil diameter, where mechanical factors could artefactually reduce pupil size variability.

Figure 2A illustrates the time course of the pupillary response averaged across participants while mean pupil changes during the stimulus presentation is shown in **Figure 2B**.

A 2×2 ANOVA for repeated measures was carried out on the mean pupil size during the stimulus interval (shown in **Figures 2C,D**) with Condition (no-CFS vs. CFS) and Image Type (sun vs. scrambled) as main factors, revealing a significant interaction ($F_{1,20} = 12.835, p < 0.01$). The statistical significance of the interaction term means that the pupil difference between sun and scrambled images varies across conditions. This indicates that the CFS procedure was able to modulate the "sun-pupil effect" and suggests that the level of conscious awareness of the images is important for determining the pupil response they evoke. Note that the same conclusions hold when analyzing pupillary responses in trials when the sun/scrambled images were seen or unseen (**Figure S1**, collapsing no_CFS trials and trials in which CFS failed to suppress awareness of the images, and comparing them with trials in which CFS was successful in suppressing awareness). The conclusions also hold when analyzing only a subset of trials where both the average luminance and the spatial profile of luminance are matched between sun and scrambled images (**Figures S2, S3**).

To further investigate the effect of suppressing images from conscious awareness, we focused on the CFS condition and analyzed pupil responses separately in trials where CFS failed to suppress awareness of the sun/phase-scrambled pictures and where it succeeded in suppressing pictures visibility. Because different participants contributed an uneven number of trials, this analysis was conducted with a Linear Mixed Model approach (see methods). **Figure 3** shows the distribution of pupil responses when the sun pictures or the phase-scrambled images were displayed for the no_CFS condition (panel A), and separately for trials where CFS was successful at making the pictures invisible (panel C) and trials where pictures remained visible despite CFS (panel B). In the latter case, like in the no_CFS condition, there was a clear and reliable difference between pupil responses to the sun pictures and their phase-scrambled versions. In line with this, the Linear Mixed Model analysis revealed a significant interaction ($F_{(2,1970)} = 7.786$, $p < 0.001$) between the factors "Image Type" (sun vs. phase-scrambled) and "Suppression Condition" (no_CFS vs. failed CFS vs. successful CFS). The same significant interaction holds when selecting only CFS trials, failed and successful ($F_{(1,956)} = 4.842$, $p < 0.05$) indicating that the sun-scrambled pupil difference depends

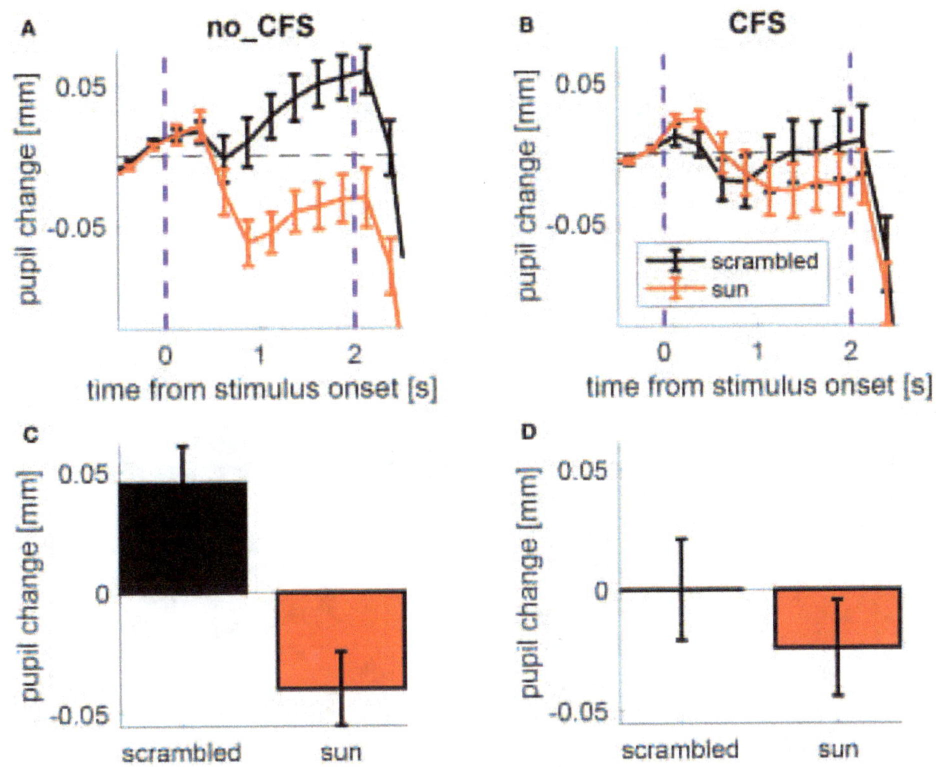

FIGURE 2 | Pupillary response to sun pictures and their phase-scrambled versions, under no_CFS (visible), and CFS conditions. **(A,B)** Baseline-corrected pupil diameter (i.e., pupil change) as a function of time from stimulus onset. **(C,D)** Mean pupil change during the last second of the stimulus interval. Error bars represent standard error of the mean (s.e.m) across our 21 observers.

on the awareness of the images. *Post-hoc t*-tests indicated a significant effect of Image type in the no-mask [two-sample *t*-test: $t_{(510,506)} = 6.71, p < 10^{-5}$] and failed CFS [$t_{(186,214)} = 3.50$, $p < 0.001$] conditions. However, there was no reliable difference between pupil responses to the sun and phase-scrambled pictures in trials where they were not consciously perceived, due to successful CFS [$t_{(295,265)} = 0.01$, $p = 0.994$]. For each of these *t*-tests, we computed the JZS Bayes Factor (49), which quantifies the amount of evidence against or in favor of the null hypothesis (i.e., that sun and phase-scrambled pictures evoke equal pupil responses): a BF smaller than 0.3 is strong evidence in favor of the null hypothesis; a BF larger than 3 is strong evidence against it. In the no-mask and the failed CFS condition, Bayes Factors were >30. In the successful CFS condition, however, the Bayes Factor was 0.094: strong evidence in support of the null hypothesis, or equal pupillary response to the sun and scrambled images.

Complementary to these *post-hoc* tests is another set of comparisons assessing the effect of CFS on pupillary responses to each image type (sun and scrambled). These indicate that the pupil dilation evoked by scrambled images was significantly reduced in successful CFS trials compared to failed CFS trials ($t_{(186,295)} = 4.71$, $p < 10^{-5}$, BF = 3903), whereas the pupil response to sun images was the same ($t_{(204,265)} = 1.00, p = 0.317$, BF = 0.166). Due to a limitation of the experimental design, this result does not lend itself to an unequivocal interpretation (as discussed below).

DISCUSSION

A growing body of evidence shows the role that extra-retinal factors exerts on the pupil diameter, challenging the notion that the pupillary light response is merely a reflex. The aim of the current study was to determine whether these modulations require visual awareness. In agreement with previous research (11, 12), we observed pupil constrictions to pictures of the sun relative to their phase-scrambled versions. However, this effect was only present when participants were aware of such stimuli, namely when the mask was replaced by a blank background (no_CFS) or when the stimuli broke through suppression and became consciously visible (failed_CFS). The effect disappeared when stimuli were made invisible (successful_CFS). Importantly, any potential difference in the luminance profile of the stimuli cannot account for the effect, implying that retinal and subcortical processing alone are insufficient to explain changes in pupil response. Instead, the pupil needs conscious (high-level) processing to be able to distinguish between sun and phase-scrambled pictures. This finding is in line with the large literature on CFS, showing that suppressing a stimulus from conscious

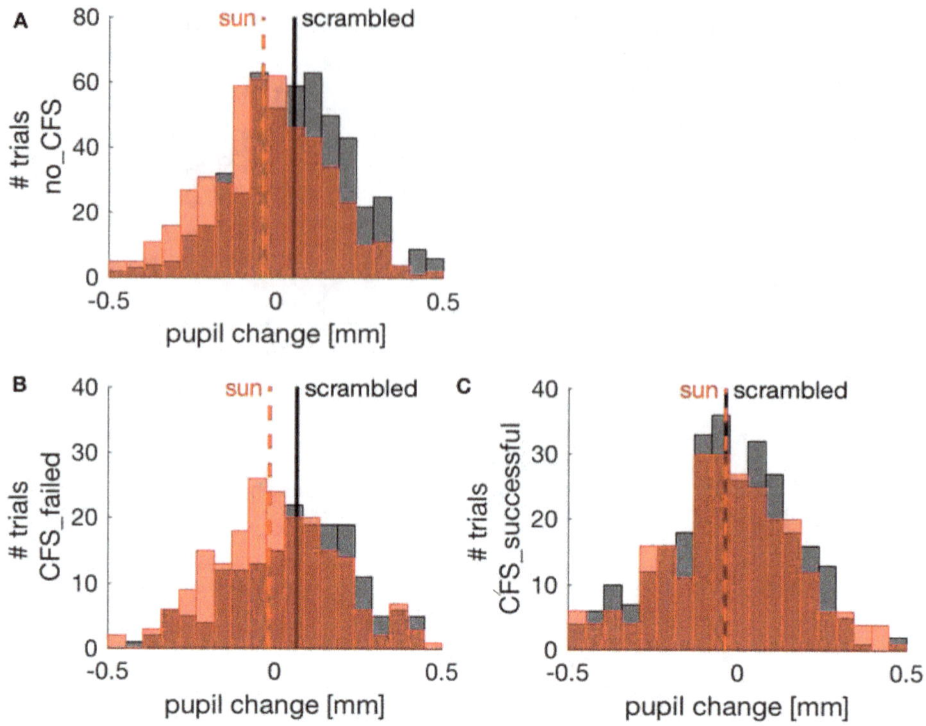

FIGURE 3 | Pupil changes (relative to the pre-stimulus baseline) in individual trials (pooled across participants). Red and black distributions show pupil responses to sun and phase scrambled pictures, respectively, with their means indicated by vertical lines. **(A)** trials from the no CFS condition; **(B)** trials where CFS failed to suppress awareness of the picture; **(C)** trials where CFS successfully made the sun/scrambled pictures unseen.

awareness limits its perceptual processing, especially for complex high-level stimulus properties (28, 37).

The hypothesis of a high-level modulation of pupil diameter is supported by numerous studies demonstrating changes in pupil response during high-level cognition, including spatial attention (6–8, 50), imagery (9), memory (51), decision-making (52), contextual (10–12), and semantic processing (13). Relevant to the present work is the observation of pupil modulations during binocular rivalry of stimuli with different luminance, whereby pupillary dilations were associated with perceptual transitions from bright to dark stimuli, and pupillary constrictions with transitions from dark to bright stimuli (15). Similar to Naber et al. (15), we found that under constant retinal illumination, pupil size adjusts according to the dominant percept. However, in our case, pupil size is independent of actual luminance of the dominant image [as was in Naber et al. (15)] but depends on high-level visual analyses producing a differential pupil response to pictorial representations of a high-luminance object (the sun) vs. a meaningless image matched in luminance and contrast (scrambled).

Note that, when images were successfully suppressed from visual awareness, the pupillary response was dominated by constriction—not dilation, as could be expected if the constriction in response to the sun image was selectively suppressed. This finding lends itself to two explanations. The first, which is hard to interpret, is that CFS only affects the pupil dilation in response to the scrambled images, leaving the response to sun images unaffected. The second, which we deem more sound, is that successful CFS trials are associated with enhanced pupil constriction because the high-contrast Mondrian mask-pattern dominates perception in these trials. This is a very reasonable scenario, given that high contrast images are known to generate pupillary constriction, provided that they are cortically processed [as reviewed in Barbur (53)], and given previous evidence shows that, when different stimuli are presented to the two eyes, pupillary responses are primarily driven by the consciously perceived stimulus (15). This constriction response to the mask-pattern confounds the interpretation of the individual pupil traces in response to the sun and scrambled images, leading to our inability to establish whether CFS interferes more with the response to one or the other image type. However, this does not confound our ability to compare the sun-scrambled difference in pupil response across conditions, and affirms that this is reduced in successful CFS trials, implying that CFS hampers the signals that differentiate sun and scrambled images for the purpose of generating a pupillary response.

What are these signals, and how do they affect pupil control? The pupillary light reflex relies on a simple subcortical system: from the retina, luminance signals are relayed to the olivary pretectal nucleus, which activates the parasympathetic neurons of the Edinger-Westphal nucleus to induce pupillary constriction

(54). Our findings along with several pupillometry studies lead to the suggestion that the pupilloconstrictor activity must incorporate input from a separate pathway: a brightness signal from the visual cortex, which is sensitive to the top-down effects described above [see also (55)]. This idea is further corroborated by a recent study on patients with Parinaud's syndrome (56), a rare condition following selective lesions of the subcortical pretectal area; although the pupillary reflex was depleted in these patients, remarkably their pupil size was modulated by attention. This indicates that pupil response may be regulated by multiple pathways, some of which are cortically-mediated. Together with the present results, this implies that pupil control incorporates information from relatively complex cortical visual processing. This conclusion is line with direct evidence from cortical lesion patients, who have atypical pupillary responses to light (e.g., 20–23) and to contrast, which are tightly linked to their residual (sometimes unconscious, e.g., blindisight) visual abilities (57).

Although a high-level cortical site appears to be the most likely origin for the signals controlling the pupil sun-scrambled differential response, we cannot exclude the possibility that both the perceptual suppression and the suppression of the pupil response in fact originate at an earlier site. Our two image categories (sun and scrambled) were matched in luminance and (for many images, see **Figures S2, S3**) in the gross spatial profile of luminance. However, many simple visual features were eliminated by the phase scrambling procedure, including local contrast at lines and edges (58). Further insight into the neural underpinning of this effect could be gained by creating alternative control images, through novel scrambling methods [e.g., (59)].

A note on the size of pupil modulations is in order. The pupil modulations we report here are 0.1 mm and less. These are similar in size to the effects of other perceptual and cognitive variables found to affect pupil size: while light responses are often in the range of 1 mm and more (2), 0.05–0.1mm is the typical size of pupil responses to equiluminant contrast (53), motion direction changes (60), spatial attention (6), and feature-based attention (61), implying that pupil modulations in this range can be reliably measured (with eye-tracking apparatus comparable to the one used here). Albeit measurable, 0.05–0.1 mm pupil change is very small compared to the full range of pupil size (2–9 mm). Appreciation of this point is important to guide speculations on the functional relevance of this and other cognitive and perceptual influences on pupil size. Some have argued that these influences could "optimize" the optics of the eye for specific perceptual and cognitive tasks, given that pupil diameter is known to affect the light adaptation state of the retina (62) and visual spatial resolution (63). However, there is no evidence that changing pupil diameter by a fraction of mm has any measurable consequence on vision. Thus, it is possible that the importance of these small pupil modulations does not lay in their impact on perception, but in their usefulness as indices to track the contents of perception or cognition. Specifically, here we have shown that pupil size is a sensitive and accessible index of visual awareness, which can precisely track the contents of consciousness on a trial-by-trial basis. As such, pupillometry may prove to be an important tool for the study of consciousness that could overcome methodological limitations of introspective reports when assessing perceptual experience.

AUTHOR CONTRIBUTIONS

IS and PB conceived the study and developed the study design. IS and NB built the experimental setup and developed the software for eye-tracking and stimulus presentation. NB performed data collection. PB analyzed the data. IS wrote the manuscript and PB provided critical revisions. All authors approved the final version of the manuscript for submission.

FUNDING

This research was supported by the European Research Council under the European Union's Seventh Framework Programme (FPT/2007-2013) under grant agreement number 338866 and by Fondazione Roma under the Grants for Biomedical Research: Retinitis Pigmentosa (RP)-Call for proposals 2013- Cortical Plasticity in Retinitis Pigmentosa: an Integrated Study from Animal Models to Humans.

REFERENCES

1. Goldwater BC. Psychological significance of pupillary movements. *Psychol Bull.* (1972) 77:340.
2. Loewenfeld I. *The Pupil: Anatomy, Physiology, and Clinical Applications.* Detroit, MI: Wayne State University Press (1993).
3. Laeng B, Sirois S, Gredebäck G. Pupillometry: a window to the preconscious? *Perspect Psychol Sci.* (2012) 7:18–27. doi: 10.1177/1745691611427305
4. Binda P, Murray SO. Keeping a large-pupilled eye on high-level visual processing. *Trends Cogn Sci.* (2015) 19:1–3. doi: 10.1016/j.tics.2014.11.002
5. Mathôt S, Van der Stigchel S. New light on the mind's eye: the pupillary light response as active vision. *Curr Dir Psychol Sci.* (2015) 24:374–8. doi: 10.1177/0963721415593725
6. Binda P, Pereverzeva M, Murray SO. Attention to bright surfaces enhances the pupillary light reflex. *J Neurosci.* (2013) 33:2199–204. doi: 10.1523/JNEUROSCI.3440-12.2013
7. Mathôt S, Van der Linden L, Grainger J, Vitu F. The pupillary light response reveals the focus of covert visual attention. *PLoS ONE* (2013) 8:e78168. doi: 10.1371/journal.pone.0078168
8. Naber M, Alvarez GA, Nakayama K. Tracking the allocation of attention using human pupillary oscillations. *Front Psychol.* 4:919. doi: 10.3389/fpsyg.2013.00919
9. Laeng B, Sulutvedt U. The eye pupil adjusts to imaginary light. *Psychol Sci.* (2014) 25:188–97. doi: 10.1177/0956797613503556
10. Laeng B, Endestad T. Bright illusions reduce the eye's pupil. *Proc Natl Acad Sci.* (2012) 109:2162–7. doi: 10.1073/pnas.1118298109

11. Binda P, Pereverzeva M, Murray SO. Pupil constrictions to photographs of the sun. *J Vis.* (2013) 13:8. doi: 10.1167/13.6.8
12. Naber M, Nakayama K. Pupil responses to high-level image content. *J Vis.* (2013) 13:7. doi: 10.1167/13.6.7
13. Mathot S, Grainger J, Strijkers K. Pupillary responses to words that convey a sense of brightness or darkness. *Psychol Sci.* (2017) 28:1116–24. doi: 10.1177/0956797617702699
14. Bárány EH, Halldén U. Phasic inhibition of the light reflex of the pupil during retinal rivalry. *J Neurophysiol.* (1948) 11:25–30.
15. Naber M, Frässle S, Einhäuser W. Perceptual rivalry: reflexes reveal the gradual nature of visual awareness. *PLoS ONE* (2011) 6:e20910. doi: 10.1371/journal.pone.0020910
16. Fahle MW, Stemmler T, Spang KM. How much of the "unconscious" is just pre-threshold? *Front Hum Neurosci.* (2011) 5:120. doi: 10.3389/fnhum.2011.00120
17. Brenner R, Charles S, Flynn J. Pupillary responses in rivalry and amblyopia. *Arch Ophthalmol.* (1969) 82:23–9. doi: 10.1001/archopht.1969.009900200 25007
18. Lowe S, Ogle K. Dynamics of the pupil during binocular rivalry. *Arch Ophthalmol.* (1966) 75:395–403. doi: 10.1001/archopht.1966.009700503 97017
19. Richards W. Attenuation of the pupil response during binocular rivalry. *Vision Res.* (1966) 6:239–40. doi: 10.1016/0042-6989(66)90044-7
20. Schmid R, Luedtke H, Wilhelm BJ, Wilhelm H. Pupil campimetry in patients with visual field loss. *Eur J Neurol.* (2005) 12:602–8. doi: 10.1111/j.1468-1331.2005.01048.x
21. Yoshitomi T, Matsui T, Tanakadate A, Ishikawa S. Comparison of threshold visual perimetry and objective pupil perimetry in clinical patients. *J Neuro Ophthalmol.* (1999) 19:89–99. doi: 10.1097/00041327-199906000-00003
22. Maeda F, Kelbsch C, Straßer T, Skorkovská K, Peters T, Wilhelm B, et al. Chromatic pupillography in hemianopia patients with homonymous visual field defects. *Graefe's Arch Clin Exp Ophthalmol.* (2017) 255:1837–42. doi: 10.1007/s00417-017-3721-y
23. Naber M, Roelofzen C, Fracasso A, Bergsma DP, van Genderen M, Porro GL, et al. Gaze-Contingent flicker pupil perimetry detects scotomas in patients with cerebral visual impairments or glaucoma. *Front Neurol.* (2018) 9:558. doi: 10.3389/fneur.2018.00558
24. Turi M, Burr DC, Binda P. Pupillometry reveals perceptual differences that are tightly linked to autistic traits in typical adults. *Elife* (2018) 7:e32399. doi: 10.7554/eLife.32399
25. Benedetto A, Binda P. Dissociable saccadic suppression of pupillary and perceptual responses to light. *J Neurophysiol.* (2016) 115:1243–51. doi: 10.1152/jn.00964.2015
26. Tsuchiya N, Koch C. Continuous flash suppression reduces negative afterimages. *Nat Neurosci.* (2005) 8:1096. doi: 10.1038/nn1500
27. Sterzer P, Stein T, Ludwig K, Rothkirch M, Hesselmann G. Neural processing of visual information under interocular suppression: a critical review. *Front Psychol.* 5:453. doi: 10.3389/fpsyg.2014.00453
28. Yang E, Brascamp J, Kang MS, Blake R. On the use of continuous flash suppression for the study of visual processing outside of awareness. *Front Psychol.* 5:724. doi: 10.3389/fpsyg.2014.00724.
29. Maruya K, Watanabe H, Watanabe M. Adaptation to invisible motion results in low-level but not high-level aftereffects. *J Vis.* (2008) 8:7.1–11. doi: 10.1167/8.11.7
30. Yang E, Hong SW, Blake R. Adaptation aftereffects to facial expressions suppressed from visual awareness. *J Vis.* (2010) 10:24. doi: 10.1167/ 10.12.24
31. Adams WJ, Gray KL, Garner M, Graf EW. High-level face adaptation without awareness. *Psychol Sci.* (2010) 21:205–10. doi: 10.1177/09567976093 59508
32. Amihai I, Deouell L, Bentin S. Conscious awareness is necessary for processing race and gender information from faces. *Conscious Cogn.* (2011) 20:269–79. doi: 10.1016/j.concog.2010.08.004
33. Bahrami B, Carmel D, Walsh V, Rees G, Lavie N. Unconscious orientation processing depends on perceptual load. *J Vis.* (2008) 8:12. doi: 10.1167/ 8.3.12
34. Shin K, Stolte M, Chong SC. The effect of spatial attention on invisible stimuli. *Attention Percept Psychophys.* (2009) 71:1507–13. doi: 10.3758/APP.71.7.1507
35. Gobbini MI, Gors JD, Halchenko YO, Rogers C, Guntupalli JS, Hughes H, et al. Prioritized detection of personally familiar faces. *PLoS ONE* (2013) 8:e66620. doi: 10.1371/journal.pone.0066620
36. Yang E, Zald DH, Blake R. Fearful expressions gain preferential access to awareness during continuous flash suppression. *Emotion* (2007) 7:882–6. doi: 10.1037/1528-3542.7.4.882
37. Gayet S, Van der Stigchel S, Paffen CL. Breaking continuous flash suppression: competing for consciousness on the pre-semantic battlefield. *Front Psychol.* (2014) 5:460. doi: 10.3389/fpsyg.2014.00460
38. Bahrami B, Vetter P, Spolaore E, Pagano S, Butterworth B, Rees G. Unconscious numerical priming despite interocular suppression. *Psychol Sci.* (2010) 21:224–33. doi: 10.1177/0956797609360664
39. Almeida J, Mahon BZ, Nakayama K, Caramazza A. Unconscious processing dissociates along categorical lines. *Proc Natl Acad Sci USA.* (2008) 105:15214–8. doi: 10.1073/pnas.0805867105
40. Almeida J, Pajtas PE, Mahon BZ, Nakayama K, Caramazza A. Affect of the unconscious: visually suppressed angry faces modulate our decisions. *Cogn Affect Behav Neurosci.* (2013) 13:94–101. doi: 10.3758/s13415-012-0133-7
41. Kang MS, Blake R, Woodman GF. Semantic analysis does not occur in the absence of awareness induced by interocular suppression. *J Neurosci.* (2011) 31:13535–45. doi: 10.1523/JNEUROSCI.1691-11.2011
42. Faivre N, Berthet V, Kouider S. Nonconscious influences from emotional faces: a comparison of visual crowding, masking, and continuous flash suppression. *Front Psychol.* (2012) 3:129. doi: 10.3389/fpsyg.2012. 00129
43. Cox E, Sperandio I, Laycock R, Chouinard PA. Conscious awareness is required for the perceptual discrimination of threatening animal stimuli: a visual masking and continuous flash suppression study. *Conscious Cogn.* (2018) 65:280–92. doi: 10.1016/j.concog.2018.09.008
44. Laycock R, Sherman JA, Sperandio I, Chouinard PA. Size aftereffects are eliminated when adaptor stimuli are prevented from reaching awareness by continuous flash suppression. *Front Hum Neurosci.* (2017) 11:479. doi: 10.3389/fnhum.2017.00479
45. Faul F, Erdfelder E, Lang AG, Buchner A. G* Power 3: a flexible statistical power analysis program for the social, behavioral, and biomedical sciences. *Behav Res Methods* (2007) 39:175–91. doi: 10.3758/BF03193146
46. Carmel D, Arcaro M, Kastner S, Hasson U. How to create and use binocular rivalry. *JoVE* (2010) 45:e2030. doi: 10.3791/2030
47. Kanai R, Tsuchiya N, Verstraten FA. The scope and limits of top-down attention in unconscious visual processing. *Curr Biol.* (2006) 16:2332–6. doi: 10.1016/j.cub.2006.10.001
48. Mudrik L, Breska A, Lamy D, Deouell LY. Integration without awareness: expanding the limits of unconscious processing. *Psychol Sci.* (2011) 22:764–70. doi: 10.1177/0956797611408736
49. Rouder JN, Speckman PL, Sun D, Morey RD, Iverson G. Bayesian t tests for accepting and rejecting the null hypothesis. *Psychonom Bull Rev.* (2009) 16:225–37. doi: 10.3758/PBR.16.2.225
50. Ebitz RB, Moore T. Selective modulation of the pupil light reflex by microstimulation of prefrontal cortex. *J Neurosci.* (2017) 37:5008–18. doi: 10.1523/JNEUROSCI.2433-16.2017
51. Bergt A, Urai AE, Donner TH, Schwabe L. Reading memory formation from the eyes. (2018) *Eur J Neurosci.* 47:1525–33. doi: 10.1111/ejn.13984
52. Urai AE, Braun A, Donner TH. Pupil-linked arousal is driven by decision uncertainty and alters serial choice bias. *Nat Commun.* (2017) 8:14637. doi: 10.1038/ncomms14637
53. Barbur J. Learning from the pupil: studies of basic mechanisms and clinical applications. Chalupa L, Werner J, editors, In: *The Visual Neurosciences*, Cambridge: The MIT Press (2004). p. 641–56.
54. Gamlin PD, Clarke RJ. The pupillary light reflex pathway of the primate. *J Am Optom Assoc.* (1995) 66:415–8.
55. Binda P, Gamlin PD. Renewed attention on the pupil light reflex. *Trends Neurosci.* (2017) 40:455–7. doi: 10.1016/j.tins.2017.06.007
56. Binda P, Straßer T, Stingl K, Richter P, Peters T, Wilhelm H, et al. Pupil response components: attention-light interaction in patients with Parinaud's syndrome. *Sci Rep.* (2017) 7:10283. doi: 10.1038/s41598-017-10816-x

57. Sahraie A, Trevethan CT, MacLeod MJ, Urquhart J, Weiskrantz L. Pupil response as a predictor of blindsight in hemianopia. *Proc Natl Acad Sci USA*. (2013) 110:18333–8. doi: 10.1073/pnas.1318395110
58. Thomson MG. Visual coding and the phase structure of natural scenes. *Netw Comput Neural Syst*. (1999) 10:123–32.
59. Stojanoski B, Cusack R. Time to wave good-bye to phase scrambling: creating controlled scrambled images using diffeomorphic transformations. *J Vis*. (2014) 14:6. doi: 10.1167/14.12.6
60. Sahraie A, Barbur JL. Pupil response triggered by the onset of coherent motion. *Graefes Arch Clin Exp Ophthalmol*. (1997) 235:494–500. doi: 10.1007/BF00947006
61. Binda P, Pereverzeva M, Murray SO. Pupil size reflects the focus of feature-based attention. *J Neurophysiol*. (2014) 112:3046–52. doi: 10.1152/jn.00502.2014
62. Campbell FW, Woodhouse JM. "Role of pupil light reflex in dark-adaptation. *J Physiol Lond*. (1975) 245:P111–2.
63. Campbell FW, Gregory AH. Effect of size of pupil on visual acuity. *Nature* (1960) 187:1121–3. doi: 10.1038/1871121c0

9

Functional Organization of the Sympathetic Pathways Controlling the Pupil: Light-Inhibited and Light-Stimulated Pathways

Elemer Szabadi*

Developmental Psychiatry, Queen's Medical Centre, University of Nottingham, Nottingham, United Kingdom

***Correspondence:**
Elemer Szabadi
elemer.szabadi@nottingham.ac.uk

Pupil dilation is mediated by a sympathetic output acting in opposition to parasympathetically mediated pupil constriction. While light stimulates the parasympathetic output, giving rise to the light reflex, it can both inhibit and stimulate the sympathetic output. Light-inhibited sympathetic pathways originate in retina-receptive neurones of the pretectum and the suprachiasmatic nucleus (SCN): by attenuating sympathetic activity, they allow unimpeded operation of the light reflex. Light stimulates the noradrenergic and serotonergic pathways. The hub of the noradrenergic pathway is the locus coeruleus (LC) containing both excitatory sympathetic premotor neurones (SympPN) projecting to preganglionic neurones in the spinal cord, and inhibitory parasympathetic premotor neurones (ParaPN) projecting to preganglionic neurones in the Edinger-Westphal nucleus (EWN). SympPN receive inputs from the SCN via the dorsomedial hypothalamus, orexinergic neurones of the latero-posterior hypothalamus, wake- and sleep-promoting neurones of the hypothalamus and brain stem, nociceptive collaterals of the spinothalamic tract, whereas ParaPN receive inputs from the amygdala, sleep/arousal network, nociceptive spinothalamic collaterals. The activity of LC neurones is regulated by inhibitory α_2-adrenoceptors. There is a species difference in the function of the preautonomic LC. In diurnal animals, the α_2-adrenoceptor agonist clonidine stimulates mainly autoreceptors on SymPN, causing miosis, whereas in nocturnal animals it stimulates postsynaptic α_2-arenoceptors in the EWN, causing mydriasis. Noxious stimulation activates SympPN in diurnal animals and ParaPN in nocturnal animals, leading to pupil dilation via sympathoexcitation and parasympathetic inhibition, respectively. These differences may be attributed to increased activity of excitatory LC neurones due to stimulation by light in diurnal animals. This may also underlie the wake-promoting effect of light in diurnal animals, in contrast to its sleep-promoting effect in nocturnal species. The hub of the serotonergic pathway is the dorsal raphe nucleus that is light-sensitive, both directly and indirectly (via an orexinergic input). The light-stimulated pathways mediate a latent mydriatic effect of light on the pupil that can be unmasked by drugs that either inhibit or stimulate SympPN in these pathways. The noradrenergic pathway has widespread connections to neural networks controlling a variety of functions, such as sleep/arousal, pain, and fear/anxiety. Many physiological and psychological variables modulate pupil function via this pathway.

Keywords: pupil, sympathetic, light, locus coeruleus, species difference, dorsal raphe nucleus, Edinger-Westphal nucleus, arousal

INTRODUCTION

The basic autonomic mechanism controlling the pupil is straightforward: pupil constriction is mediated via parasympathetic activation of the circular sphincter pupillae muscle, and dilation via sympathetic activation of the radial dilator pupillae muscle (1). The autonomic pathways regulating the pupil are illustrated in **Figure 1**. Both the sympathetic and parasympathetic controls are organized in a hierarchical fashion, in an ascending order from the periphery, to the spinal cord, brainstem, hypothalamus, and finally cerebral cortex (not shown). The autonomic output pathways have the general structure of autonomic efferents: two serially connected neurones synapsing in autonomic ganglia. Both the ganglia and the pre-ganglionic neurones projecting to them are well defined for pupillary control. Sympathetic preganglionic neurones in the "ciliospinal center" in the intermedio-lateral nuclear column (IML) of the cervico-thoracic spinal cord [segments C8-T2] project to the superior cervical ganglion (SCG), and parasympathetic preganglionic neurones in the Edinger-Westphal nucleus (EWN) of the midbrain project to the ganglion ciliare (GC). It should be noted that the EWN is not a homogenous structure: apart from preganglionic parasympathetic cholinergic neurones (EWpg) innervating the GC, there is also a population of centrally-projecting urocortin-containing neurones (EWcp) in the nucleus (2). Autonomic outflow to the iris is modulated by central autonomic pathways projecting to the preganglionic neurones via premotor autonomic neurones. Sympathetic promotor nuclei are the paraventricular nucleus (PVN) in the hypothalamus and the locus coeruleus (LC) and dorsal raphe nucleus (DRN) in the brainstem; parasympathetic premotor nuclei are the olivary pretectal nucleus (OPN) and the LC (see **Figure 2**). Some of the premotor nuclei are light-sensitive, either directly (DRN, OPN) or indirectly (PVN, LC), receiving luminance information from light-sensitive areas (see sections Pretectum/Periaqueductal Gray Pathway, Suprachiasmatic Nucleus/Paraventricular Nucleus Pathway, Dorsomedial Hypothalamus, and **Figure 2**, below).

In order to unravel the complexity of central autonomic regulation, it has been suggested to consider central autonomic control in terms of the functional organization of autonomic pathways (3–5, 7). Organizing principles have been suggested, such as target (5) or sensory input (4). Examples of functional organization have been presented (3, 7). However, the autonomic control of the pupil receives only patchy treatment in these papers.

As the fundamental function of the autonomic innervation of the pupil is to transmit the effect of light, it is proposed that the effect of light be used as the organizational principle in the case of pupil-controlling autonomic pathways. While light has a robust stimulatory effect on parasympathetic outflow, it has a dual (inhibitory/stimulatory) effect on sympathetic outflow. Thus the parasympathetic output is controlled by a light-stimulated pathway, whereas the sympathetic outflow is controlled by separate light-inhibited and light-stimulated pathways. The light-inhibited sympathetic pathway is yoked to the light-stimulated parasympathetic pathway mediating the pupillary light reflex: as the pupil is constricted by stimulation of the parasympathetic pathway, sympathetically mediated pupil dilation is withdrawn (8). The activity of the light-stimulated sympathetic pathways is less obvious since it is masked by sympatho-inhibition evoked by light. This masked effect can be revealed by pharmacological means, as discussed below (see section Noradrenergic Pathway). These pathways operate via more than one sympathetic premotor nucleus, and play an important role in mediating the effects of a number of physiological (arousal, pain, high temperature) and psychological (attention, mood, anxiety) variables on the pupil.

LIGHT-INHIBITED SYMPATHETIC PATHWAYS

Early work has shown that light inhibits neuronal activity in efferent peripheral sympathetic fibers, recorded from both preganglionic ("sympathetic nerves") (9–11) and postganglionic (long ciliary nerves) (12, 13) fibers, in cats. The reduction in discharge is linearly related to the intensity of the light stimulus (10). The sympathetic pathways conveying the effect of light originate from retina-receptive light-sensitive sites in the brain that project to the ciliospinal center (10, 12) Two possible candidates for the sites of origin of light-inhibited sympathetic pathways are the pretectum and the suprachiasmatic nucleus (SCN) of the hypothalamus. These pathways are displayed in

---

Abbreviations: CFFF, critical flicker fusion frequency; CRF, corticotropin-releasing factor; DMH, dorsomedial hypothalamus; DRN, dorsal raphe nucleus; IML, intermedio-lateral column (of spinal cord); EWN, Edinger-Westphal nucleus; GABA, y-aminobutyric acid; GC, ganglion ciliare; 5-HT, 5-hydrytryptamine (serotonin); LC, locus coeruleus; LHA, lateral hypothalamic area; OPN, olivary pretectal nucleus; PAG, periaqueductal gray (matter); PFA, perifornical area; PVN, paraventricular nucleus; SCG, superior cervical ganglion; SCN, suprachiasmatic nucleus; SPN, sleep-promoting neurones; TMN, tuberomamillary nucleus; VLPO, ventrolateral preoptic nucleus; VMAT, vesicular monoamine transporter; VTA, ventral tegmental area; WPN, wake-promoting neurones.

Figure 1 (for detailed description of the figure, see section Introduction, above).

Pretectum/Periaqueductal Gray Pathway

Early work by Okada et al. (13) provided experimental evidence in support of the hypothesis that the light-inhibited sympathetic pathway to the pupil, like the light reflex pathway (14), might originate from the pretectum. These authors introduced serial brainstem lesions to disrupt this putative pathway in an anesthetized cat preparation. On the basis of the effects of the lesions on light-inhibited sympathetic activity in long ciliary nerves, they concluded that there was a neural connection running from the pretectum to the cervical sympathetic. As the output from the pretectum to the parasympathetic preganglionic neurones in the Edinger-Westphal nucleus is excitatory, it remains to be explained how an inhibitory sympathetic pathway originates from the same area.

Two groups of light-sensitive neurones have been identified in the pretectum: one group in the olivary pretectal nucleus ("luminance detectors") that is stimulated by light, and another one ("darkness detectors") in the posterior pretectal nucleus that is inhibited by light (15). An attractive possibility may be that the light-stimulated parasympathetic and light-inhibited sympathetic pathways originate from these two different populations of light-sensitive pretectal neurones: the parasympathetic pathway from the luminance detectors, and the sympathetic pathway from the darkness detectors. However, there is no evidence to support this hypothesis.

More recent experimental evidence supports the existence of a neural link between the pretectal area and sympathetic premotor neurones. A direct link has been identified between the anterior pretectal nucleus and the rostral ventrolateral medulla (16), a major location of sympathetic premotor neurones in the brainstem (17). However, there is no evidence that the anterior pretectal nucleus is light-sensitive, and the rostral ventrolateral medulla is involved mainly in cardiovascular regulation (17). Therefore, it is likely that the inhibitory effect of light on sympathetic outflow to the iris is transmitted indirectly via the periaqueductal gray matter (PAG) of the midbrain. It has been shown that a projection from the OPN reaches sympathetic preganglionic neurones in the upper thoracic spinal cord and postganglionic neurones in the SCG via the PAG (18).

The PAG functions as an integrative relay nucleus (19). Sympathetic premotor neurones innervated by the PAG include the C1 (adrenergic) neurones in the rostral ventrolateral medulla, noradrenergic neurones in the A5 and A6 (locus coeruleus) nuclei, serotonergic neurones in the medullary raphe nuclei, and the PVN (20). Interestingly, the synapses of the PAG neurones on sympathetic premotor neurones have the morphological features of inhibitory synapses, and, therefore, it is assumed that the PAG may exert an inhibitory influence on the innervated postsynaptic cells (18, 21, 22).

Therefore, it is likely that, in the case of this light-inhibited sympathetic pathway, an excitatory output from the light-sensitive cells of the pretectum is converted into an inhibitory signal by the PAG (**Figure 1**).

Suprachiasmatic Nucleus/Paraventricular Nucleus Pathway

The PVN has been identified as a major sympathetic premotor nucleus (23), and its roles in the regulation of cardiac (24, 25) renal, (24) and liver functions, and melatonin synthesis (26, 27) are well documented in experiments conducted in rodents. It has been shown that the PVN exerts an excitatory effect on sympathetic preganglionic neurones via the neuropeptides vasopressin and oxytocin (28, 29). The PVN receives an input from the retina-recipient light-sensitive cells of the SCN of the hypothalamus, the "biological clock of the brain." It has been shown that, via this connection, light exerts a marked circadian influence on some sympathetic functions controlled by the PVN, such as melatonin synthesis (27) and glucose metabolism (30).

There is an overlap between the sympathetic controls of melatonin synthesis by the pineal gland and that of pupil dilation by the dilator muscle of the iris. In the case of both functions, the preganglionic neurones are located in the C8-T2 segments of the IML, and project to the SCG. This overlap is highlighted by a clinical observation: bilateral oculo-sympathetic paresis (Horner's syndrome) resulting from injury to the lower cervical/upper thoracic spinal cord leads to the cessation of nocturnal melatonin secretion (31).

The neuronal pathway controlling melatonin synthesis is well established: it runs from the SCN to the PVN, that projects to the preganglionic neurones in the IML (26) (**Figure 1**). Light exerts an inhibitory influence on melatonin synthesis via stimulation of an inhibitory GABAergic output from the SCN to the PVN. Two GABAergic inhibitory mechanisms have been identified in the SCN: (1) a time-of-day-dependent circadian mechanism that switches off the premotor neurones in the PVN during daytime, leading to the cessation of melatonin synthesis for the day phase of the day/night cycle; and (2) a light-activated inhibitory mechanism that becomes operational at night-time, when melatonin synthesis is released from its circadian inhibition, leading to acute suppression of melatonin synthesis (32).

Premotor neurones in the PVN involved in pupillary control are likely to be separate from those controlling melatonin synthesis since there is no evidence that pupil control is subject to the same circadian regulation as melatonin synthesis. However, these neurones, like those controlling melatonin synthesis, may also be susceptible to the direct inhibitory effect of light relayed via the SCN. Thus the SCN may give rise to a light-inhibited sympathetic pathway controlling pupillary function (**Figure 1**). On the other hand, the light-inhibited projection from the pretectum controlling pupil dilation (see Pretectum/Periaqueductal Gray Pathway), via inhibiting PVN activity, may contribute to the suppression of melatonin synthesis by light.

LIGHT-STIMULATED SYMPATHETIC PATHWAYS

It is well established that light constricts the pupil by stimulating the parasympathetic output to the constrictor pupillae muscle via

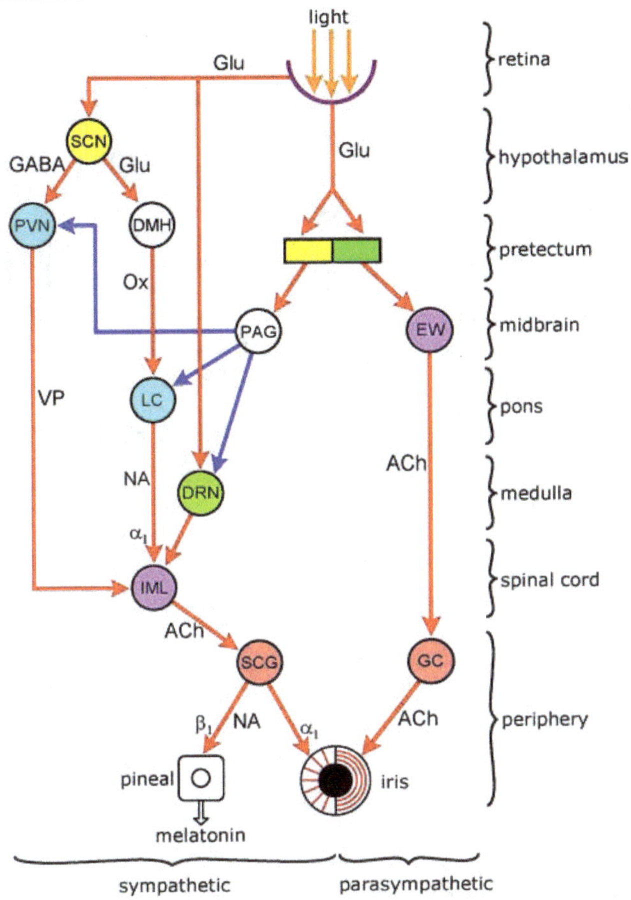

FIGURE 1 | Functional organization of autonomic pathways controlling the pupil. The encircled areas represent nuclei and ganglia. *Retinoreceptive light-sensitive relay nuclei* (yellow): SCN (suprachiasmatic nucleus); pretectum. *Retinoreceptice light-sensitive premotor autonomic nuclei* (green): parasympathetic–OPN (olivary pretectal nucleus); sympathetic–DRN (dorsal raphe nucleus). *Premotor autonomic nuclei* (blue): PVN (paraventricular nucleus); LC (locus coeruleus). *Preganglionic nuclei* (purple): parasympathetic–EW (Edinger-Westphal nucleus); sympathetic–IML (intermedio-lateral column). *Integrative relay nuclei* (white): DMH (dorso-medial hypothalamus); PAG (periaqueductal gray. *Autonomic ganglia* (pink): sympathetic–SCG (superior cervical ganglion); parasympathetic–GC (ganglion ciliare). *Connections* are shown by arrows: red-excitatory; blue-inhibitory. *Neurotransmitters*: Glu (glutamate); GABA (γ-amino-butyric acid); Ox (orexin); VP (vasopressin); NA (noradrenaline); ACh (acetylcholine). *Adrenoceptors* (postsynaptic): α_1 (excitatory); β_1 (excitatory). There are 5 *light-modulated autonomic pathways*: (1) parasympathetic (light-stimulated): OPN → EW → GC → sphincter pupillae muscle; (2) sympathetic (light-inhibited): pretectum → PAG → sympathetic premotor nuclei (PVN, LC, DR) → IML→ SCG → dilator pupillae muscle; (3) sympathetic (light-inhibited): SCN → PVN → IML→ SCG → dilator pupillae muscle; (4) sympathetic (light-stimulated): SCN → DMH → LC → IML → SCG → dilator pupillae muscle; (5) sympathetic (light-stimulated): DR → IML → SCG → dilator pupillae muscle. Please note overlap of pathway 3 with control of melatonin synthesis. See text for details.

the light reflex pathway, and that pupil constriction is facilitated by the concurrent inhibition of the sympathetic output to the dilator pupillae muscle (1). Indeed, when recording from pre- or post-ganglionic sympathetic fibers innervating the iris, an inhibition of impulse flow in response to light has been detected (see section Light-Inhibited Sympathetic Pathways). Therefore, any increase in impulse flow in response to light would be masked by the dominant inhibitory effect. A stimulatory effect of light on the sympathetic control of the pupil, using pupil dilation as its corollary, could be unmasked by drugs modulating the activity of potential light-stimulated sympathetic pathways (see Pharmacological Unmasking of Light-Evoked Latent Pupil Dilation).

Noradrenergic Pathway

This pathway, with some of its connections, is shown in **Figure 2**. This Figure, like **Figure 1**, displays the basic autonomic control of the pupil, the sympathetic output projecting to the dilator pupillae muscle and the parasympathetic output to the sphincter pupillae muscle of the iris. The figure also shows the light reflex pathway (retina → OPN → EWN → GC → sphincter pupillae muscle). The hub of the noradrenergic pupil-control pathway is the LC. The LC functions as both a sympathetic and parasympathetic premotor nucleus. Anatomical studies in rats have shown that the LC (A6 noradrenergic nucleus), together with the A5 and A7 noradrenergic nuclei, projects to the spinal cord where noradrenergic axon terminals reach sympathetic preganglionic neurones [(33, 34), see also Figure 4 in (35)]. Furthermore, this projection is likely to be excitatory via postsynaptic α_1-adrenoceptors (36). The LC also projects to parasympathetic preganglionic neurones in the EWN (see Outputs) and the salivatory nuclei (SN) (37, 38). The LC exerts an inhibitory influence on preganglionic parasympathetic neurones via the stimulation of α_2-adrenoceptors (39, 40). The LC sends a rich ascending excitatory projection to the cerebral cortex, and functions as a major wake-promoting nucleus (41–44). Inputs to the LC include an indirect excitatory connection from the retina-recipient light-sensitive neurones of the SCN via the dorsomedial hypothalamus (DMH) (see Dorsomedial hypothalamus), excitatory inputs from the wake-promoting neurones (WPN) of the sleep-arousal network and inhibitory inputs from sleep-promoting neurones (SPN) of the sleep-arousal network (see Association With Sleep/Arousal Network), an excitatory input from the amygdala to parasympathetic premotor neurones (see Amygdala), and an excitatory input from the spinothalamic pathway conveying pain sensation (see Collaterals From Spinothalamic Tract).

The anatomical basis for the classification of the noradrenergic pathway as a light-sensitive pathway is an indirect connection from the retina to the LC via the SCN and DMH, identified by Aston-Jones and his colleagues [(45, 46); for a recent review see (47)]. There is evidence that light activates the LC both in humans and diurnal animals. It has been shown in humans by fMRI that light causes activation in a brain area corresponding to the LC (48), and in Nile grass rats, a species of diurnal rodents, increases the expression of cFOS, a marker of neuronal activity (49), both in the SCN and the LC (50). Furthermore, light exerts effects consistent with LC activation. It increases the level of arousal in both humans (51, 52) and diurnal animals (50, 53), and enhances sympathetic activity in both humans (51, 54), and animals, such as mice (55, 56).

The involvement of the LC in pupil control is well established. When recording simultaneously the firing rate of LC neurones and the diameter of the pupil in monkeys, a close parallelism could be observed between fluctuations in firing rate and pupil diameter (57). More recently, it has been reported that electrical microstimulation of the LC in monkeys (58) and rodents (59, 60) leads to pupil dilation. In humans, it has been shown with fMRI that pupil dilation responses to psychological stimuli correlate with activation in a brain area overlapping with the LC (61, 62).

Pharmacological Unmasking of Light-Evoked Latent Pupil Dilation

As light apparently constricts the pupil, any latent dilation of the pupil resulting from sympathetic activation via the noradrenergic pathway would be masked by pupil constriction resulting from sympathetic inhibition via the pretectum/PAG and SCN/PVN pathways, and parasympathetic stimulation via the OPN/EWN/GC pathway. The latent pupil dilation evoked by light can be unmasked by drugs that modulate the activity of the noradrenergic pathway via LC activity. The activity of central noradrenergic neurones is regulated by inhibitory α2-adrenoceptors on the noradrenergic neurones themselves ("autoreceptors"): α2-adrenoceptor agonists (e.g., clonidine) "switch off" the activity of these neurones, whereas α2-adrenoceptor antagonists (e.g., yohimbine) enhance it [see (44, 63)] (see α2-Adrenoceptors Associated With Premotor Autonomic Neurones).

Clonidine, by switching off the LC neurones in the noradrenergic sympatho-excitatory pathway to the pupil, causes pupil constriction in man. Interestingly, this effect is light-dependent: the reduction in pupil diameter in response to clonidine is greater in light than in darkness (64). This is likely to reflect a "baseline effect" (65): in darkness the baseline (i.e., sympathetic activity) is low, leading to an attenuated response to the sympatholytic drug clonidine; increasing latent sympathetic activity by light, and thus elevating the baseline, would enhance the response to the sympatholytic drug. A corollary to the potentiation of the miotic effect of clonidine by light is the potentiation of light-evoked pupil constriction by clonidine. When pupil diameter in light is used as a measure of pupil constriction, the light stimulus intensity/pupil diameter curve (pupil diameter plotted against logarithm of light intensity) is shifted to the left (66, 67). Thus the same light intensity evokes a larger response, or the same response is evoked by a lower intensity stimulus, indicative of potentiation. On the other hand, the α2-adrenoceptor antagonist yohimbine has the opposite effect: it shifts the light intensity/pupil diameter curve to the right, consistent with antagonism. Furthermore, when applied together, there is evidence of mutual antagonism between the effects of clonidine and yohimbine (66).

An alternative explanation for the light-dependent effect of clonidine may be that it is due to attenuation of the noradrenergic inhibition of the EWN, leading to potentiation of the light reflex (63, 68). However, potentiation of the light reflex response by clonidine is reported only rarely (see Pupillary Effects of Noradrenergic Drugs), and usually it cannot be observed at a time when there is evidence of the potentiation of light-evoked

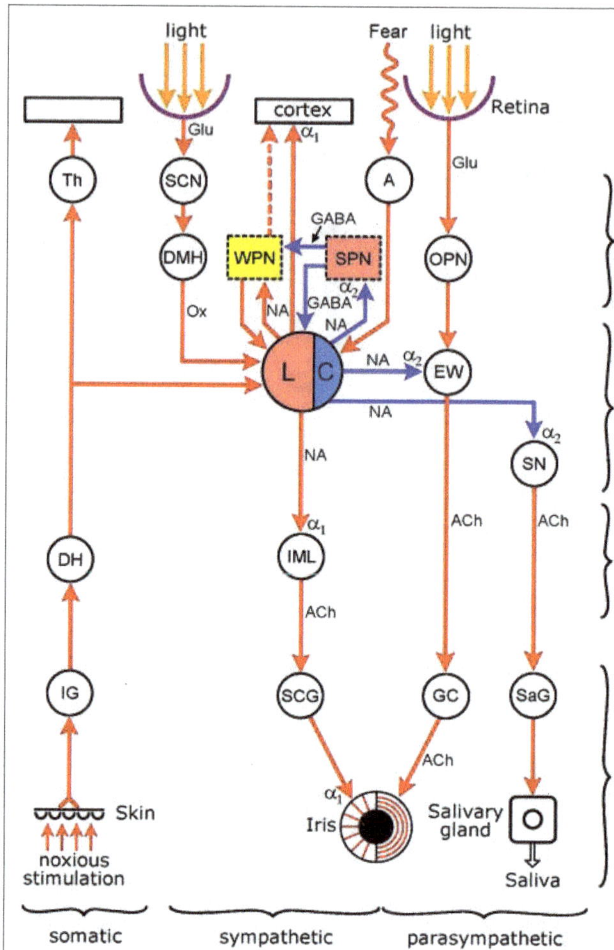

FIGURE 2 | Connections of the light-stimulated noradrenergic pathway. The encircled areas represent nuclei and ganglia. *Diencephalon* Th (thalamus); SCN (suprachiasmatic nucleus of hypothalamus); DMH (dorso-medial hypothalamus). WPN (yellow): wake-promoting nuclei (basal forebrain, thalamus, pedunculopontine tegmental nucleus, tuberomamillary nucleus. ventral tegmental area, dorsal raphe nucleus); SPN (pink): sleep-promoting nuclei (ventrolateral preoptic nucleus of hypothalamus, basal forebrain). A, amygdala; OPN, olivary pretectal nucleus. *Brainstem*: LC, locus coeruleus (pink: excitatory sympathetic premotor neurones, blue: inhibitory parasympathetic premotor neurones); EW (EWN in text: Edinger-Westphal nucleus); SN, salivatory nucleus. *Spinal cord*: DH (dorsal horn); IML (intermedio-lateral column). *Peripheral ganglia*: IG (intervertebral somatosensory ganglion); SCG (superior cervical ganglion); GC (ganglion ciliare); SaG (salivatory ganglion). *Connections* are shown by arrows: red–excitatory; blue–inhibitory. *Neurotransmitters*: Glu (glutamate); GABA (γ-amino-butyric acid); Ox (orexin); NA (noradrenaline); ACh (acetylcholine). *Adrenoceptors* (postsynaptic): α_1 (excitatory); α_2 (inhibitory). The *excitatory sympathetic premotor neurones in the LC* are stimulated by light (via the retina → SCN → DMH → LC pathway), by pain (via collaterals from the spino-thalamic tract), and via inputs from WPN during wakefulness; this would lead to an increase in sympathetic outflow to the iris (LC → IML → SCG → dilator pupillae muscle), manifesting as pupil dilation. The excitatory sympathetic premotor neurones in the LC are inhibited by SPN during sleep, leading to a reduction in sympathetic outflow to the iris, manifesting as pupil constriction. The *inhibitory parasympathetic premotor neurones in the LC* can be activated by fear and anxiety, via an input from the amygdala, leading to enhancement of the inhibition of parasympathetic preganglionic neurones in the EW (inhibition of light reflex: retina → OPN → GC → sphincter pupillae muscle pathway) and in the SN (reduction in salivary output: SN → SaG → salivary gland pathway). For WPN and SPN, see Szabadi (6). See text for details.

pupil constriction (67). Therefore, although occasionally there may be a parasympathetic contribution to the potentiation of light-evoked pupil constriction by clonidine, it is likely to be largely due to sympathetic inhibition.

Drugs indirectly modulating LC activity also have effects consistent with the unmasking of latent pupil dilation. The LC is activated by inputs from wake-promoting nuclei of the sleep/arousal network, such as the dopaminergic ventral tegmental area (VTA) of the midbrain (69, 70); and the histaminergic tuberomamillary nucleus (TMN) of the hypothalamus (71, 72) [for reviews, see (6, 44)]. The stimulant drug modafinil, by blocking the reuptake of dopamine at excitatory dopaminergic synapses on LC neurones (73), increases LC activity, and thus also the latent mydriatic effect of light. Indeed, modafinil shifts the light intensity/pupil diameter curve to the right, consistent with antagonism of light-evoked pupil constriction (67). Histamine, the excitatory neurotransmitter of wake-promoting tuberomamillary neurones, excites LC neurones via stimulation of H_1 histamine receptors (6), and this excitation is blocked by H_1 receptor antagonists (72). The H_1 receptor antagonists would decrease LC activity and thus potentiate latent pupil dilation. Indeed, diphenhydramine, a H_1 histamine receptor antagonist, has been shown to potentiate light-evoked pupil constriction (74). There is also evidence of antagonism between the effects of drugs that potentiate and antagonize light-evoked pupil constriction: the effect of modafinil is antagonized by clonidine (67), and the effect of diphenhydramine is antagonized by modafinil (74).

In conclusion, drugs modifying LC activity reveal the operation of a latent mydriatic effect of light that acts to attenuate light-evoked pupil constriction.

Functional Organization of Noradrenergic Premotor Autonomic Neurones in the Locus Coeruleus

Central noradrenergic neurones are dual function neurones: by stimulating both postsynaptic excitatory α_1-adrenoceptors and inhibitory α_2-adreneceptors at their postsynaptic projection targets, they can mediate both excitatory and inhibitory effects (44). This feature of the individual neurones underlies the dual function of the LC as a premotor autonomic nucleus. The LC contains both sympathetic and parasympathetic premotor neurones. The sympathetic premotor neurones send excitatory projections to the IML where they stimulate α_1-adrenoceptors on sympathetic preganglionic neurones (34, 36), while the parasympathetic premotor neurones project to inhibitory preganglionic neurones in the EWN (see Outputs) and salivatory nuclei (38) where they stimulate α_2-adrenoceptors (39, 40). For further details, see Noradrenergic Pathway, above, and for reviews, see 40, 41, 43. Although individual central noradrenergic neurones may have a dual excitatory/inhibitory role, projecting to several targets where they can stimulate either excitatory or inhibitory adrenoceptors, it is likely that the preautonomic neurones in the LC segregate into separate populations of excitatory sympathetic and inhibitory parasympathetic premotor neurones. These two populations are defined not only by their separate outputs but also by their separate inputs and their distinct susceptibility to physiological (light, pain) and psychological (threat) variables (41–43). Interestingly, recently two subpopulations of LC neurones have been identified on a genetic/developmental basis (75); however, there is no evidence to date whether these separate populations correspond to sympathetic and parasympathetic premotor neurones.

α_2-Adrenoceptors Associated With Premotor Autonomic Neurones

Inhibitory α_2-adrenoceptors are located at two sites: on the noradrenergic neurones themselves ("autoreceptors") (76, 77) and on the innervated target cells (neurone, glia cell or smooth muscle of blood vessels: postsynaptic receptors) (78, 79) [for reviews, see (44, 63, 80, 81)]. The inhibitory autoreceptors operate a negative feedback mechanism dampening the activity of the noradrenergic neurone. Somatodendritic autoreceptors, stimulated by noradrenaline released from dendrites and/or recurrent axon collaterals synapsing with the cell body/dendrites, attenuate the firing of the neurone (82), whereas presynaptic receptors on nerve terminals reduce the release of the neurotransmittter (83). Stimulation of postsynaptic α_2-adrenoceptors initiates inhibition of the cell receiving noradrenergic innervation.

There are three populations of α_2-adrenoceptor in/or associated with the preautonomic LC: autoreceptors on (1) sympathetic, and (2) parasympathetic premotor neurones, and (3) postsynaptic receptors innervated by parasympathetic premotor neurones. Drugs interacting with α_2-adrenoceptors can have differential effects on the three receptor populations,

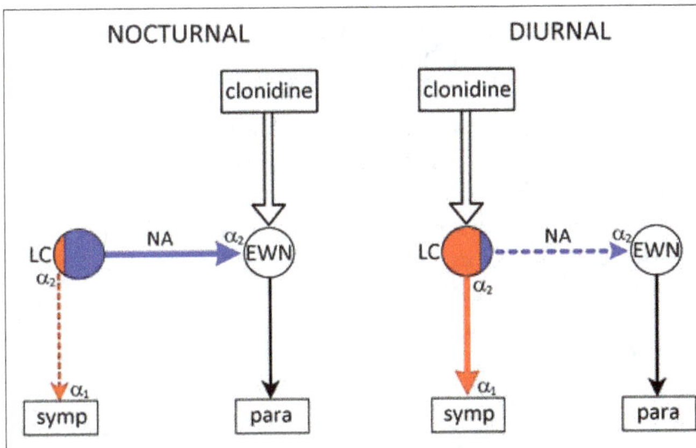

FIGURE 3 | Species-specific effect of the α_2-adrenoceptor agonist clonidine on the pupil. *Nuclei*: LC–locus coeruleus (red area: sympathetic premotor neurones; blue area: parasympathetic premotor neurones); EWN, Edinger-Westphal nucleus. symp: target of output from LC (sympathetic preganglionic neurones); para: target of output from EWN (ganglion ciliare). *Connections* are shown by arrows: red–excitatory; blue–inhibitory. *Adrenoceptors*: α_2 in LC–presynaptic inhibitory autoreceptor; α_2 in EWN–inhibitory postsynaptic receptor; α_1 on sympathetic preganglionic neurones–excitatory postsynaptic receptor. *Nocturnal animals*: clonidine stimulates inhibitory postsynaptic receptors in the EWN–inhibition of the EWN leads to mydriasis. *Diurnal animals:* clonidine stimulates inhibitory autoreceptors on sympathetic premotor neurones in the LC–attenuation of sympathetic outflow leads to miosis. See text (α2-Adrenoceptors Associated With Premotor Autonomic Neurones) for details.

due to their differential sensitivities. Interestingly, there is a species difference in the sensitivities of the three receptor populations: diurnal and nocturnal animals are affected differently by α_2-adrenoceptor agonists and antagonists.

In diurnal species (man, monkey, dog), the α_2-adrenoceptor agonist clonidine evokes miosis and sedation, consistent with a sympatholytic effect resulting from stimulation of inhibitory autoreceptors on sympathetic premotor neurones in the LC (42, 43, 63) (**Figure 3**). This is a selective effect: the other two populations of α_2-adrenoceptor remain largely unaffected. This may be due partly to the greater sensitivity of autoreceptors than postsynaptic receptors (84, 85), and partly the higher activity of sympathetic, compared to parasympathetic, premotor neurones. Sympathetic premotor neurones are likely to be more active due to their preferential stimulation by light (see Dorsomedial hypothalamus), and autoreceptor activity is a function of neuronal activity (81).

In contrast to diurnal animals, clonidine causes mydriasis in nocturnal (mouse, rat) and crepuscular (cat) animals (42, 43, 63) (**Figure 3**). This is consistent with the selective stimulation of postsynaptic inhibitory α_2-adrenoceptors in the EWN (40), innervated by a noradrenergic output from parasympathetic premotor neurones in the LC (see Outputs). The lack of evidence of autoreceptor stimulation in these neurones may be due to their presumed low baseline activity in the absence of stimulation by light.

Connections of Excitatory Sympathetic Premotor Neurones

Outputs

There is a robust projection from the LC to the spinal cord (coeruleo-spinal pathway), demonstrated in the rat (86). This pathway innervates all three contingents of spinal neurones: autonomic preganglionic neurones in the IML (87), sensory neurones in the dorsal horn (88), and motor neurones in ventral horn (89). The ciliospinal center receives its noradrenergic innervation via this pathway (41, 44).

Excitatory LC neurones also operate in the sleep/arousal network: they project to other wake-promoting neurones and the cerebral cortex (see Association With Sleep/Arousal Network).

Inputs

Latero-posterior hypothalamus. The orexinergic neurones in the lateral hypothalamic area/perifornical area (LHA/PFA) play an important role in the control of both arousal (6) and autonomic regulation (90): they mediate wake-promoting (91) and sympatho-excitatory (92) effects. The sympatho-excitatory effects of these neurones are mediated either directly by their projections to sympathetic preganglionic neurones (92), or indirectly via projections to sympathetic premotor neurones in the rostral ventrolateral medulla (RVLM) (90) and PVN (93). By projections to sympathetic premotor neurones in the LC (94), the orexinergic neurones of the LHA/ PFA stimulate sympathetic outflow to the iris. Interestingly, the hypothalamus, and in particular the latero-posterior hypothalamus containing the orexinergic neurones, has been implicated for a long time in the sympathetic control of the pupil (78, 95). Pupil dilatory responses reported in response to the electrical stimulation of the latero-posterior hypothalamus [see Table 6–19 in (96)] are likely to have been due to activation of orexinergic neurones projecting to the LC. Furthermore, the "tonic inhibition" of the EWN observed following hypothalamic stimulation may reflect the activation of parasympathetic premotor neurones in the LC in response to stimulation of the orexinergic input (see Connections of Inhibitory Parasympathetic Premotor Neurones).

There is also clinical evidence highlighting the importance of the lateral hypothalamus in the sympathetic control of the pupil. It is recognized that lesions of the postero-lateral hypothalamus can cause central type ipsilateral Horner's syndrome, characterized by miosis, blepharoptosis, and facial anhidrosis. This reflects the loss of the sympathetic output from the hypothalamus channeled through a descending pathway, via the SCG, to the iris (97).

Dorsomedial hypothalamus. The DMH projects to the LC (45) that sends excitatory outputs to the IML, wake-promoting neurones in the sleep/arousal network, and the cerebral cortex (see Noradrenergic Pathway, para 1). Via these connections light increases both the level of arousal and sympathetic activity in diurnal animals, including man (50, 51, 98, 99). This direct effect of light is separate from the effect of light on the entrainment of circadian rhythmicity to the day/night cycle, and is often referred

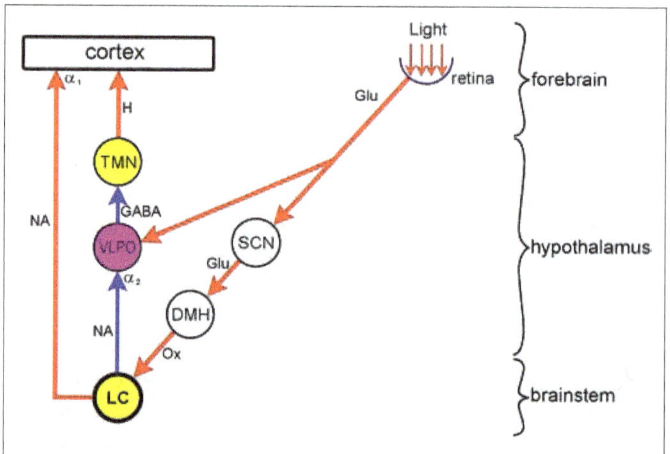

FIGURE 4 | Dual effect of light on arousal *Nuclei*: wake-promoting (yellow)–LC (locus coeruleus); TMN (tuberomamillary nucleus); sleep-promoting (purple)–VLPO (ventrolateral preoptic nucleus; relay (white)–SCN (suprachiasmatic nucleus); DMH (dorsomedial hypothalamus. *Connections* are shown by arrows: red–excitatory; blue–inhibitory. *Neurotransmitters*: Glu (glutamate); GABA (y-amino-butyric acid); Ox (orexin); H (histamine); NA (noradrenaline). *Adrenoceptors* (postsynaptic): α_1 (excitatory), α_2 (inhibitory). Light exerts a sleep-promoting effect by directly stimulating the sleep-promoting nucleus VLPO. This effect is largely mediated by inhibition of the wake-promoting nucleus TMN. Light also exerts a wake-promoting effect by indirectly stimulating, via the SCN and DMH, the wake-promoting nucleus LC. This effect is mediated by the direct stimulation of the cerebral cortex and the inhibition of the VLPO, thereby disinhibiting the wake-promoting TMN. In nocturnal animals the sleep-promoting, and in diurnal animals the wake-promoting, effect of light predominates. See text (Dorsomedial Hypothalamus) for details.

to as "masking," since it used to be regarded as a side-effect in the study of circadian regulation (50).

In contrast to diurnal animals, light is sleep-promoting ("somnogenic"), and darkness is wake-promoting in nocturnal animals, including rodents used in laboratory research (50, 100–102). Interestingly, in nocturnal animals the wake-promoting orexinergic neurones in the hypothalamus are activated by darkness (103), whereas in diurnal animals they are activated by light (104). The dual effect of light on arousal is likely to reflect the opposite effects of light on two hypothalamic nuclei: stimulation of the SCN leads to an alerting effect via the DMH and LC, whereas the stimulation of the ventrolateral preoptic nucleus (VLPO), a major sleep-promoting nucleus, leads to a sedative effect (43, 44, 102, 105) (**Figure 4**). In diurnal animals light would activate predominantly the SCN, while in nocturnal animals the predominant effect of light would be the activation of the VLPO. It has been suggested that the basis for the "temporal niche" (i.e., diurnality or nocturnality) may lie in the retina (106, 107). This suggestion has received experimental support recently (105). It has been shown that blue light has an alerting and green light a sedative effect. Therefore diurnal animals may show a higher sensitivity to blue in the spectrum, and retinal ganglion cells stimulated by blue light may project preferentially to the SCN. On the other hand, nocturnal animals' retinae may be more sensitive to green in the spectrum, and retinal ganglion cells stimulated by green light, may project preferentially to the VLPO (53, 105, 108).

In diurnal animals, luminance information is channeled via the SCN → DMH route to the LC leading to activation of not only wake-promoting but also sympathetic premotor neurones. The latter activation leads to an increase in sympathetic outflow in general, including cardiovascular activity, and increased sympathetic stimulation of the iris manifesting as pupil dilation [see Figure 9 in (44)]. Activation of the wake-promoting neurones in the LC leads to activation of the cerebral cortex, both directly via the coeruleo-cortical pathway (41, 44), and indirectly via shifting the overall activity of the subcortical sleep-arousal network in the direction of wake-promotion (6). Interestingly, cortical activation may involve areas associated with processing non-luminance-related information, such as cognitive load. As these cortical areas are known to project to the LC (58, 59, 109), their activation would provide reinforcing positive feedback to luminance-evoked LC activation.

Collaterals from spinothalamic tract. Pain signals are carried, via the somatosensory nucleus of the thalamus, to the somatosensory area of the cerebral cortex, by the spinothalamic (110, 111) and trigemino-thalamic (112) pathways (for review, see 42). Both pathways send collaterals to the LC, as demonstrated in the cat and monkey (113) (**Figure 2**). Pain signals increase LC activity, as shown in the rat by recording the electrical discharge of LC neurones (114, 115), expression of cFos (116), and noradrenaline release (117). Noxious stimulation also leads to pupil dilation, referred to as "reflex dilation." There is evidence that reflex dilation in humans and other diurnal species (e.g., rabbit) is related to sympathetic activation, suggesting that the collaterals from pain pathways synapse with excitatory sympathetic premotor neurones in the LC (**Figure 5**).

In humans, reflex dilation can be evoked by noxious cold (plunging one hand into ice-cold water: "cold pressor test") (118, 119), or electric shock (120, 121). Pupil dilation evoked by acute pain is a pure sympathetic response: the amplitude of the light reflex response, an index of parasympathetic activity, is unaffected (118, 119, 122) Reflex dilation can be antagonized by sympatholytics: α_1-adrenoceptor antagonists (e.g., dapiprazole) applied topically to the cornea (119, 121), or α_2-adrenoceptor agonists (e.g., dexmedetomidine) applied systemically (120).

In rabbits, another diurnal species, the noxious stimulus used was electrical stimulation of the sciatic nerve (123). Reflex dilation was antagonized by α_1-adrenoceptor antagonists (phentolamine, phenoxybenzamine, and prazosin), and potentiated by the α_2-adrenoceptor antagonist RS79948, administered systemically (123). The α_1-adrenoceptor antagonists may have blocked α_1-adrenoceptors at two sites (IML and iris) in the noradrenergic sympathetic pathway originating from the LC, whereas the α_2-adrenoceptor antagonist may have antagonized inhibitory autoreceptors in the LC. The α_1- and α_2-adrenoceptor antagonists failed to affect reflex dilation in the eye whose sympathetic input had been sectioned (124). Therefore, reflex dilation in the rabbit, like in man, is likely to be mediated by sympathetic excitation originating in sympathetic premotor neurones in the LC.

In contrast to diurnal species, in nocturnal animals, reflex dilation seems to reflect parasympathetic inhibition rather than sympathetic stimulation (**Figure 5**). Reflex dilation in cats (crepuscular animals) and rats was studied extensively by Michael Koss and his colleagues in the 1980s (40, 78, 125, 126). They found that pupil dilation evoked by painful electrical stimulation of the sciatic nerve was not affected by sympathectomy, was antagonized by monoamine depletion by reserpine or α-methyl-para-tyrosine and α_2-adrenoceptor antagonists (e.g., yohimbine),

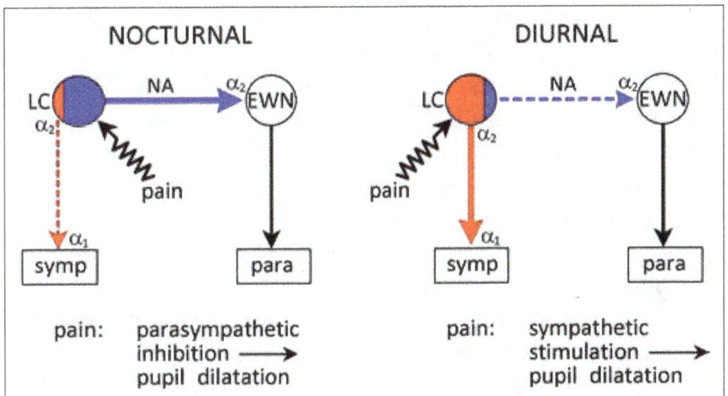

FIGURE 5 | Species-specific effects of noxious stimulation on the pupil. Conventions are as in **Figure 3**. Pain signals arising from noxious (painful) stimulation are conveyed to the LC via collaterals from the spinothalamic tract. Pain signals evoke pupil dilation ("reflex dilation") in both nocturnal and diurnal animals. However, the mechanisms are different. In nocturnal animals pain signals stimulate parasympathetic premotor neurones in the LC that project to the EWN to stimulate inhibitory α_2-adrenoceptors, mediating a parasympatholytic effect. On the other hand, in diurnal animals pain signals stimulate sympathetic premotor neurones in the LC, leading to a sympatho-excitatory effect. See text (Collaterals From Spinothalamic Tract) for details.

and potentiated by α_2-adrencoptor agonists (e.g., clonidine). They concluded that noxious stimulation in cats and rats activated a noradrenergic pathway inhibiting the EWN, leading to a reduction in parasympathetic outflow, appearing as pupil dilation (40) (see Collaterals From Spinothalamic Tract).

The differential effect of noxious stimulation on the noradrenergic control of pupil function in diurnal and nocturnal animals suggests that while in diurnal animals pain signals may preferentially activate excitatory sympathetic premotor neurones in the LC, in nocturnal animals they may activate mainly inhibitory parasympathetic premotor neurones projecting to the EWN (**Figure 5**).

Connections of Inhibitory Parasympathetic Premotor Neurones

Outputs

It has been shown in cats and rats that there is a central noradrenergic pathway that exerts an inhibitory influence on the EWN by stimulating inhibitory α_2-adrenoceptors (40). Moreover, it has been proposed that the inhibitory noradrenergic pathway to the EWN may originate from the LC, and that the LC could exert dual influence on pupillary activity via an excitatory output to the IML and an inhibitory output to the EWN (63) This model of the dual noradrenergic control of pupillary activity by the LC is elaborated further in the present review. An anatomical link has been described from the LC to the EWN (127, 128). Furthermore, it has been shown recently that this link operates via stimulation of α_2-adrenoceptors in the EWN. Liu et al. (60) found that pupil dilation evoked by the electrical microstimulation of the LC, following removal of the SCG, was abolished dose-dependently by the α_2-adrenoceptor antagonist yohimbine, applied to the EWN. This finding is also consistent with the existence of a direct link between the LC and the EWN, and thus has bearing on a controversy regarding the connection between the LC and the EWN (129). Nieuwenhuis et al. (130) argued that there was no direct connection between the LC and the EWN, and suggested a number of possible "alternative anatomical routes." However, direct and indirect connections are not mutually exclusive: such parallel connections between autonomic nuclei are known to exist in the autonomic nervous system (131). An example is the projection from the retina to the DRN: both a direct and an indirect connection have been described (see Retinal Inputs to the Dorsal Raphe Nucleus, and **Figure 6**).

Apart from sending an inhibitory output to the EWN, the LC also inhibits other parasympathetic preganglionic brainstem nuclei (salivatory nuclei, vagal nuclei) (44).

Inputs

Latero-posterior hypothalamus. Orexinergic neurones in the LHA/PFA project to the LC where they innervate both sympathetic and parasympathetic premotor neurones (see Connections of Excitatory Sympathetic Premotor Neurones). Electrical stimulation of the lateral hypothalamus in experimental animals leads to pupil dilation due to inhibition of the EWN via an inhibitory noradrenergic input (78). The likely mechanism underlying this observation is the activation of parasympathetic premotor neurones in the LC via an excitatory orexinergic input from the hypothalamus, leading to inhibition of the EWN via the stimulation of α_2-adrenoceptors.

Amygdala. The central nucleus of the amygdala sends an excitatory peptidergic projection to the LC; the neuropeptide involved is corticotrophin-releasing factor (CRF) (132). Both the amygdala (133) and the LC (134) have been implicated in the generation of anxiety. Furthermore, there is likely to be a synergistic interaction between these two nuclei in mediating anxious responses: stress-induced activation of the central amygdala is transmitted to the LC by a CRF-containing output from the amygdala (135, 136).

Anxious states amenable for experimental study can be generated by the paradigm of fear conditioning: pairing of a noxious stimulus (e.g., electric shock) with a neutral stimulus (e.g., light, sound) leads to the development of the ability of the neutral stimulus to evoke the response to the noxious stimulus. Using this paradigm, it was possible to modulate two physiological reflexes, the acoustic startle reflex and the pupillary light reflex, by the anticipatory anxiety associated with the procedure (43). Interestingly, the two reflexes are changed in opposite directions: the acoustic startle reflex is potentiated, whereas the pupillary light reflex is inhibited by conditioned fear.

In the case of the modulation of both reflexes by fear ("anticipatory anxiety"), the amygdala and the LC play a joint role. The activation of the amygdala by stressful stimulation is transmitted to the LC, leading to potentiation of the noradrenergic facilitation of striated muscle contraction, in the startle reflex paradigm, and enhancement of the noradrenergic inhibition of the EWN, leading to inhibition of the light reflex (43). As the inhibition of the light reflex by fear cannot be antagonized by the topical application of the α_1-adrenoceptor antagonist dapiprazole, while a small associated increase in pupil diameter can (137), the fear-inhibited light reflex is likely to be mediated entirely by the parasympathetic output to the iris, consistent with the predominant activation of parasympathetic premotor neurones in the LC by fear. The sensitivity of the accompanying mydriasis to antagonism by dapiprazole would indicate the associated involvement of the sympathetic output, probably arising from the activation of sympathetic premotor neurones in the LC.

Collaterals from spinothalamic tract. Collaterals from the spinothalamic tract project to parasympathetic premotor neurones in the LC in nocturnal animals, such as rats (40, 125, 126), and in crepuscular animals, such as cats (40, 78). Via this pathway, pain signals cause excitation of parasympathetic premotor neurones projecting to the EWN, where stimulation of inhibitory postsynaptic α_2-adenoceptors would lead to parasympathetic inhibition and pupil dilation (**Figure 5**).

Association With Sleep/Arousal Network

The sleep/arousal network is an assembly of interacting nuclei in the hypothalamus and brainstem, responsible for the control of arousal (6). The network consists of functionally antagonistic

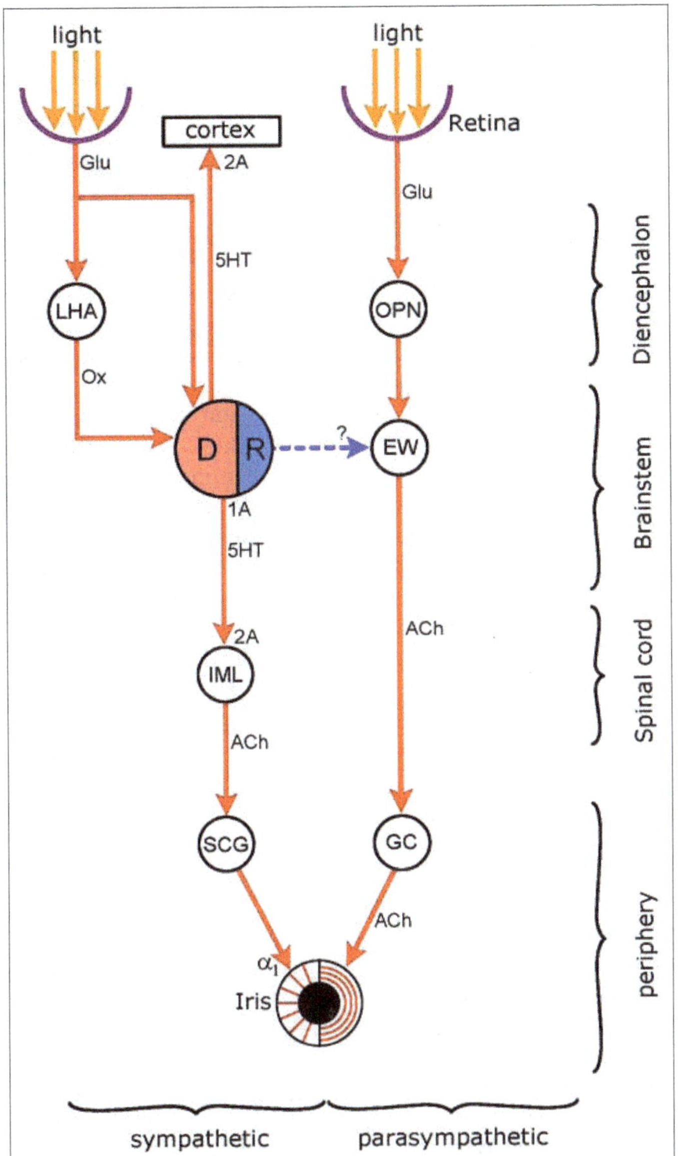

FIGURE 6 | Connections of the light-stimulated serotonergic pathway. *Nuclei*: DR (DRN in text: dorsal raphe nucleus; pink: excitatory sympathetic premotor neurones, blue: inhibitory parasympathetic premotor neurones); EW (EWN in text: Edinger-Westphal nucleus); OPN (olivary pretectal nucleus); LHA (lateral hypothalamic area), IML (intermedio-lateral column of spinal cord). *Ganglia*: SCG (superior cervical ganglion), GC (ganglion ciliare). *Connections* are shown by arrows: red-excitatory; blue-inhibitory (putative). *Neurotransmitters*: Glu (glutamate); Ox (orexin), 5HT (5-hydroxytryptamine, serotonin), ACh (acetylcholine). *Receptors*: α_1-excitatory postgsynaptic adrenoceptors; 2A–excitatory postsynaptic 5-HT_{2A} receptors; 1A–inhibitory 5-HT_{1A} autoreceptors. The DR receives both a direct and an indirect input from the retina; the indirect connection involves hypothalamic orexinergic neurones. The possibility of an inhibitory output from the DR to the EW, stimulating inhibitory postsynaptic 5-HT_{1A} receptors, has been investigated (see 5-HT1A Receptors).

wake-promoting nuclei (WPN) and sleep-promoting nuclei (SPN). WPN are active during wakefulness and quiescent during sleep, whereas SPN display the opposite pattern of activity. Each nucleus in the network is defined by its connections and the neurotransmitter used. WPN neurones use glutamate, the neuropeptide orexin, acetylcholine, and the monoamines noradrenaline, dopamine, serotonin (5-hydroxytryptamine [5-HT]), and histamine. The neurotransmitters of SPN neurones are γ-amino-butyric acid (GABA) and galanin. WPN send excitatory outputs to the cerebral cortex, whereas SPN function mainly by inhibiting WPN.

The LC is in the hub of this network. It receives inputs from all nuclei of the network, both WPN and SPN, and thus is a major integrator of sleep/arousal-related neuronal activity. It sends excitatory outputs, that operate via α_1-adrenoceptors, to the cerebral cortex and other wake-promoting nuclei, and inhibitory outputs, that operate via α_2-adrenoceptors, to the SPN (**Figure 2**). The LC has a two-way, mutually antagonistic relationship with the VLPO of the hypothalamus, a major sleep-promoting nucleus. The LC inhibits the VLPO, thus releasing other wake-promoting nuclei (e.g., tuberomamillary nucleus, TMN) from GABAergic inhibition, and consequently promoting waking, whereas the VLPO inhibits the LC, and thus facilitates sleep (**Figure 4**) (42).

Arousal-modifying drugs (sedatives, anesthetics, stimulants) may influence LC activity either directly or indirectly via inputs from the sleep/arousal network. Directly acting sedative drugs are the α_2-adrenoceptor agonists (e.g., clonidine, dexmedetomidine) and the μ opiod receptor agonists (e.g., morphine, heroin). The α_2-adrenoceptor agonists "switch off" LC activity by stimulating inhibitory autoreceptors on LC neurones (see α2-Adrenoceptors Associated With Premotor Autonomic Neurones). The μ opiod receptor agonists also suppress LC activity since μ opiod receptors are co-localized with α_2-adrenoceptors in the membrane of LC neurones and operate via a shared signaling mechanism (i.e., blockade of potassium channels) (138). Examples of drugs indirectly influencing LC activity and thus leading to alterations in the level of arousal are the stimulant modafinil and the sedative drug pramipexole. Both drugs act via an excitatory dopaminergic pathway from the VTA to the LC ("mesocoerulear pathway"). Modafinil increases dopaminergic excitation of LC neurones via blocking the uptake of dopamine into dopaminergic nerve terminals, leading to stimulation of excitatory postsynaptic D_2 dopamine receptors (67), whereas pramipexole reduces LC activity by attenuating the dopaminergic activation of LC neurones via stimulating inhibitory D_2 dopamine autoreceptors on the dopaminergic neurones (139).

As the LC is not only a wake-promoting, but also a pre-autonomic nucleus, it couples arousal and autonomic activity ("arousal/autonomic activity interphase") (42, 68). Consequently, alterations in the level of arousal are transmitted to the pupil. In general, an increase in alertness is associated with an increase in sympathetic output and pupil dilation, whereas sedation is linked to a decrease in sympathetic output and pupil constriction.

During transition from wakefulness to sleep (drowsiness or sleepiness), there is likely to be instability between opposing excitatory wake-promoting and inhibitory sleep-promoting inputs impinging on the LC, leading to fluctuations in LC activity. Due to the close association between LC activity and pupillary diameter (see Noradrenergic Pathway), the drowsiness-related fluctuations of LC activity are transmitted to the pupil, leading to fluctuations in pupil diameter. Thus instability between opposing excitatory and inhibitory inputs may be the basis for the appearance of pupillary oscillations in darkness, termed "fatigue waves" or "sleepiness waves" (140, 141). These oscillations increase as the level of arousal decreases. The Pupillographic Sleepiness Test (PST) provides quantitative measures of the oscillations that can be used as indices of the degree of sedation (142, 143). Indeed, the two measures of pupil diameter fluctuations generated by the PST (total power, Pupillary Unrest Index), correlate with electroencephalographic and subjective measures of sedation (144, 145).

The PST has also been used to assess the sedative and alerting properties of centrally acting drugs (74, 119, 139, 146–148), and the PST measures correlate well with other measures of alertness, such as critical flicker fusion frequency (CFFF) and visual analog scales. It would be expected that drug-induced changes in arousal would affect both pupillary indices of alertness: in the case of sedation, an increase in sleepiness waves would be paralleled by miosis, and in the case of stimulation, a decrease in sleepiness waves would be paralleled by mydriasis. Although this prediction has been confirmed in the case of some drugs (e.g., clonidine, yohimbine, modafinil), there are also exceptions to this general pattern. Examples of a dissociation between the effects of sedation on pupillary oscillations and pupil diameter are two highly sedative drugs: diazepam and pramipexole. While both drugs enhance pupillary oscillations in darkness, and display sedative effects on CFFF and visual analog scales, diazepam-induced sedation is associated with no change in pupil diameter (119), whereas pramipexole-induced sedation is accompanied by mydriasis (139). The possible explanation for the dissociation may lie in some actions of these drugs outside the sleep/arousal network or the LC. Such extraneous actions may either compromise the transmission of sympatho-excitatory signals from the LC to the SCG, or change the balance between sympathetic and parasympathetic outputs to the iris, by interfering with the parasympathetic output.

Diazepam, like all benzodiazepines, enhances the effect of endogenously released GABA at inhibitory $GABA_A$ receptors (149). Although the LC is richly endowed with GABA receptors, these receptors are insensitive to benzodiazepines (150). Therefore, benzodiazepines would induce sedation by stimulating inhibitory $GABA_A$ receptors elsewhere in the sleep/arousal network, leading to a reduction in the activity of wake-promoting neurones. However, the resultant decrease in LC activity is not passed on to the pupil by the sympathetic output from the LC. The possibility that diazepam may alter the relationship between the sympathetic and parasympathetic outputs to the iris has been excluded: it does not affect the parameters of the light reflex response or the diameter of the pupil dilated by the cholinoceptor antagonist tropicamide, applied topically (119). Therefore it is likely that diazepam interferes with sympathetic outflow "downstream" from the LC, most probably at the level of the IML.

Preganglionic sympathetic neurones in the IML integrate inputs from supraspinal premotor neurones, including those in the LC, and an intricate network of intraspinal interneurones (151). GABA receptors have been identified on bulbospinal neurones, projecting to sympathetic preganglionic neurones in the IML, on presynaptic terminals of such neurones, and on interneurones in the IML (152). Indeed, GABAergic neurotransmission plays an important role in controlling sympathetic outflow (153). Benzodiazepines may increase the activity of sympathetic preganglionic neurones via disinhibiting some of their excitatory inputs, and this increase in activity may mask the effect of the sedation-induced reduction in the excitatory input from the LC (119). However, further experimental work would be needed to confirm this hypothesis.

Pramipexole is a dopamine D_2/D_3 receptor agonist with a high affinity for inhibitory D_2 autoreceptors on dopaminergic neurones. It is highly sedative due to inhibiting an excitatory input to the LC from dopaminergic neurones located in the VTA. As expected, pramipexole-induced sedation is associated with enhancement of pupillary sleepiness waves. However, paradoxically, this is paralleled by mydriasis, rather than miosis (139, 148). This paradoxical effect of pramipexole may be due to the unexpected finding that it attenuates the pupillary light reflex response. As pramipexole has no affinity for cholinoceptors, a central mechanism has been postulated. Pramipexole, by stimulating inhibitory D_2 receptors on dopaminergic neurones in a putative excitatory pathway projecting to the EWN ("meso-pupillomor pathway"), may withdraw the dopaminergic activation of EWN neurones. Consistent with this model, it has been shown that amisulpiride, a D_2 dopamine autoreceptor antagonist, evokes an effect opposite to that of pramipexole: it potentiates the light reflex (148). Therefore, in the case of pramipexole-induced sedation, miosis resulting from a reduction in sympathetic outflow to the iris, as a consequence of reduced LC activity, may have been superseded by mydriasis, due to parasympathetic inhibition.

In conclusion, a change in pupil diameter may be a reliable index of drug-induced sedation only in the case of drugs that reduce sympathetic outflow to the iris by selectively reducing LC activity, such as the α_2-adrenoceptor agonists (e.g., clonidine, dexmedetomidine) (63) However, as many sedative drugs also influence sympathetic output by actions outside the LC, and/or also affect parasympathetic output to the iris, sedation-induced pupil diameter changes should not be used to draw conclusions about the sedative properties of centrally acting drugs. On the other hand, as alterations in pupillary oscillations ("sleepiness waves") are likely to be linked directly to LC activity, they may provide a reliable measure of sedation.

Connections Between Sympathetic and Parasympathetic Premotor Neurones

As discussed above (see Functional Organization of Noradrenergic Premotor Autonomic Neurones in the Locus Coeruleus), there is evidence supporting the view that sympathetic and parasympathetic premotor neurones in the LC form separate populations, and, in many situations, operate independently. However, the sympathetic and parasympathetic divisions of the autonomic nervous system do not function in isolation. Examples of cross-talk between the two divisions have been described in the medulla oblongata and the PVN in the hypothalamus (154).

There is also evidence of cross-talk between the two populations of premotor autonomic neurones in the LC. The anatomical basis of such cross-talk may be the gap junctions between LC neurones, through which cells can communicate with each other via eletrotonic transmission (155). Electrotonic coupling of LC neurones has been implicated in the synchronization of spontaneous firing and the generation of endogenous rhythmic activity (156, 157). An alternative mechanism may be the activation of noradrenergic parasympathetic premotor neurones from recurrent excitatory axon terminals of sympathetic premotor neurones. Indeed, such a mechanism has been described to operate in the LC (158).

The following two subsections discuss how two variables, light (Dual Modulation of Autonomic Activity by Light) and noradrenergic drugs (monoamine depletors, reuptake inhibitors, α_2-adrenoceptor agonists) (Pupillary Effects of Noradrenergic Drugs), may influence autonomic function by interacting with both contingents of noradrenergic premotor neurones in the LC.

Dual Modulation of Autonomic Activity by Light

Light is a powerful activator of sympathetic activity, consistent with light-evoked stimulation of sympathetic premotor neurones in the LC (see Dorsomedial hypothalamus). However, in addition to its sympatho-excitatory effect, light has also been reported to evoke a parasympatholytic effect (55, 159). The possible mechanism for this dual effect of light on autonomic outflow, affecting both divisions of the autonomic nervous system, may be the simultaneous activation of both sympathetic and parasympathetic premotor neurones in the LC. Parasympathetic premotor neurones may have been activated either directly or indirectly, via the spread of sympathetic premotor neuronal activity to parasympathetic premotor neurones via electorotonic transmission or recurrent axon collateras.

Pupillary Effects of Noradrenergic Drugs

Drugs acting at noradrenergic neurones may modify the activity and/or the transmitted effects of both sympathetic and parasympathetic premotor neurones, leading to alterations in both sympathetic and parasympathetic pupil control. Three classes of such drugs will be considered: vesicular monoamine transporter (VMAT) inhibitors ("monoamine depletors"), noradrenaline reuptake inhibitors, and α_2-adrenoceptor agonists.

Monoamines are accumulated in synaptic vesicles of the nerve terminals by an active membrane pump, the vesicular monoamine transporter (VMAT). The form of VMAT accumulating noradrenaline is termed VMAT2. Drugs that inhibit VMAT2 in noradrenergic nerve terminals, such as reserpine and tetrabenazine, lead to depletion of noradrenergic neurones of noradrenaline (160). These drugs are not selective for either sympathetic or parasympathetic premotor neurones in the LC: they deplete both populations of noradrenergic premotor neurones of noradrenaline. Depletion of noradrenaline of sympathetic premotor neurones leads to a sympatholytic effect (sedation, miosis, hypotension), whereas depletion of noradrenaline of parasympathetic premotor neurones results in a parasympathomimetic effect (potentiation of the light reflex response, increase in salivation) (161). The parasympathomimetic effect is likely to be due to removal of the noradrenergic inhibition of the EWN by the LC.

Noradrenaline reuptake inhibitors, including a number of antidepressants, enhance the effect of released noradrenaline, by blocking its reuptake into noradrenergic nerve terminals (44). They, like the VMAT inhibitors, are not selective for either population of pre-autonomic noradrenergic neurones in the LC, and potentiate the effects of noradrenaline at all the different targets of noradrenergic projection. The antidepressants desipramine, reboxetine, and venlafaxine enhance both the sympatho-excitatory and parasympatholytic effects mediated by noradrenergic autonomic outputs. These drugs cause mydriasis and shortening of the recovery time of the light reflex response, due to potentiation of noradrenergic stimulation of preganglionic sympathetic neurones in the IML and of the dilator pupillae muscle in the iris. They also attenuate the pupillary light reflex response and reduce salivary output, due to potentiation of the noradrenergic inhibition of preganglionic parasympathetic neurones in the EWN and the salivatory nuclei (162–165). It should be noted that while the parasympatholytic effect of desipramine could be due to the blockade of cholinoceptors in the iris, this explanation cannot be applied to the parasympatholytic effects of venlafaxine and reboxetine since these drugs have little affinity for cholinoceptors (164).

In contrast to the VMAT inhibitors and noradrenaline reuptake inhibitors, α_2-adrenoceptor agonists, like clonidine and dexmedetomidine, are selective for sympathetic premotor neurones in man and other diurnal species (see α2-Adrenoceptors Associated With Premotor Autonomic Neurones). The basis for this selectivity is likely to be a difference in the baseline activities of sympathetic and parasympathetic premotor neurones. Sympathetic premotor neurones are likely to have high baseline activity due to their stimulation by light via an input from the retina (see Dorsomedial hypothalamus), whereas the baseline activity of parasympathetic premotor neurones is likely to be low. Therefore, while inhibitory α_2 adrenergic autoreceptors are likely to occur on both populations of premotor autonomic neurones, the low baseline of parasympathetic premotor neurones does not allow the conversion of their stimulation into an inhibitory response (65). Indeed, while α_2-adrenoceptor agonists consistently evoke miosis, reflecting sympatho-inhibition in man, they do not usually affect the parasympathetically mediated light reflex response. However, there are exceptions to this general pattern: α_2-adrenoceptor agonists may occasionally potentiate the light reflex response (120, 166), consistent with the attenuation of the inhibition of the EWN by the LC. It is likely that in these cases the baseline activity of parasympathetic premotor neurones was high enough to allow autoreceptor stimulation to be converted into an observable response. The baseline activity of parasympathetic premotor neurones may have been raised by the spread of activity from the sympathetic premotor neurones to the parasympathetic premotor neurones via electronic transmission through gap junctions. An alternative mechanism may be stimulation of postsynaptic α_2-adrenoceptors on postsynaptic neurones in the EWN by clonidine, leading to disinhibition of the light reflex, as seen in nocturnal animals (see α2-Adrenoceptors Associated With Premotor Autonomic Neurones).

Serotonergic Pathway

This pathway is displayed in **Figure 6**. The figure shows the dual sympathetic/parasympathetic innervation of the iris, including the light reflex pathway via the parasympathetic output. The hub of the serotonergic pathway is the dorsal raphe nucleus (DRN) which contains serotonergic neurones, some of which function as sympathetic premotor neurones. These neurones send an excitatory projection to preganglionic neurones in the IML where it stimulates $5HT_{2A}$ receptors. The premotor autonomic neurones in the DRN contain inhibitory $5HT_{1A}$ receptors: the stimulation of these receptors by serotonin, released from recurrent serotonergic axon terminals, inhibits the activity of the serotonergic neurones. The existence of parasympathetic premotor neurones has been postulated: these neurones, via an inhibitory output to the EWN, would inhibit the light reflex. However, although the DRN inhibits the parasympathetic output to the pupil, this is likely to be via an indirect route (see 5-HT1A Receptors, below). The DRN also sends an excitatory output to the cerebral cortex where it stimulates $5HT_{2A}$ receptors. The DRN receives afferents from the retina, both directly and indirectly, via the LHA/PFA.

Serotonergic Neurones

Serotonin (5-hydroxytryptamine, 5-HT) is one of the major monamine neurotransmitters that, like noradrenaline, is involved in the regulation of both arousal (6, 167) and autonomic function (168, 169). Serotonergic neurones are located in nine nuclei (B1–B9) in the midline raphe of the brainstem, and project widely throughout the neuraxis (170, 171). Largest of these nuclei is B7, corresponding to the DRN, that is responsible for the serotonergic control of arousal (172). Several serotonergic nuclei are involved in autonomic regulation, including the DRN and a number of caudal raphe nuclei. These nuclei project to the IML of the spinal cord (171), where they are likely to stimulate excitatory $5HT_2$ receptors on sympathetic preganglionic neurones (152). There is also a population of serotonergic interneurones in the IML (173).

Serotonin interacts with a large array of presynaptic (auto) and postsynaptic receptors that can mediate both excitatory and inhibitory effects. $5\text{-}HT_1$ receptors are inhibitory, and occur both in presynaptic and postsynaptic locations, whereas $5HT_2$ and $5\text{-}HT_3$ receptors are excitatory, and occur postsynaptically (174). The most common and best studied receptor sub-types are the $5\text{-}HT_{1A}$ and the $5\text{-}HT_{2A}$ receptor (175). Inhibitory $5\text{-}HT_{1A}$ autoreceptors on serotonergic neurones play an important role in the regulation of serotonergic neurotransmission (176).

Retinal Inputs to the Dorsal Raphe Nucleus

Direct Link

During the past decade or so, an anatomical link has been identified between the retina and the DRN ("retino-raphe projection") in a number of rodent species. These species include the rat (177–179), the mouse (180); the Mongolian gerbil (179, 181, 182), and the Chilean degus (183). It has been shown that stimulation of this pathway by light can modulate the expression of cFos, an index of neuronal activity, in the DRN (182). Furthermore, stimulation of the DRN by light can lead to alterations in complex behaviors, such as affective (184) and defensive (180) behaviors. It has been shown that both conventional and melanopsin-containing retinal ganglion cells project to the DRN (185). The majority of retinal ganglion cells projecting to the DRN are conventional alpha-like ganglion cells with Y-like physiological properties (186, 187).

Indirect Link

Apart from the direct link described above, an indirect link via the orexinergic neurones of the LHA/PFA has also been reported. Orexinergic neurones may be directly light-sensitive via an input from the retina (188), or may be activated indirectly by light via the SCN (189). It has been found that, in the diurnal rodent Nile grass rat, a light pulse evoked an increase in the expression of cFos, in both the LHA/PFA and the DRN. Pretreatment of the animals with the orexin receptor type 1 (OXR1) antagonist SB-334867 prevented the activation of the DRN by light, leading to the conclusion that "in the diurnal brain light induces excitatory responses in the 5-HTergic DRN through activating orexinergic pathways" (104). For the role of the orexinergic system in pupillary control, see Latero-Posterior Hypothalamus.

5-HT Receptors Modulating Pupil Function

Serotonergic neurones in the DRN operate via stimulating serotonin receptors both in the DRN and the targets innervated by it. The two most important receptor types are the $5\text{-}HT_{1A}$ and $5\text{-}HT_2$ receptor. The role of these receptors in controlling pupil function has been explored using selective $5\text{-}HT_{1A}$ receptor agonists and $5\text{-}HT_2$ receptor antagonists.

$5\text{-}HT_{1A}$ Receptors

$5\text{-}HT_{1A}$ receptors occur both presynaptically (autoreceptors) and postsynatically where they mediate an inhibitory action. The autoreceptors are usually more sensitive than the postsynaptic receptors, and their role in controlling serotonergic neuronal function is analogous to that of the α_2-adrenoeptors in controlling noradrenergic neurone function (see α2-Adrenoceptors Associated With Premotor Autonomic Neurones). $5\text{-}HT_{1A}$ autoreceptors are abundant on serotonergic neurones in the DRN (190). The stimulation of these receptors on sympathetic premotor neurones would mediate a sympatholytic effect by switching off the activity of these neurones, and thus attenuating their excitatory influence on sympathetic preganglionic neurones (152). Postsynaptic $5\text{-}HT_{1A}$ receptors also play a role in autonomic regulation: by inhibiting sympathetic premotor neurones in the RVLM they mediate a sympatholytic effect on cardiovascular function (168). It has been postulated that, like α_2-adrenoceptors, $5\text{-}HT_{1A}$ receptors may occur on parasympathetic preganglionic neurones in the EWN (191) (**Figure 6**).

$5\text{-}HT_{1A}$ receptor agonists have marked effects on pupil function that are, like the effects of the α_2-adrenoceptor agonists, species-specific (see α2-Adrenoceptors Associated With Premotor Autonomic Neurones). In diurnal species, these drugs evoke miosis, whereas in nocturnal animals they cause mydriasis.

The 5-HT_{1A} receptor agonists buspirone, lesopitron, and 8-OH-DPAT evoked dose-dependent miotic responses in rabbit (192), monkey (193), and man (194–196). As in man, the buspirone-induced miosis was unaffected by the topical application of the cholinoceptor antagonist homatropine, it was concluded that the miotic response was likely to be due to sympathetic inhibition (194). Miotic responses to buspirone and lesopitron were also light-dependent: responses were larger in light than in darkness. As miotic responses to the α_2-adrenoceptor agonist clonidine show the same light-dependence, a similar mechanism was postulated, probably involving the noradrenergic inhibition of the EWN (see Pharmacological Unmasking of Light-Evoked Latent Pupil Dilation) (195). The light-dependence of the miotic responses to the 5-HT_{1A} receptor agonists is consistent with the operation of a serotonergic light-stimulated sympathetic pathway.

The 5-HT_{1A} receptor agonist 8-OH-DPAT evoked consistent dose-dependent mydriatic responses in mice (197) and rats (191). The pupillary responses could be antagonized by not only 5-HT_{1A} receptor antagonists (e.g., WAY-100135 and WAY 100635), but also by α_2-adrenoceptor antagonists (e.g., yohimbine and RS 79948). These observations argue against the existence of a direct serotonergic inhibitory input to the EWN operating via 5-HT_{1A} receptors (**Figure 6**). It was proposed that 8-OH-DPAT might have acted indirectly via the noradrenergic system: activation of noradrenergic neurones in the LC by the drug would have increased the release of noradrenaline onto inhibitory α_2-adrenoceptors in the EWN (191). Indeed, an intricate neuronal network has been proposed to operate within the LC modulating the firing of noradrenergic neurones. In this network, the noradrenergic neurones may be under tonic inhibition by GABAergic interneurones that in turn may be inhibited by a serotonergic input operating via inhibitory 5-HT_{1A} receptors. Therefore, disinhibition of the noradrenergic neurones by $5HT_{1A}$ receptor stimulation could lead to an increase in noradrenergic neuronal firing (198).

5-HT_2 receptors

An ascending output from the DRN to the cerebral cortex stimulates excitatory 5-HT_{2A} receptors, and thereby increases arousal (6), and a descending output to the sympathetic preganglionic neurones in the IML stimulates 5-HT_{2A} receptors, leading to sympathetic stimulation (**Figure 6**). It has been shown that the 5-HT_2 receptor antagonists ICI 169,369 and ICI 170,809 have dose-dependent miotic and sedative effects in man (199, 200), consistent with the attenuation of 5-HT_2 receptor-mediated functions. The dose-dependent miosis suggests that the 5-HT_2 receptors in the IML may mediate a tonic sympatho-excitatory effect on the pupil.

CONCLUSIONS

Light has robust effects on the autonomic control of the pupil: it stimulates the parasympathetic output and inhibits the sympathetic output. Stimulation of the parasympathetic output results in the light reflex mediating a constrictor response, whereas sympathetic inhibition, working "in the background," allows unimpeded expression of light-evoked pupil constriction (1). While the mechanisms underlying the light reflex have been the subject of intensive investigation, especially since the discovery of the role of melanopsin-containing retinal ganglion cells in its initiation (201), there has been relatively less interest in the sympathetic control of the pupil by light.

Interestingly, there may be multiple sympathetic pathways mediating the effect of light on the pupil: two pathways mediating an inhibitory effect ("light-inhibited sympathetic pathways") and two pathways mediating a paradoxical stimulatory effect ("light-stimulated sympathetic pathways") are described.

While the inhibitory effect of light on the sympathetic output to the pupil was demonstrated in the 1960s and 1970s, little experimental work has been done since then. Okada et al. (13) demonstrated a connection between the pretectal area and the sympathetic preganglionic neurones projecting to the iris. The course of this pathway has not been investigated since then. However, review of the literature of experimental work investigating the connections of the pretectum to autonomic nuclei, allows filling in the missing gaps. This has led to the proposal of the pretectum/periaqueductal gray pathway (see Pretectum/Periaqueductal Gray Pathway). A second putative light-inhibited sympathetic pathway is the suprachiasmatic nucleus/paraventricular nucleus pathway (see Suprachiasmatic Nucleus/Paraventricular Nucleus Pathway). This pathway overlaps with the pathway controlling melatonin synthesis, as sympathetic preganglionic neurones in the same segments (C8-T2) of the IML innervate, via the SCG, both the pineal gland and the dilator pupillae muscle in the iris. Although the role of this pathway in mediating the effect of light on the sympathetic control of melatonin synthesis is well established, its role in mediating the inhibitory effect of light on the sympathetic output to the pupil has not been studied experimentally.

The two light-stimulaed sympathetic pathways are based on well-established connections of their "hub" nuclei, the LC and the DRN. Both these nuclei are light sensitive, either directly (DRN) and/or indirectly (DRN and LC), and there is evidence of their roles in both the sympathetic and parasympathetic controls of the pupil. Light has a manifest sympatho-excitaroy effect on functions (e.g., cardiovascular or renal activity) controlled by the thoraco-lumbar sympathetic outflow. However, at the levels of C8-T2, the sympatho-excitatory effect of light may be superseded by its powerful inhibitory effect required for the operation of the light reflex and control of melatonin synthesis. Therefore, pupil dilation resulting from the stimulation of the sympathetic output to the iris would be masked by the pupil-constricting effect of light. The latent mydriasis can be unmasked by drugs that modulate the activity of the hub nuclei. Drugs that inhibit LC activity (e.g., clonidine, diphenhydramine) or DRN activity (e.g., buspirone) potentiate light-evoked pupil constriction, while drugs that enhance LC activity (e.g., yohimbine, modafinil) antagonize light-evoked pupil constriction. The light-stimulated sympathetic pathways, by attenuating light-evoked pupil constriction, may enable diurnal animals to function in daylight, when light may cause pinpoint pupils in nocturnal animals (202).

The activity of the light-stimulated pathways appears to be related to age. The monotonic decline in pupil diameter with increasing age in humans (203–205) may reflect the gradual withdrawal of the activity of the light-stimulated sympathetic pathways since the decline in pupil diameter is paralleled by the age-dependent decline in the number of noradrenergic neurones in the LC (42). The effect of age on the pupil is accentuated in Alzheimer's disease (206) when the loss of noradrenergic neurones in the LC exceeds that seen in old age (207).

The noradrenergic light-stimulated sympathetic pathway has widespread connections via sympathetic and parasympathetic premotor neurones in the LC, and via these connections it is integrated into the wider central autonomic network (41, 44). It is also integrated with the sleep/arousal network, and participates in the processing of pain signals and fear/anxiety. Many drugs (sedatives, stimulants, antidepressants, anxiolytics) modify pupil function by actions via the noradrenergic light-stimulated sympathetic pathway. Through its multiple inputs the noradrenergic light-stimulated sympathetic pathway is amenable to modulation by a wide range of physiological and psychological variables, and via its outputs it can transmit sympathetically and parasympathetically mediated alterations in pupil function.

There is a remarkable species difference in the operation of light-stimulated sympathetic pathways: diurnal animals respond differently from nocturnal animals to light, noxious stimulation, and autoreceptor agonist drugs (e.g., clonidine in the noradrenergic, buspirone in the serotonergic light-stimulated sympathetic pathway). A tentative explanation for the species difference may be that it is related to regular exposure to light in diurnal animals that may lead to proliferation and/or a raised baseline activity of sympathetic premotor neurones in the LC and DRN. Therefore autoreceptor agonists and pain signals may affect sympathetic premotor neurones preferentially, as compared to parasympathetic premotor neurones, in diurnal animals. These observations suggest that the effects of some non-luminance-related variables (monoaminergic autoreceptor agonists, noxious stimuli) may be influenced by the luminance-exposure history of the species, determined by the "temporal niche."

Apart from transmitting slow time-course ("tonic") changes in pupil diameter in response to light, the LC is also involved in mediating non-luminance-related fast time-course ("phasic") pupil dilations in response to cognitive load (57). It has been shown in the monkey (58, 109) and in the mouse and rat (59) that cognitive load, applied using different paradigms, evokes fast transient changes in the firing rate and pattern of LC neurones. Furthermore, corresponding changes can be observed in neuronal firing in different areas of the cerebral cortex and colliculi.

Unraveling the multiple sympathetic pathways controlling the pupil suggests that the sympathetic has roles beyond fading away in the background when the light reflex operates. While the parasympathetic pathway mediating the light reflex has one robust dedicated function, the sympathetic pathways, through their connections, are multifunctional, integrating pupil function with a wide range of autonomic, neuroendocrine, physiological, and psychological functions.

AUTHOR CONTRIBUTIONS

The author confirms being the sole contributor of this work and has approved it for publication.

ACKNOWLEDGMENTS

The author is grateful to Mr. RW Langley for drawing the figures.

REFERENCES

1. McDougall DH, Gamlin PD. Autonomic control of the eye. *Compr Physiol.* (2015) 5:439–73. doi: 10.1002/cphy.c140014
2. Kozicz T, Bittencourt JS, May P, Reiner A, Gamlin PDR, Palkovits M, et al. The Edinger-Westphal nucleus: a historical, structural and functional perspective on a dichotomous terminology. *J Comp Neurol.* (2011) 519:1413–34. doi: 10.1002/cne.22580
3. Janig W, McLachlan EM. Specialized functional pathways are the building blocks of the autonomic nervous system. *J Auton Nerv Syst.* (1992) 41:3–13. doi: 10.1016/0165-1838(92)90121-V
4. Saper CB. The central autonomic nervous system: conscious visceral perception and autonomic pattern generation. *Annu Rev Neurosci.* (2002) 25:433–69. doi: 10.1146/annurev.neuro.25.032502.111311
5. Janig W, Häbler HJ. Neurophysiological analysis of target-related sympathetic pathways – from animal to human: similarities and differences. *Acta Physiol Scand.* (2002) 177:255–74. doi: 10.1046/j.1365-201X.2003.01088.x
6. Szabadi E. Neuronal networks regulating sleep and arousal: effect of drugs. In: Guglietta A, editor. *Drug Treatment of Sleep Disorders* (Cham: Springer) (2015), p. 25–70.
7. Gibbins I. Functional organization of autonomic neural pathways. *Organogenesis* (2013) 9:169–75. doi: 10.4161/org.25126
8. Loewy AD. Autonomic control of the eye. In: Loewy AD and Spyer KM. *Central Regulation of Autonomic Functions*, Oxford: Oxford University Press. (1990) p. 268–85.
9. Passatore M. Physiological characterization of efferent cervical sympathetic fibers influenced by changes in illumination. *Exp Neurol.* (1976) 53:71–81. doi: 10.1016/0014-4886(76)90282-X
10. Passatore M, Pettorossi VE. Efferent fibers in the cervical sympathetic nerve influenced by light. *Exp Neurol.* (1976) 52:66–82. doi: 10.1016/0014-4886(76)90201-6
11. Passatore M, Pettorossi VE, Casoni RP. Sympathetic preganglionic pupillodilator fibres in the light reflex. *Experientia* (1977) 15:218–9. doi: 10.1007/BF02124076
12. Nisida I, Okada H, Nakano O. The activity of the cilio-spinal centers and their inhibition in pupillary light reflex. *Jap J Physiol.* (1960) 10:73–84. doi: 10.2170/jjphysiol.10.73
13. Okada H, Nakano O, Okamoto K, Nakayama K, Nisida I. The central path of the light reflex via the sympathetic nerve in the cat. *Jap J Physiol.* (1960) 10:646–58. doi: 10.2170/jjphysiol.10.646
14. Ranson SW, Magoun HW. The central path of the pupilloconstrictor reflex in response to light. *Arch Neurol Psychiat.* (1933) 30:1193–204. doi: 10.1001/archneurpsyc.1933.02240180015001

15. Clarke RJ, Ikeda H. Luminance and darkness detectors in the olivary and posterior pretectal nuclei and their relationship to the pupillary light reflex in the rat. I. Studies with steady luminance levels. *Exp Brain Res.* (1985) 57:224:232.
16. Zagon A, Terenzi MG, Roberts MHT. Direct projections from the anterior pretectal nucleus to the ventral medulla oblongata in rats. *Neuroscience* (1995) 65:253–72. doi: 10.1016/0306-4522(94)00468-K
17. Guyenet PG. Role of the ventral medulla oblongata in blood pressure regulation. In: AD Loewy and KM Spyer, editors. *Central Regulation of Autonomic Functions* (Oxford: Oxford University Press) (1990) p. 145–67.
18. Klooster J, Vrensen GFJM. New indirect pathways subserving the pupillary light reflex: projections of the accessory oculomotor nuclei and the periaqueductal gray to the Edinger-Westphal nucleus and the thoracic spinal cord in rats. *Anat Embryol.* (1998) 198:123–32. doi: 10.1007/s004290050170
19. Dampney RA, Furlong TM, Horiuchi J, Iigaya K. Role of dorsolaral periaqueductal grey in the coordinated regulation of cardiovascular and respiratory function. *Auton Neurosci.* (2013) 175:17–25. doi: 10.1016/j.autneu.2012.12.008
20. Farkas E, Jansen ASP, Loewy AD. Periaqueductal gray matter input to cardiac-related sympathetic premotor neurones. *Brain Res.* (1998) 792:179–92. doi: 10.1016/S0006-8993(98)00029-8
21. Bajic D, Proudfit HK, van Bockstaele EJ. Periaqueductal gray neurons monosynaptically innervate extranuclear noradrenergic dendrites in the rat pericoerulear region. (2000). *J Comp Neurol.* 427:649–662. doi: 10.1002/1096-9861(20001127)427:4<649::AID-CNE11>3.0.CO;2-M
22. Bajic D, van Bockstaele EJ, Proudfit HK. Ultrastructural analysis of rat ventrolateral periaqueductal gray projections to the A5 cell group. *Neuroscience* (2012) 224:145–59. doi: 10.1016/j.neuroscience.2012.08.021
23. Nunn N, Womack M, Dart C, Barrett-Jolley R. Function and pharmacology of spinally-projecting sympathetic pre-autonomic neurones in the paraventricular nucleus of the hypothalamus. *Curr Neuropharmacol.* (2011) 9:262–77. doi: 10.2174/157015911795596531
24. Coote JH. A role for the paraventricular nucleus in the hypothalamus in the autonomic control of heart and kidney. *Exp Physiol.* (2005) 90:169–73. doi: 10.1113/expphysiol.2004.029041
25. Pyner S. The paraventricular nucleus and heart failure. *Exp Physiol.* (2014) 99:332–9. doi: 10.1113/expphysiol.2013.072678
26. Moore RY. Neural control of the pineal gland. *Behav Brain Res.* (1996) 73:125–30. doi: 10.1016/0166-4328(96)00083-6
27. Kalsbeek A, Garidou ML, Palm IF, Van Der Vliet J, Simonneaux V, Pévet P, et al. Melatonin sees the light: blocking GABA-ergic transmission in the paraventricular nucleus induces daytime secretion of melatonin. *Eur J Neurosci.* (2000) 12:3146–54. doi: 10.1046/j.1460-9568.2000.00202.x
28. Pyner S. Neurochemistry of the paraventricular nucleus of the hypothalamus: implications for cardiovascular regulation. *J Chem Neuroanat.* (2009) 38:197–208. doi: 10.1016/j.jchemneu.2009.03.005
29. Japundzic-Zigon N. Vasopressin and oxytocin control of the cardiovascular system. *Curr Neuropharmacol.* (2013) 11:218–30. doi: 10.2174/1570159X11311020008
30. Kalsbeek A, La Fleur S, Van Heijningen C, Buijs RM. Suprachiasmatic GABAergic inputs to the paraventricular nucleus control plasma glucose concentrations in the rat via sympathetic innervation of the liver. *J Neurosci.* (2004) 24:7604–13. doi: 10.1523/JNEUROSCI.5328-03.2004
31. Zeitzer JM, Ayas NT, Wu AD, Czeisler CA, Brown R. Bilateral oculosumpathetic paresis associated with loss of nocturnal melatonin secretion in patients with spinal cord injury. *J Spinal Cord Med.* (2005) 28:55–9. doi: 10.1080/10790268.2005.11753798
32. Kalsbeek A, Cutrera RA, Van Heerikhuize JJ, Van DerVliet J, Buijs RM. GABA release from suprachiasmatic nucleus terminals is necessary for the light-induced inhibition of nocturnal melatonin release in the rat. *Neurosience* (1999) 91:453–61. doi: 10.1016/S0306-4522(98)00635-6
33. Clark FM, Proudfitt H. The projection of locus coeruleus neurons to the spinal cord in the rat determined by anterograde tracing combined with immunocytochemistry. *Brain Res.* (1991) 538:231–45. doi: 10.1016/0006-8993(91)90435-X
34. Bruinstroop E, Cano G, VanderHorst VGJM, Cavalcante JC, Wirth J, Sena-Esteves M, et al. Spinal projections of the A5, A6 (locus coeruleus), and A7 noradrenergic cell groups in rats. *J Comp Neurol.* (2012) 520:1985–2001. doi: 10.1002/cne.23024
35. Pacak K, Palkovits M. Stressor specificity of central neuroendocrine rseponses: implications for stress-related disorders. *Endocr Rev.* (2001) 22:502–48. doi: 10.1210/edrv.22.4.0436
36. Lewis DI, Coote JH. Excitation and inhibition of rat sympathetic preganglionic neurones by catecholamines. *Brain Res.* (1990) 530:229–34. doi: 10.1016/0006-8993(90)91287-Q
37. Spencer SE, Sawyer WB, Wada H, Platt KB, Loewy AD. CNS projections to the pterygopalatine parasympathetic preganglionic neurons in the rat: a retrograde transneuronal viral cell body labelling study. *Brain Res.* (1990) 534:149–69. doi: 10.1016/0006-8993(90)90125-U
38. Jansen AS, Ter Horst GJ, Mettenlleiter TC, Loewy AD. CNS cell groups projecting to the submandibular parasympathetic preganglionic neurons in the rat: a retrograde transneuronal viral cell body labelling study. *Brain Res.* (1992) 572:253–60. doi: 10.1016/0006-8993(92)90479-S
39. Unnerstall JR, Kopajtic TA, Kuhar MJ. Distribution of alpha 2 agonist binding sites in the rat and human central nervous system: analysis of some functional, anatomic correlates of the pharmacologic effects of clonidine and related adrenergic agents. *Brain Res.* (1984) 319:69–101. doi: 10.1016/0165-0173(84)90030-4
40. Koss MC. Pupillary dilation as an index of central nervous system α_2-adrenoeptor activation. *J Pharmacol Met.* (1986) 15:1–19. doi: 10.1016/0160-5402(86)90002-1
41. Samuels ER, Szabadi E. Functional neuroanatomy of the locus coeruleus: its role in the regulation of arousal an autonomic function. Part I: Principles of functional organisation. *Curr Neuropharmacol.* (2008) 6:235–53. doi: 10.2174/157015908785777229
42. Samuels ER, Szabadi E. Functional neuroanatomy of the locus coeruleus: its role in the regulation of arousal an autonomic function. Part II: Physiological and pharmacological manipulations and pathological alterations of locus coeruleus activity in humans. *Curr Neuropharmacol.* (2008) 6:25–285. doi: 10.2174/157015908785777193
43. Szabadi E. Modulation of physiological reflexes by pain: role of the locus coeruleus. *Front Integr Neurosci.* (2012) 6:94. doi: 10.3389/fnint.2012.00094
44. Szabadi E. Functional neuroanatomy of the central noradrenergic system. *J Psychopharmacol.* (2013) 27:659–93. doi: 10.1177/02698811134 90326
45. Aston-Jones G, Chen S, Zhu Y, Oshinsky ML. A neural circuit for circadian regulation of arousal. *Nat Neurosci.* (2001) 4:732–8. doi: 10.1038/89522
46. Gonzalez MM, Aston-Jones G. Circadian regulation of arousal: role of the noradrenergic locus coeruleus system and light exposure. *Sleep* (2006) 29:1327–36. doi: 10.1093/sleep/29.10.1327
47. Bowrey HE, James MH, Aston-Jones G. New directions for the treatment of depression: Targeting the photic regulation of arousal and mood (PRAM pathway). *Depress Anxiety* (2017) 34:588–95. doi: 10.1002/da.22635
48. Vandewalle G, Schmidt C, Albouy G, Sterpenich V, Darsaud A, Rauchs G, et al. Brain responses to violet, blue, and green monochromatic light exposures in humans: prominent role of blue light and the brainstem. *PLoS ONE* (2007) 2:e1247. doi: 10.1371/journal.pone.0001247
49. Bullitt E. Expression of c-fos-like protein as a marker for neuronal activity following noxious stimulation in the rat. *J Comp Neurol.* (1990) 296:517–30. doi: 10.1002/cne.902960402
50. Shuboni DD, Cramm SL, Yan L, Ramanathan BL, Nunez AA, Smale L. Acute effects of light on the brain and behaviour of diurnal *Arvicanthis niloticus* and nocturnal *Mus musculus*. *Physiol Behav.* (2015) 138:75–86. doi: 10.1016/j.physbeh.2014.09.006
51. Cajochen C, Münch M, Kobialka S, Krauchi K, Steiner R, Oelhafen P, et al. High sensitivity of human melatonin, alertness, thermoregulation, and heart rate to short wavelength light. *J Clin Endocrin Metab.* (2005) 90:1311–6. doi: 10.1210/jc.2004-0957
52. Rodriguez-Morilla B, Madrid JA, Molina E, Correa A. Blue-enriched white light enhances physiological arousal but not behavioral performance during simulated driving at early night. *Front Psychol.* (2017) 8:997. doi: 10.3389/fpsyg.2017.00997
53. Bourgin P, Hubbard J. Alerting or somnogenic light: pick your color. *PLoS Biol.* (2016) 14:8. doi: 10.1371/journal.pbio.2000111

54. Scheer FA, van Doornen LJ, Buijs RM. Light and diurnal cycle affect human heart rate: possible role for the circadian pacemaker. *J Biol Rhythms* (1999) 14:202–12. doi: 10.1177/074873099129000614
55. Mutoh T, Shibata S, Korf H-W, Okamura H. Melatonin modulates the light-induced sympathoexciation and vagal suppression with participation of the suprachiasmatic nuicleus in mice. *J Physiol.* (2003) 547(Pt 1):317–32. doi: 10.1113/jphysiol.2002.028001
56. Kiessling S, Sollars PJ, Pickard GE. Light stimulates the mouse adrenal through a retinohypothalamic pathway independent of an effect on the clock in the suprchiasmatic nucleus. *PLoS ONE* (2014) 9:3. doi: 10.1371/journal.pone.0092959
57. Aston-Jones G, Cohen JD. An integrative theory of locus coeruleus-norepinephrine function: adaptive gain and optimal performance. *Annu Rev Neurosci.* (2005) 28:40450. doi: 10.1146/annurev.neuro.28.061604.135709
58. Joshi S, Li Y, Kalwani R, Gold JI. Relationships between pupil diameter and neuronal activity in the locus coeruleus, colliculi, and cingulate cortex. *Neuron* (2016) 89:221–34. doi: 10.1016/j.neuron.2015.11.028
59. Reimer J, McGinley MJ, Liu Y, Rodenkirch C, Wang Q, McCormick DA, et al. Pupil fluctuations track rapid changes in adrenergic and cholinergic activity in cortex. *Nat Commun.* (2016) 7:13289. doi: 10.1038/ncomms13289
60. Liu Y, Rodenkirch C, Moskowitz N, Schriver B, Wang Q. Dynamic lateralization of pupil dilation evoked by locus coeruleus activation results from sympathetic not parasympathetic contributions. *Cell Rep.* (2017) 20:3099–112. doi: 10.1016/j.celrep.2017.08.094
61. Murphy PR, O'Connell RG, O'sullivan M, Robertson IH, Balsters JH. Pupil dimeter covaries with BOLD activity in human locus coeruleus. *Hum Brain Mapp.* (2014) 35:4140–54. doi: 10.1002/hbm.22466
62. de Gee JW, Colizoli O, Kloosterman NA, Knapen T, Nieuwenhuis S, Donner TH. Dynamic modulation of decision biases by brainstem arousal systems. *Elife* (2017) 6:e23232. doi: 10.7554/eLife.23232
63. Szabadi E, Bradshaw CM. Autonomic pharmacology of α_2-adrenoceptors. *J Psychopharmacol.* (1996) 10(Suppl. 3):6–18.
64. Bitsios P, Langley RW, Szabadi E, Bradshaw CM. Comparison of the effects of clonidine on tyramine- and methoxamine-evoked mydriasis in man. *Br J Clin Pharmacol.* (1996) 41:269–75. doi: 10.1046/j.1365-2125.1996.03202.x
65. Szabadi E. The influence of the baseline on the size of pharmacological responses: a theoretical model. *Br J Clin Pharmacol.* (1977) 61:492–3.
66. Phillips MA, Szabadi E, Bradshaw CM. Comparison of the effects of clonidine and yohimbine on pupillary diameter at different illumination levels. *Br J Clin Pharmacol.* (2000) 50:65–8. doi: 10.1046/j.1365-2125.2000.00225.x
67. Hou RH, Freeman C, Langley RW, Szabadi E, Bradshaw CM. Does modafinil activate the locus coeruleus in man? Comparison of modafinil and clonidine on arousal and autonomic functions in human volunteers Psychopharmacology. (2005) 181:537–49. doi: 10.1007/s00213-005-0013-8
68. Szabadi E. The integrated control of arousal and pupil function: role of the noradrenergic locus coeruleus. *Neuro-ophthalmol Jpn.* (2008) 25:176–89.
69. Deutch AY, Goldstein M, Roth RH. Activation of the locus coeruleus induced by selective stimulation of the ventral tegmental area. *Brain Res.* (1986) 363:307–14. doi: 10.1016/0006-8993(86)91016-4
70. Ornstein K, Milon H, McRae-Degueurce A, Alvarez C, Berger B, Würzner HP. Biochemical and radioautographic evidence for dopaminergic afferents of the locus coeruleus originating in the ventral tegmental area. *J Neural Transm.* (1987) 70:183–91. doi: 10.1007/BF01253597
71. Lee HS, Lee BY, Waterhouse BD. Retrograde study of projections from the tuberomammillary nucleus to the dorsal raphe and the locus coeruleus in the rat. *Brain Res.* (2005) 1043:65–75. doi: 10.1016/j.brainres.2005.02.050
72. Korotkova TM, Sergeva OA, Ponomarenko AA, Haas HL. Histamine excites noradrenergic neurones in locus coeruleus in rats. *Neuropharmacology* (2005) 49:129–34. doi: 10.1016/j.neuropharm.2005.03.001
73. Niepel G, Bibani RH, Vilisaar J, Langley RW, Bradshaw CM, Szabadi E, et al. Association of a deficit of arousal with fatigue in multiple sclerosis: effect of modafinil. *Neuropharmacology* (2013) 64:380–8. doi: 10.1016/j.neuropharm.2012.06.036
74. Hou RH, Langley RW, Szabadi E, Bradshaw CM. Comparison of diphenhydramine and modafinil on arousal and autonomic functions in healthy volunteers. *J Psychopharmacol.* (2007) 21:567–78. doi: 10.1177/0269881106071022
75. Plummer NW, Scappini EL, Smith KG, Tuckder CJ, Jensen P. Two subpopulations of noradrenergic neurons in the locus coeruleus complex distinguished by expression of the dorsal neural tube marker *Pax7. Front Neuroanat.* (2017) 11:60. doi: 10.3389/fnana.2017.00060
76. Williams JT, Henderson G, North RA. Characterization of α_2-adrenoceptors which increase potassium conductance in rat locus coeruleus neurones. *Neuroscience* (1985) 14:95–101. doi: 10.1016/0306-4522(85)90166-6
77. Fernández-Pastor B, Mateo Y, Gómez-Urquijo S, Meana JJ. Characterization of noradrenaline release in the rat cortex of freely moving awake rats by *in vivo* microdialysis. *Psychopharmacology* (2005) 180:570–9. doi: 10.1007/s00213-005-2181-y
78. Koss MC, Gherezghiher T, Nomura A. CNS adrenergic inhibition of parasympathetic oculomotor tone. *J Auton Nerv Syst.* (1984) 10:55–68. doi: 10.1016/0165-1838(84)90067-5
79. Heal DJ, Cheetham SC, Butler SA, Gosden J, Prow MR, Buckett WR. Receptor binding and functional evidence suggest that postsynaptic α_2-adrenoceptors are of the α_{2D} subtype. *Eur J Pharmacol.* (1995) 277:25–221. doi: 10.1016/0014-2999(95)00078-Y
80. Gilsbach R, Hein L. Are the pharmacology and physiology of α_2-adrenoceptors determined by α_2-heteroreceptors and autoreceptors respectively? *Br J Pharmacol.* (2012) 165:90–102. doi: 10.1111/j.1476-5381.2011.01533.x
81. Szabadi E. GHB for cataplexy: Possible mode of action. *J Psychopharmacol.* (2015) 29:744–9. doi: 10.1177/0269881115573807
82. Huang HP, Zhu FP, Chen XW, Xu ZQ, Zhang CX, Zhou Z. (2012). Physiology of quantal norepinephrine release from somatodendritic sites of neurons in locus coeruleus. *Front. Mol. Neurosci.* 5:29. doi: 10.3389/fnmol.2012.00029
83. Starke K. Presynaptic autoreceptors in the third decade: focus on α_2-adrenoceptors. *J Neurochem.* (2001) 78:685–93. doi: 10.1046/j.1471-4159.2001.00484.x
84. Charney DS, Heninger GR, Sternberg DE. Alpha-2 adrenergic receptor sensitivity and the mechanism of action of antidepressant therapy. The effect of long-term amitriptyline treatment. *Br J Psychiatry* (1983) 142:265–75. doi: 10.1192/bjp.142.3.265
85. Jeziorski M, White FJ. Dopamine agonists at repeated "autoreceptor-selective" doses: effects upon the sensitivity of A10 dopamine autoreceptors. *Synapse* (1989) 4:267–80.
86. Guyenet PG. The couruleospinal noradrenergic neurons: anatomical and electrophysiological studies in the rat. *Brain Res.* (1980) 189:121–33.
87. Yoon SY, Kwon YB, Kim HW, Roh DH, Seo HS, Han HJ, et al. Peripheral bee venom's anti-inflammatory effect involves activation of the coeruleospinal pathway and sympathetic preganglionic neurons. *Neurosci Res.* (2007) 59:51–9. doi: 10.1016/j.neures.2007.05.008
88. Tsuruoka M, Maeda M, Nagasawa I, Inoue T. Spinal pathways mediating coeruleospinal antinociception in the rat. *Neurosci Lett.* (2004) 362:236–9. doi: 10.1016/j.neulet.2004.03.026
89. Fung SJ, Manzoni D, Chan JY, Pompeiano O, Barnes CD. Locus coeruleus control of spinal motor output. *Prog Brain Res.* (1991) 88:395–409. doi: 10.1016/S0079-6123(08)63825-X
90. Nattie E, Li A. Respiration and autonomic regulation and orexin. *Prog Brain Res.* (2012) 198:25–46. doi: 10.1016/B978-0-444-59489-1.00004-5
91. Ohno K, Sakurai T. Orexin neuronal circuitry: role in the regulation of sleep and wakefulness. *Front Neuroendocrin.* (2008) 29:70–87. doi: 10.1016/j.yfrne.2007.08.001
92. Van den Top M, Nola MF, Lee K, Richardson OJ, Buijs RM, Davies CH, et al. Orexins induce increased excitability and synchronisation of rat sympathetic preganglionic neurones. *J Physiol.* (2003) 549(Pt 3):809–21. doi: 10.1113/jphysiol.2002.033290
93. Dergacheva O, Yamanaka A, Schwartz AR, Polotsky VY, Mendelowitz D. Optogenetic identification of hypothalamic orexin neuron projections to paraventricular spinally projecting neurons. *Am J Physiol Heart Circ Physiol.* (2017) 312:H808–17. doi: 10.1152/ajpheart.00572.2016
94. Horvath TL, Peyron C, Diano S, Ivanov A, Aston-Jones G, Kilduff TS, et al. Hypocretin (orexin) activation and synaptic innervation of the

locus coeruleus noradrenergic system. *J Comp Neurol.* (1999). 415:145–59. doi: 10.1002/(SICI)1096-9861(19991213)415:2<145::AID-CNE1>3.0.CO;2-2

95. Loewenfeld IE. Mechanism of reflex dilation of the pupil. Historical review and experimental analysis. *Documenta Ophthalmol.* (1958) 12:185–448. doi: 10.1007/BF00913471
96. Loewenfeld IE. *The Pupil Anatomy, Physiology, and Clinical Applications.* Ames, IA: Iowa State University Press (1993).
97. Lee JH, Lee HK, Lee DH, Choi CG, Kim SJ, Suh DC. Neuroimaging strategies for three types of Horner syndrome with emphasis on anatomic location. *Am J Roentgenol.* (2007) 188:W74–81. doi: 10.2214/AJR.05.1588
98. Cajochen C. Alerting effects of light. *Sleep Med Rev.* (2007) 11:453–64. doi: 10.1016/j.smrv.2007.07.009
99. Souman JL, Tingha AM, Te Pas SF, van Ee R, Vlaskamp BNS. Acute alerting effects of light: a systematic review. *Behav Brain Res.* (2018) 337:228–39. doi: 10.1016/j.bbr.2017.09.016
100. Tsai JW, Hannibal J, Hagiware G, Colas D, Ruppert E, Ruby NF, et al. Melanopsin as a sleep modulator: circadian gating of the direct effects of light on sleep and altered homeostasis in *Opn4*$^{-/-}$ mice. *PLoS Biol.* (2009) 7:e1000125. doi: 10.1371/journal.pbio.1000125
101. Muindi F, Zeitzer JM, Colas D, Heller HC. The acute effects of light on murine sleep during the dark phase: importance of melanopsin for maintenance of light-induced sleep. *Eur J Neurosci.* (2013) 37:1727–36. doi: 10.1111/ejn.12189
102. Muindi F, Zeitzer JM, Heller HC. Retino-hypothalamic regulation of light-induced murine sleep. *Front Syst Neurosci.* (2014) 8:135. doi: 10.3389/fnsys.2014.00135
103. Marston OJ, Williams RH, Canal MM, Samuels RE, Upton N, Piggins HD. Circadian and dark-pulse activation of orexin/hypocretin neurons. *Mol Brain* (2008) 1:19. doi: 10.1186/1756-6606-1-19
104. Adidharma W, Leach G, Yan L. Orexinergic signalling mediates light-induced neuronal activation in the dorsal raphe nucleus. *Neuroscience* (2012) 220:201–7. doi: 10.1016/j.neuroscience.2012.06.020
105. Pilorz V, Tam SKE, Hughes S, Pothecary CA, Jagannath A, Hankins MW, et al. Melanopsin regulates both sleep-promoting and arousal-promoting responses to light. *PLoS Biol.* (2016) 14:e1002482. doi: 10.1371/journal.pbio.1002482
106. Doyle SE, Yoshikawa T, Hillson H, Menaker M. Retinal pathways influence temporal niche. *Proc Natl Acad Sci USA.* (2008) 105:13133–8. doi: 10.1073/pnas.0801728105
107. McNeill DS, Altimus CM, Hattar S. Retina-clock relations dictate nocturnal to diurnal behaviours. *Proc Natl Acad Sci USA.* (2008) 105:12645–6. doi: 10.1073/pnas.0806878105
108. Cajochen V, Chellappa SL. Commentary: melanopsin regulates both sleep-promoting and arousal promoting response to light. *Front Neural Circuits* (2016) 10:94. doi: 10.3389/fncir.2016.00094
109. Wang C-A, Munoz DP. A circuit for pupil orienting responses: implications for cognitive modulation of pupil size. *Curr Opin Neurobiol.* (2015) 33:134–40. doi: 10.1016/j.conb.2015.03.018
110. Applebaum AE, Beall JE, Foreman RD, Willis WD. Organization and receptive fields of primate spinothalamic tract neurons. *J Neurophysiol.* (1975) 38:572–86. doi: 10.1152/jn.1975.38.3.572
111. Davidson S, Truong H, Giesler GJ Jr. Quantitative analysis of spinothalamic tract neurons in adult and developing mouse. *J Comp Neurol.* (2010) 518:3193–204. doi: 10.1002/cne.22392
112. Nash PG, Macefield VG, Klineberg IJ, Gustin SM, Murray GM, Henderson LA. Bilateral activation of the trigeminothalamic tract by acute orofacial cutaneous and muscle pain in humans. *Pain* (2010) 151:384–93. doi: 10.1016/j.pain.2010.07.027
113. Craig AD. Spinal and trigeminal lamina I input to the locus coeruleus anterogradely labeled with Phaseolus vulgaris leucoagglutinin (PHA-L) in the cat and monkey. *Brain Res.* (1992) 584:325–28.
114. Hirata H, Aston-Jones G. A novel long-latency response of locus coeruleus neurons to noxious stimuli: mediation by peripheral C-fibers. *J Neurophysiol.* (1994) 71:1752–61. doi: 10.1152/jn.1994.71.5.1752
115. Sugiyama D, Hur SW, Pickering AE, Kase D, Kim SJ, Kawamata M, et al. *In vivo* patch-clamp recording from locus coeruleus neurones in the rat brainstem. *J Physiol.* (2012) 590:2225–31. doi: 10.1113/jphysiol.2011.226407
116. Voisin DL, Guy N, Chalus M, Dallel R. Nociceptive stimulation activates locus coeruleus neurones projecting to the somatosensory thalamus in the rat. *J Physiol.* (2005) 566:929–37. doi: 10.1113/jphysiol.2005.086520
117. Singewald N, Kaehler ST, Philippu A. Noradrenaline release in the locus coeruleus of conscious rats triggered by drugs, stress and blood pressure changes. *Neuroreport* (1999) 10:1583–7. doi: 10.1097/00001756-199905140-00035
118. Tavernor SJ, Abduljawad KA, Langley RW, Bradshaw CM, Szabadi E. Effects of pentagastrin and the cold pressor test on the acoustic startle response and pupillary function in man. *J Psychopharmacol.* (2000) 14:387–94. doi: 10.1177/026988110001400407
119. Hou RH, Samuels ER, Langley RW, Szabadi E, Bradshaw CM. Arousal and the pupil: why diazepam-induced sedation is not accompanied by miosis. *Psychopharmacology* (2007) 195:41–59. doi: 10.1007/s00213-007-0884-y
120. Larson MD, Talke PO. Effect of dexmedetomidine, an α_2-adrenoceptor agonist, on human pupillary reflexes during general anaesthesia. *Brit J Clin Pharmacol.* (2001) 51:27–33. doi: 10.1046/j.1365-2125.2001.01311.x
121. Yang LL, Niemann CU, Larson MD. Mechanism of pupillary reflex dilation in awake volunteers and organ donors. *Anesthesiology* (2003) 99:1281–6. doi: 10.1097/00000542-200312000-00008
122. Davis BC, Daluwatte C, Colona NC, Yao DG. Effects of cold-pressor test and mental arithmetic on pupillary light reflex. *Physiol Meas.* (2013) 34:873–82. doi: 10.1088/0967-3334/34/8/873
123. Yu Y, Koss MC. Studies of alpha adrenoceptor antagonists on sympathetic mydriasis in rabbits. *J Ocul Pharmacol Ther.* (2003) 19:255–63. doi: 10.1089/108076803321908374
124. Yu Y, Koss MC. Alpha2-adrenoceptors do not mediate reflex mydriasis in rabbits. *Ocul Pharmacol Ther.* (2004) 20:479–88. doi: 10.1089/jop.2004.20.479
125. Hey JA, Gherezghiher T, Koss MC. Studies on the mechanism of clonidine-induced mydriasis in the rat. *Naunyn Schmiedebergs Arch Pharmacol.* (1985) 328:258–63. doi: 10.1007/BF00515551
126. Hey JA, Koss MC. Alpha-1- and alpha-2-adrenoceptor antagonists produce opposing mydriatic effects by a central action. *J Auton Pharmacol.* (1988) 8:229–39. doi: 10.1111/j.1474-8673.1988.tb00186.x
127. Breen LA, Burde RM, Loewy AD. Brainstem connections to the Edinger-Westphal nucleus of the cat: a retrograde tracer study. *Brain Res.* (1983) 261:303–6. doi: 10.1016/0006-8993(83)90633-9
128. Da Silva AV, Torres KR, Haemmerle CA, Céspedes IC, Bittencourt JC. The Edinger-Westphal nucleus II: hypothalamic afferents in the rat. *J Chem Neuroanat.* (2013) 54:5–19. doi: 10.1016/j.jchemneu.2013.04.001
129. Larsen RL, Waters J. Neuromodulatory correlates of pupil dilation. *Front Neural Circuits* (2018) 12:21. doi: 10.3389/fncir.2018.00021
130. Nieuwenhuis S, De Geus EJ, Aston-Jones G. The anatomical and functional relationship between the P3 and autonomic components of the orienting response. *Psychophysiology* (2011) 48:162–75. doi: 10.1111/j.1469-8986.2010.01057.x
131. Gebber GL. Central determinants of sympathetic nerve discharge. In: *Central Regulation of Autonomic Functions.* Loewy AD, Spyer KM editors, (Oxford: Oxford University Press) (1990) p. 126–44.
132. Van Bockstaele EJ, Colago EE, Valentino RJ. Amygdaloid corticotropin-releasing factor targets locus coeruleus dendrites: substrate for the co-ordination of emotional and cognitive limbs of the stress response. *J Neuroendocrinol.* (1998) 10:743–57. doi: 10.1046/j.1365-2826.1998.00254.x
133. Tasan RO, Nguyen NK, Weger S, Sartori SB, Singewald N, Heilbronn R, et al. The central and basolateral amygdala are critical sites of neuropeptide Y/Y2 receptor-mediated regulation of anxiety and depression. *J Neurosci.* (2010) 30:6282–90. doi: 10.1523/JNEUROSCI.0430-10.2010
134. Tanaka M, Yoshida M, Emoto H, Ishii H. Noradrenaline systems in the hypothalamus, amygdala and locus coeruleus are involved in the provocation of anxiety: basic studies. *Eur J Pharmacol.* (2000) 405:397–406. doi: 10.1016/S0014-2999(00)00569-0
135. McCall JG, Al-Hasani R, Siuda E, Hong DY, Norris AJ, Ford CP, et al. CRH engagement of the locus coeruleus noradrenergic

system mediates stress-induced anxiety. *Neuron* (2015) 87:605–20. doi: 10.1016/j.neuron.2015.07.002
136. Sun Y, Hunt S, Sah P. Norepinephrine and corticotropin-releasing hormone: partners in the neural circuits that underpin stress and anxiety. *Neuron* (2015) 87:468–70. doi: 10.1016/j.neuron.2015.07.022
137. Giakoumaki SG, Hourdaki E, Grinakis V, Theou K, Bitisos P. Effects of peripheral sympathetic blockade with dapiprazole on the fear-inhibited light reflex. *J Psychopharmacol.* (2005) 19:139–48. doi: 10.1177/0269881105048994
138. Christie MJ. Mechanism of opioid actions on neurons in the locus coeruleus. *Prog Brain Res.* (1991) 88:197–205. doi: 10.1016/S0079-6123(08)63809-1
139. Samuels ER, Hou RH, Langley RW, Szabadi E, Bradshaw CM. Comparison of pramipexole and modafinil on arousal, autonomic, and endocrine functions in healthy volunteers. *J Psychopharmacol.* (2006) 20:756–70. doi: 10.1177/0269881106060770
140. Lowenstein O, Feinberg R, Loewenfeld IE. Pupillary movements during acute and chronic fatigue. *Invest Ophthalmol.* (1963) 2:138–57.
141. Yoss RE, Moyere NJ, Hollenurst RW. Pupil size and spontaneous pupillary waves associated with alertness, drowsiness, and sleep. *Neurology* (1970) 20:545–54. doi: 10.1212/WNL.20.6.545
142. Lüdtke H, Wilhelm B, Adler M, Schaeffel F, Wilhelm H. Mathematical procedures in data recording and processing of pupillary fatigue waves. *Vision Res.* (1998) 38:2889–96. doi: 10.1016/S0042-6989(98)00081-9
143. Wilhelm B, Wilhelm H, Lüdtke H, Streicher P, Adler M. Pupillogrphic assessment of sleepiness in sleep-deprived healthy subjects. *Sleep* (1998) 31:258–65.
144. Regen F, Dorn H, Danker-Hopfe H. Association between pupillary unrest index and waking electroencephalogram activity in sleep-deprived healthy adults. *Sleep Med.* (2013) 14:902–12. doi: 10.1016/j.sleep.2013.02.003
145. Landwehr R, Liszka R. Pupillographic sleepiness tests and polysomnography in nondemented patients with ischemic white matter lesions. *J Geriatr.* (2015) 2015:150927. doi: 10.1155/2015/150927
146. Phillips MA, Bitsios P, Szabadi E, Bradshaw CM. Comparison of the antidepressants reboxetine, fluvoxamine and amitriptyline upon spontaneous pupillary fluctuations in healthy human volunteers. *Psychopharmacology* (2000) 149:72–6. doi: 10.1007/s002139900334
147. Phillips MA, Szabadi E, Bradshaw CM. Comparison of the effects of clonidine and yohimbine on pupillary fluctuations in healthy human volunteers. *Psychopharmacology* (2000) 150:85–9. doi: 10.1007/s002130000398
148. Samuels ER, Hou RH, Langley RW, Szabadi E, Bradshaw CM. Comparison of pramipexole and amisulpride on alertness, autonomic, and endocrine functions in healthy volunteers. *Psychopharmacology* (2006) 187:498–510. doi: 10.1007/s00213-006-0443-y
149. Sigel E, Steinmann ME. Structure, function and modulation of $GABA_A$ receptors. *J Biol Chem.* (2012) 287:40224–31. doi: 10.1074/jbc.R112.386664
150. Chen CL, Yang YR, Chiu TH. (1999). Activation of rat locus coeruleus neuron GABAA receptors by propofol and its potentiation by pentobarbital or alphaxalone. *Eur Pharmacol.* 386:201–10.
151. Weaver LC, Polosa C. Spinal cord circuits providing control of sympathetic preganglionic neurons. In: Jordan D, editor. *Central Nervous Control of Autonomic Function* (Amsterdam: Harwood) (1997), p. 29–61.
152. Gilbey MP. Fundamental aspects of the control of sympathetic preganglionic neuronal discharge. In: Jordan D, editor. *Central Nervous Control of Autonomic Function* (Amsterdam: Harwood) (1997), p. 1–28.
153. Llewellyn-Smith IJ. GABA in the control of sympathetic preganglionic neurons. *Clin Exp Pharmacol Physiol.* (2002) 29:507–13. doi: 10.1046/j.1440-1681.2002.03664.x
154. Ondicova K, Mravec B. Multilevel interactions between sympathetic and parasympathetic nervous systems: a minireview. *Endocr. Regul.* (2010) 44:69–75. doi: 10.4149/endo_2010_02_69
155. Balllantyne D, Andrzejewski M, Mückenhoff K, Scheid P. Rhythms, synchrony and electrical coupling in the Locus coeruleus. *Respir Physiol Neurobiol.* (2004) 143:199–214. doi: 10.1016/j.resp.2004.07.018
156. Alvarez VA, Chow CC, Van Bockstaele EJ, Williams JT. Frequency-dependent synchrony in locus ceruleus: role of electrotonic coupling. *Proc Natl Acad Sci USA.* (2002) 99:4032–6. doi: 10.1073/pnas.062716299
157. De Carvalho D, Patrone LG, Taxini CL, Biancardi V, Vicente MC, Gargaglioni LH. Neurochemical and electrical modulation of the locus coeruleus: contribution to CO_2drive to breathe. *Front Physiol.* 5:288. doi: 10.3389/fphys.2014.00288
158. Nakamura S, Sakaguchi T, Kimura F, Aoki F. The role of alpha$_1$-adrenoceptor-medicated collateral excitation in the regulation of the electrical activity of locus coeruleus neurons. *Neuroscience* (1988) 27:921–9. doi: 10.1016/0306-4522(88)90195-9
159. Niijima A, Nagai K, Nagai N, Nakagawa H. Light enhances sympathetic and suppresses vagal outflows and lesions including the suprachiasmatic nucleus eliminate these changes in rats. *J Auton Nerv Syst.* (1992) 40:155–60. doi: 10.1016/0165-1838(92)90026-D
160. Zheng G, Dwoskin LP, Crooks PA. Vesicular monoamine transporter 2: role as a novel target for drug development. *AAPS J.* (2006) 8:E682–92. doi: 10.1208/aapsj080478
161. Bogdanski DF, Sulser F, Brodie BB. Comparative action of reserpine, tetrabenazine and chlorpromazine on central parasympathetic activity; effects on pupillary size and lacrimation in rabbit and on salivation in dog. *J Pharmacol Exp Ther.* (1961) 132:176–82.
162. Theofilopulos N, McDade G, Szabadi E, Bradshaw CM. Effects of reboxetine and desipramine on the kinetics of the pupillary light reflex. *Br J Clin Pharmacol.* (1995) 39:251–5. doi: 10.1111/j.1365-2125.1995.tb04444.x
163. Bitsios P, Szabadi E, Bradshaw CM. Comparison of the effects of venlafaxine, paroxetine and desipramine on the pupillary light reflex in man. *Psychopharmacology* (1999) 143:286–92. doi: 10.1007/s002130050949
164. Szabadi E, Bradshaw CM. Mechanisms of action of reboxetine. *Rev Contemp Pharmacother.* (2000) 11:267–82.
165. Siepmann T, Ziemssen T, Mueck-Wymann M, Kirch W, Siepmann M. The effects of venlafaxine on autonomic functions in healthy volunteers. *J Clin Psychopharmacol.* (2007) 27:687–91. doi: 10.1097/jcp.0b013e31815a255b
166. Bitsios P, Szabadi E, Bradshaw CM. The effects of clonidine on the fear-inhibited light reflex. *J Psychopharmacol.* (1998) 12:137–45. doi: 10.1177/026988119801200204
167. Monti JM. Serotonin control of sleep-wake behaviour. *Sleep Med Rev.* (2011) 15:269–81. doi: 10.1016/j.smrv.2010.11.003
168. Ramage AG, Villalón CM. 5-Hydroxytryptamine and cardiovascular regulation. *Trends Pharmacol Sci.* (2008) 29:472–81. doi: 10.1016/j.tips.2008.06.009
169. Watts SW, Morrison SF, Davis RP, Barman SM. Serotonin and blood pressure regulation. *Pharmacol Rev.* (2012) 64:359–88. doi: 10.1124/pr.111.004697
170. Nieuwenhuys R. *Chemoarchitecture of the Brain.* Berlin: Springer (1985).
171. Hornung J-P. The human raphe nuclei and the serotonergic system. *J Chem Neuroanat.* (2003) 26:331–43. doi: 10.1016/j.jchemneu.2003.10.002
172. Monti JM. The structure of the dorsal raphe nucleus and its relevance to the regulation of sleep and wakefulness. *Sleep Med Rev.* (2010) 14:307–17. doi: 10.1016/j.smrv.2009.11.004
173. Newton BW, Maley BE, Hamill RW. Immunohistochemical demonstration of serotonin neurons in autonomic regions of the rat spinal cord. *Brain Res.* (1986) 376:155–63. doi: 10.1016/0006-8993(86)90910-8
174. Hoyer D, Hannon JP, Martin GR. Molecular, pharmacological and functional diversity of 5-HT receptors. *Pharmacol Biochem Behav.* (2002) 71:533–54. doi: 10.1016/S0091-3057(01)00746-8
175. Carhart-Harris RL, Nutt DJ. Serotonin and brain function: a tale of two receptors. *J Psychopharmacol.* (2017) 31:1091–120. doi: 10.1177/0269881117725915
176. McDevitt RA, Neumaier JF. Regulation of dorsal raphe nucleus function by serotonin autoreceptors: a behavioral perspective. *J Chem Neuroanat.* (2011) 41:234–46. doi: 10.1016/j.jchemneu.2011.05.001
177. Shen H, Semba K. A direct retinal projection to the dorsal raphe nucleus in the rat. *Brain Res.* (1994) 635:159–68. doi: 10.1016/0006-8993(94)91435-4
178. Kawano H, Decker K, Reuss S. Is there a direct retina-raphe-suprachiasmatic nucleus pathway in the rat? *Neurosci Lett.* (1996) 212:143–6.

179. Fite KV, Janusonis S, Foote W, Bengston L. Retinal afferents to the dorsal raphe nucleus in rats and *Mongolian gerbils*. *J Comp Neurol.* (1999) 414:469–84. doi: 10.1002/(SICI)1096-9861(19991129)414:4<469::AID-CNE4>3.0.CO;2-P
180. Huang L, Yuan T, Tan M, Xi Y, Hu Y, Tao O, et al. A retionoraphe projection regulates serotonergic activity and looming-evoked defensive behaviour. (2017) *Nat Commun.* 8:14908. doi: 10.1038/ncomms14908
181. Fite KV, Birkett MA, Smith A, Janusonis S, McLaughlin S. Retinal ganglion cells projecting to the dorsal raphe and lateral geniculate complex in *Mongolian gerbils*. *Brain Res.* (2003) 973:146–50. doi: 10.1016/S0006-8993(03)02549-6
182. Fite KV, Wu PS, Bellemer A. Photostmulation alters c-Fos expression in the dorsal raphe nucleus. *Brain Res.* (2005) 1031:245–52. doi: 10.1016/j.brainres.2004.10.054
183. Fite KV, Janusonis S. Retinal projection to the dorsal raphe nucleus in the Chilean degus (*Octodon degus*). *Brain Res.* (2001) 895:139–45. doi: 10.1016/S0006-8993(01)02061-3
184. Ren C, Wui-Man Lau B, Huang X, Yang J, Zhou Y, Wu X, et al. Direct retino-raphe projection alters serotonergic tone and affective behaviour. *Neuropsychopharmacology* (2013) 38:1163–75. doi: 10.1038/npp.2013.35
185. Li X, Ren C, Huang L, Lin B, Pu M, Pickard GE, et al. The dorsal raphe nucleus receives afferents from alpha-like retinal ganglion cells and intrinsically photosensitive retinal ganglion cells in the rat. *Invest Ophthalmol Vis Sci.* (2015) 56:8373–81. doi: 10.1167/iovs.15-16614
186. Pickard GE, So KF, Pu M. Dorsal raphe nucleus projecting retinal ganglion cells: why Y cells? *Neurosci Biobehav Rev.* (2015) 57:118–31. doi: 10.1016/j.neubiorev.2015.08.004
187. Zhang T, Huang L, Zhang L, Tan M, Pu M, Pckard GE, et al. ON and OFF retinal ganglion cells differentially regulate serotonergic and GABAergic activity in the dorsal raphe nucleus. *Sci. Rep.* (2016). 6:26060. doi: 10.1038/srep26060
188. Hattar S, Kumar M, Park A, Tong P, Yau KW, Tong P, et al. Central projections of melanopsin-expressing retinal ganglion cells in the mouse. *J Comp Neurol.* (2006) 497:326–49. doi: 10.1002/cne.20970
189. Abrahamson EE, Leak RK, Moore RY. The suprachiasmatic nucleus projects to posterior hypothalamic arousal systems. *Neuroreport* (2001) 12:435–40. doi: 10.1097/00001756-200102120-00048
190. Montalbano A, Corradetti R, Mlinar B. Pharmacological characterization of 5-HT$_{1A}$ autoreceptor-coupled GIRK channels in rat dorsal raphe neurons. *PLoS ONE* (2015) 10:e0140369. doi: 10.1371/journal.pone.0140369
191. Yu Y, Ramage AG, Koss MC. Pharmacological studies of 8-OH-DPAT-induced pupillary dilation in anaesthetized rats. *Eur J Pharmacol.* (2004) 489:207–13. doi: 10.1016/j.ejphar.2004.03.007
192. Chidlow G, Nash MS, De Santis LM, Osborne NN. The 5-HT(1A)receptor agonist 8-OH-DPAT lowers intraocular pressure in normotensive NZW rabbits. *Exp Eye Res.* (1999) 69:587–93. doi: 10.1006/exer.1999.0756
193. Kotani M, Urushino M, Natsutani I, Ogi Y, Ikeda K. Effects of the 5HT$_{1A}$ receptor agonists buspirone and 8-OH-DPAT on pupil size in common marmosets. *Behav Pharmacol.* (2017) 28:313–7. doi: 10.1097/FBP.0000000000000275
194. Fanciullacci M, Sicuteri R, Alessandri M, Geppetti P. Buspirone, but not sumatriptan, induces miosis in humans: relevance for a serotonergic pupil control. *Clin Pharmacol Ther.* (1995) 57:349–55. doi: 10.1016/0009-9236(95)90161-2
195. Phillips MA, Szabadi E, Bradshaw CM. The effects of the novel anxiolytic drug lesopitron, a full and selective 5-HT$_{1A}$ receptor agonist, on pupil diameter and oral temperature in man: comparison with buspirone. *J Psychopharmacol.* (1999) 13:391–7. doi: 10.1177/026988119901300410
196. Koudas V, Nikolaou A, Hourdaki E, Giakoumaki SG, Rousos P, Bitsios P. Comparison of ketanserin, buspirone and propranolol on arousal, pupil size and autonomic function in healthy volunteers. *Psychopharmacology* (2009) 205:1–9. doi: 10.1007/s00213-009-1508-5
197. Prow MR, Martin KF, Heal DJ. 8-OH-DPAT-induced mydriasis in mice: a pharmacological characterisation. *Eur J Pharmacol.* (1996) 317:21–8. doi: 10.1016/S0014-2999(96)00693-0
198. Szabo ST, Blier P. Functional and pharmacological characterization of the modulatory role of serotonin on the firing activity of locus coeruleus norepinephrine neurons. *Brain Res.* (2001) 922:9–20. doi: 10.1016/S0006-8993(01)03121-3
199. Millson DS, Jessup CL, Swaisland A, Haworth SJ, Rushton A, Harry J. The effects of a selective 5-HT$_2$ receptor antagonist (ICI 170,809) on platelet aggregation and pupillary responses in healthy volunteers. *Br J Clin Pharmacol.* (1992) 33:281–8. doi: 10.1111/j.1365-2125.1992.tb04036.x
200. Millson DS, Haworth SJ, Rushton A, Wilkinson D, Hobson S, Harry J. The effects of the 5-HT$_2$ receptor antagonist (ICI 169,369) on changes in waking EEG, pupillary responses and state of arousal in human volunteers. *Br J Clin Pharmacol.* (1991) 32:447–54. doi: 10.1111/j.1365-2125.1991.tb03929.x
201. Joyce DS, Feigl B, Cao D, Zele A. Temporal characteristics of melanopsin inputs to the human pupil light reflex. *Vision Res.* (2015) 107:58–66. doi: 10.1016/j.visres.2014.12.001
202. Güler AD, Ecker JL, Lall GS, Haq S, Altimus CM, Liao HW, et al. Melanopsin cells are the principal conduits for rod-cone input to non-image forming vision. *Nature* (2008) 453:102–6. doi: 10.1038/nature06829
203. Smith SA. Pupil function: tests and disorders. In: Bannister R, Mathias CJ, editors. *Autonomic Failure* (Oxford: Oxford University Press) (1992) p. 393–412.
204. Guillon M, Dumbleton K, Theodoratos P, Gobbe M, Wooley CB, Moody K. The effects of age, refractive status, and luminance on pupil size. *Optom Vis Sci.* (2016) 93:1093–100. doi: 10.1097/OPX.0000000000000893
205. Bitsios P, Prettyman R, Szabadi E. Changes in autonomic function with age: a study of pupillary kinetics in healthy young and old people. *Age Ageing* (1996) 25:432–8. doi: 10.1093/ageing/25.6.432
206. Prettyman R, Bitsios P, Szabadi E. Altered pupillary size and darkness and light reflexes in Alzheimer's disease. *J Neurol Neurosurg Psychiatry* (1997) 62:665–8.
207. Lyness SA, Zarow C, Chui HC. Neuron loss in key cholinergic and aminergic nuclei in Alzheimer disease: a meta-analysis. *Neurobiol Aging* (2003) 24:1–23. doi: 10.1016/S0197-4580(02)00057-X

10

Light-Induced Pupillary Responses in Alzheimer's Disease

*Pratik S. Chougule [1], Raymond P. Najjar [1,2], Maxwell T. Finkelstein [1], Nagaendran Kandiah [3,4] and Dan Milea [1,2,5]**

[1] Department of Visual Neurosciences, Singapore Eye Research Institute, Singapore, Singapore, [2] The Ophthalmology & Visual Sciences ACP, Duke-National University of Singapore (NUS) Medical School, Singapore, Singapore, [3] Department of Neurology, National Neuroscience Institute, Singapore, Singapore, [4] Duke-National University of Singapore (NUS), Singapore, Singapore, [5] Singapore National Eye Centre, Singapore, Singapore

***Correspondence:**
Dan Milea
dan.milea@snec.com.sg

The impact of Alzheimer's disease (AD) on the pupillary light response (PLR) is controversial, being dependent on the stage of the disease and on the experimental pupillometric protocols. The main hypothesis driving pupillometry research in AD is based on the concept that the AD-related neurodegeneration affects both the parasympathetic and the sympathetic arms of the PLR (cholinergic and noradrenergic theory), combined with additional alterations of the afferent limb, involving the melanopsin expressing retinal ganglion cells (mRGCs), subserving the PLR. Only a few studies have evaluated the value of pupillometry as a potential biomarker in AD, providing various results compatible with parasympathetic dysfunction, displaying increased latency of pupillary constriction to light, decreased constriction amplitude, faster redilation after light offset, decreased maximum velocity of constriction (MCV) and maximum constriction acceleration (MCA) compared to controls. Decreased MCV and MCA appeared to be the most accurate of all PLR parameters allowing differentiation between AD and healthy controls while increased post-illumination pupillary response was the most consistent feature, however, these results could not be replicated by more recent studies, focusing on early and pre-clinical stages of the disease. Whether static or dynamic pupillometry yields useful biomarkers for AD screening or diagnosis remains unclear. In this review, we synopsize the current knowledge on pupillometric features in AD and other neurodegenerative diseases, and discuss potential roles of pupillometry in AD detection, diagnosis and monitoring, alone or in combination with additional biomarkers.

Keywords: Alzheimer's disease, dementia, pupillary light response, chromatic pupillometry, melanopsin expressing intrinsically photosensitive retinal ganglion cells, Parkinson's disease, post -llumination pupil response, cholinergic deficit

INTRODUCTION

Dementia is a global epidemic and has become a public health priority. Alzheimer's disease (AD) is the most common cause for dementia worldwide (1), accounting for 50–70% of dementia cases. The two major neuropathological landmarks of AD are deposition of insoluble amyloid-β (Aβ) plaques and formation of neurofibrillary tangles, composed of hyperphosphorylated *tau* proteins. These pathologic abnormalities are found in the central nervous system, as well as in the retina (2–4). The pathophysiology of AD is poorly understood, but a common hypothesis postulates that aggregation of Aβ is a pre-requisite for tau accumulation, neurodegeneration, and ultimately, to clinical manifestations. Clinical features of AD include progressive cognitive decline, affecting memory, learning, language, visuospatial abilities, and executive functions, but also deterioration of sleep and normal circadian rhythms (5). Most often extensive and largely irreversible neuronal histopathological changes precede clinical features of AD (6), which may explain the current failure of all disease modifying agents in this condition. For these reasons, it is believed that early diagnosis of AD is crucial for early and effective therapeutic interventions, improving AD outcomes.

Several *in vivo* biomarkers have been proposed for early identification of AD pathology, including brain imaging biomarkers (positron emission tomography after Aβ labeling) (7), as well as fluid biomarkers (within the cerebrospinal fluid and, possibly, in the blood) (8). These, and other novel genetic, biological, deep-learning based, or behavioral biomarkers aim to surpass the current performance of classical clinical evaluations in AD, which are subjective, time-consuming and deliver variable results. The eye, which is embryologically, anatomically, and physiologically an extension of the brain, has been an early explored target for identification of neurodegeneration biomarkers in AD (9, 10). Functionally, various ocular biomarkers have been tested for detection and evaluation of AD, such as eye movement recordings and pupillary responses to light or to cognitive load (9–11). Several studies have suggested that AD may be associated with altered pupillary light responses (PLR), as a consequence of abnormalities in the retina and/or the efferent pupillary system. Several arguments support the possible pupillary involvement in AD, including pathological changes in the retina, as well as existence of parasympathetic (cholinergic) and sympathetic (adrenergic) dysfunctions in the disease. Indeed, neurodegeneration commonly affects the locus coeruleus (LC), located in pons and involved in the sympathetic control of pupil size and PLR (2, 12), as well as the Edinger Westphal nucleus (EWN) (4, 13), involved in the parasympathetic control of the pupil. Pupillometry is an easy, non-invasive and affordable tool, allowing the evaluation of the PLR in AD and other ocular and neurological diseases. Whether static or dynamic pupillometry yields useful biomarkers for AD screening or diagnosis remains unclear. In this review, we synopsize the current knowledge on pupillometric features in AD and other neurodegenerative diseases, and discuss potential roles of pupillometry in AD detection, diagnosis and monitoring, alone or in combination with additional biomarkers.

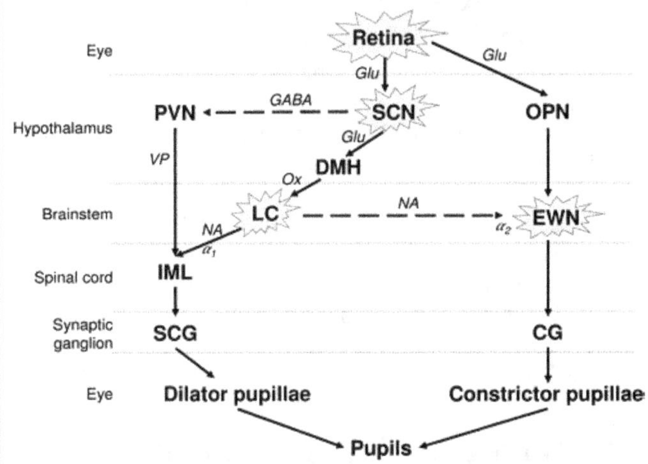

FIGURE 1 | Neuronal control of the PLR and affected structures in AD. The pupil size depends on the interplay between antagonistic parasympathetic and sympathetic impulses. The photoreceptors in retina, including the melanopsin expressing retinal ganglion cells (mRGCs), stimulate the OPN, connected to the parasympathetic EWN. mRGCs also project to the SCN, which is connected to the sympathetic LC. EWN is the major cholinergic center subserving the pupillary constriction to light. Light has an inhibitory effect on sympathetic activity and PVN via SCN. This inhibitory effect is attenuated by sympatho-excitation, which is mediated via the SCN and LC (14). The encircled structures are affected in AD. Solid lines, excitatory connections; dashed lines, inhibitory connections; Hypothalamic nuclei: SCN, suprachiasmatic nucleus; PVN, paraventricular nucleus; DMH, dorsomedial hypothalamus. Autonomic premotor nuclei: OPN, olivary pretectal nucleus; LC, locus coeruleus. Parasympathetic nucleus/ganglion: EWN, Edinger Westphal nucleus; CG, Cilliary ganglion. Sympathetic nucleus/ganglion: IML, intermedio-lateral column of spinal cord; SCG, superior cervical ganglia. Neurotransmitters: Glu, glutamate; GABA, γ-amino-butyric acid; VP, vasopressin; Ox, orexin; Ach, acetylcholine; NA, noradrenaline. Adrenoceptors: α1, excitatory; α2, inhibitory.

THE NEUROPHYSIOLOGY OF THE PUPILLARY LIGHT RESPONSE

Afferent and Efferent Pathways Governing the Pupillary Light Response

The pupil size is under the control of a closed autonomic loop. The pupil constrictor and dilator muscles receive antagonistic impulses from the parasympathetic (cholinergic) and sympathetic (adrenergic) autonomic nervous systems, respectively (**Figure 1**). The PLR is also dependent on the integrity of the retina, and in particular on the integrity of the intrinsically photosensitive melanopsin expressing retinal ganglion cells (mRGCs) (15). Although the mRGCs are activated by rods and cones, they are also intrinsically photosensitive through the melanopsin photopigment, subserving the PLR via central projections to the olivary pretectal nucleus (OPN) (16), which projects to the EWN, as demonstrated in non-human primates. The parasympathetic EWN is a cholinergic nucleus in the oculomotor complex, at the origin of preganglionic efferent neurons which synapse in the ciliary ganglion, subsequently innervating the constrictor pupillae (14, 17). The mRGCs also project to the central circadian clock located in the hypothalamic suprachiasmatic nucleus (SCN), which governs various bodily circadian rhythms and projects to the sympathetic locus coeruleus (LC), located in pons (**Figure 1**) (18, 19) [for review see (20)]. The sympathetic efferent system, including LC and SCN, regulates the resting pupil size at different levels of background illumination (17), by controlling the tone of the dilator muscle. Beyond the intervention of these motor structures, the pupillary size and function can be modulated by supranuclear neuronal influences. Other possible confounding factors, affecting the size of the pupils include the respiration rate (21), emotional status (22), vigilance (23), and age (24).

Retinal Photoreception and Chromatic Pupillometry

Recorded using an infra-red pupilometer, the PLR is governed by rods, cones and mRGCs. The intrinsically photosensitive mRGCs, located in the inner retina, produce a sustained constriction of the pupil in response to bright blue light which persists even after light offset; in addition to integrating signals from rods and cones (25). Different light wavelengths, at different intensities stimulate specifically different retinal photoreceptors (26–29). Thus, chromatic pupillometry, using different wavelengths and light intensities has been used for the evaluation of inner and outer retina integrity, in various conditions (26–29).

PATHOPHYSIOLOGY OF LIGHT-INDUCED PUPILLARY RESPONSES IN AD

Cholinergic Deficit in AD

Loss of cholinergic neurons is a common event in AD, possibly leading to alteration of cognitive processes. Specific loss of cholinergic neurons, mainly located in the medial septum and in the para-hippocampal area, is associated with memory impairment (30), but also with other cognitive deficits seen in AD (31, 32). The hypothesis of cholinergic deficit fails however, to explain other impairments in AD, i.e., disruption of circadian rhythms, sleep, and executive functions.

AD affects the cholinergic EWN, which is the central brainstem sub-nucleus of the oculomotor complex, involved in the control of the pupil constriction. Pathologic studies have shown that the EWN is affected even at early stages of AD, displaying deposition of Aβ amyloid plaques and neurofibrillary tangles (4, 13, 33). AD is associated with increased glutaminyl cyclase activity, resulting in formation of highly neurotoxic Aβ amyloid precursors (pyroglutamate Aβ peptide), identified in the EWN and in the preganglionic cholinergic PLR-governing neurons, as well as in other cholinergic neurons in the nucleus basalis of Meynert (34). In AD, the EWN neurons, display a decrease in their total dendritic length per neuron as well as a severe loss of distal dendritic branches and dendritic spines, leading to severe decrease in synaptic contacts (35). It has been suggested that these pathological changes of the EWN may be an early and specific feature of AD and they may result in decreased cholinergic control of pupillary responses (35). Unfortunately, little is known about the involvement of other parasympathetic structures involved in the PLR, i.e., the olivary pretectal nucleus and ciliary ganglia.

Adrenergic Deficit in AD

The LC modulates pupil size in 2 possible ways; by direct stimulation of preganglionic sympathetic neurons, as well as by inhibitory regulation of the EWN (**Figure 1**) (17, 36). Various factors stimulating the LC may modulate the PLR. For example, anxiety, associated with excitation of the LC (37, 38) or drugs increasing noradrenergic output to the EWN like noradrenaline re-uptake inhibitors (14, 39), lead to an increased sympathetic response on PLR like prolonged latency, reduced amplitude of constriction and faster redilation. Conversely, drugs inhibiting LC activity like clonidine (α2-adrenoceptor agonist) cause pupillary miosis and reduce the sympathetic effect on PLR (40–42). In monkeys, an electrophysiologically detectable activity in LC has been associated with mydriasis at rest (43).

Patients with AD and mild cognitive impairment (MCI), considered as the pre-clinical stage for AD, undergo significant loss of noradrenergic neurons in the LC (55 and 30%, respectively), compared to healthy controls, a finding which may impact the PLR (44). Neuronal loss in the LC of patients with AD may lead to decreased sympathetic supply to the iris and reduce the baseline pupil size (45).

Retinal Changes in AD

Aging is associated with optical (46, 47) photoreceptoral and retinal neuronal changes (48–50). Optically, in spite of decreased lens transmittance for short wavelength blue light in aging and cataract, the mRGCs induced pupillary response by blue light are well-preserved (51–53), and the pupillary responses are reduced irrespective of the wavelength of light. Although, aging has been associated with axonal and retinal ganglion cell loss (54), AD has been associated with greater thinning of retinal nerve fiber layer compared to age matched healthy controls (55–57), suggesting an accelerated loss of RGCs in AD patients. Pathological studies have shown presence of Aβ amyloid plaques in the retina of AD patients (58, 59) including in the inner layers of retina (3). These changes were often associated with blood vessel abnormalities and areas of cellular degeneration, similar to what is seen histologically in the brain of patients with AD (60, 61).

Moreover, retinas of patients with advanced AD display not only histological evidence of mRGC loss, but also selective deposition of Aβ amyloid plaques within these cells, which subserve the PLR (3). Less is known about the early selective loss of mRGC and possible mRGC Aβ deposition, occurring in AD. Occurrence of such a phenomenon should allow discrimination between normal aging patients and AD, using chromatic pupillometry. Chromatic pupillometry has been used in other conditions as a marker of mRGC integrity (62). In primary open angle glaucoma, a condition associated with histological mRGC loss (63), abnormal melatonin secretion profile (64) and sleep and circadian rhythm dysfunction (65), various pupillometric studies have shown abnormal PLR responses (28, 66–70). Conversely, in mitochondrial hereditary optic neuropathies, mRGCs are resistant to neurodegeneration, explaining the relatively preserved chromatic pupillometry parameters (71–73) and melatonin profiles (74). It is possible that mRGC loss, alone or combined with neuronal loss occurring in the suprachiasmatic nuclei, may be associated with circadian rhythm dysfunctions which can occur even at early stages of AD (3, 5).

FEATURES OF THE PUPILLARY LIGHT RESPONSES IN AD

Baseline Pupil Diameter

The consequence of AD on the pupillary diameter at rest has been controversial in various studies, probably due to methodological differences, i.e., measurement conditions and sample sizes. A few

TABLE 1 | Summary of studies on PLR in AD.

Study (n = sample size)*	Light paradigm	BPD	LoC	AC	MCV	MCA	Redilation velocity	Comments and features of parasympathetic (PSD) and sympathetic (SD) deficiencies
Prettyman et al. (45), (n = 9)	11 × 200 ms 565 nm flashlights at 8.5×10^{-3} and 7×10^{-2} mW/cm^{-2}, 0.43 and 1.84 mW/cm^{-2} at 1 cm from the eye	↓	↔	↓	NA	NA	↑	PSD features: ↓ AC and ↑redilation SD features: In darkness, pupillary dilation amplitude and velocity decreased, along with decreased BPD.
Ferrario et al. (80), (n = 20)	1 s of 660 nm flashlight	↑	↑	↔	↔	↑	↔	PSD: ↑BPD and ↑LoC SD: ↑MCA Limitations: Age of different groups not mentioned.
Fotiou et al. (81), (n = 5)	20 ms flashlight delivered using a xenon lamp at 30 cm from the eye	↑	↔	NA	NA	NA	NA	PSD: ↑BPD. Cholinergic medications reduced BPD close to controls.
Granholm et al. (79), (n = 15)	16 × 150 ms pulses of light at 20 and 40 lux from a computer screen at 77 cm	↔	NA	↓	NA	NA	NA	PLR checked after diluted tropicamide test. 9 AD patients were using cholinergic medications and 5 were using anti-depressant medications.
Fotiou et al. (75, 76), (n = 23)	20 ms flashlight delivered using a xenon lamp at 30 cm from the eye	↓	↑	↓	↓	↓	↑	PSD: ↓AC, ↓MCV, ↓MCA, ↑LoC, ↑redilation SD: ↓BPD
Frost et al. (77), (n = 19)	31 ms white flash at 180 μW	↓	↔	↓	↓	↓	↑	PSD: ↓ Mean constriction velocity, ↓MCV, ↓MCA, ↓AC and ↑% redilation at 3.5 s SD: ↓BPD
Bittner et al. (78), (n = 66AD, 42MCI)	40 × 200 ms pulse of 585 nm light at 200 cd/m^2	↔	↔	↔	NA	NA	NA	Controls were younger than AD and MCI patients and had greater constriction amplitude on repetitive stimulations
Fotiou et al. (82), (n = 42)	20 ms flashlight at 24.6 cd/m^2	NA	↑	NA	↓	↓	NA	PSD: ↓ MCV, ↓MCA, ↑LC MCV and MCA correlated well with MMSE scores.
Frost et al. (83), (n = 14)	31 ms white flashlight at 180 μW	NA	NA	↓	↓	↓	NA	Limitations: Controls were younger than AD patients.
Van Stavern et al. (84), (n = 24)	3 × 525 ms white flashlight at 180 W	NA	↔	↔	NA	NA	↔	Preclinical AD patients with no cognitive impairment were studied.

*BPD, baseline pupillary diameter in mm; LoC, latency of constriction in seconds; AC, amplitude of constriction; MCV, Maximum constriction velocity; MCA, maximum constriction acceleration; AD, Alzheimer's disease; PSD, Parasympathetic deficiency; SD, Sympathetic deficiency; ↓, decreased; ↑, increased; ↔, Not significant; NA, Not applicable/available; PLR, pupillary light response; MMSE, Mini-Mental State Examination; *n, Sample size of patients included in the study (excluding controls).*

studies with small sample size (range 9 to 23 AD patients) have reported reduced baseline pupillary diameters in AD compared to those of healthy subjects (45, 75–77). Other studies did not find any difference in baseline pupil diameters between AD, MCI and controls (78, 79), however, the groups were not age-matched in the study with largest sample size (n = 66 AD, 42 MCI) (78), while AD patients in the other study were using cholinergic and anti-depressant medications which may alter the baseline pupil size (n = 15 AD) (79). An increased baseline pupillary diameter has also been reported in AD (n = 20 AD), but no details of age of the two groups were mentioned (80) (**Table 1**).

Constriction Phase

Most pupillometric studies in patients with AD have reported results compatible with parasympathetic deficiency, translating to increased latency of pupillary constriction to light, decreased constriction amplitude, reduced mean constriction velocity and faster redilation after light offset (45, 75, 76, 83, 85) (**Table 1**). Pupil constriction velocity is obtained as the first derivative of change in pupil size with respect to time and acceleration as the second derivative (change in constriction velocity with respect to time) (**Figure 2**). Patients with AD typically display decreased maximum velocity of constriction (MCV) and maximum constriction acceleration (MCA) compared to controls, suggesting a parasympathetic deficiency. Amongst all pupillometric features, MCA and MCV have been reported as the most accurate parameters to differentiate AD patients from healthy controls (75, 76, 83). Nonetheless, other studies have failed to find such differences between AD patients and healthy individuals (78, 80). These differences may be the result of the different illumination protocols used, since studies using white light typically are associated with larger constriction amplitudes and shorter latencies (24), compared to studies using red light at 660 nm (80) or 585 nm (78). Considering that different studies have used different intensity and wavelength stimuli, this effect cannot be completely attributed to the wavelength alone.

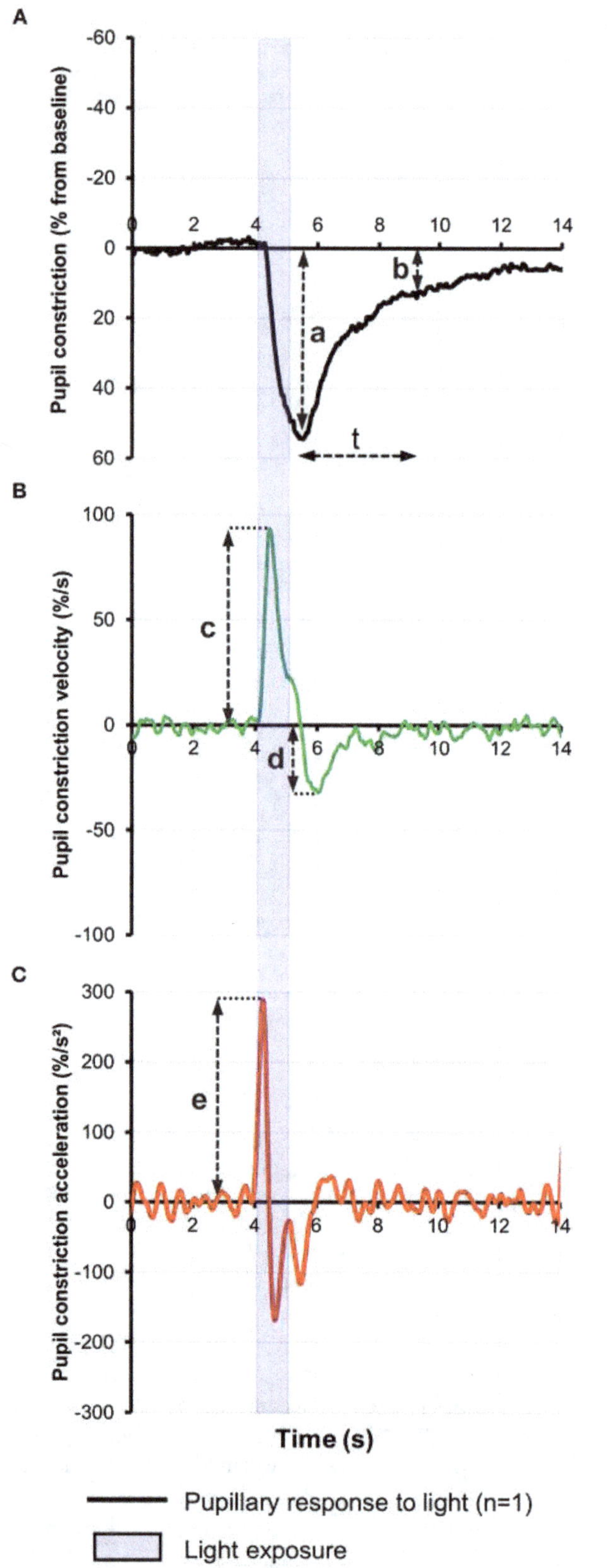

FIGURE 2 | (A) Representative baseline-adjusted pupillary response to a 1-s bright blue light (480 nm) stimulus of 13.0 Log photons/cm²/s in a healthy

(Continued)

FIGURE 2 | individual. Pupil constriction velocity **(B)** and acceleration **(C)** curves were computed, respectively, from the trace in **(A)** as the first and second derivatives of change in pupil constriction with respect to time. Pupillometric features extracted include: a, amplitude of pupillary constriction; b, post-illumination pupillary response after (t) seconds from light offset; c, Maximum constriction velocity (MCV); d, maximum redilation velocity; e, Maximum constriction acceleration (MCA).

However, other studies have demonstrated that when photon density is kept constant, shorter wavelength light produced greater constriction amplitude than longer wavelength (86, 87).

In a recent study in cognitively normal pre-clinical AD subjects, diagnosed on the basis of high cortical binding potential of Aβ amyloid on PET imaging and/or low CSF Aβ amyloid levels, there was no significant difference in any of the pupillary parameters in response to light emitting diodes (LEDs) producing a white flash of 180 W for 525 ms, compared to healthy controls (84). Only a marginal difference was observed in PLR in pre-clinical stages, suggesting that the effect of AD on PLR in pre-clinical stages is very small and may not be detectable. This suggests that PLR using achromatic light stimulus may be a valid biomarker for established Alzheimer's disease but it may have limited clinical utility in screening for AD in pre-clinical stages, perhaps due to the very small disease effect on PLR (84).

A pupillometric study, using non-Maxwellian retinal stimulation with repetitive, brief, long wavelength light (585 nm), aimed to compare patients with MCI, AD and normal controls, but failed to find inter-group differences (evaluating baseline diameters, constriction amplitudes, and constriction latencies), after adjustment for age (78). However, the use of specific repetitive light stimuli induced stronger pupillary responses in controls in terms of relative constriction amplitude (difference in the PLR measurements of the first and last stimuli), compared to AD and MCI patients, suggesting that repetitive pupillary stimulation might be a more appropriate stimulus to discriminate patients with AD and MCI from controls (78). It was proposed that repetitive stimuli caused a fatigue of the sympathetic inhibitory system to the parasympathetic pathway revealing the true effect of parasympathetic system alone on PLR. Smaller relative miosis and amplitude of constriction in AD patients suggests a decreased parasympathetic innervation to the pupillary system which may not be detected in the presence of inhibitory sympathetic system. Although relative amplitude was independent of age, the difference between MCI and control groups was not statistically significant while between AD and controls may fail to reach statistical significance if Bonferroni correction is applied. Moreover, its definition and calculation is not clearly explained in the study. Constriction phase due to different wavelength light stimuli in AD patients has not been studied yet.

Pupillary Redilation Phase

The pupillary redilation phase has been explored in several studies, but these results are sometimes difficult to compare, given the variable definitions of this parameter such as (i) percentage of pupillary redilation after 3.5 s of white flash light offset (75–77), (ii) 75% redilation time (45, 77), and (iii) average dilation velocity (77, 84). The majority of these studies have reported a faster pupillary redilation phase [analogous to decreased Post-illumination pupil response (PIPR)] in AD patients compared to controls, making it the most consistent PLR feature in AD patients (45, 75–77). In a study which extensively studied the redilation phase, the percentage recovery at 3.5 s and the 75% redilation time was significantly greater in AD patients compared to aging controls. Although the mean dilation velocity (mm/sec) was slower in AD patients, it can be ignored since the pupil size was not calculated as a percentage of baseline pupil diameter which was significantly smaller in AD (77). A recent study in preclinical AD alone did not find a significant increase in dilation velocity compared to controls following an achromatic light stimulus, however, it is not clear whether the measurements were adjusted to baseline pupil diameter (84). The faster pupillary redilation after light offset has been attributed to the diminished parasympathetic tonus associated with the cholinergic deficit, translating into failure to maintain a tonic pupillary constriction. An alternative explanation, which was not yet considered in previous studies, is that the accelerated pupillary redilation may be the result of selective mRGC loss in AD, causing an abnormal, faster PIPR as seen in other conditions affecting the mRGC, such as glaucoma (66). This hypothesis is in line with the findings of another study, which did not find any difference of the redilation phase between a group of AD patients and controls, after exposure to red light (660 nm) (80). Indeed, red light at medium high intensities is less prone to stimulate the mRGC and might have failed to explore their dysfunction. Although, redilation was not found to be different in preclinical AD patients in a recent study using a 180 W achromatic stimulus for 525 ms (84), chromatic pupillometry studying different parameters like constriction amplitude or PIPR to blue light, can still be a viable option in such cases due to selective mRGCs loss as reported in AD patients (3). No study till date has investigated pupillometric signs of mRGC dysfunction or impaired PIPR to blue light in AD patients and needs to be explored in the future. However, these interpretations are speculative, it is well-possible that the faster redilation in AD patients may be the result of an interplay between the two factors, i.e., the mRGC loss and the cholinergic deficit. It is noticeable that mRGC loss in AD should result in selective faster redilation after offset of blue light (460 nm), which specifically stimulates the mRGCs. On the opposite, faster redilation due to cholinergic deficiency should be independent of wavelength of stimulus used, occurring after offset of both blue and red light. Future studies taking into account these factors, should be able to disentangle the respective role of the afferent vs. efferent system in the pupillary redilation phase.

A POTENTIAL ROLE FOR PUPILLOMETRY IN A MULTI-MODAL APPROACH FOR DETECTING AD?

Generic Screening and Diagnostic Tests for AD

The gold standard for AD diagnosis is still based on pathology findings. However, in clinical practice, screening for AD or cognitive impairment uses various questionnaires and interactive tests, including the Mini Mental Scoring Examination (MMSE) or the Montreal cognitive assessment test (MoCA). These tests have numerous limitations, including language barriers, geographical adaptability, subjectivity, long implementation time, and the necessity for constant supervision by trained and skilled personnel. Several objective tests have been developed for early AD detection and diagnosis including cerebro-spinal fluid (CSF) analysis to measure beta amyloid (Aβ), total tau proteins and phosphorylated tau peptides quantification (8, 88), and magnetic resonance imaging (MRI) imaging of the brain and positron emission tomography (PET) scan measuring the brain Aβ plaque burden (6, 7, 89). These modalities are expensive, invasive and potentially dangerous (90, 91). In addition, they detect only structural and not functional changes in AD.

From the published studies, pupillometric evaluations may not suffice for early AD detection. However, they may constitute an adjunctive method in a, multimodal approach, combining (i) novel, cognitive, visuospatial, and memory tests involving portable virtual reality devices, (ii) retinal imaging for detection of neuronal loss and/or amyloid deposition, and (iii) objective functional outcomes provided by targeted color pupillometry.

PLR and Genetic Mutations

Apolipoprotein E is a fat-binding protein involved in the metabolism of fat, produced by APOE gene found on chromosome 19, being the only genetic factor associated with the common late onset AD. APOE mutation is not a causative mutation, but is rather considered as a risk factor for AD (92, 93). Although the PLR is not directly influenced by the APOE ε4 carrier status (78), their combination may increase the area under the curve for the combined test performance (83).

A pupillometric study has evaluated participants from a single family harboring an Amyloid-Beta Precursor Protein genetic mutation (APPGlu693Gln) (6 carriers with no cognitive impairment and 6 non-carriers) (94). This mutation results in a rare form of autosomal dominant Alzheimer's disease with phenotypical penetration approaching 100% and which is responsible for an early onset of AD. The pupillometric assessment yielded a slower pupil 75% recovery time in mutation carriers compared to non-mutation carriers. Globally, pupillometric changes were detected in pre-symptomatic carriers of the mutations, but were not statistically significant.

PLR and Cognitive Assessment Tools

MMSE is routinely used to screen elderly subjects for dementia and has a AUROC of 0.89 (95). PLR in patients with AD having higher MMSE and Wechsler Memory Scale (better cognition) scores correlated moderately with MCV, MCA and latency of constriction (82). On repetitive pupillary stimulation, higher MMSE correlated with larger increase in amplitude and relative amplitude and greater decrease in the latency ($p < 0.05$) of constriction (78). These outcomes suggest that the pupillary light response may depend on the severity of the disease and can be used for monitoring the disease progression. However, combined efficacy of MMSE and PLR has not been explored as both tools are practical, easy, non-invasive, and affordable and may yield better accuracy if combined together, compared to individual outcomes.

PLR and CSF Abnormalities

Decrease in pupillary constriction amplitude with repetitive stimulation in AD patients correlated with lower Aβ42 protein levels ($p = 0.01$) and a trend with higher tau levels in CSF ($p = 0.08$) (78). This suggests a possible association between cholinergic deficit, decreased Aβ42 protein levels and a trend with higher tau levels in CSF which supports a causative role of Aβ amyloid plaques in central cholinergic deficit (92). To date, the efficacy of a combined PLR-CSF screening method remains unknown.

PLR and Topical Weak Anticholinergic Eye Drops

In a highly controversial study, Scinto et al. reported that patients with AD exhibit larger pupil dilation compared to age-matched controls after instillation of diluted anticholinergic eyedrops (Tropicamide 0.01%) (96) Several studies have contradicted this finding (97–99) which could be due to ethnicity, age, ocular penetration of drug, properties of the solution and background luminance (79). A combination of topical weak anticholinesterase and PLR showed significant reduction in constriction amplitude for AD and Parkinson's patients compared to controls, but no significant difference between Alzheimer's and Parkinson's patients was found, while latency of constriction was similar within the 3 groups (79). However, others did not find any such significant difference in PLR pre or post weak anticholinergic eyedrops use, between AD patients and controls (80). Hence, the use of weak anticholinergic eyedrops may not improve the efficacy of PLR in detecting AD, since it may not give consistent results and decrease in amplitude of constriction is noted in AD even without using topical anticholinesterase.

LIMITATIONS OF PREVIOUS PUPILLOMETRIC STUDIES IN AD

Most of the previously published pupillometric studies in AD have various methodologic limitations. The intensity, light wavelength and duration of light exposure were variable in all the above mentioned studies. Yet, these parameters can affect, independently, or in combination, the PLR outcomes (24, 100). Therefore, there is a high need for standardization of experimental conditions in AD studies, similar to what has been described in studies using light therapy (101) and in other animal studies (102). Most current pupillometric studies agree of the need for standardized analysis of baseline pupil diameters (103, 104). Interestingly, most of the previous PLR studies in AD have not normalized the baseline diameter in their subjects, making any comparison very difficult. In a few studies evaluating pupillometric results in AD, there was no age-matching between the groups of patients and controls (78, 79, 83). Indeed, the decreased pupillary diameter with age (105, 106) may constitute a confounding factor. Last, but not least, the severity of AD was rarely taken into account in the evaluation of the PLR.

Effect of Cholinergic Medications

Only a few, small sample studies have reported the effect on the PLR of cholinergic drugs, commonly used in AD (79, 81). Thus, AD patients without cholinergic medications displayed larger baseline pupillary diameter, reduced pupillary miosis and higher number of oscillations at rest, compared to AD patients on cholinergic treatments and to healthy controls. Patients on medications had a greater latency of onset of constriction compared to both the controls and the medication free AD patients (81). However, other study in AD patients, have not found an effect of cholinergic medications on pupillary miosis but supported the increase in latency of constriction (79). PLR in AD patients on cholinergic medications behaved more like controls with no significant difference in constriction amplitude and baseline pupil diameter than their medication free counterparts (81). Taken together, these findings suggest that cholinergic medications might improve the pupillary responses in AD patients. Due to the very small sample size of these studies, it is difficult to conclude regarding a possible effect of cholinergic medications on the PLR in these patients. Additional studies are needed to understand the effect of cholinergic medications on PLR.

Effect of Ocular Co-morbidities

The most common ocular condition associated with aging is cataract which can attenuate the PLR response to both red and blue light. But the senescence of the lens does not selectively reduce the mRGCs responses to intense blue light and is well-preserved, in spite of its decreased lens transmittance in aging and cataract (51). Different retinal and optic nerve conditions can affect PLR and using chromatic pupillometry it is possible to localize the loss of photoreceptoral function i.e., inner or outer retina (107). Primary open angle glaucoma is associated with decreased PLR in response to exposure to both red and blue light with decreased PIPR for blue light (28, 70), while retinal dystrophies affecting rods and cones lead to decreased PLR responses to red and low intensity blue light with an increased PIPR to bright blue light stimulus (108, 109). Diabetic retinopathy and age-related macular degeneration can also affect the PLR (110, 111), but there is little indication to what extent these PLR alterations might be disease-specific, or whether they may confound co-existence of AD in the aging population.

PLR IN OTHER NEURODEGENERATIVE DISORDERS

Autonomic nervous system dysfunction has been described in Parkinson's disease (PD) (112), including cholinergic deficit (113), Various PLR abnormalities have been described in PD, including reduced amplitude of constriction, increased latency and decreased velocity and acceleration of constriction, while the baseline pupil diameter may be increased or not significantly different compared to healthy controls (**Table 2**) (76, 114). Pupillary unrest has also been increased in PD patients which were not on medications compared to healthy individuals or in treated patients (115), Pupillary redilation has not been

TABLE 2 | Summary of studies on PLR in PD.

Study (n = sample size)*	Light paradigm		BPD	LoC	AC	MCV	MCA	Redilation velocity	Comments and features of parasympathetic (PSD) and sympathetic (SD) deficiencies
Micieli et al. (114), (n = 23)	500 ms flashes of white light at 1,400 lux		↔	↑	↓	NA	NA	↔	BPD in dark was not significantly different from controls but in photopic conditions, pupillary diameter was significantly larger in PD patients. PSD: ↑LoC, ↓AC
Granholm et al. (79), (n = 15)	16 × 150 ms pulses of light at 20 and 40 lux from a computer screen at 77 cm		↔	NA	↓	NA	NA	NA	PLR checked before and after diluted tropicamide test.
Fotiou et al. (76), (n = 22)	20 ms flashlight delivered using a xenon lamp at 30 cm from the eye		↔	↑	↓	↓	↓	NA	PSD: ↓AC, ↓MCV, ↓MCA, ↑LoC, ↑redilation SD: ↓BPD
Jain et al. (115), (n = 17)	11 × 1 s white flashlight at 13 cd/m^2, subtending a visual angle of 4.60° at a distance of 73 cm		NA	NA	NA	↔	NA	↔	Pupillary unrest was significantly higher suggestive of autonomic dysfunction. Five patients were on dopaminergic medications.
Joyce et al. (116), (n = 17)	8 s pulsed and 12 s 0.5 Hz sinusoidal stimulations using 465 nm and 638 nm lights at 15.1 log photons/cm^2.s at the corneal level	Blue	NA	NA	↔	NA	NA	↑	Selective faster redilation to short wavelength light suggests mRGC dysfunction.
		Red	NA	NA	↓	NA	NA	↔	

*BPD, baseline pupillary diameter in mm; LoC, latency of constriction in seconds; AC, amplitude of constriction; MCV, Maximum constriction velocity; MCA, maximum constriction acceleration; PD, Parkinson's disease; PSD, Parasympathetic deficiency; SD, Sympathetic deficiency; ↓, decreased; ↑, increased; ↔, Not significant; NA, Not applicable/available; mRGC, Melanopsin expressing retinal ganglion cells; PLR, pupillary light response; *n, Sample size of patients included in the study (excluding controls).*

significantly different in PD studies using white flash light stimuli (114, 115). However, a recent chromatic pupillometry study in PD patients has suggested that the PIPR following a short wavelength blue light elicits a faster redilation compared to healthy controls. This finding is consistent with loss of mRGCs in PD (116), possibly related to deposition of α-synuclein in the retinal ganglion cells in the inner plexiform layer of the retina (117, 118). An alternative explanation might be related to reduction in the dopamine expression in the amacrine cells which relay information from rods and cones to mRGCS.

Autonomic nervous system dysfunction has also been described in dementia with Lewy bodies and to a lesser extent in fronto-temporal dementia, which can be associated with retinal abnormalities (119, 120). However, the specific effects of autonomic dysfunctions and retinal changes on pupillary light reflexes have not yet been studied in these disorders.

SUMMARY

In summary, MCV and MCA appear to be the most accurate PLR features, but also the least studied, while redilation velocity/rate (corresponding to PIPR) appears to be the most consistently altered PLR feature in AD. In conjunction with other features (baseline pupillary diameter, amplitude and latency of constriction), these parameters predominantly suggest parasympathetic deficiency, associated with mRGCs dysfunction. Longitudinal and adequately designed studies are necessary to validate the use of pupillometry in the early detection and follow-up of AD. Further studies are needed to establish the respective contribution of retinal (afferent) vs. efferent pupillary pathways in the alteration of the pupillary responses, for which chromatic pupillometry can potentially be used and translated into clinical application. Studies may also be designed to investigate the effect of cholinergic medication on PLR in AD patients and the potential use of artificial intelligence on pupillometric traces and video recordings. Using low-cost hardware, pupillometry can now easily be implemented in both remote tele-ophthalmology settings (121), as well as in continuous home monitoring (122). Combined with cognitive game-based investigations and wearables (123, 124), pupillometry may allow a more accurate screening, follow-up, and management of patients with AD.

AUTHOR CONTRIBUTIONS

PC conducted the review of literature. PC, DM, and RN wrote the manuscript. All authors (PC, RN, DM, MF, and NK) reviewed and approved the manuscript.

FUNDING

This work was supported by the National Medical Research Council, Singapore (NMRC/CIRG/1401/2014) to DM.

REFERENCES

1. Prince M, Jackson MJ, Ferri DCP, Sousa R, Albanese DE, Ribeiro MWS, et al. *World Alzheimer Report 2009*. Alzheimer's Disease International (2009).
2. Bondareff W, Mountjoy CQ, Roth M, Rossor MN, Iversen LL, Reynolds GP, et al. Neuronal degeneration in locus ceruleus and cortical correlates of Alzheimer disease. *Alzheimer Dis Assoc Disord.* (1987) 1:256–62. doi: 10.1097/00002093-198701040-00005
3. La Morgia C, Ross-Cisneros FN, Koronyo Y, Hannibal J, Gallassi R, Cantalupo G, et al. Melanopsin retinal ganglion cell loss in Alzheimer disease. *Ann Neurol.* (2016) 79:90–109. doi: 10.1002/ana.24548
4. Scinto LF, Wu CK, Firla KM, Daffner KR, Saroff D, Geula C. Focal pathology in the Edinger-Westphal nucleus explains pupillary hypersensitivity in Alzheimer's disease. *Acta Neuropathol.* (1999) 97:557–64.
5. Wu Y-H, Swaab DF. Disturbance and strategies for reactivation of the circadian rhythm system in aging and Alzheimer's disease. *Sleep Med.* (2007) 8:623–36. doi: 10.1016/j.sleep.2006.11.010
6. Villemagne VL, Burnham S, Bourgeat P, Brown B, Ellis KA, Salvado O, et al. Amyloid β deposition, neurodegeneration, and cognitive decline in sporadic Alzheimer's disease: a prospective cohort study. *Lancet Neurol.* (2013) 12:357–67. doi: 10.1016/s1474-4422(13)70044-9
7. Morris JC, Roe CM, Grant EA, Head D, Storandt M, Goate AM, et al. Pittsburgh compound B imaging and prediction of progression from cognitive normality to symptomatic Alzheimer disease. *Arch Neurol.* (2009) 66:1469–75. doi: 10.1001/archneurol.2009.269
8. Blennow K, Hampel H, Weiner M, Zetterberg H. Cerebrospinal fluid and plasma biomarkers in Alzheimer disease. *Nat Rev Neurol.* (2010) 6:131–44. doi: 10.1038/nrneurol.2010.4
9. Leruez S, Annweiller C, Etcharry-Bouyx F, Verny C, Beauchet O, Milea D. Les troubles visuels au cours de la maladie d'Alzheimer. *J Français Ophtalmol.* (2012) 35:308–11. doi: 10.1016/j.jfo.2011.11.003
10. Javaid FZ, Brenton J, Guo L, Cordeiro MF. Visual and ocular manifestations of Alzheimer's disease and their use as biomarkers for diagnosis and progression. *Front Neurol.* (2016) 7:55. doi: 10.3389/fneur.2016.00055
11. Granholm EL, Panizzon MS, Elman JA, Jak AJ, Hauger RL, Bondi MW, et al. Pupillary responses as a biomarker of early risk for Alzheimer's disease. *J Alzheimer Dis.* (2017) 56:1419–28. doi: 10.3233/jad-161078
12. Tomlinson BE, Irving D, Blessed G. Cell loss in the locus coeruleus in senile dementia of Alzheimer type. *J Neurol Sci.* (1981) 49:419–28. doi: 10.1016/0022-510X(81)90031-9
13. Scinto LF, Frosch M, Wu CK, Daffner KR, Gedi N, Geula C. Selective cell loss in Edinger-Westphal in asymptomatic elders and Alzheimer's patients. *Neurobiol Aging.* (2001) 22:729–36. doi: 10.1016/s0197-4580(01)00235-4
14. Samuels ER, Szabadi E. Functional neuroanatomy of the noradrenergic locus coeruleus: its roles in the regulation of arousal and autonomic function part II: physiological and pharmacological manipulations and pathological alterations of locus coeruleus activity in humans. *Curr Neuropharmacol.* (2008) 6:254–85. doi: 10.2174/157015908785777193
15. Hattar S, Liao H-W, Takao M, Berson DM, Yau K-W. Melanopsin-containing retinal ganglion cells: architecture, projections, and intrinsic photosensitivity. *Science.* (2002) 295:1065–70. doi: 10.1126/science.1069609
16. Hannibal J, Kankipati L, Strang CE, Peterson BB, Dacey D, Gamlin PD. Central projections of intrinsically photosensitive retinal ganglion cells in the macaque monkey. *J Comp Neurol.* (2014) 522:Spc1. doi: 10.1002/cne.23555
17. Szabadi E. Modulation of physiological reflexes by pain: role of the locus coeruleus. *Front Integr Neurosci.* (2012) 6:94. doi: 10.3389/fnint.2012.00094
18. Gooley JJ, Lu J, Fischer D, Saper CB. A broad role for melanopsin in nonvisual photoreception. *J Neurosci.* (2003) 23:7093–106. doi: 10.1523/JNEUROSCI.23-18-07093.2003
19. Lu J, Shiromani P, Saper CB. Retinal input to the sleep-active ventrolateral preoptic nucleus in the rat. *Neuroscience.* (1999) 93:209–14. doi: 10.1016/S0306-4522(99)00094-9
20. Najjar RP, Zeitzer JM. Chapter 2—anatomy and physiology of the circadian system. In: Miglis MG, editor. *Sleep and Neurologic Disease.* San Diego: Academic Press (2017). p. 29–53. Available online at: http://www.sciencedirect.com/science/article/pii/B9780128040744000029
21. Ohtsuka K, Asakura K, Kawasaki H, Sawa M. Respiratory fluctuations of the human pupil. *Exp Brain Res.* (1988) 71:215–7. doi: 10.1007/BF00247537
22. Bradley MM, Miccoli L, Escrig MA, Lang PJ. The pupil as a measure of emotional arousal and autonomic activation. *Psychophysiology.* (2008) 45:602–7. doi: 10.1111/j.1469-8986.2008.00654.x
23. Brink RL van den, Murphy PR, Nieuwenhuis S. Pupil diameter tracks lapses of attention. *PLoS ONE.* (2016) 11:e0165274. doi: 10.1371/journal.pone.0165274
24. Lobato-Rincón L-L, Cabanillas-Campos M del C, Bonnin-Arias C, Chamorro-Gutiérrez E, Murciano-Cespedosa A, Sánchez-Ramos Roda C. Pupillary behavior in relation to wavelength and age. *Front Hum Neurosci.* (2014) 8:221. doi: 10.3389/fnhum.2014.00221
25. Hattar S, Lucas RJ, Mrosovsky N, Thompson S, Douglas RH, Hankins MW, et al. Melanopsin and rod-cone photoreceptive systems account for all major accessory visual functions in mice. *Nature.* (2003) 424:75–81. doi: 10.1038/nature01761
26. Kardon R, Anderson SC, Damarjian TG, Grace EM, Stone E, Kawasaki A. Chromatic pupil responses: preferential activation of the melanopsin-mediated versus outer photoreceptor-mediated pupil light reflex. *Ophthalmology.* (2009) 116:1564–73. doi: 10.1016/j.ophtha.2009.02.007
27. Kawasaki A, Crippa SV, Kardon R, Leon L, Hamel C. Characterization of pupil responses to blue and red light stimuli in autosomal dominant retinitis pigmentosa due to NR2E3 mutation. *Invest Ophthalmol Vis Sci.* (2012) 53:5562–9. doi: 10.1167/iovs.12-10230
28. Rukmini AV, Milea D, Baskaran M, How AC, Perera SA, Aung T, et al. Pupillary responses to high-irradiance blue light correlate with glaucoma severity. *Ophthalmology.* (2015) 122:1777–85. doi: 10.1016/j.ophtha.2015.06.002
29. Park JC, Moura AL, Raza AS, Rhee DW, Kardon RH, Hood DC. Toward a clinical protocol for assessing rod, cone, and melanopsin contributions to the human pupil response. *Invest Ophthalmol Vis Sci.* (2011) 52:6624–35. doi: 10.1167/iovs.11-7586
30. Craig LA, Hong NS, Kopp J, McDonald RJ. Selective lesion of medial septal cholinergic neurons followed by a mini-stroke impairs spatial learning in rats. *Exp Brain Res.* (2009) 193:29–42. doi: 10.1007/s00221-008-1592-5
31. Bartus RT. On neurodegenerative diseases, models, and treatment strategies: lessons learned and lessons forgotten a generation following the cholinergic hypothesis. *Exp Neurol.* (2000) 163:495–529. doi: 10.1006/exnr.2000.7397
32. Bartus RT, Dean RL, Beer B, Lippa AS. The cholinergic hypothesis of geriatric memory dysfunction. *Science.* (1982) 217:408–14. doi: 10.1126/science.7046051
33. Hunter S. The rostral mesencephalon in Parkinson's disease and Alzheimer's disease. *Acta Neuropathol.* (1985) 68:53–8.
34. Morawski M, Hartlage-Rübsamen M, Jäger C, Waniek A, Schilling S, Schwab C, et al. Distinct glutaminyl cyclase expression in Edinger-Westphal nucleus, locus coeruleus and nucleus basalis Meynert contributes to pGlu-Abeta pathology in Alzheimer's disease. *Acta Neuropathol.* (2010) 120:195–207. doi: 10.1007/s00401-010-0685-y
35. Mavroudis IA, Manani MG, Petrides F, Petsoglou C, Njau SN, Costa VG, et al. Dendritic and spinal alterations of neurons from Edinger-Westphal nucleus in Alzheimer's disease. *Folia Neuropathol.* (2014) 52:197–204. doi: 10.5114/fn.2014.43791
36. Samuels ER, Szabadi E. Functional neuroanatomy of the noradrenergic locus coeruleus: its roles in the regulation of arousal and autonomic function part i: principles of functional organisation. *Curr Neuropharmacol.* (2008) 6:235–53. doi: 10.2174/157015908785777229
37. Bakes A, Bradshaw CM, Szabadi E. Attenuation of the pupillary light reflex in anxious patients. *Br J Clin Pharmacol.* (1990) 30:377–81. doi: 10.1111/j.1365-2125.1990.tb03787.x
38. Bitsios P, Szabadi E, Bradshaw CM. The inhibition of the pupillary light reflex by the threat of an electric shock: a potential laboratory model of human anxiety. *J Psychopharmacol.* (1996) 10:279–87. doi: 10.1177/026988119601000404
39. Theofilopoulos N, McDade G, Szabadi E, Bradshaw CM. Effects of reboxetine and desipramine on the kinetics of the pupillary light reflex. *Br J Clin Pharmacol.* (1995) 39:251–5. doi: 10.1111/j.1365-2125.1995.tb04444.x
40. Abercrombie ED, Jacobs BL. Microinjected clonidine inhibits noradrenergic neurons of the locus coeruleus in freely moving cats. *Neurosci Lett.* (1987) 76:203–8.

41. Bitsios P, Szabadi E, Bradshaw CM. The effects of clonidine on the fear-inhibited light reflex. *J Psychopharmacol.* (1998) 12:137–45. doi: 10.1177/026988119801200204
42. Clifford JM, Day MD, Orwin JM. Reversal of clonidine induced miosis by the alpha 2-adrenoreceptor antagonist RX 781094. *Br J Clin Pharmacol.* (1982) 14:99–101. doi: 10.1111/j.1365-2125.1982.tb04941.x
43. Joshi S, Li Y, Kalwani RM, Gold JI. Relationships between pupil diameter and neuronal activity in the locus coeruleus, colliculi, and cingulate cortex. *Neuron.* (2016) 89:221–34. doi: 10.1016/j.neuron.2015.11.028
44. Kelly SC, He B, Perez SE, Ginsberg SD, Mufson EJ, Counts SE. Locus coeruleus cellular and molecular pathology during the progression of Alzheimer's disease. *Acta Neuropathol Commun.* (2017) 5:8. doi: 10.1186/s40478-017-0411-2
45. Prettyman R, Bitsios P, Szabadi E. Altered pupillary size and darkness and light reflexes in Alzheimer's disease. *J Neurol Neurosurg Psychiatry.* (1997) 62:665–8.
46. Najjar RP, Teikari P, Cornut P-L, Knoblauch K, Cooper HM, Gronfier C. Heterochromatic flicker photometry for objective lens density quantification. *Invest Ophthalmol Vis Sci.* (2016) 57:1063–71. doi: 10.1167/iovs.15-18642
47. Teikari P, Najjar RP, Knoblauch K, Dumortier D, Cornut P-L, Denis P, et al. Refined flicker photometry technique to measure ocular lens density. *J Opt Soc Am A.* (2012) 29:2469–78. doi: 10.1364/JOSAA.29.002469
48. Freund PR, Watson J, Gilmour GS, Gaillard F, Sauvé Y. Differential changes in retina function with normal aging in humans. *Doc Ophthalmol.* (2011) 122:177–90. doi: 10.1007/s10633-011-9273-2
49. Gerth C, Garcia SM, Ma L, Keltner JL, Werner JS. Multifocal electroretinogram: age-related changes for different luminance levels. *Graefes Arch Clin Exp Ophthalmol.* (2002) 240:202–8. doi: 10.1007/s00417-002-0442-6
50. Song H, Chui TYP, Zhong Z, Elsner AE, Burns SA. Variation of cone photoreceptor packing density with retinal eccentricity and age. *Invest Ophthalmol Vis Sci.* (2011) 52:7376–84. doi: 10.1167/iovs.11-7199
51. Rukmini AV, Milea D, Aung T, Gooley JJ. Pupillary responses to short-wavelength light are preserved in aging. *Sci Rep.* (2017) 7:43832. doi: 10.1038/srep43832
52. Najjar RP, Chiquet C, Teikari P, Cornut P-L, Claustrat B, Denis P, et al. Aging of non-visual spectral sensitivity to light in humans: compensatory mechanisms? *PLoS ONE.* (2014) 9:e85837. doi: 10.1371/journal.pone.0085837
53. Daneault V, Vandewalle G, Hébert M, Teikari P, Mure LS, Doyon J, et al. Does pupil constriction under blue and green monochromatic light exposure change with age? *J Biol Rhythms.* (2012) 27:257–64. doi: 10.1177/0748730412441172
54. Esquiva G, Lax P, Pérez-Santonja JJ, García-Fernández JM, Cuenca N. Loss of melanopsin-expressing ganglion cell subtypes and dendritic degeneration in the aging human retina. *Front Aging Neurosci.* (2017) 9:79. doi: 10.3389/fnagi.2017.00079
55. Berisha F, Feke GT, Trempe CL, McMeel JW, Schepens CL. Retinal abnormalities in early Alzheimer's disease. *Invest Ophthalmol Vis Sci.* (2007) 48:2285–9. doi: 10.1167/iovs.06-1029
56. Chan VTT, Sun Z, Tang S, Chen LJ, Wong A, Tham CC, et al. Spectral-domain OCT measurements in Alzheimer's disease: a systematic review and meta-analysis. *Ophthalmology.* (2018) 126:497-510. doi: 10.1016/j.ophtha.2018.08.009
57. Cunha JP, Proença R, Dias-Santos A, Almeida R, Águas H, Alves M, et al. OCT in Alzheimer's disease: thinning of the RNFL and superior hemiretina. *Graefes Arch Clin Exp Ophthalmol.* (2017) 255:1827–35. doi: 10.1007/s00417-017-3715-9
58. Alexandrov PN, Pogue A, Bhattacharjee S, Lukiw WJ. Retinal amyloid peptides and complement factor H in transgenic models of Alzheimer's disease. *Neuroreport.* (2011) 22:623–7. doi: 10.1097/wnr.0b013e32834 97334
59. Koronyo-Hamaoui M, Koronyo Y, Ljubimov AV, Miller CA, Ko MK, Black KL, et al. Identification of amyloid plaques in retinas from Alzheimer's patients and noninvasive in vivo optical imaging of retinal plaques in a mouse model. *Neuroimage.* (2011) 54 (Suppl. 1):S204–17. doi: 10.1016/j.neuroimage.2010.06.020
60. Koronyo Y, Biggs D, Barron E, Boyer DS, Pearlman JA, Au WJ, et al. Retinal amyloid pathology and proof-of-concept imaging trial in Alzheimer's disease. *JCI Insight.* (2017) 2:93621. doi: 10.1172/jci.insight.93621
61. Tsai Y, Lu B, Ljubimov AV, Girman S, Ross-Cisneros FN, Sadun AA, et al. Ocular changes in TgF344-AD rat model of Alzheimer's disease. *Invest Ophthalmol Vis Sci.* (2014) 55:523–34. doi: 10.1167/iovs.13-12888
62. Lucas RJ, Hattar S, Takao M, Berson DM, Foster RG, Yau K-W. Diminished pupillary light reflex at high irradiances in melanopsin-knockout mice. *Science.* (2003) 299:245–7. doi: 10.1126/science.1077293
63. Obara EA, Hannibal J, Heegaard S, Fahrenkrug J. Loss of melanopsin-expressing retinal ganglion cells in severely staged glaucoma patients. *Invest Ophthalmol Vis Sci.* (2016) 57:4661–7. doi: 10.1167/iovs.16-19997
64. Kim JY, Jeong AR, Chin HS, Kim NR. Melatonin levels in patients with primary open-angle glaucoma with high or low intraocular pressure. *J Glaucoma.* (2019) 28:154–60. doi: 10.1097/IJG.0000000000001130
65. Gubin DG, Malishevskaya TN, Astakhov YS, Astakhov SY, Cornelissen G, Kuznetsov VA, et al. Progressive retinal ganglion cell loss in primary open-angle glaucoma is associated with temperature circadian rhythm phase delay and compromised sleep. *Chronobiol Int.* (2019) 36:564–77. doi: 10.1080/07420528.2019.1566741
66. Kankipati L, Girkin CA, Gamlin PD. The post-illumination pupil response is reduced in glaucoma patients. *Invest Ophthalmol Vis Sci.* (2011) 52:2287–92. doi: 10.1167/iovs.10-6023
67. Feigl B, Mattes D, Thomas R, Zele AJ. Intrinsically photosensitive (melanopsin) retinal ganglion cell function in glaucoma. *Invest Ophthalmol Vis Sci.* (2011) 52:4362–7. doi: 10.1167/iovs.10-7069
68. Nissen C, Sander B, Milea D, Kolko M, Herbst K, Hamard P, et al. Monochromatic pupillometry in unilateral glaucoma discloses no adaptive changes subserved by the ipRGCs. *Front Neurol.* (2014) 5:15. doi: 10.3389/fneur.2014.00015
69. Adhikari P, Zele AJ, Thomas R, Feigl B. Quadrant field pupillometry detects melanopsin dysfunction in glaucoma suspects and early glaucoma. *Sci Rep.* (2016) 6:33373. doi: 10.1038/srep33373
70. Najjar RP, Sharma S, Atalay E, Rukmini AV, Sun C, Lock JZ, et al. Pupillary responses to full-field chromatic stimuli are reduced in patients with early-stage primary open-angle glaucoma. *Ophthalmology.* (2018) 125:1362-1371. doi: 10.1016/j.ophtha.2018.02.024
71. Kawasaki A, Herbst K, Sander B, Milea D. Selective wavelength pupillometry in Leber hereditary optic neuropathy. *Clin Experiment Ophthalmol.* (2010) 38:322–4. doi: 10.1111/j.1442-9071.2010.02212.x
72. Moura ALA, Nagy BV, La Morgia C, Barboni P, Oliveira AGF, Salomão SR, et al. The pupil light reflex in Leber's hereditary optic neuropathy: evidence for preservation of melanopsin-expressing retinal ganglion cells. *Invest Ophthalmol Vis Sci.* (2013) 54:4471–7. doi: 10.1167/iovs.12-11137
73. Loo JL, Singhal S, Rukmini AV, Tow S, Amati-Bonneau P, Procaccio V, et al. Multiethnic involvement in autosomal-dominant optic atrophy in Singapore. *Eye.* (2017) 31:475–80. doi: 10.1038/eye.2016.255
74. La Morgia C, Ross-Cisneros FN, Sadun AA, Hannibal J, Munarini A, Mantovani V, et al. Melanopsin retinal ganglion cells are resistant to neurodegeneration in mitochondrial optic neuropathies. *Brain.* (2010) 133 (Pt 8):2426–38. doi: 10.1093/brain/awq155
75. Fotiou DF, Brozou CG, Haidich A-B, Tsiptsios D, Nakou M, Kabitsi A, et al. Pupil reaction to light in Alzheimer's disease: evaluation of pupil size changes and mobility. *Aging Clin Exp Res.* (2007) 19:364–71. doi: 10.1007/bf03324716
76. Fotiou DF, Stergiou V, Tsiptsios D, Lithari C, Nakou M, Karlovasitou A. Cholinergic deficiency in Alzheimer's and Parkinson's disease: evaluation with pupillometry. *Int J Psychophysiol.* (2009) 73:143–9. doi: 10.1016/j.ijpsycho.2009.01.011
77. Frost S, Kanagasingam Y, Sohrabi H, Bourgeat P, Villemagne V, Rowe CC, et al. Pupil response biomarkers for early detection and monitoring of Alzheimer's disease. *Curr Alzheimer Res.* (2013) 10:931–9. doi: 10.2174/15672050113106660163
78. Bittner DM, Wieseler I, Wilhelm H, Riepe MW, Müller NG. Repetitive pupil light reflex: potential marker in Alzheimer's disease? *J Alzheimers Dis.* (2014) 42:1469–77. doi: 10.3233/jad-140969
79. Granholm E, Morris S, Galasko D, Shults C, Rogers E, Vukov B. Tropicamide effects on pupil size and pupillary light reflexes in

Alzheimer's and Parkinson's disease. *Int J Psychophysiol.* (2003) 47:95–115. doi: 10.1016/s0167-8760(02)00122-8

80. Ferrario E, Molaschi M, Villa L, Varetto O, Bogetto C, Nuzzi R. Is videopupillography useful in the diagnosis of Alzheimer's disease? *Neurology.* (1998) 50:642–4.
81. Fotiou F, Fountoulakis KN, Tsolaki M, Goulas A, Palikaras A. Changes in pupil reaction to light in Alzheimer's disease patients: a preliminary report. *Int J Psychophysiol.* (2000) 37:111–20. doi: 10.1016/s0167-8760(00)00099-4
82. Fotiou D, Kaltsatou A, Tsiptsios D, Nakou M. Evaluation of the cholinergic hypothesis in Alzheimer's disease with neuropsychological methods. *Aging Clin Exp Res.* (2015) 27:727–33. doi: 10.1007/s40520-015-0321-8
83. Frost S, Robinson L, Rowe CC, Ames D, Masters CL, Taddei K, et al. Evaluation of cholinergic deficiency in preclinical alzheimer's disease using pupillometry. *J Ophthalmol.* (2017) 2017:7935406. doi: 10.1155/2017/7935406
84. Van Stavern GP, Bei L, Shui Y-B, Huecker J, Gordon M. Pupillary light reaction in preclinical Alzheimer's disease subjects compared with normal ageing controls. *Br J Ophthalmol.* (2018). doi: 10.1136/bjophthalmol-2018-312425. [Epub ahead of print].
85. Tales A, Troscianko T, Lush D, Haworth J, Wilcock GK, Butler SR. The pupillary light reflex in aging and Alzheimer's disease. *Aging.* (2001) 13:473–8.
86. Gamlin PDR, McDougal DH, Pokorny J, Smith VC, Yau K-W, Dacey DM. Human and macaque pupil responses driven by melanopsin-containing retinal ganglion cells. *Vis Res.* (2007) 47:946–54. doi: 10.1016/j.visres.2006.12.015
87. Mure LS, Cornut P-L, Rieux C, Drouyer E, Denis P, Gronfier C, et al. Melanopsin bistability: a fly's eye technology in the human retina. *PLoS ONE.* (2009) 4:e5991. doi: 10.1371/journal.pone.0005991
88. Sunderland T, Linker G, Mirza N, Putnam KT, Friedman DL, Kimmel LH, et al. Decreased beta-amyloid1-42 and increased tau levels in cerebrospinal fluid of patients with Alzheimer disease. *JAMA.* (2003) 289:2094–103. doi: 10.1001/jama.289.16.2094
89. Rowe CC, Ellis KA, Rimajova M, Bourgeat P, Pike KE, Jones G, et al. Amyloid imaging results from the Australian Imaging, Biomarkers and Lifestyle (AIBL) study of aging. *Neurobiol Aging.* (2010) 31:1275–83. doi: 10.1016/j.neurobiolaging.2010.04.007
90. Hays MT, Watson EE, Thomas SR, Stabin M. MIRD dose estimate report no. 19: radiation absorbed dose estimates from (18)F-FDG. *J Nucl Med.* (2002) 43:210–4.
91. Santana P do C, Mourão AP, de Oliveira PMC, Bernardes FD, Mamede M, da Silva TA. Dosimetry of patients submitted to cerebral PET/CT for the diagnosis of mild cognitive impairment. *Radiol Bras.* (2014) 47:350–4. doi: 10.1590/0100-3984.2013.1800
92. McDonald RJ. Multiple combinations of co-factors produce variants of age-related cognitive decline: a theory. *Can J Exp Psychol.* (2002) 56:221–39. doi: 10.1037/h0087399
93. Strittmatter WJ, Saunders AM, Goedert M, Weisgraber KH, Dong LM, Jakes R, et al. Isoform-specific interactions of apolipoprotein E with microtubule-associated protein tau: implications for Alzheimer disease. *Proc Natl Acad Sci USA.* (1994) 91:11183–6. doi: 10.1073/pnas.91.23.11183
94. Frost SM, Kanagasingam Y, Sohrabi HR, Taddei K, Bateman R, Morris J, et al. Pupil response biomarkers distinguish amyloid precursor protein mutation carriers from non-carriers. *Curr Alzheimer Res.* (2013) 10:790–6. doi: 10.2174/15672050113109990154
95. O'Bryant SE, Humphreys JD, Smith GE, Ivnik RJ, Graff-Radford NR, Petersen RC, et al. Detecting dementia with the mini-mental state examination (MMSE) in highly educated individuals. *Arch Neurol.* (2008) 65:963–7. doi: 10.1001/archneur.65.7.963
96. Scinto LF, Daffner KR, Dressler D, Ransil BI, Rentz D, Weintraub S, et al. A potential noninvasive neurobiological test for Alzheimer's disease. *Science.* (1994) 266:1051–4.
97. FitzSimon JS, Waring SC, Kokmen E, McLaren JW, Brubaker RF. Response of the pupil to tropicamide is not a reliable test for Alzheimer disease. Arch Neurol. (1997) 54:155–9. doi: 10.1001/archneur.1997.00550140031009
98. Kurz A, Marquard R, Fremke S, Leipert KP. Pupil dilation response to tropicamide: a biological test for Alzheimer's disease? *Pharmacopsychiatry.* (1997) 30:12–5.
99. Loupe DN, Newman NJ, Green RC, Lynn MJ, WIlliams KK, Geis TC, et al. Pupillary response to tropicamide in patients with Alzheimer disease. *Ophthalmology.* (1996) 103:495–503. doi: 10.1016/S0161-6420(96)30666-0
100. Winn B, Whitaker D, Elliott DB, Phillips NJ. Factors affecting light-adapted pupil size in normal human subjects. *Invest Ophthalmol Vis Sci.* (1994) 35:1132–7.
101. Aarts MPJ, Rosemann ALP. Towards a uniform specification of light therapy devices for the treatment of affective disorders and use for non-image forming effects: radiant flux. *J Affect Disorders.* (2018) 235:142–9. doi: 10.1016/j.jad.2018.04.020
102. Bullough JD, Rea MS, Figueiro MG. Of mice and women: light as a circadian stimulus in breast cancer research. *Cancer Causes Control.* (2006) 17:375–83. doi: 10.1007/s10552-005-0574-1
103. Adhikari P, Pearson CA, Anderson AM, Zele AJ, Feigl B. Effect of age and refractive error on the melanopsin mediated post-illumination pupil response (PIPR). *Sci Rep.* (2015) 5:17610. doi: 10.1038/srep17610
104. Kankipati L, Girkin CA, Gamlin PD. Post-illumination pupil response in subjects without ocular disease. *Invest Ophthalmol Vis Sci.* (2010) 51:2764–9. doi: 10.1167/iovs.09-4717
105. Herbst K, Sander B, Lund-Andersen H, Broendsted AE, Kessel L, Hansen MS, et al. Intrinsically photosensitive retinal ganglion cell function in relation to age: a pupillometric study in humans with special reference to the age-related optic properties of the lens. *BMC Ophthalmol.* (2012) 12:4. doi: 10.1186/1471-2415-12-4
106. Sharma S, Baskaran M, Rukmini AV, Nongpiur ME, Htoon H, Cheng C-Y, et al. Factors influencing the pupillary light reflex in healthy individuals. *Graefes Arch Clin Exp Ophthalmol.* (2016) 254:1353–9. doi: 10.1007/s00417-016-3311-4
107. Rukmini AV, Milea D, Gooley JJ. Chromatic pupillometry methods for assessing photoreceptor health in retinal and optic nerve diseases. *Front Neurol.* (2019) 10:76. doi: 10.3389/fneur.2019.00076
108. Kardon R, Anderson SC, Damarjian TG, Grace EM, Stone E, Kawasaki A. Chromatic pupillometry in patients with retinitis pigmentosa. *Ophthalmology.* (2011) 118:376–81. doi: 10.1016/j.ophtha.2010.06.033
109. Lorenz B, Strohmayr E, Zahn S, Friedburg C, Kramer M, Preising M, et al. Chromatic pupillometry dissects function of the three different light-sensitive retinal cell populations in RPE65 deficiency. *Invest Ophthalmol Vis Sci.* (2012) 53:5641–52. doi: 10.1167/iovs.12-9974
110. Feigl B, Zele AJ, Fader SM, Howes AN, Hughes CE, Jones KA, et al. The post-illumination pupil response of melanopsin-expressing intrinsically photosensitive retinal ganglion cells in diabetes. *Acta Ophthalmol.* (2012) 90:e230-234. doi: 10.1111/j.1755-3768.2011.02226.x
111. Park JC, Chen Y-F, Blair NP, Chau FY, Lim JI, Leiderman YI, et al. Pupillary responses in non-proliferative diabetic retinopathy. *Sci Rep.* (2017) 7:44987. doi: 10.1038/srep44987
112. Dewey RB. Autonomic dysfunction in Parkinson's disease. *Neurol Clin.* (2004) 22 (Suppl. 3):S127–39. doi: 10.1016/j.ncl.2004.05.006
113. Perez-Lloret S, Barrantes FJ. Deficits in cholinergic neurotransmission and their clinical correlates in Parkinson's disease. *NPJ Parkinsons Dis.* (2016) 2:16001. doi: 10.1038/npjparkd.2016.1
114. Micieli G, Tassorelli C, Martignoni E, Pacchetti C, Bruggi P, Magri M, et al. Disordered pupil reactivity in Parkinson's disease. Clinical Autonomic Research. (1991) 1:55–8.
115. Jain S, Siegle GJ, Gu C, Moore CG, Ivanco LS, Jennings JR, et al. Autonomic insufficiency in pupillary and cardiovascular systems in Parkinson's disease. *Parkinson Relat Disorders.* (2011) 17:119–22. doi: 10.1016/j.parkreldis.2010.11.005
116. Joyce DS, Feigl B, Kerr G, Roeder L, Zele AJ. Melanopsin-mediated pupil function is impaired in Parkinson's disease. *Sci Rep.* (2018) 8:7796. doi: 10.1038/s41598-018-26078-0
117. Beach TG, Carew J, Serrano G, Adler CH, Shill HA, Sue LI, et al. Phosphorylated α-synuclein-immunoreactive retinal neuronal elements in Parkinson's disease subjects. *Neurosci Lett.* (2014) 571:34–8. doi: 10.1016/j.neulet.2014.04.027
118. Bodis-Wollner I, Kozlowski PB, Glazman S, Miri S. α-synuclein in the inner retina in Parkinson disease. *Ann Neurol.* (2014) 75:964–6. doi: 10.1002/ana.24182

119. Ferrari L, Huang S-C, Magnani G, Ambrosi A, Comi G, Leocani L. Optical coherence tomography reveals retinal neuroaxonal thinning in frontotemporal dementia as in Alzheimer's disease. *J Alzheimers Dis.* (2017) 56:1101–7. doi: 10.3233/jad-160886
120. Kim BJ, Irwin DJ, Song D, Daniel E, Leveque JD, Raquib AR, et al. Optical coherence tomography identifies outer retina thinning in frontotemporal degeneration. *Neurology.* (2017) 89:1604–11. doi: 10.1212/WNL.0000000000004500
121. DeBuc DC. The role of retinal imaging and portable screening devices in tele-ophthalmology applications for diabetic retinopathy management. *Curr Diab Rep.* (2016) 16:132. doi: 10.1007/s11892-016-0827-2
122. Roesch K, Swedish T, Raskar R. Automated retinal imaging and trend analysis—a tool for health monitoring. *Clin Ophthalmol.* (2017) 11:1015–20. doi: 10.2147/OPTH.S116265
123. Coughlan G, Coutrot A, Khondoker M, Minihane AM, Spiers H, Hornberger M. Impact of sex and APOE status on spatial navigation in pre-symptomatic Alzheimer's disease. *bioRxiv.* (2018). doi: 10.1101/287722. [Epub ahead of print].
124. Katz S, Marshall BL. Tracked and fit: FitBits, brain games, and the quantified aging body. *J Aging Stud.* (2018) 45:63–8. doi: 10.1016/j.jaging.2018.01.009

11

Localization of Neuronal Gain Control in the Pupillary Response

Corinne Frances Carle[1,2*], *Andrew Charles James*[1], *Yanti Rosli*[3] *and Ted Maddess*[1]

[1] *John Curtin School of Medical Research, Eccles Institute of Neuroscience, The Australian National University, Canberra, ACT, Australia,* [2] *ANU Medical School, The Australian National University, Canberra, ACT, Australia,* [3] *Diagnostic and Applied Health Sciences, Biomedical Science Program, Faculty of Health Science, Universiti Kebangsaan Malaysia, Kuala Lumpur, Malaysia*

Correspondence:
Corinne Frances Carle
corinne.carle@anu.edu.au

Multifocal pupillographic objective perimetry (mfPOP) is being developed as an alternative to standard visual perimetry. In mfPOP, pupil responses to sparse multifocal luminance stimuli are extracted from the overall composite response. These individual test-region responses are subject to gain-control which is dependent on the temporal and spatial density of stimuli. This study aimed to localize this gain within the pupil pathway. Pupil constriction amplitudes of 8 subjects (41.5 ±12.7 y, 4 male) were measured using a series of 14 mfPOP stimulus variants. The temporal density of stimulus signal at the levels of retina, pretectal olivary nuclei (PON), and Edinger-Westphal nuclei (EWN) were controlled using a combination of manipulation of the mean interval between stimulus presentations (3 or 6 stimuli/s/hemiretina) and the restriction of stimuli to specific subsets of the 24 visual field test-regions per eye (left or right eye, left or right hemifield, or nasal or temporal hemifield). No significant difference was observed between mfPOP variants with differing signal density at the retina or PON but matched density at the other levels. In contrast, where signal density differed at the EWN but was the same at the retinal and PON levels e.g., between 3 stim/s *homonymous hemifield* and *all test-region* variants, significant reductions in constriction amplitudes were observed [$t_{(30)} = -2.07$ to -2.50, all $p < 0.05$]. Similar, although more variable, relationships were seen using nasal, and temporal hemifield stimuli. Results suggest that the majority of gain-control in the subcortical pupillary pathway occurs at the level of the EWN.

Keywords: pupil, gain-control, neural pathways, visual fields, perimetry, pupillometry, multifocal

INTRODUCTION

Far from being the product of a simple reflex arc, the pupillary luminance response has been shown to reflect quite complex processing of visual information. In addition to the diversity of signal arising from intrinsically photosensitive retinal ganglion cells (1–3) and various regions of visual cortex (4–7), non-linear gain-control acts within these pathways to modulate the size of the resulting pupillary constrictions. We have previously reported on the segregation and summation of pupillary visual signal (8) and have observed that constriction amplitudes are modulated on the basis of a combination of luminance intensity and temporal and spatial density of inputs (9–11). Presenting a number of stimuli simultaneously, or in close temporal proximity, to different areas of the visual-field does not produce a constriction that is equivalent to the product of the response to a single stimulus and the number of test-regions stimulated. The overall summed response is instead somewhat less than this, and therefore the shared response attributed to each of numerous stimuli will be less than that obtained to a single isolated stimulus. This is likely to be the effect of a divisive or subtractive gain mechanism (12) however the location of this neuronal gain-control within the pupillary pathway is at present unclear.

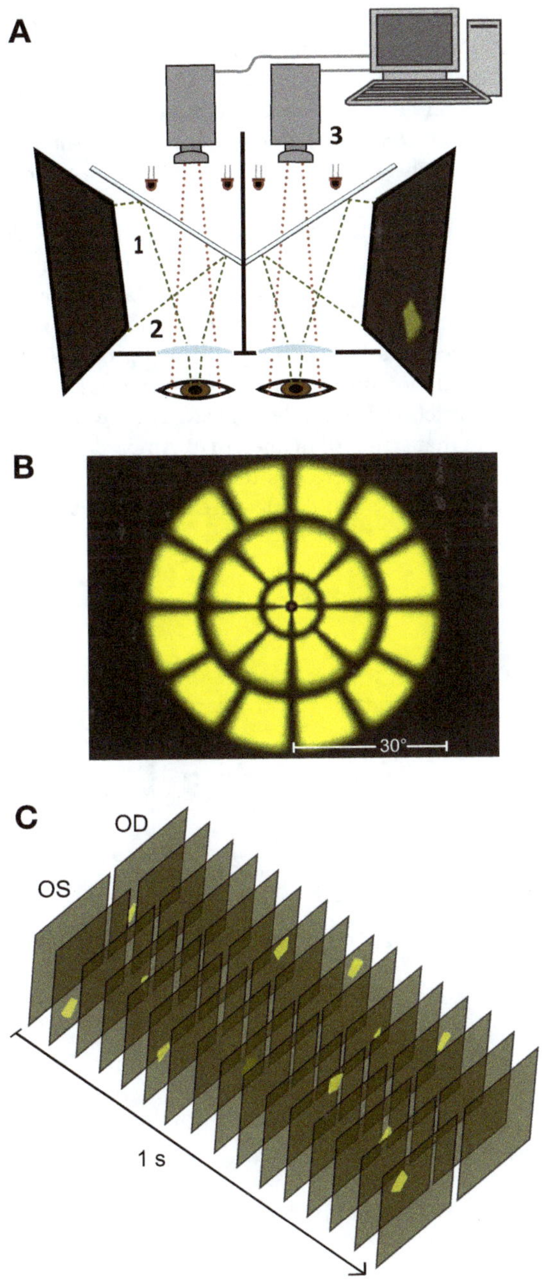

FIGURE 1 | Stimulus presentation. **(A)** Stimuli are presented on two liquid crystal displays (LCDs, 1) with viewing distance set to optical infinity (2). Cold dichroic mirrors reflect the LCDs while allowing infrared light to illuminate subjects' eyes. Responses in both pupils are monitored using two infrared video cameras (3). **(B)** All the stimulus variants used in this study (**Table 1**) employed sub-sets of a basic 24 test-region per eye array. The array comprised 3 rings of stimuli extending ± 30° from fixation. **(C)** A 1 second duration representative excerpt of the stimulus sequence showing temporally and spatially sparse multifocal presentation for left (OS) and right (OD) eyes. This sample is consistent with the All test-regions both eyes 3 stimuli/s/hemiretina stimulus variant (**Table 1**, top row).

Localizing pupillary gain is an important goal because the pupil response is commonly used in the clinical detection and assessment of pathological conditions affecting both afferent and efferent pathways. It will allow for better interpretation of results and for tests to be designed that produce more accurate representations of function within different parts of the pupillary pathway. Our recent development of multifocal pupillographic objective perimetry (mfPOP) provides a unique means to achieve this aim. This technique measures the composite response of the pupils to sparse multifocal luminance stimuli that are presented concurrently to left and right eyes (13–15). In this study we aim to manipulate the temporal density of visual signal within the retina, PON, and Edinger-Westphal nuclei (EWN) using a combination of differences in the mean interval between stimulus presentations (either 3 or 6 stimuli/s/hemiretina) and by the restriction of stimuli to specific areas of the visual field (left or right eye, left or right hemifield, or nasal or temporal hemifield). Comparison between conditions in which the density of visual signal is the same with those in which it differs will therefore allow the assessment of gain at each of the levels of the pupillary pathway.

METHODS

Subjects

Participants in this study were 8 subjects (4 male) with corrected to normal vision (mean age 41.5 ± 12.7 y). Each subject underwent testing with 14 different mfPOP variants across 5 sessions (2 or 3 variants per session) over a period of three days. Visual acuity was checked and visual fields were assessed using Humphrey FDT C-20 full threshold perimetry (Carl Zeiss Meditec, Inc., Dublin, CA, USA). Exclusion criteria included evidence of other ocular pathology or previous ocular surgery,

TABLE 1 | Stimulus protocol parameters for the 14 variants used in this study.

Active test-regions	Presentation rate (stimuli/s/hemiretina)	Summed signal at each PON/s	Summed signal at each EWN/s
All test-regions both eyes	3	6	12
	6	12	24
Left or right eye only*	3	3	6
	6	6	12
Left or right	3	6	6
homonymous hemifields*	6	12	12
Bitemporal hemifields	3	3	6
	6	6	12
Binasal hemifields	3	3	6
	6	6	12

*Subjects were tested with two protocols, at presentation rates of either 3 or 6 stimuli/second/hemiretina, for each of the active test-region variants. *These active test-region variants had separate versions for each eye or hemifield i.e., left and right versions at each presentation rate, making four stimulus protocols each.*

refractive errors greater than ±6 diopters or more than 2 diopters of cylinder, or systemic disease or medication that might impair vision or pupillary responses. Subjects were requested not to consume caffeine or alcohol for 1 h before testing. Informed written consent was given by all participants after the nature and possible consequences of the study were explained, under ANU Human Experimentation Ethics Committee approval 238/04. All research adhered to the tenets of the Declaration of Helsinki.

Multifocal Infrared Pupillography

Presentation of stimuli and monitoring of pupil diameter were carried out using a prototype of the objectiveFIELD Analyzer (Konan Medical Inc., Irvine, CA, USA). This device uses concurrent, dichoptic presentation of sparse multifocal stimuli at 60 frames/s (9, 11, 16, 17). Infrared light is used to illuminate subjects' eyes and their pupillary responses are video monitored at 30 frames/s/eye (**Figure 1A**). Stimuli are presented at optical infinity to minimize accommodative responses. During testing, subjects fixated a small cross in the center of the viewing field. Binocular fusion of the two images was aided by large crosshairs. Gaze was monitored online, and data during blinks and fixation losses were deleted. Corrective lenses compensated for refractive errors to within 1.5 diopters; the stimuli contained no spatial frequencies above 2 cycles/degree, making them tolerant of this degree of misrefraction (18).

Processing of pupillary signal utilized custom-designed software developed using Matlab (release R2016b; MathWorks Inc., Natick, MA, USA). Response waveforms for each test-region were extracted from raw pupillary responses using multiple linear regression as previously described (19, 20). This method provided a set of 96 response estimates (waveforms) for each subject and stimulus variant i.e., direct and consensual responses for left and right eyes for each of the 24 test-regions. Thus, for each test-region, these response estimates are effectively the mean of the responses to either 60 or 120 individual stimulus presentations to that region, depending on the temporal density of the stimuli. As in previous studies, pupil measurements were normalized to a baseline pupil diameter of 3,500 μm (the estimated population mean) and are referred to as **AmpStd**. This provides constriction amplitudes for each eye of each subject that are relative to that standard diameter i.e., AmpStd = constriction amplitude *(3,500/c) where c is the mean value of a trend line through the baseline pupil diameter record for each eye of each subject (9, 11, 15, 16).

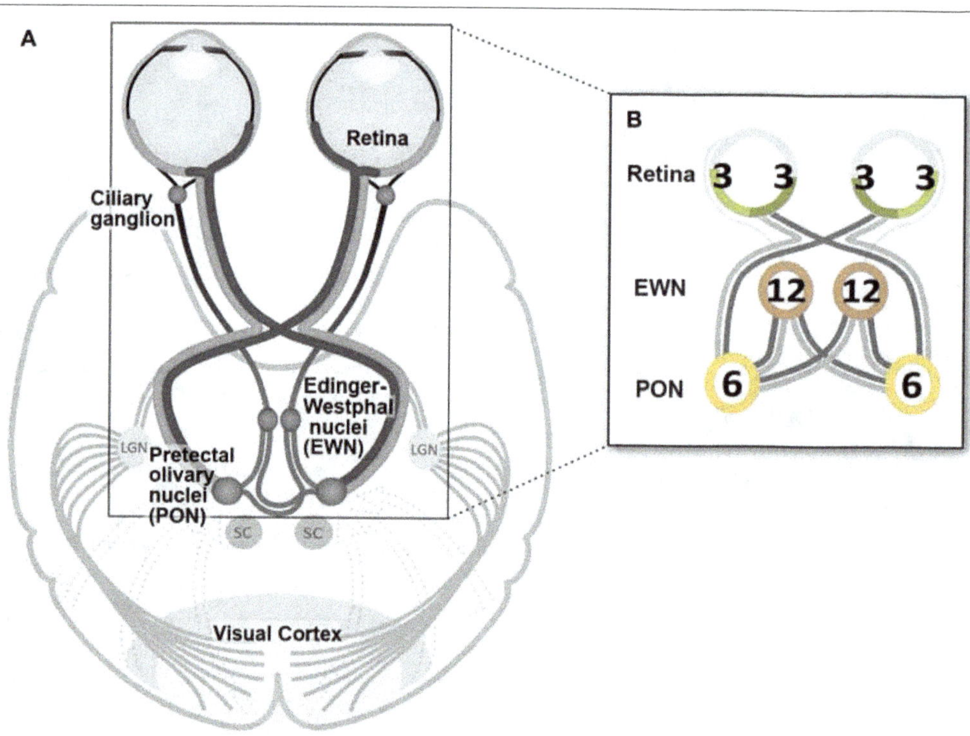

FIGURE 2 | (A) Decussating and non-decussating input from retinal neurons arrives at the pretectal olivary nucleus (PON) via the brachium of the superior colliculus (SC) as well as from various regions of visual cortex. Axons of PON neurons project bilaterally to left and right Edinger-Westphal nuclei (EWN) forming a second hemi-decussation in the pathway. Parasympathetic fibers originating in the EWN travel within the inferior branch of the oculomotor nerve to the ciliary ganglion from where the fibers of the short ciliary nerves project to innervate the pupil constrictor muscle. **(B)** In the Results section, the temporal density of the luminance signal is indicated at each synapse in the pathway as shown in this example. Numerals reflect the amount of input arriving at each nucleus as the sum of the average total stimuli presented to each individual hemiretina (nasal or temporal) during a one second interval. Color coding reflects this: signal from 3 stimuli s^{-1} is shown in green, 6 stimuli s^{-1} hemiretina^{-1} in yellow, and 12 stimuli s^{-1} in orange. These signal densities are manipulated in the different experimental conditions (**Table 1**). As shown in this cartoon, lighter and darker hemiretinas, and projections as far as the EWN indicate the presence of temporal and nasal retinal signal, respectively, for each specific experimental condition.

Stimuli

Stimulus layouts were based on a 24 region dartboard layout extending ±30° from fixation (**Figure 1B**). Yellow luminance-balanced stimuli of 33 ms duration were displayed on a 10 cd/m^2 background at a maximum luminance of 150 cd/m^2. Luminance-balancing involves lowering the luminance of stimuli relative to the inherent sensitivity of that test-region. This reduces topographic variation in constriction amplitudes and increases overall signal quality (21, 22). Multifocal stimulus presentation in this experiment was spatially as well as temporally sparse (**Figure 1C**) in contrast to the newer Clustered Volleys method (17, 19, 20). The mfPOP tests were of 4 min duration, broken into eight 30 s segments separated by short breaks.

The fourteen stimulus variants differed by the specific eye or visual hemifield in which stimuli were presented, as well as in the presentation rate of stimuli (**Table 1**, **Figure 1C**). Because ganglion cell axons from nasal and temporal retina follow different trajectories at the optic chiasm, the summed luminance signal arriving at each PON, and subsequently each EWN, will differ depending on the hemiretina of origin (**Figure 2A**). Comparisons were made between stimulus variants with estimates of signal density by linear summation as shown in **Figure 2B**. For example, compare a variant with stimuli presented in both hemifields of a single eye with another having stimuli restricted to homonymous hemifields of both eyes: both variants will have the same signal density within each stimulated hemiretina as well as at the EWN (which receives projections from both PON), but the second variant will have twice the signal density at the PON due to hemidecussation at the chiasm (this example is illustrated in **Figure 5B**). Using the differences in summed signal density between stimulus variants (**Table 1**), it is possible to construct comparisons such as this for retina, PON and EWN. Specific comparisons used will be described in the Results. The presentation rate condition, stimuli/s/hemiretina will be abbreviated to ***n/s/hr*** in the text, with *n* representing the number of stimuli presented.

Data Analysis

Data analysis was undertaken using Matlab (R2016b; MathWorks Inc., Natick, MA, USA). Summary statistics are presented as the AmpStd median and median absolute deviation in the figures. Linear models were used for parametric testing of differences in constriction amplitudes between stimulus variants. In these regression models, the distribution of variance in responses was stabilized using a generalized logarithmic transform using a lambda (λ) value of 6 as described previously (14). Inputs to these regression models were based on the conservative assumption of complete within-subjects correlation. Thus, regressions were performed on the mean amplitudes across pupils, test-regions and, in the All Regions condition, eyes. This dataset was not large enough to accurately fit effects for factors such as sex or age so these were not included in the analysis.

To enable placement of specific comparisons within the overall dataset, the median amplitudes in **Figures 5**, **6** are presented in the context of the data from comparable conditions. The data pertaining to the comparisons illustrated in the accompanying cartoons are highlighted by a gray bar. For example in **Figure 5A** the comparison is between the 3/s/hr All Regions condition and the 6/s/hr Left and Right Eye conditions. The subsets of these data that were entered into the regression models are indicated by individual brackets for each comparison.

RESULTS

Median test-region amplitudes across pupils and subjects ranged from below zero in regions in which stimuli were not presented

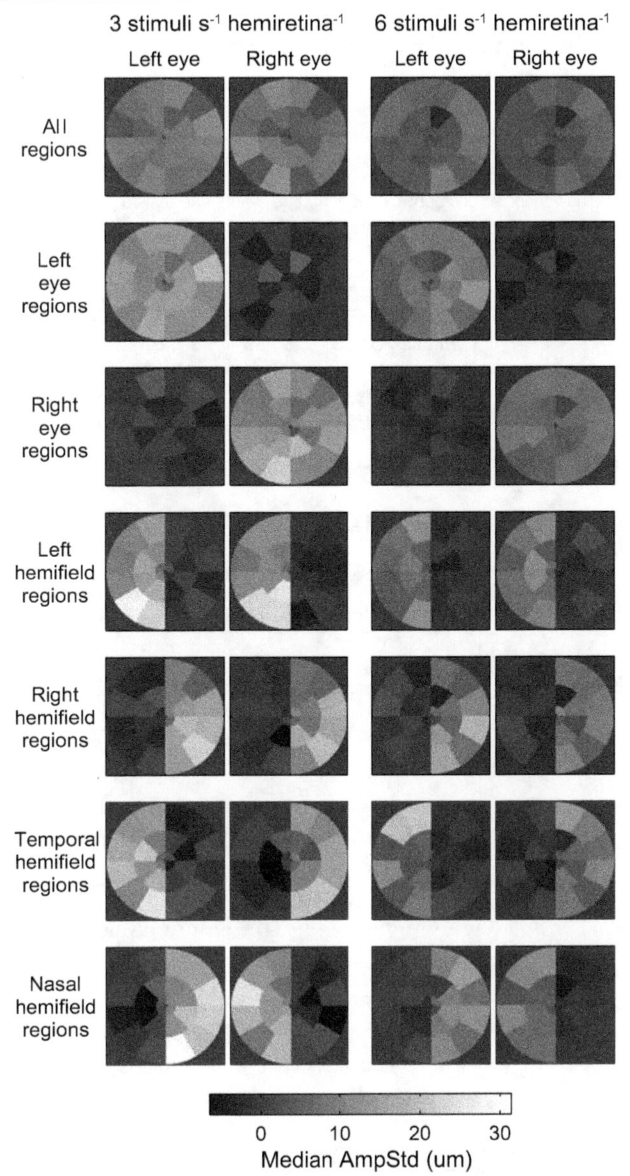

FIGURE 3 | Median standardized constriction amplitudes (AmpStd) across pupils and subjects for each test-region and eye of each of the 14 stimulus variants. The rows of **Table 1** correspond to the rows here.

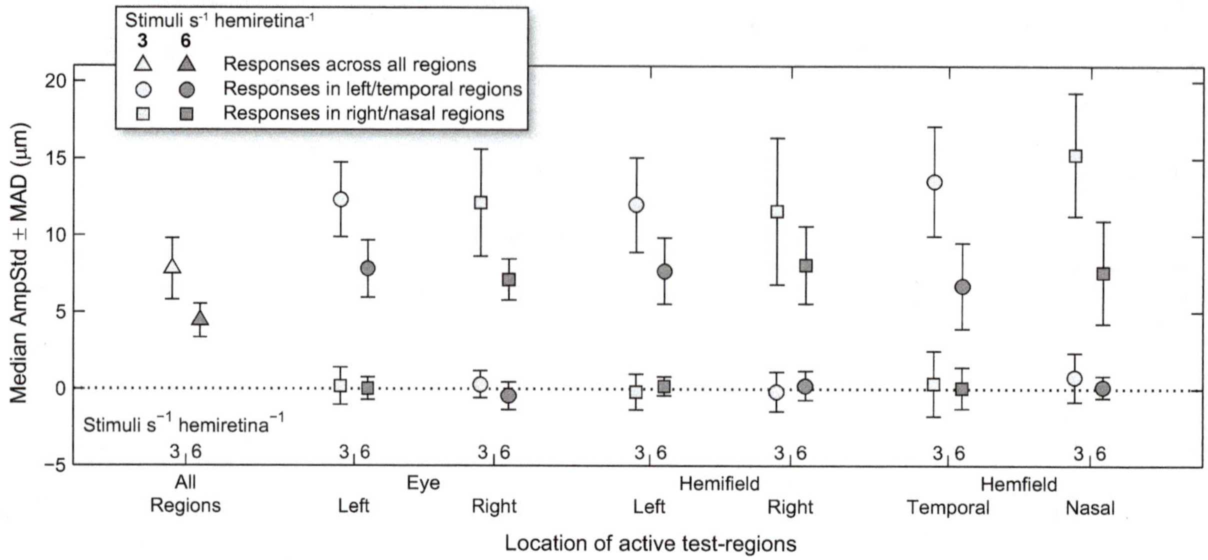

FIGURE 4 | Median and median-absolute-deviation (MAD) of standardized constriction amplitudes (AmpStd) for the active and inactive subsets of test-regions in each stimulus variant across pupils, eyes (where relevant), and test-regions of all subjects.

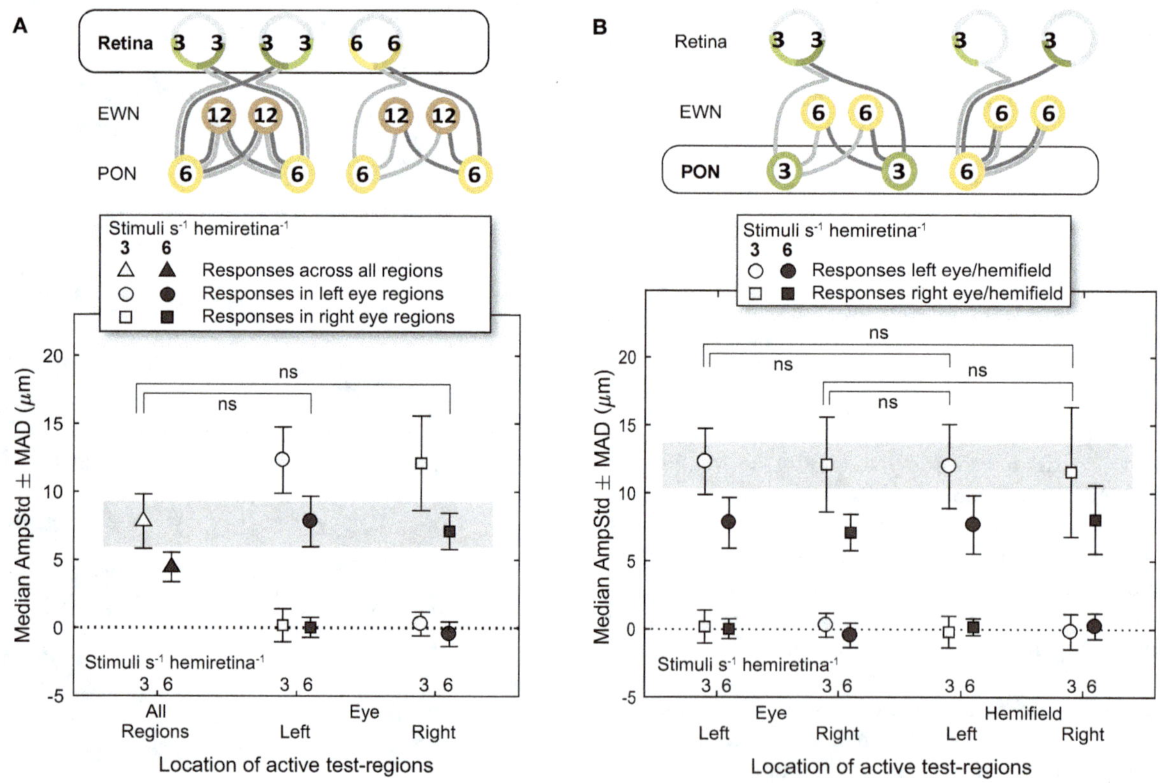

FIGURE 5 | Effect of different stimulus presentation rates at the retinal and PON levels. In the cartoons at top, numerals represent the estimated summed signal density at each level of the pathway and the black outline the level of the pathway where the signal density differs between conditions. The gray bars indicate the data points relevant to these comparisons. **(A)** Doubling the signal density at the retina, while holding it the same in the pretectal olivary nuclei (PON) and Edinger-Westphal nuclei (EWN), did not significantly affect constriction amplitudes (AmpStd). **(B)** Doubling the signal density at the PON, while holding it the same in the retina and Edinger-Westphal nuclei (EWN), also did not significantly affect constriction amplitudes (AmpStd). "ns," comparison not significant: $p > 0.05$.

to 31.4 μm AmpStd in stimulated regions (**Figure 3**). Within stimulated regions, constriction amplitudes varied according to the total number of regions stimulated as well as the temporal density of stimuli. These patterns can perhaps be seen more clearly in **Figure 4**, in which an overview of the medians across subsets of test-regions is presented. The median AmpStd for subsets where no stimuli were presented, e.g., right eye regions in variants where stimuli were presented to the left eye only, are close to zero in all instances. Of the region subsets where stimuli *were* presented, variants with a stimulus presentation rate of 6/s/hr produced smaller median amplitudes than the equivalent 3/s/hr variants in all cases. This is the expected outcome given the higher temporal density, and therefore larger summed signal and lower response gain, of the 6/s/hr variants. Selected data from this overview will be used to facilitate the comparison of constriction amplitudes under conditions of differing signal density at the retina, PON, and EWN.

Retina

Analysis of constriction amplitudes for variants in which the signal density differed at the level of the retina comprised a comparison between the 3/s/hr All Regions variant and the two 6/s/hr single eye variants (**Figure 5A**). Note that although the retinal signal density differs (3/s/hr vs. 6/s/hr), the summed signal at the PON (6/s/hr) and EWN (12/s/hr) are the same for each of these three variants. There was very little difference between constriction amplitudes for the All Regions variant and either of the Left or Right Eye variants; the small differences that were present were found to be non-significant [$t_{(21)} = 0.22, p = 0.83$, $t_{(21)} = 0.46, p = 0.65$, respectively]. This suggests that increasing the pooled signal density at the retinal level alone is unlikely to have any effect on constriction amplitudes.

Pretectal Olivary Nuclei

The first comparison where signal density was manipulated to differ at the PON utilized 3/s/hr Left Eye (LE) and Right Eye (RE) variants contrasted against 3/s/hr Left and Right Homonymous Hemifield (LHH, RHH) variants (**Figure 5B**). In this comparison retinal (3/s/hr) and EWN (6/s/hr) signal are the same, but the signal density varies at the PON (3/s/hr vs. 6/s/hr). Amplitudes were very similar with none found to be significantly different (LE vs. LHH: $t_{(14)} = 0.27$, $p = 0.79$, LE vs. RHH: $t_{(14)} = 0.03$, $p = 0.998$, RE vs. LHH: $t_{(14)} = 0.35$, $p = 0.73$, RE vs. RHH: $t_{(14)} = 0.10$, $p = 0.92$). These results suggest that, as with the retina, doubling the signal density at the PON does not affect constriction amplitudes.

Edinger-Westphal Nuclei

Comparisons between different signal densities at the EWN firstly involved the 3/s/hr LHH and RHH variants, contrasted against the 3/s/hr All Regions variant (**Figure 6A**). Here, retinal (3/s/hr) and PON (6/s/hr) signal density were the same, and the EWN differed (6/s/hr vs. 12/s/hr). In contrast to the earlier

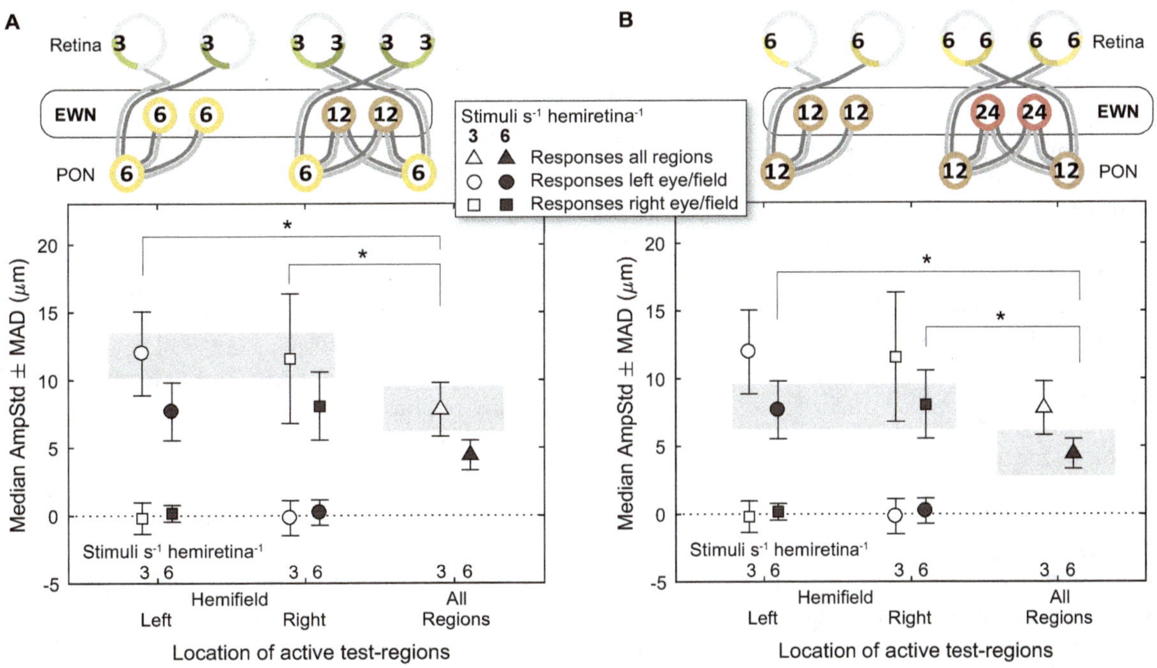

FIGURE 6 | Effect of differing summed signal density at the Edinger-Westphal nuclei (EWN). In the cartoons at top, numerals represent the estimated summed signal density at each level of the pathway and the black outline the level of the pathway where the signal density differs between conditions. The gray bars indicate the data points relevant to these comparisons. **(A)** Increasing the signal density at the EWN, while holding it the same in the retina and pretectal olivary nuclei (PON), significantly reduced constriction amplitudes (AmpStd) in the 3/s/hr variants. **(B)** The 6/s/hr variants produced the same outcome, with significant differences in amplitude due to differing signal density at the EWN. *$p < 0.05$.

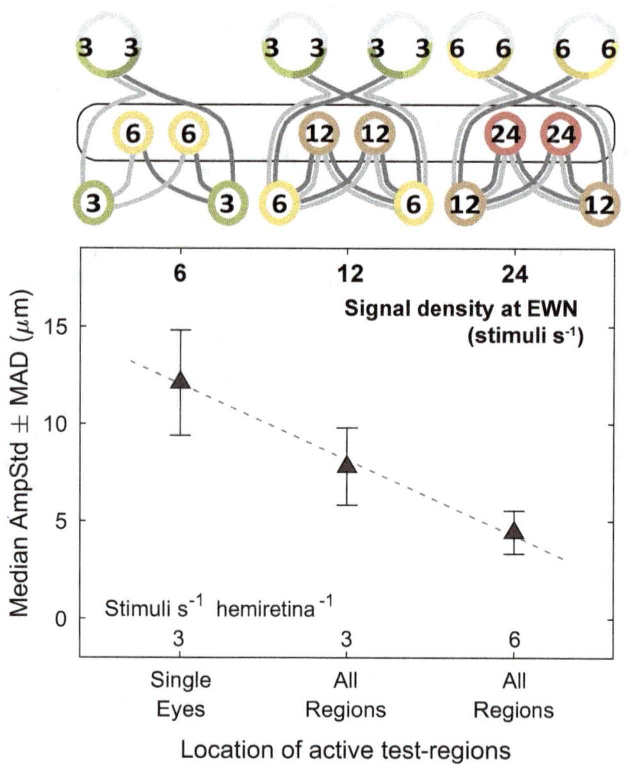

FIGURE 7 | Effect of increasing the summed signal density at the Edinger-Westphal nuclei (EWN). In the cartoons at top, numerals represent the estimated summed signal density at each level of the pathway and the black outline the level of the pathway where the signal density differs between conditions. Doubling the summed signal density, equivalent to logarithmic increments of 0.301, resulted in a linear decrease in median pupil constriction amplitudes (AmpStd).

results, the mean amplitude of the variant with the higher EWN signal density (3/s/hr All Regions) was significantly smaller than that of each of the other two variants [$t_{(30)} = -2.26, p < 0.05$, $t_{(30)} = -2.28, p < 0.05$). A similar comparison (**Figure 6B**) for the 6/s/hr variants also produced significant differences ($t_{(30)} = -2.50, p < 0.05$, $t_{(30)} = -2.07, p < 0.05$).

These results lend support to the hypothesis that modulation of pupillary responses due to changes in summed signal density occurs at the level of the EWN or later. As shown in **Figure 7**, progressively doubling the density of the visual signal at the EWN results in a linear decrease in constriction amplitudes within the range tested.

Nasal and Temporal Hemifields

Looking back at **Figure 4**, it can be seen that the regular pattern that has been seen so far does not appear to extend to variants in which Temporal and Nasal hemifield test-regions were stimulated in isolation from the opposite hemifield. The more sparse 3/s/hr condition responses are slightly larger than homonymous hemifield or individual eye variants, and the 6/s/hr conditions slightly smaller. In order to gain some insight into this irregularity, the medians of direct and consensual responses were estimated separately (**Figure 8**). Although not significant, consistent patterns emerged. On stimulation of the temporal hemifield, consensual responses appeared slightly smaller than direct. The opposite pattern occurred in the nasal hemifield. Although these results reveal at most a small trend, the direction of this trend is consistent with observations in the literature (23, 24). Further investigations targeting this specifically may yield useful information regarding the nature of the pooling of retinal signal.

DISCUSSION

In multifocal testing, many stimuli are presented in close temporal proximity. This means that the overall pupillary response at any given time will comprise temporally overlapping response components from a number of individual stimuli at different visual-field locations. Individual responses therefore, reflect just a proportion of this overall response. The actual number of stimuli that are summed will depend on the temporal density of the stimuli i.e., the stimulus presentation rate, as well as the time-constant, or memory, of the system. In this experiment, where very few stimuli were presented simultaneously (**Figure 1C**), it is clear that the gain of the system incorporates a temporal component since smaller amplitudes are obtained to the higher density 6/s/hr stimuli than 3/s/hr in all variants. Determining the location of this gain-control process within the pupillary pathway was the overarching aim of this project.

Gain-Control Occurs in the Edinger-Westphal Nuclei

Responses were compared between stimulus variants having differing gain-states at a specific level of the pathway (retina, PON, EWN) while other levels of the system were subjected to equivalent gain. This experiment produced strong evidence for the Edinger-Westphal nuclei being the location of this gain-control mechanism, and no evidence of gain occurring at the retina or PON. This outcome may seem incongruous with the presence of GABAergic neurons in the rat PON (25) and the considerable degree of pooling of retinal inputs that occurs in the PON of primates (26); these two findings could point to the PON as a possible location for pupillary gain. PON luminance neuron outputs however, more closely resemble retinal signal than the pupillary response (27), leading to the alternative proposal that the EWN is the site of this signal modulation. Our results lend support to this latter hypothesis.

Binocular vs. Monocular Summation

It is interesting to note that no difference was observed between summation of retinal signal across the two eyes and within the retina of a single eye (e.g., **Figure 5B**). Thompson in 1947 (28) reported that the area of monocular stimulation required to produce an equivalent constriction was four times that of the same area stimulated binocularly. There is no sign of this binocular amplification occurring in this study: our findings were more in line with those of Clarke et al. (29) in which binocular responses were slightly less than double the size of responses to otherwise identical monocular stimulation.

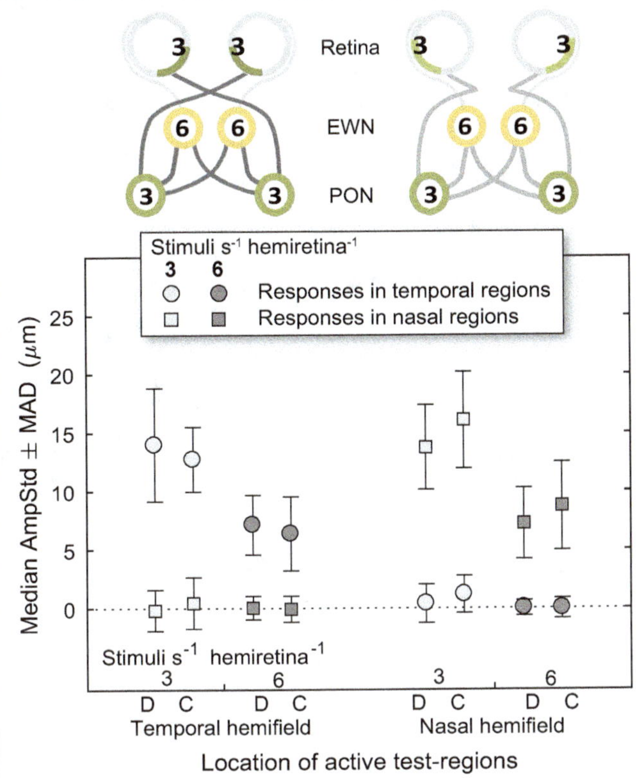

FIGURE 8 | Direct and consensual responses for stimulus protocols with active test-regions in temporal or nasal hemifields. (On the abscissa, the letter D is used to indicate direct responses, C indicates consensual). In the cartoons at top, numerals represent the estimated summed signal density at each level of the pathway. Amplitudes for both 3/s/hr and 6/s/hr variants are plotted although only the 3/s/hr variants are represented in the cartoons.

Models of Gain and Integrity of Signal Within Pathways

It would appear from our results that pretectal large field luminance neurons likely pool information from the retina rather than modulate it, although the possibility exists that GABAergic PON neurons utilize a different time constant and e.g., may only modulate concurrent inputs. Varju (30) proposed a model of shunting inhibition for binocular summation but could only speculate as to where this might occur. His model proposes that the input from each retina is reduced proportionally by increases in input from the other i.e., maximal response is only obtained from stimulation of one retina when the other is in the dark. From our results it would seem likely that this same pattern may also apply for signal originating within the same eye. This point raises the question of how far along the pupillary pathway the retinotopy of signal is maintained. Our proposed model for signal summation and segregation in contraction anisocoria (8) would suggest that, at the least, pooling appears to maintain the separation of signal originating in different hemifields and eyes.

These experiments may have been somewhat limited by their use of an older version of mfPOP stimulus presentation than is currently used in our research (17); this is reflected by the relatively small stimulus amplitudes and variability of the results. The finding that constriction amplitudes were linear with the log of the stimulus presentation rate however, is consistent with Atchison's observations (31) that stimulus area is the reciprocal of luminance, given that pupil constrictions increase linearly with the log of the stimulus luminance over much of their range. Of course, these results do not preclude the existence of gain-control in other locations such as retinal adaptation of photoreceptors (32). The relatively small number of subjects in this study unfortunately prevented any exploration of variation in gain with age or across different populations. The localization of this gain-control to the EWN however, will act to inform the development of future pupillary stimuli and multifocal response extraction methods therefore leading to more accurate and reliable perimetric assessments. The findings also provide a starting point for further investigations into the precise nature of the pooling, segregation, and modulation of retinal signal within this nucleus, and broaden the knowledge surrounding the complexities of the pupillary response in humans.

AUTHOR CONTRIBUTIONS

CC designed the study, undertook data acquisition and processing, designed and created the stimulus variants, analyzed the data and wrote the manuscript. AJ created the software for signal processing and stimulus generation. YR undertook data acquisition. TM provided scientific advice and oversight of the study and revised the manuscript.

FUNDING

This work was supported by the Australian Research Council through the ARC Centre of Excellence in Vision Science (CE0561903).

REFERENCES

1. Gamlin PD, McDougal DH, Pokorny J, Smith VC, Yau KW, Dacey DM. Human and macaque pupil responses driven by melanopsin-containing retinal ganglion cells. *Vision Res.* (2007) 47:946–54. doi: 10.1016/j.visres.2006.12.015
2. Dacey DM, Liao HW, Peterson BB, Robinson FR, Smith VC, Pokorny J, et al. Melanopsin-expressing ganglion cells in primate retina signal colour and irradiance and project to the LGN. *Nature.* (2005) 433:749–54. doi: 10.1038/nature03387
3. McDougal DH, Gamlin PD. The influence of intrinsically-photosensitive retinal ganglion cells on the spectral sensitivity and response dynamics

of the human pupillary light reflex. *Vision Res.* (2010) 50:72–87. doi: 10.1016/j.visres.2009.10.012

4. Barbur JL, Harlow AJ, Sahraie A. Pupillary responses to stimulus structure, colour and movement. *Opthalmic Physiol Opt.* (1992) 12:137–41. doi: 10.1111/j.1475-1313.1992.tb00276.x
5. Heywood CA, Nicholas JJ, LeMare C, Cowey A. The effect of lesions to cortical areas V4 or AIT on pupillary responses to chromatic and achromatic stimuli in monkeys. *Exp Brain Res.* (1998) 122:475–80. doi: 10.1007/s002210050536
6. Sahraie A, Barbur JL. Pupil response triggered by the onset of coherent motion. *Graefes Arch Clin Exp Ophthalmol.* (1997) 235:494–500. doi: 10.1007/BF00947006
7. Gamlin PD. The pretectum: connections and oculomotor-related roles. *Prog Brain Res.* (2006) 151:379–405. doi: 10.1016/S0079-6123(05)51012-4
8. Carle CF, Maddess T, James AC. Contraction anisocoria: segregation, summation, and saturation in the pupillary pathway. *Invest Ophth Vis Sci.* (2011) 52:2365–71. doi: 10.1167/iovs.10-6335
9. Maddess T, Ho YL, Wong SS, Kolic M, Goh XL, Carle CF, et al. Multifocal pupillographic perimetry with white and colored stimuli. *J Glaucoma.* (2011) 20:336–43. doi: 10.1097/IJG.0b013e3181efb097
10. Sabeti F, James AC, Maddess T. Spatial and temporal stimulus variants for multifocal pupillography of the central visual field. *Vision Res.* (2011) 51:303–10. doi: 10.1016/j.visres.2010.10.015
11. Carle CF, James AC, Kolic M, Loh YW, Maddess T. High-resolution multifocal pupillographic objective perimetry in glaucoma. *Invest Ophthalmol Vis Sci.* (2011) 52:604–10. doi: 10.1167/iovs.10-5737
12. Ayaz A, Chance FS. Gain modulation of neuronal responses by subtractive and divisive mechanisms of inhibition. *J Neurophysiol.* (2009) 101:958–68. doi: 10.1152/jn.90547.2008
13. James AC, Kolic M, Bedford SM, Maddess T. Stimulus parameters for multifocal pupillographic objective perimetry. *J Glaucoma.* (2012) 21:571–8. doi: 10.1097/IJG.0b013e31821e8413
14. Carle CF, James AC, Maddess T. The pupillary response to color and luminance variant multifocal stimuli. *Invest Ophthalmol Vis Sci.* (2013) 54:467–75. doi: 10.1167/iovs.12-10829
15. Maddess T, Bedford SM, Goh XL, James AC. Multifocal pupillographic visual field testing in glaucoma. *Clin Exp Ophthalmol.* (2009) 37:678–86. doi: 10.1111/j.1442-9071.2009.02107.x
16. Bell A, James AC, Kolic M, Essex RW, Maddess T. Dichoptic multifocal pupillography reveals afferent visual field defects in early type 2 diabetes. *Invest Ophthalmol Vis Sci.* (2010) 51:602–8. doi: 10.1167/iovs.09-3659
17. Sabeti F, Maddess T, Essex RW, Saikal A, James A, Carle C. Multifocal pupillography in early age-related macular degeneration. *Optom Vis Sci.* (2014) 91:904–15. doi: 10.1097/OPX.0000000000000319
18. Anderson AJ, Johnson CA. Frequency-doubling technology perimetry and optical defocus. *Invest Ophth Vis Sci.* (2003) 44:4147–52. doi: 10.1167/iovs.02-1076
19. James AC. The pattern-pulse multifocal visual evoked potential. *Invest Ophthalmic Visual Sci.* (2003) 44:879–90. doi: 10.1167/iovs.02-0608
20. James AC, Ruseckaite R, Maddess T. Effect of temporal sparseness and dichoptic presentation on multifocal visual evoked potentials. *Visual Neurosci.* (2005) 22:45–54. doi: 10.1017/S0952523805221053
21. Carle CF, James AC, Kolic M, Essex RW, Maddess T. Blue multifocal pupillographic objective perimetry in glaucoma. *Invest Ophthalmic Visual Sci.* (2015) 56:6394–403. doi: 10.1167/iovs.14-16029
22. Carle CF, James AC, Kolic M, Essex RW, Maddess T. Luminance and colour variant pupil perimetry in glaucoma. *Clin Exp Ophthalmol.* (2014) 42:815–24. doi: 10.1111/ceo.12346
23. Cox TA, Drewes CP. Contraction anisocoria resulting from half-field illumination. *Am J Ophthalmol.* (1984) 97:577–82. doi: 10.1016/0002-9394(84)90375-1
24. Martin TL, Kardon R, Thompson HS. Unequal direct and consensual pupillary responses to hemiretinal stimuli. *Invest Ophth Vis Sci.* (1991) 32:1124.
25. Campbell G, Lieberman AR. The olivary pretectal nucleus: experimental anatomical studies in the rat. *Philos Transac R Soc Lond B Biol Sci.* (1985) 310:573. doi: 10.1098/rstb.1985.0132
26. Clarke RJ, Zhang H, Gamlin PD. Primate pupillary light reflex: receptive field characteristics of pretectal luminance neurons. *J Neurophysiol.* (2003) 89:3168–78. doi: 10.1152/jn.01130.2002
27. Pong M, Fuchs AF. Characteristics of the pupillary light reflex in the macaque monkey: discharge patterns of pretectal neurons. *J Neurophysiol.* (2000) 84:964–74. doi: 10.1152/jn.2000.84.2.964
28. Thomson LC. Binocular summation within the nervous pathways of the pupillary light reflex. *J Physiol.* (1947) 106:59–65. doi: 10.1113/jphysiol.1947.sp004192
29. Clarke RJ, Zhang H, Gamlin PD. Characteristics of the pupillary light reflex in the alert rhesus monkey. *J Neurophysiol.* (2003) 89:3179–89. doi: 10.1152/jn.01131.2002
30. Varju D. Human pupil dynamics. In: *Proceedings of the International School of Physics "Enrico Fermi".* New York, NY: Academic Press (1969). p. 442–64.
31. Atchison DA, Girgenti CC, Campbell GM, Dodds JP, Byrnes TM, Zele AJ. Influence of field size on pupil diameter under photopic and mesopic light levels. *Clin Exp Optometry.* (2011) 94:545–8. doi: 10.1111/j.1444-0938.2011.00636.x
32. Shapley R, Enroth-Cugell C, Bonds AB, Kirby A. Gain control in the retina and retinal dynamics. *Nature.* (1972) 236:352. doi: 10.1038/236352a0

12

Effect of Single and Combined Monochromatic Light on the Human Pupillary Light Response

Maria A. Bonmati-Carrion[1,2], *Konstanze Hild*[3], *Cheryl M. Isherwood*[4], *Stephen J. Sweeney*[3], *Victoria L. Revell*[5], *Juan A. Madrid*[1,2], *Maria A. Rol*[1,2] and *Debra J. Skene*[4*]

[1] Chronobiology Laboratory, Department of Physiology, IMIB-Arrixaca, University of Murcia, Murcia, Spain, [2] Ciber Fragilidad y Envejecimiento Saludable, Madrid, Spain, [3] Advanced Technology Institute and Department of Physics, University of Surrey, Guildford, United Kingdom, [4] Chronobiology, Faculty of Health and Medical Sciences, University of Surrey, Guildford, United Kingdom, [5] Surrey Clinical Research Centre, Faculty of Health and Medical Sciences, University of Surrey, Guildford, United Kingdom

***Correspondence:**
Debra J. Skene
d.skene@surrey.ac.uk

The pupillary light reflex (PLR) is a neurological reflex driven by rods, cones, and melanopsin-containing retinal ganglion cells. Our aim was to achieve a more precise picture of the effects of 5-min duration monochromatic light stimuli, alone or in combination, on the human PLR, to determine its spectral sensitivity and to assess the importance of photon flux. Using pupillometry, the PLR was assessed in 13 participants (6 women) aged 27.2 ± 5.41 years (mean ± SD) during 5-min light stimuli of purple (437 nm), blue (479 nm), red (627 nm), and combinations of red+purple or red+blue light. In addition, nine 5-min, photon-matched light stimuli, ranging in 10 nm increments peaking between 420 and 500 nm were tested in 15 participants (8 women) aged 25.7 ± 8.90 years. Maximum pupil constriction, time to achieve this, constriction velocity, area under the curve (AUC) at short (0–60 s), and longer duration (240–300 s) light exposures, and 6-s post-illumination pupillary response (6-s PIPR) were assessed. Photoreceptor activation was estimated by mathematical modeling. The velocity of constriction was significantly faster with blue monochromatic light than with red or purple light. Within the blue light spectrum (between 420 and 500 nm), the velocity of constriction was significantly faster with the 480 nm light stimulus, while the slowest pupil constriction was observed with 430 nm light. Maximum pupil constriction was achieved with 470 nm light, and the greatest AUC_{0-60} and $AUC_{240-300}$ was observed with 490 and 460 nm light, respectively. The 6-s PIPR was maximum after 490 nm light stimulus. Both the transient (AUC_{0-60}) and sustained ($AUC_{240-300}$) response was significantly correlated with melanopic activation. Higher photon fluxes for both purple and blue light produced greater amplitude sustained pupillary constriction. The findings confirm human PLR dependence on wavelength, monochromatic or bichromatic light and photon flux under 5-min duration light stimuli. Since the most rapid and high amplitude PLR occurred within the 460–490 nm light range (alone or combined), our results suggest that color discrimination should be studied under total or partial substitution of this blue light range (460–490 nm) by shorter wavelengths (~440 nm). Thus for nocturnal lighting, replacement of blue light with purple light might be a plausible solution to preserve color discrimination while minimizing melanopic activation.

Keywords: pupillometry, light, pupillary light reflex, ipRGC, melanopsin, human melanopic lux

INTRODUCTION

The pupillary light reflex (PLR) is a neurological reflex characterized by a reduction in pupil diameter in response to an increase in retinal illumination, as well as the subsequent redilation of the pupil after light cessation. Its main function is to increase the depth of field and image sharpness in bright light conditions.

Rods and cones were the only known mammal photoreceptors until the discovery of melanopsin (1), a photopigment with a peak of sensitivity (λ_{max}) at 480 nm, which is expressed in the intrinsically photosensitive retinal ganglion cells (ipRGCs) (2). These ipRGCs project to the suprachiasmatic nuclei (SCN), the circadian pacemaker, and other non-image forming brain areas, such as the olivary pretectal nucleus (OPN), a control center for the PLR (3–7). Thus, ipRGCs participate in a common pathway for the PLR and other processes such as circadian entrainment, either by themselves (intrinsically) or through their connections with the outer retinal photoreceptors (extrinsically), the most efficient wavelengths (humans, λ_{max} 446–477 nm) to both entrain the circadian timing system and inhibit melatonin synthesis (8, 9) being those closer to the maximal sensitivity for ipRGCs. In addition, a relationship between circadian status and PLR has recently been reported (10), indicating a complex inverse relationship between both systems. Once this common pathway and its interactions are further studied, it may be plausible to assess the effect of different lights on the human circadian system through their effects on the PLR.

The human PLR follows a general dynamic (11–14), that can be affected by the intensity, spectral composition (15, 16) and duration of the light stimulus. When the stimulus starts, the pupil shows a rapid constriction until it reaches a minimum size (maximal constriction amplitude). After this early transient response, a pupillary re-dilatation occurs (escape), reaching a more sustained state of partial pupil constriction, which lasts until the end of the light stimulus (17) as well as after termination (post-illumination pupil response, PIPR) (12). According to some studies in primates and humans, the early transient pupil constriction is predominantly driven by cones, while control of the sustained and persistent PIPR seems to correspond to a melanopsin-mediated intrinsic response (12, 18–20). Recent studies, however, have suggested that the outer retinal photoreceptors could also participate in this sustained (21–23) and post-illumination pupil response (PIPR) (24, 25). Despite some limitations of pupillometry, it is possible to infer rod and cone function and the intrinsic activation of ipRGCs independently by analyzing the transient, sustained, and persistent (or PIPR) pupillary response to light stimuli of different wavelengths, intensities, and durations (17).

Apart from their relative specificity on the PLR dynamics, each human retinal photoreceptor exhibits different wavelength sensitivities, based on their corresponding photopigments: λ_{max} 498 nm for rods, λ_{max} 420 nm for S-cones, λ_{max} 530 nm for M-cones, λ_{max} 559 nm for L-cones (26). The maximum sensitivity for melanopsin-containing ipRGCs has been established at 480 nm (2, 6, 27), although other PLR studies in humans indicate peak sensitivities around 490 nm (28), based on ocular photoresponses. In primates intensity thresholds for each photoreceptor are also different, being higher for ipRGCs (~10–11 log quanta/cm^2/s) (23, 29) than for the classical photoreceptors [cones 2.30 log quanta/cm^2/s; rods 1.70 log quanta /cm^2/s, at the cornea level (30)]. Furthermore, it has been proposed that melanopsin's spatial conformation and thus its wavelength sensitivity can switch back from the M to R state by absorbing longer wavelength photons, so-called melanopsin bistability (31, 32). This has also been associated with the PLR, exhibiting increased pupil constriction when the light stimulus was preceded by longer wavelength light (32). Tristability (with two silent and one signaling state) has also been suggested as a mechanism for ipRGC to integrate both time and wavelength (33). However, not all studies have been able to demonstrate this long wavelength potentiation of blue light responses (34, 35), while some studies have proposed the existence of retinal pigment epithelium (RPE)-derived regeneration in melanopsin (36, 37), which could be interpreted as a complementary mechanism [reviewed in (38)].

The study of possible interactions between two monochromatic wavelengths when administered simultaneously, as well as assessment of PLR sensitivity over a high resolution short wavelength range will help to provide knowledge on the effect of polychromatic lights on the PLR.

The aim of this study was thus to achieve a more precise picture of the effects of 5-min monochromatic light stimuli, alone or in combination [long (red) combined with short (blue and purple) wavelength lights], on the human PLR (including PIPR), to determine its spectral sensitivity and to confirm the importance of photon flux as a determinant of the human PLR.

Based on previous knowledge, we hypothesized that blue or purple light would produce different responses when combined with red light as a result of melanopsin bistability, probably increasing the sustained response (greater amplitude) due to the conformational change of melanopsin by red light. Regarding monochromatic short wavelength light, we expected greater pupillary responses under the 460–490 nm light range, and under higher light intensities.

MATERIALS AND METHODS

Participants

This study was approved by the University of Surrey Ethics Committee. Volunteers received appropriate information about the study protocol, signed a written informed consent form (in compliance with the Declaration of Helsinki) before being enrolled and were compensated for their participation.

In both experimental conditions participants were healthy, non-smoking volunteers: 13 (6 women) between 19 and 35 years (27.2 ± 5.41 years, mean ± SD) for Study A, and 15 (8 women) between 19 and 35 years (25.7 ± 8.90 years) for Study B. Data from three participants from Study A were excluded from analysis because of very noisy PLR signals that were not interpretable.

All participants declared no medical or mental health disorders and were not taking any medication that could affect circadian rhythms, according to the general health questionnaires completed during the screening period. None of them were shift workers nor had crossed more than two time zones in the 2 months prior to study admission. They kept regular sleep-wake cycles with no reported sleep disorders (Pittsburgh Sleep Quality Index ≤5) (39), and were not extreme morning or evening types (40). A full ophthalmic examination including uncorrected vision, near vision corrected, ophthalmoscopy, pupil reactions, Henson Field Test, refraction, intra-ocular pressure, oculomotor status, stereo acuity, accommodation, and color vision by the Ishihara test, was performed to confirm they all were free from any ocular disorders.

Pre-study Measurements

The protocol used was similar to that previously described (41) with participants maintaining a regular, actigraphically (AWL, Cambridge Neurotechnology, UK) monitored sleep/wake schedule for at least 7 days before and throughout the in-laboratory sessions. For 72 h before and during each laboratory session, participants refrained from caffeinated drinks, alcohol, excessive exercise, bright lights, and non-steroidal anti-inflammatory drug intake.

In-laboratory Protocol

Protocol for Light Stimuli Presentation

A randomized, within-subject design was performed. In both experimental conditions A and B, all the sessions were carried out in the morning. In Study A (**Figure 1A**) the participants (3 per session) arrived at the laboratory and remained seated in dim light (<5 lux) for 30 min in order to progressively adapt their vision to the dark conditions. Then, he or she received a drop of tropicamide [Minims Tropicamide (1.0%, Chauvin Pharmaceuticals, Romford, UK)] in the right eye to dilate the pupil. After that, the participant remained in darkness (0 lux + eye mask) for an hour prior to pupil recording in order to avoid any confounding effect due to prior light exposures (42). Once this dark adaptation schedule was completed, pupil recording started. For this, the left non-dilated pupil was recorded [220 frames per second] in darkness for 60 s to obtain a baseline, which was later used as a control to normalize the pupil diameter. Then, the light source was turned on and the right eye (pupil dilated) received a light stimulus for 5 min (**Figure 1A**) while recording the left pupil, thus assessing the consensual reflex. Only one light condition was tested per laboratory session.

The protocol for light stimuli presentation and administration of tropicamide in Study B is shown in **Figure 1B** and has been detailed in a previous study (10). The pupillary recording followed the same protocol as described for Study A, except that pupil recording continued for 60 s after light offset.

Light Stimuli Characteristics

A 5-min light stimulus was administered to the participant's right eye (dilated) through a specially constructed Ganzfeld sphere (Apollo Lighting, Leeds, UK) coated with white reflectance paint (WRC-680 Labsphere, Pro-Lite Technology, Bedfordshire, UK) to produce patternless illumination. An ultra high-pressure mercury lamp (Focus 100LS3, 100 W, Philips Lighting, Eindhoven, The Netherlands) illuminated the sphere via a fiber optic cable connected to a light box (10, 35, 41)

In Study A, monochromatic light (purple, blue, and red) was produced using narrow bandwidth interference filters (Coherent Ealing Europe Ltd., Watford, UK) peaking at 440, 480, and 630 nm (half maximal bandwidth of 10 nm), respectively. The spectra measured at eye level, exhibited peaks at 437, 479, and 627 nm (**Figure 2A**), respectively, as measured by a calibrated spectrometer (Ocean Optics BV, Dunedin, Florida, USA). Light irradiances were adjusted using neutral density filters (0.10, 0.60, 0.90) (Kodak, Hemel Hempsted, UK) and were verified at the participant's eye level (cornea) using a calibrated radiometer (R203, Macam Photometrics Ltd., Livingston, Scotland) before and after each light exposure.

Purple (437 nm), blue (479 nm), and red (627 nm) monochromatic lights were administered alone or in combination [monochromatic purple + monochromatic red (PR) and monochromatic blue + monochromatic red (BR)] (**Figures 2A,B**). Both purple and blue lights were administered at photopic light intensities of 1.2×10^{13} photons/cm^2/s (13.1 log quanta/cm^2/s), while 5 x 10^{13} photons/cm^2/s (13.7 log quanta/cm^2/s) was selected for red light administration (**Figure 2A**). The photon densities for each light stimulus were chosen based on the previously determined irradiance response curves to monochromatic light for melatonin suppression (8, 9). In addition, since bistability was demonstrated in human PLR experiments using a higher irradiance of red light (32), a similar decision was made for the current study.

In Study B, 9 × 10 nm increment monochromatic lights (420, 430, 440, 450, 460, 470, 480, 490, and 500 nm), each with a half maximal bandwidth of 7 nm, were obtained using a Bentham M300 monochromator (**Figures 3A,B**). Technical characteristics of this system have been previously described (10). Due to the narrower spectral range selected and the wavelength dependent grating response of the monochromator, the photon densities tested (**Figure 3A**) were 10-fold lower than the ones achieved in Study A (**Figure 2A**). The achieved photon density was approximately 11.9 log quanta/cm^2/s at the level of the cornea. Considering a 0.3 correction for optical media, all the photon fluxes tested would have been applied above 11 log quanta/cm^2/s,

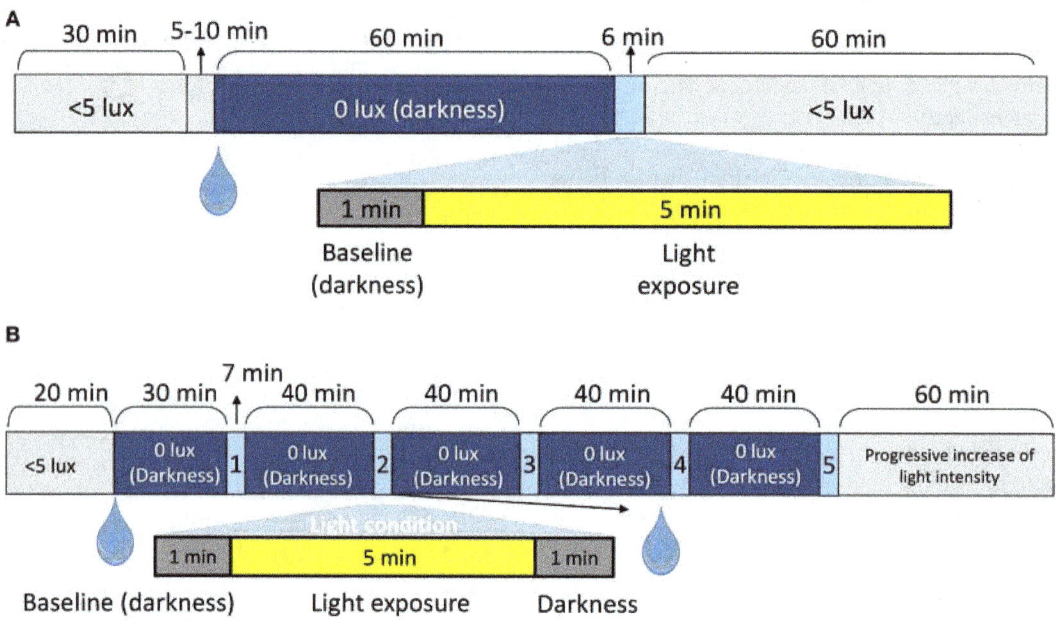

FIGURE 1 | In-laboratory protocol for Study A **(A)** and Study B **(B)**. The drop symbol shows the time when the pupil dilator was administered. The up arrows point to the duration (mins) of the shorter periods.

A

Peak of emission (nm)	437	479	627	437 + 627	479 + 627
Name	Purple	Blue	Red	Purple + Red	Blue + Red
Photon flux (10^{13} photons/cm^2/s)	1.2	1.2	5.13	6.33	6.33

B

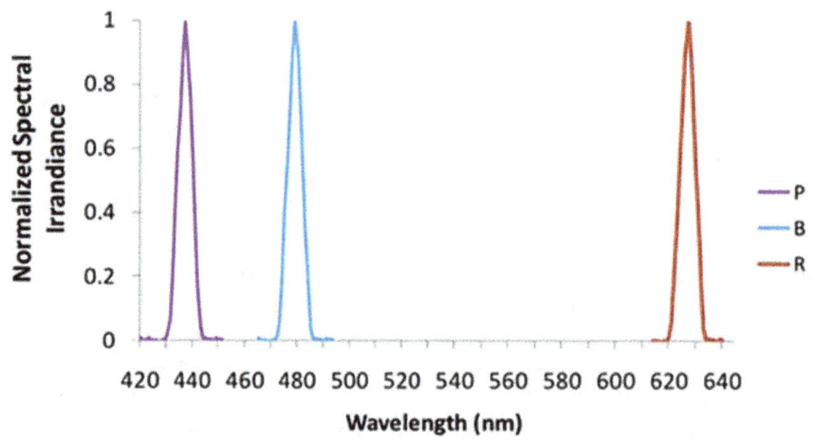

FIGURE 2 | Light wavelengths tested in Study A and their corresponding photon fluxes **(A)**, and normalized spectra **(B)**.

thus being above the photopic threshold (43) and within the limits for melanopsin activation (18). Identical photon fluxes could not be obtained for all the wavelengths tested due to technical limitations of the instrumentation. Some data from Study B have already been published as part of a previous study in which they were correlated with different aspects of the circadian system (10).

The tested range of wavelengths were selected according to previous studies on short wavelength sensitivity of the human circadian system (8, 9, 44–46). In addition, assessing the effects of

A

Peak of emission (nm)	420	430	440	450	460	470	480	490	500
Photon flux (10^{11} photons/cm^2/s)	8.87	8.82	9.17	8.58	8.14	8.31	7.99	7.85	7.39

B

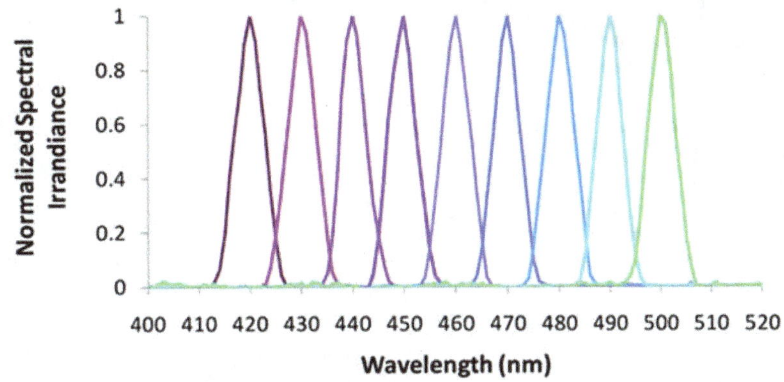

FIGURE 3 | Light wavelengths tested in Study B and their corresponding photon fluxes **(A)**, and normalized spectra **(B)**.

wavelengths shorter than the melanopsin λ_{max} peak on the PLR could help to clarify the role of very short wavelength light.

Since two of the lights in Study A and B were almost identical in terms of maximum spectral emission (peak at 437 nm in Study A vs. 440 nm in Study B and peak at 479 nm in Study A vs. 480 nm in Study B), comparison between a higher (1.2×10^{13} photons/cm^2/s) and a lower ($8–9 \times 10^{11}$ photons/cm^2/s) photon density at those wavelengths was performed.

Pupil Recording

To assess the consensual PLR, a pupillometer system was used. The pupil size was tracked from the infrared illuminated (left) eye through a video pupil tracking system (ViewPoint Eye Tracker®, Arrington Research Inc., Scottsdale, AZ). The researcher helped the participants to be seated in front of the sphere in darkness, resting their forehead and chin on the pupillometer system support while the left eye was focussed by the infrared camera. The system recorded 220 data per second [see (10) for further technical details].

Data Analysis

Data Pre-processing

Pupil diameter was analyzed using software specifically designed by the Chronobiology Laboratory and the Artificial Intelligence Group at the University of Murcia (Pupilabware®), as already described (10). This processing included the determination of baseline (mean pupil diameter during the 60 s in darkness prior to the light stimulus) and normalized pupil size (NPS), i.e., ratio of the measured pupil diameter divided by the baseline pupil size.

Primary Pupil Outcome Parameters

Minimum diameter (expressed as relative maximum rapid pupil constriction), time to minimum (time required to achieve the relative maximum rapid pupil constriction), velocity of pupil constriction as $(\frac{\text{maximum constriction}}{\text{time to minimum}})$ and area under the curve $(AUC = AUC\sum_{t0}^{t1} 100 - NPS)$, where t_0 is the initial time point of pupil response and t_1 is the end time, 100 is the baseline pupil size, and NPS is normalized pupil size. Two AUCs were calculated: AUC_{0-60}, corresponding to the first minute of light exposure and $AUC_{240-300}$ that corresponds to the last minute of light exposure within a 5 min light stimulus. AUC was expressed as "arbitrary units" (A.U./AU) (**Figure 4**). Pupil diameter 6-s after light offset (6-s PIPR) was calculated in Study B.

Statistical Analysis

All statistical analyses were carried out using SPSS 25 (SPSS Inc., Chicago, IL, USA). When not all participants received all light conditions, missing parameters were replaced by the average parameter under that light condition. For parameters that did not have a normal distribution Friedman's non-parametric test for related samples (*post-hoc* Wilcoxon) was performed instead of repeated measures ANOVA (Bonferroni *post-hoc*). The significance level was set at $p < 0.05$. Bonferroni correction was applied after *post-hoc* pairwise comparisons. When only two conditions were compared, a paired or unpaired Student's *t*-test (or Mann-Whitney U) was performed. All the results were expressed as mean ± standard error of the mean (SEM).

Photoreceptor Activation

The photoreceptor activation was assessed for each light condition using the Irradiance Toolbox (v1.), developed by Lucas et al. (47), that calculates the α-opic lux parameter, which in turn represents the excitation of each of the 5 photoreceptors under different light spectra. This calculation is based on the estimated sensitivity curves for each photoreceptor (47). Both absolute values (obtained directly from the toolbox) and the relative and absolute contribution for each photoreceptor were assessed.

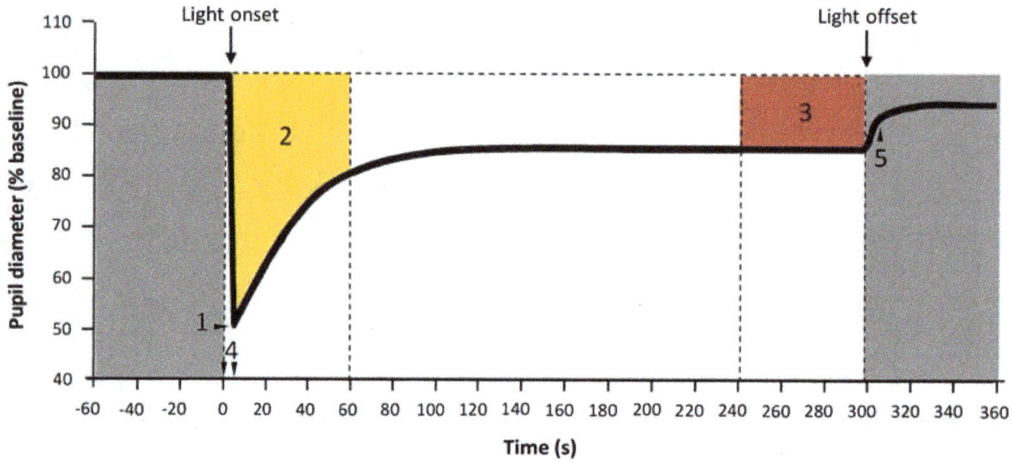

FIGURE 4 | Parameters assessed for PLR. 1: Maximum constriction; 2: Area under the curve from 0 to 60 s of light exposure (AUC_{0-60}, yellow); 3: Area under the curve from 240 to 300 s of light exposure ($AUC_{240-300}$, red), expressed in A.U.; 4: Time from light onset to the minimum pupil diameter reached during constriction; 5: 6-s PIPR. Gray areas indicate lights off.

RESULTS

Study A

Monochromatic purple (437 nm; $n = 3$), blue (479 nm; $n = 9$), and red (627 nm; $n = 8$) light stimuli and the combinations "purple + red" (PR; $n = 7$) and "blue + red" (BR; $n = 9$), were tested (photon densities indicated in **Figure 2A**). **Figures 5A,B** show the average pupil recordings for each light condition. As expected, under all tested light conditions, pupil constriction reached its minimum relative diameter within the first 10-s after light onset (transient response) (**Figure 5C**), re-dilating in a rapid manner during the following 50-s (escape), followed by the sustained part (steady state photoequilibrium) of the PLR.

There were no significant differences in the maximum pupil constriction following the light stimuli. Constriction under blue 479 nm light (57.5 ± 3.7%) > red 627 nm light (54.4 ± 2.3%) ≈ purple 437 nm light (54.2 ± 3.7%). Although the time needed to reach the minimum diameter tended to be shorter under the blue light condition, there were no significant differences between the different light stimuli. The velocity of pupil constriction, however, was significantly faster (one-way repeated measures ANOVA, $F = 51.168$, $df = 2.065$, $p < 0.001$) with blue light (27.9 ± 10.3%/s) than with the red (14.6 ± 1.7%/s) and purple (15.7 ± 1.1%/s) light (Bonferroni *post-hoc* test, $p < 0.001$).

The AUC of two PLR periods (first, AUC_{0-60}, and last, $AUC_{240-300}$, minute of light exposure) was calculated (**Figure 6A**), to evaluate the transient and sustained response, respectively. As expected AUC_{0-60} was always higher (thus, smaller diameter during the transient response) than the $AUC_{240-300}$ for all light conditions (Wilcoxon *post-hoc*, $p < 0.017$). There were no significant differences in the AUC_{0-60} (transient response) between the light conditions, with the highest value found under the blue + red light condition (2,720 ± 223 A.U.). Similarly, in the sustained response ($AUC_{240-300}$) there were no significant differences between the different light conditions (although significant overall effect, Friedman's test, $\chi^2 = 10.8$, $df = 4$, $p = 0.029$), although blue light alone or in combination tended to produce a more sustained higher amplitude response (blue, 1,908 ± 241 A.U.; blue + red, 2,076 ± 260) than purple (purple 1,350 ± 191 A.U.; purple + red 1,740 ± 222 A.U.) or red (1,456 ± 311 A.U.) light wavelengths.

The retinal photoreceptor excitations were obtained for each light condition (**Figure 6B**) by calculating the α-opic lux parameter, a parameter which represents each photoreceptor excitation [Irradiance Toolbox (47)]. In the case of purple light, the highest activation was for S-cones (67.3 cyanopic lux, absolute value; 68.4% of the total), while for blue light, melanopic excitation was highest (39.0 melanopic lux, absolute value; 35.2% of the total). For red light, as expected, the predominant excitation corresponded to L-cones (41.8 erythropic lux, absolute value; 78.7% of the total) with less excitation of M-cones (10.7 chloropic lux, absolute value; 20.1% of the total). Rod activation was also highest under blue light, both alone (B) (27.7 rhodopic lux, absolute value; 25% of the total) and in combination with red light (BR) (28.2 rhodopic lux, absolute value; 17.2% of the total).

Study B

Nine monochromatic light stimuli in 10 nm increments peaking between 420 and 500 nm were tested (peaks of emission at 420 ($n = 15$), 430 ($n = 14$), 440 ($n = 15$), 450 ($n = 15$), 460 ($n = 15$), 470 ($n = 15$), 480 ($n = 13$), 490 ($n = 14$), and 500 ($n = 13$) nm) at the photon densities indicated in the Table (**Figure 3A**). The average PLR for each light condition is shown in **Figure 7** (for clarity, the nine wavelengths tested have been represented in two separate graphs, **Figures 7A,B**). As expected, typical PLR dynamics were obtained in all cases, reaching the maximum pupil constriction within the first 10-s of light exposure (**Figure 7C**).

The maximum relative rapid pupil constriction under the light stimuli was achieved with the longer light wavelengths (one-way repeated measures ANOVA, $F = 5.204$, $df = 5.841$, $p < 0.001$), reaching the greatest pupil constriction at 470 nm (50.2

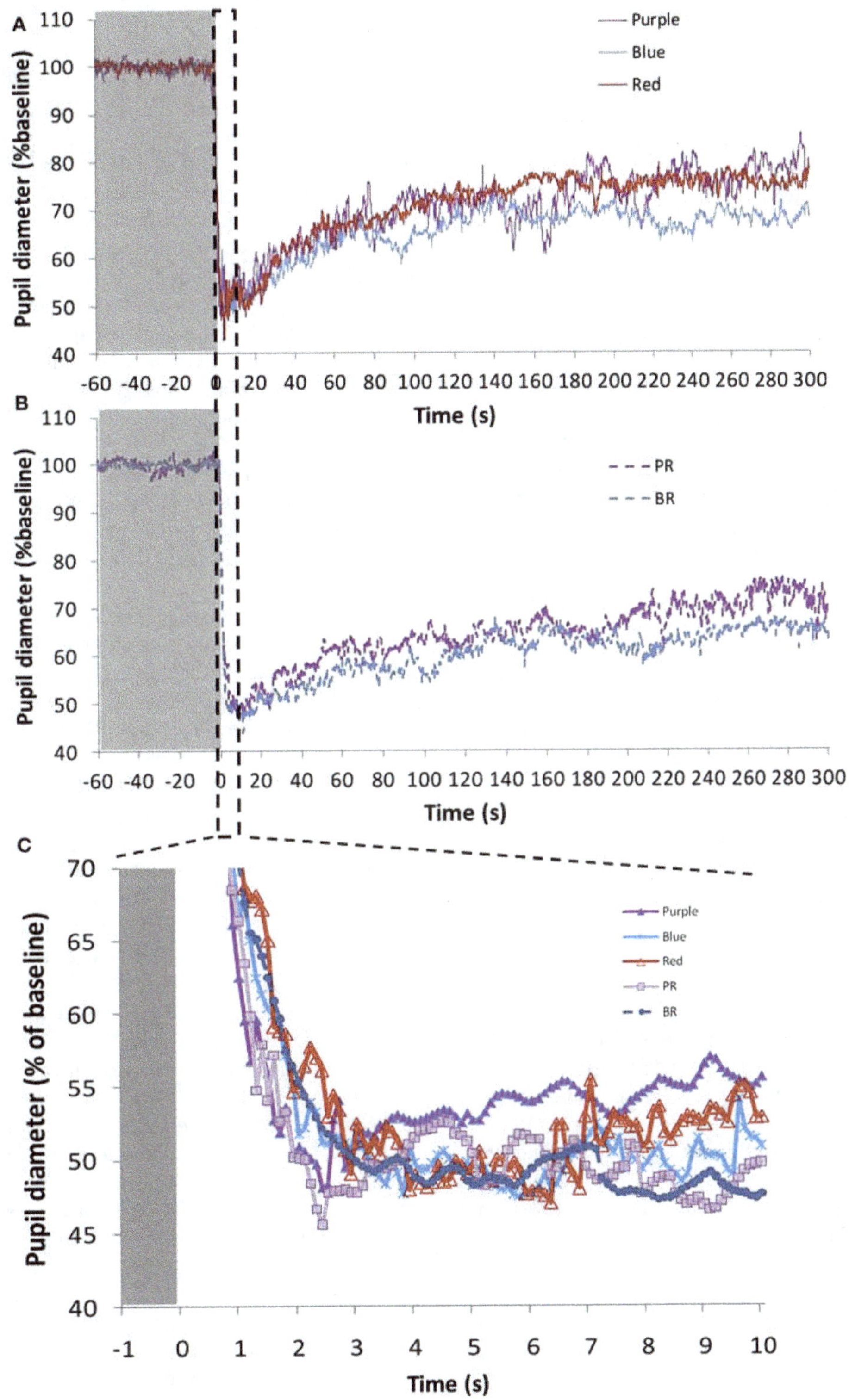

FIGURE 5 | Average pupil recordings **(A)** for purple (437 nm; $n = 3$), blue (479 nm; $n = 9$), and red (627 nm; $n = 8$) light at 1.2×10^{13} photons/cm^2/s (purple and blue), and 5.13×10^{13} photons/cm^2/s (red), and **(B)** for purple + red (PR; $n = 7$) and blue + red (BR; $n = 9$) at 6.33×10^{13} photons/cm^2/s. SEM bars have been omitted for clarity. Averaged first 10 s of pupil constriction **(C)** with error bars omitted for clarity.

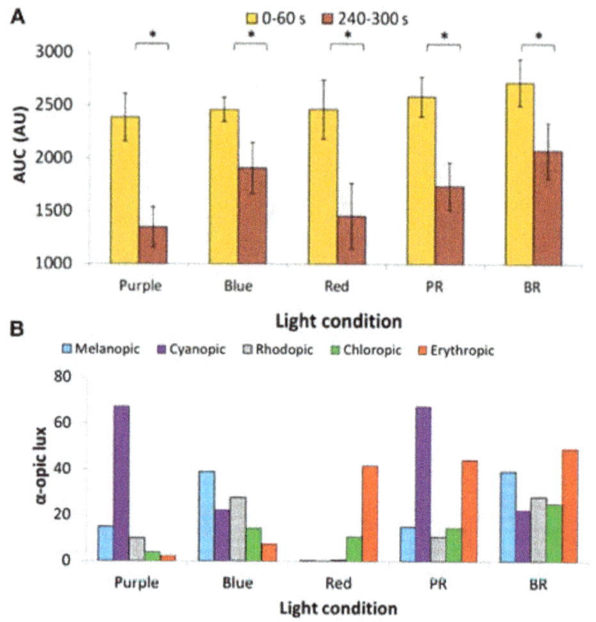

FIGURE 6 | Area under the curve (AUC, expressed in A.U.) during two time windows: from 0 to 60 s of light exposure (0–60 s; first minute of light exposure, in yellow) and from 240 to 300 s of light exposure (240–300 s; last minute of 5-min light exposure, in red). Two-way repeated measures ANOVA showed an overall significant difference between 0–60 and 240–300 s ($p < 0.05$), but not between wavelengths nor interaction between both factors. Paired-sample *t*-tests revealed significant differences (indicated by *) between AUC_{0-60} and $AUC_{240-300}$ under all the light conditions ($p < 0.05$) **(A)**. Activation of the different photoreceptors under each light condition used, assessed by the α-opic lux parameter calculated by the Irradiance toolbox (47) **(B)**. P indicates purple (437 nm; $n = 3$); B indicates blue (479 nm; $n = 9$); R indicates red (627 nm; $n = 8$); PR indicates purple + red ($n = 7$); and BR indicates blue + red ($n = 9$).

± 1.6%), and the smallest constriction at 430 nm (42.7 ± 1.9%). According to pairwise comparisons (Bonferroni *post-hoc*, $p < 0.05$), only the constriction at 430 nm (not at 420 nm nor 440 nm) was significantly smaller than that found at 470 nm (50.2 ± 1.6%), 480 nm (49.9 ± 1.8%), 490 nm (49.4 ± 1.8%), and 500 nm (49.7 ± 1.2 %).

It took less time to reach the minimum pupil diameter with 480 nm (3.7 ± 0.2 s) and 490 nm (3.8 ± 0.4 s) light than with 420 nm (4.6 ± 0.5 s) light, although these differences were not statistically significant. However, the velocity of constriction was different (Friedman test, $\chi^2 = 29.417$, $df = 8$, $p < 0.001$) with the 480 nm light stimulus eliciting the most rapid pupil constriction (14.3 ± 0.9%/s), while the slowest pupil constriction was observed with 430 nm light (9.9 ± 1.1%/s) (Wilcoxon *post-hoc*, $p = 0.002$).

Regarding the AUC (A.U.) during the transient (first minute of light exposure, AUC_{0-60}), and sustained response (last minute of light exposure, $AUC_{240-300}$) (**Figure 8A**), again as expected, AUC_{0-60} was always greater than $AUC_{240-300}$ for all light conditions and wavelengths (Wilcoxon *post-hoc*, $p = 0.001$), although an interaction between both factors was evident ($p = 0.032$). Accordingly, transient and sustained responses were analyzed separately. The transient response (AUC_{0-60}) tended to increase from 420 nm (1,517 ± 141 A.U.) to 490 nm (2,007 ± 147 A.U.), decreasing again at 500 nm (1,778 ± 108 A.U.) (one-way repeated measures ANOVA, $F = 4.861$, $df = 8$, $p < 0.001$). By contrast the greatest $AUC_{240-300}$ occurred with 460 nm (880 ± 131 A.U.) and 480 nm (838 ± 100 A.U.) light (Friedman test, $\chi^2 = 17.102$, $df = 8$, $p = 0.029$), the latter being significantly different when compared to the 420 nm light stimulus (lowest, with 567 ± 100 A.U.) (Wilcoxon *post-hoc*, $p = 0.005$).

The 6-s PIPR could only be measured in Study B, since no recording of the post-illumination response was performed in Study A. The pupil constriction 6 s after the end of light stimulus was greater at the longer wavelengths within the 420–500 nm range (Friedman test, $\chi^2 = 17.227$, $df = 8$, $p = 0.028$), being maximum at 490 nm (6.82 ± 1.88%) vs. the minima at 420 (1.61 ± 1.93%) (Wilcoxon *post-hoc*, $p = 0.001$) and 440 nm (1.37 ± 1.82%).

Retinal photoreceptor activation was assessed [Irradiance Toolbox, (47)] as shown in **Figure 8B**. Melanopic activation was lowest when exposed to 420 nm (0.3 melanopic lux, absolute value; 8.7%), increasing at every exposure, reaching its peak at 490 nm light (2.6 melanopic lux, absolute value; 38.2%), after which it decreased again at 500 nm (2.4 melanopic lux, absolute value; 35.5%), thus showing the same pattern as the transient response (AUC_{0-60}) ($R = 0.924$, $p < 0.01$). There was also a significant correlation between the sustained response ($AUC_{240-300}$) and melanopic activation ($R = 0.699$, $p = 0.036$).

Photon Flux Comparison

The effect of light intensity on the PLR was compared for purple (~440 nm) and blue (~480 nm) light considering the highest (Study A, 1.2×10^{13} photons/cm²/s or ~13 log quanta/cm²/s) and lowest (Study B, 8×10^{11} and 9.2×10^{11} photons/cm²/s, respectively or ~12 log quanta/cm²/s) photon fluxes.

Figure 9 represents the average PLR recording for each wavelength (**Figure 9A**, purple light; **Figure 9B**, blue light) at ~13 log quanta/cm²/s and ~12 log quanta/cm²/s photon fluxes. As expected, higher photon fluxes produced a greater transient and sustained pupillary constriction for both wavelengths than lower photon fluxes. The rapid pupil constriction was greater at higher compared to lower photon fluxes for both purple (54.2 ± 3.7 vs. 46.8 ± 2.3%, differences not statistically significant) and blue (57.5 ± 3.7 vs. 49.9 ± 1.8%, Mann-Whitney U test, $Z = -2.147$, $p = 0.032$) lights (**Figure 9**, central panel). Also as expected, it tended to take less time to reach the minimum pupil diameter under higher compared to lower photon flux for both purple (3.75 ± 0.62 vs. 4.10 ± 0.40 s) and blue (3.58 ± 1.36 vs. 3.74 ± 0.24 s) light conditions, although the differences did not reach statistical significance.

The integrative parameter "velocity of constriction" was significantly faster under higher photon fluxes for blue light (27.9 ± 10.3 higher vs. 14.3 ± 0.9%/s lower photon flux, $p = 0.035$). Purple light also tended to be faster, although statistical significance was not reached (15.7 ± 1.1 higher vs. 12.2 ± 1.4 %/s lower photon flux, $p = 0.207$). The velocity of pupil constriction was significantly affected by both wavelength (one-way repeated measures ANOVA, $F = 5.007$, $df = 1$, $p = 0.038$)

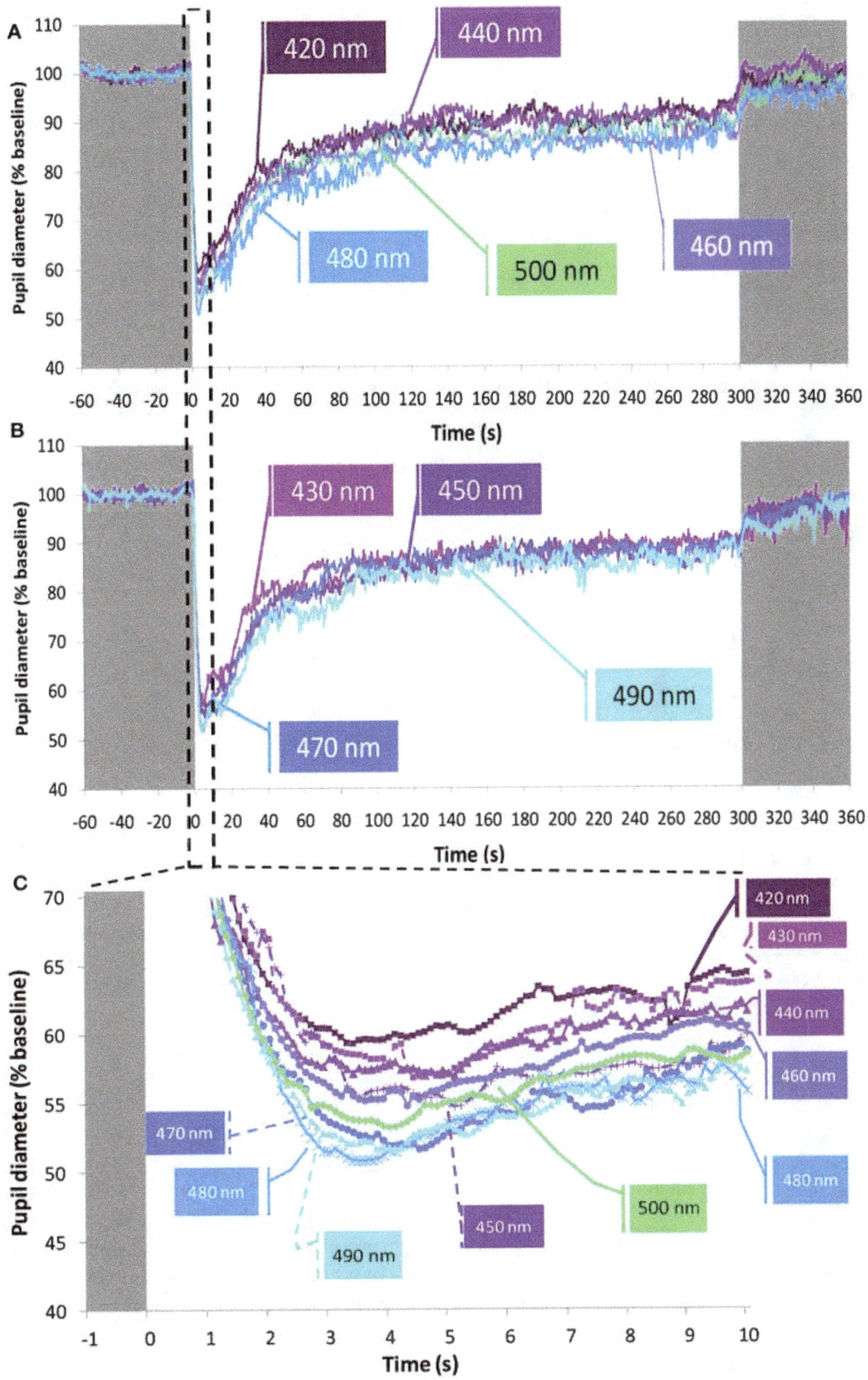

FIGURE 7 | Average pupil recordings at 420 nm ($n = 15$), 440 nm ($n = 15$), 460 nm ($n = 15$), 480 nm ($n = 13$), and 500 nm ($n = 13$) light **(A)** and at 430 nm ($n = 14$), 450 nm ($n = 15$), 470 nm ($n = 15$), and 490 nm ($n = 14$) light **(B)**. SEM bars have been omitted for clarity. See Methods and **Figure 3A** for photon flux details of the light stimuli. Averaged first 10 s of pupil constriction **(C)** with error bars omitted for clarity.

and photon flux ($F = 5.466$, $df = 1$, $p = 0.031$), interaction between these factors was not significant (one-way mixed design ANOVA).

Both the transient (AUC_{0-60}; **Figure 10A**) and sustained ($AUC_{240-300}$; **Figure 10B**) responses were greater under higher photon fluxes for both the purple and blue

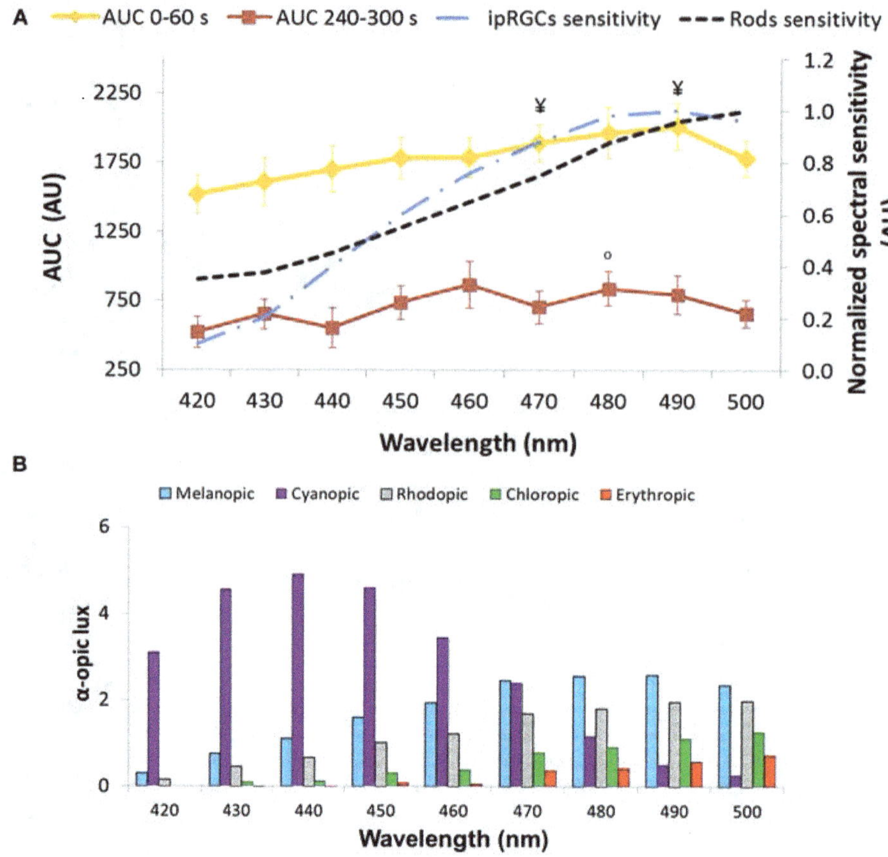

FIGURE 8 | Area under the curve (AUC, expressed in A.U.) over two time windows: from 0 to 60 s of light exposure (0–60 s; first minute of light exposure, in yellow) and from 240 to 300 s of light exposure (240–300 s; last minute of light exposure, in red). Paired-sample *t*-tests revealed significant differences between AUC_{0-60} and $AUC_{240-300}$ for all the wavelengths tested ($p < 0.05$). Two-way repeated measures ANOVA showed an overall significant difference between 0–60 and 240–300 s ($p < 0.001$), wavelength ($p < 0.001$), and a significant interaction between both factors for all light conditions. ¥ indicates statistically significant differences (Wilcoxon *post-hoc*, $p \leq 0.001$) in AUC_{0-60} vs. 430 nm. °indicates a statistically significant differences (Wilcoxon *post-hoc*, $p < 0.005$) in $AUC_{240-300}$ vs. 420 nm. Plots of the ipRGC and rod normalized sensitivities are superimposed **(A)**. Activation of the different photoreceptors according to each light tested, determined by the α-opic lux parameter calculated by the Irradiance toolbox (47) **(B)**.

light conditions (Mann-Whitney *U*-test, $Z = -2.371$, $p < 0.016$).

DISCUSSION

We aimed to better characterize the human PLR under high resolution, 5-min monochromatic light stimuli (10 nm increments) alone and in combination. Our results show higher responsiveness of the pupil to blue light stimuli, alone or in combination with red light, considering rapid pupil constriction, transient, sustained and post-illumination pupil responses, and velocity of pupil constriction. Higher light intensities also produced, as expected, higher responsiveness.

Traditionally when evaluating the PLR, single monochromatic lights have been tested. Some studies, however, have used combined monochromatic light stimuli (LEDs of various bandwidths) or spectrally tunable light sources, that have provided good evidence to understand the contributions and interactions of the retinal photoreceptors in the PLR (13, 15, 16, 20, 48–54), as well as regarding light-induced melatonin suppression (35). In the present study blue and purple monochromatic lights were combined with red at the same final intensity. In agreement with previous reports (32, 55) the smallest pupil diameter tended to occur in the presence of blue light (~480 nm alone or combined with red). According to the hypothesis of bistability, melanopsin may switch from a M state (not responsive to 480 nm light) to a R state (responsive to 480 nm light) by absorbing longer wavelength photons (32, 56, 57), the retinal epithelium being required for melanopsin regeneration (58). Thus, it may be plausible that red light (627 nm), when present, could elicit this conformational change, increasing the sustained response, not only due to the increased light intensity, but also to its effect on melanopsin. Although the differences did not reach statistical significance, red light tended to produce a greater effect in combination with purple light (compared to purple light alone) than with blue light (compared to blue light alone), probably because blue light can elicit the maximal intrinsic photoresponse on its own, while with

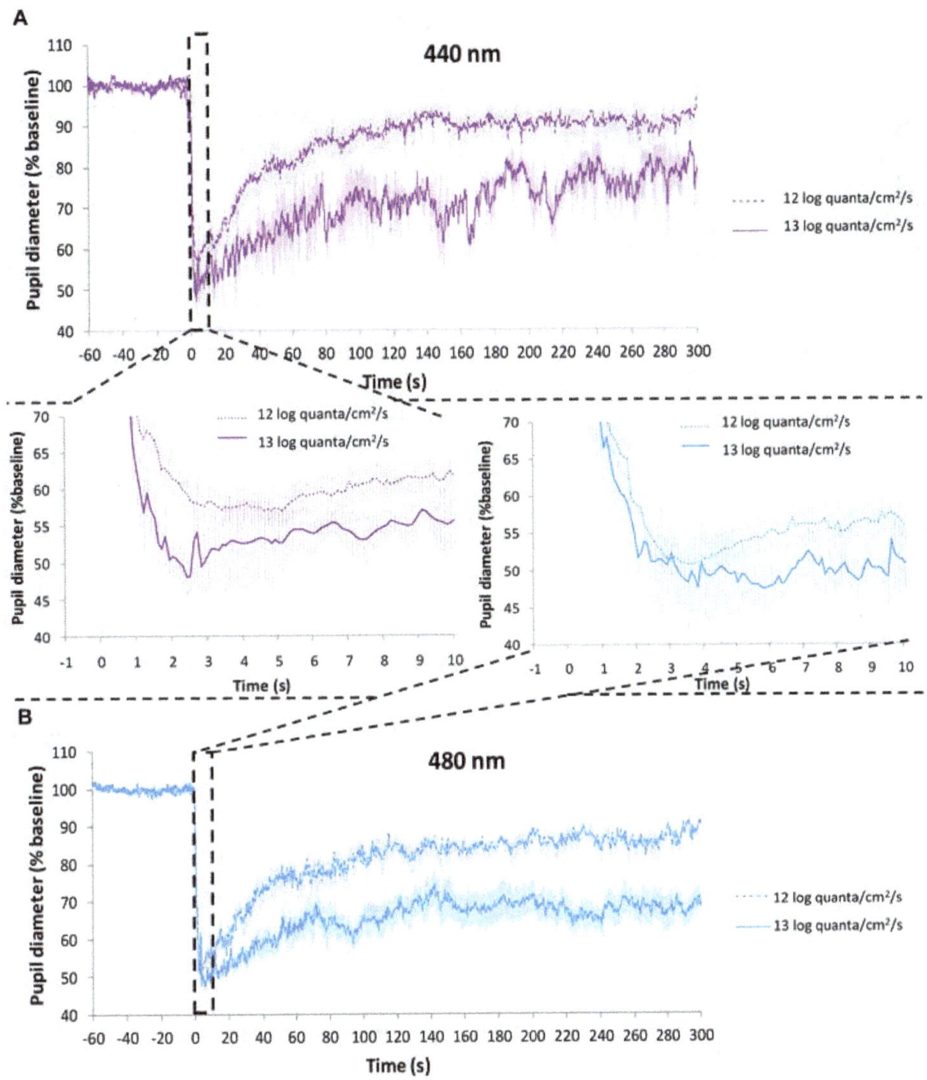

FIGURE 9 | Average PLR recordings under purple light (~440 nm) at 9.2 × 10^{11} photons/cm^2/s (~12 log quanta/cm^2/s, discontinuous line) and 1.2 × 10^{13} photons/cm^2/s (~13 log quanta/cm^2/s, continuous line) **(A)**. Average PLR recordings under blue light (~480 nm) at 8.0 × 10^{11} photons/cm^2/s (~12 log quanta/cm^2/s, discontinuous line) and 1.2 × 10^{13} photons/cm^2/s (~13 log quanta/cm^2/s, continuous line) **(B)**. Error bars indicate SEM. Averaged first 10 s of pupil constriction are shown in the central panel.

purple 440 nm light, although the melanopsin is stimulated, its activation is not maximal (45, 59). This tendency, however, could also be explained by the previously described spectral opponency between S-cones and both L- cones and ipRGCs (49, 50, 54). Thus, red (activating L-cones) plus blue (activating melanopsin) light would produce a summation in the pupil constriction (13), while the combination red plus purple light would activate L- and S-cones, respectively, thus producing opponency instead of summation, resulting in smaller constriction amplitude (49, 50, 54). Other studies, however, suggest linear/non-linear summation of the 5 types of photoreceptors stimulation (51), which contradicts the opponency hypothesis. Although both light combinations were delivered at the same photon flux, the differences in pupil response due to different colors (driven by chromatic pathways) have been previously described as being 3-fold larger than those driven by luminance pathways (16).

In our study, the velocity of pupil constriction was significantly faster under blue light than under red and purple light stimuli. However, based on previous studies, the melanopsin-ipRGCs intrinsic photoresponse would produce slow and sustained pupil constrictions, while the extrinsic pathway (mainly cone-driven) would produce fast and relatively transient responses (22, 25). The findings with blue light are thus not in agreement with the expected slow response produced by the melanopsin-ipRGCs (22, 25). The delayed response previously attributed to melanopsin-ipRGCs has also been questioned in a study using a square-wave pulse,

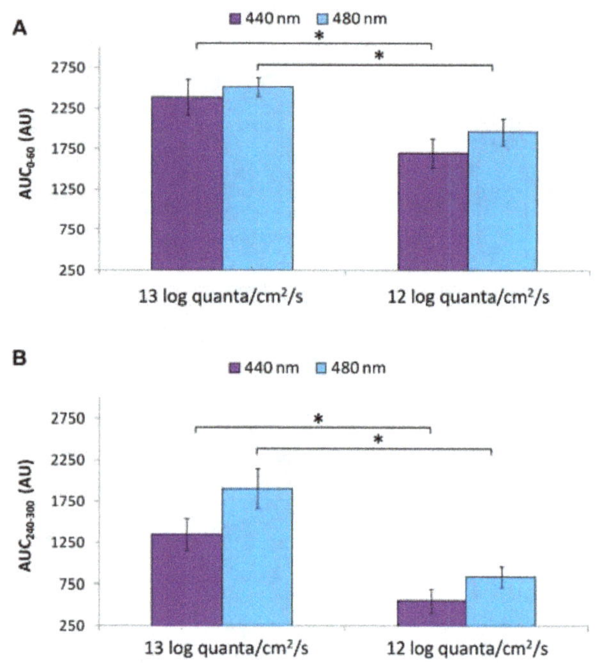

FIGURE 10 | Area under the curve (AUC, expressed in A.U.) over two time windows: from 0 to 60 s of light exposure (0–60 s; first minute of light exposure) **(A)** and from 240 to 300 s of light exposure (240–300 s; last minute of light exposure) **(B)** at higher (~13 log quanta/cm^2/s) and lower (~12 log quanta/cm^2/s) intensity purple (440 nm) and blue (480 nm) light. Error bars indicate SEM. *statistically significant differences (Mann Whitney *U*-test, $p < 0.016$).

suggesting a mechanism possibly associated with cone-mediated signals (20). In addition, we could speculate that an overlapping action of S-cones may produce this more rapid response, although considering the previously described S-cone opponency, this may not be a plausible explanation (49, 50, 54).

The post-illumination pupil response (PIPR) after short light stimuli (e.g., 1-s) has been suggested as a good marker for estimating the melanopsin function (12). However, in this study we used longer duration light stimuli (5-min) in order to assess the overall PLR dynamics. Thus in order to assess the contribution of each photoreceptor we used mathematical modeling [Irradiance Toolbox (v1) application, developed by Lucas et al. (47)], which provided the theoretical photoreceptor activation under each light condition. From these results we observed that under blue light stimuli there appears to be a summation of intrinsic (melanopsin-ipRGCs) and extrinsic (rods and cones) activation, which may explain the faster pupil constriction under blue light than under red or purple light stimuli, since the latter mainly involves cone activation with little intrinsic melanopsin activation.

When evaluating the PLR under a high resolution wavelength range (namely every 10 nm) from 420 to 500 nm, the highest pupil responsiveness was observed between 470–490 nm (depending on the PLR parameter analyzed). When looking at the transient response (AUC_{0-60}) a progressive increase (i.e., greater pupillary constriction) was observed from 420 to 490 nm. These PLR results are in agreement with Gooley et al. (28), who found in a blind subject with degeneration of the outer retina while the inner retina remained intact, that pupillary constriction was short-wavelength sensitive with a fitted peak sensitivity of 490 nm. The shorter (purple) wavelengths (420–440 nm) would activate S-cones so the lower amplitude pupil response found with these wavelengths may also be due to spectral opponency (49, 50, 54), these lights thus producing less constriction than the longer wavelengths with melanopsin activation. The 6-s PIPR parameter, calculated after 5-min light stimuli, also showed greater constriction (smaller diameters) with longer wavelengths, again the maximum pupil constriction being at 490 nm. 6-s PIPR has previously been found to be a good marker for melanopsin activation after 1-s light stimuli (12), so for the first time, as far as we know, this parameter has been calculated after longer light exposures. Our results also support the hypothesis that ipRGCs contribute significantly, not only to the pupillary sustained response ($AUC_{240-300}$) (23, 28) (which tended to be greater at 460 nm), but also to the transient part of the reflex (AUC_{0-60}). The transient responses showing a similar pattern to the theoretical melanopic activation further supports this idea.

The role of rods, however, cannot be excluded since rods (i) have been found to contribute to the sustained response (23) [as well as to the PIPR (24)], (ii) have a peak of sensitivity at 498 nm (60), and (iii) are partially activated under 480 nm light (as presented in **Figure 8B**). Cones, however, according to previous studies, contribute little to the sustained response (23, 28), since they quickly adapt to long duration light stimuli.

The PLR has been widely shown to increase with higher light intensities (18, 61, 62). In our studies (A and B) the light stimuli were similar, allowing us to compare very close wavelengths at different photon fluxes (13.08 vs. 11.93 log quanta/cm^2/s from Study A and B, respectively). Thus, at ~440 and ~480 nm, as expected, higher photon fluxes produced a greater sustained pupillary response at both wavelengths and faster velocity of pupil constriction. Overall these results are in accordance with a higher contribution of ipRGCs at higher photon fluxes (since their activation threshold is higher) and at longer duration light stimuli (23), while cone photoreceptors would contribute to non-visual light responses at the beginning of light exposure (63).

Although pupillometry has become a useful tool to evaluate non-visual light responses, it is not problem free. The PLR has been shown to depend on wake and circadian phase (64). Thus, experiments need to be controlled for time of day, wake up time and circadian phase of the participants. In the present study performing experiments during the morning at the same clock time for each participant, as well as controlling the sleep/wake cycle of the participants 7 days prior to the PLR assessments, was designed to minimize the differences between different days, time of day and wake status. PLR could also be influenced by other processes such as changes in accommodation states, in the state of arousal or even cognitive activity (23), thus even when participants are instructed to refrain from alcohol, caffeinated drinks, bright lights, excessive exercise, and non-steroidal anti-inflammatory drug intake as in the present study, there may be additional confounding factors. Despite these limitations, a close association between the observed pupillary responses and the melatonin suppression response with monochromatic lights has been reported (9, 35, 41, 46). In addition, a relationship between circadian status and PLR has been recently proposed (10). Overall this suggests that pupillometry may, in future with more evidence from different approaches, become a practical tool to evaluate the efficiency of light sources on circadian system activation in a quick, non-invasive, and relatively inexpensive way [reviewed in (65)].

Thus, if we consider pupillometry as a proxy to evaluate circadian effects of light and considering that monochromatic blue light is most effective at suppressing melatonin (8, 9, 44), we propose that substitution of blue light by purple light in polychromatic light sources may be a solution for nocturnal illumination to minimize non-visual light responses. In order to test this it will be necessary to determine, not only whether the color discrimination is acceptable under these spectra, but also the specific effects of purple light on melatonin synthesis, sleep and alertness in humans, not only isolated, (9, 46) or in combination with blue (66) or red (35) light, but also by replacing blue light within more complex light spectra (67). In this sense, further studies about the potential risks of using purple light at the intensities required should also be conducted.

AUTHOR CONTRIBUTIONS

MB-C, KH, SS, VR, JM, MR, and DS conception and design of the study. MB-C, KH, CI, and VR data acquisition. MB-C, VR, JM, and MR data analysis. MB-C, JM, MR, and DS wrote first draft of manuscript. All authors contributed to manuscript revision, read and approved the submitted version.

FUNDING

This work was supported by the Instituto de Salud Carlos III, the Ministry of Economy and competitiveness through a CIBERFES grant (CB16/10/00239), and grant 19899/GERM/15 awarded to JM (co financed by FEDER). Research fellowship granted to MB-C [AP2009 1051] awarded by Spanish Ministry of Education and Science and [20401/SF/17] by Fundación Séneca. The work was partly funded by a UK EPSRC MILES grant [EP/1000992/1]. SS gratefully acknowledges EPSRC Leadership Fellowship funding under project [EP/H005587/1]. DS is a Royal Society Wolfson Research Merit Award holder.

ACKNOWLEDGMENTS

We thank Dr. Benita Middleton for her assistance with administration of the pupil dilator.

REFERENCES

1. Provencio I, Jiang G, De Grip WJ, Hayes WP, Rollag MD. Melanopsin: an opsin in melanophores, brain, and eye. *Proc Natl Acad Sci USA.* (1998) 95:340–5.
2. Berson DM, Dunn FA, Takao M. Phototransduction by retinal ganglion cells that set the circadian clock. *Science* (2002) 295:1070–3. doi: 10.1126/science.1067262
3. Berson DM. Strange vision: ganglion cells as circadian photoreceptors. *Trends Neurosci.* (2003) 26:314–20. doi: 10.1016/S0166-2236(03)00130-9
4. Gooley JJ, Lu J, Fischer D, Saper CB. A broad role for melanopsin in nonvisual photoreception. *J Neurosci.* (2003) 23:7093–106. doi: 10.1523/JNEUROSCI.23-18-07093.2003
5. Hannibal J, Fahrenkrug J. Target areas innervated by PACAP-immunoreactive retinal ganglion cells. *Cell Tissue Res.* (2004) 316:99–113. doi: 10.1007/s00441-004-0858-x
6. Hattar S, Liao HW, Takao M, Berson DM, Yau KW. Melanopsin-containing retinal ganglion cells: architecture, projections, and intrinsic photosensitivity. *Science* (2002) 295:1065–70. doi: 10.1126/science.1069609
7. Hattar S, Kumar M, Park A, Tong P, Tung J, Yau K-W, et al. Central projections of melanopsin-expressing retinal ganglion cells in the mouse. *J Comp Neurol.* (2006) 497:326–49. doi: 10.1002/cne.20970
8. Brainard GC, Hanifin JP, Greeson JM, Byrne B, Glickman G, Gerner E, et al. Action spectrum for melatonin regulation in humans: evidence for a novel circadian photoreceptor. *J Neurosci.* (2001) 21:6405–12. doi: 10.1523/JNEUROSCI.21-16-06405.2001
9. Thapan K, Arendt J, Skene DJ. An action spectrum for melatonin suppression: evidence for a novel non-rod, non-cone photoreceptor system in humans. *J Physiol.* (2001) 535:261–7. doi: 10.1111/j.1469-7793.2001.t01-1-00261.x
10. Bonmati-Carrion MA, Hild K, Isherwood C, Sweeney SJ, Revell VL, Skene DJ, et al. Relationship between human pupillary light reflex and circadian system status. *PLoS ONE* (2016) 11:e0162476. doi: 10.1371/journal.pone.0162476
11. Löwenstein O. Pupillographic studies. *Arch Ophthalmol.* (1942) 27:969. doi: 10.1001/archopht.1942.00880050139010
12. Adhikari P, Zele AJ, Feigl B. The Post-Illumination Pupil Response (PIPR). *Invest Ophthalmol Vis Sci.* (2015) 56:3838–49. doi: 10.1167/iovs.14-16233
13. Barrionuevo PA, Nicandro N, McAnany JJ, Zele AJ, Gamlin P, Cao D. Assessing rod, cone, and melanopsin contributions to human pupil flicker responses. *Invest Ophthalmol Vis Sci.* (2014) 55:719–27. doi: 10.1167/iovs.13-13252
14. Joyce DS, Feigl B, Zele AJ. Melanopsin-mediated post-illumination pupil response in the peripheral retina. *J Vis.* (2016) 16:5. doi: 10.1167/16.8.5
15. Tsujimura S, Wolffsohn JS, Gilmartin B. A linear chromatic mechanism drives the pupillary response. *Proc Biol Sci.* (2001) 268:2203–9. doi: 10.1098/rspb.2001.1775
16. Tsujimura S, Wolffsohn JS, Gilmartin B. Pupil response to color signals in cone-contrast space. *Curr Eye Res.* (2006) 31:401–8. doi: 10.1080/02713680600681327
17. Kawasaki A, Kardon RH. Intrinsically photosensitive retinal ganglion cells. *J Neuroophthalmol.* (2007) 27:195–204. doi: 10.1097/WNO.0b013e31814b1df9
18. Gamlin PDR, McDougal DH, Pokorny J, Smith VC, Yau K-W, Dacey DM. Human and macaque pupil responses driven by melanopsin-containing retinal ganglion cells. *Vision Res.* (2007) 47:946–54. doi: 10.1016/j.visres.2006.12.015
19. Feigl B, Zele AJ. Melanopsin-expressing intrinsically photosensitive retinal ganglion cells in retinal disease. *Optom Vis Sci.* (2014) 91:894–903. doi: 10.1097/OPX.0000000000000284
20. Tsujimura S, Tokuda Y. Delayed response of human melanopsin retinal ganglion cells on the pupillary light reflex. *Ophthalmic Physiol Opt.* (2011) 31:469–79. doi: 10.1111/j.1475-1313.2011.00846.x
21. Drouyer E, Rieux C, Hut RA, Cooper HM. Responses of suprachiasmatic nucleus neurons to light and dark adaptation: relative contributions of melanopsin and rod-cone inputs. *J Neurosci.* (2007) 27:9623–31. doi: 10.1523/JNEUROSCI.1391-07.2007
22. Wong KY, Dunn FA, Graham DM, Berson DM. Synaptic influences on rat ganglion-cell photoreceptors. *J Physiol.* (2007) 582:279–96. doi: 10.1113/jphysiol.2007.133751
23. McDougal DH, Gamlin PD. The influence of intrinsically-photosensitive retinal ganglion cells on the spectral sensitivity and response dynamics

of the human pupillary light reflex. *Vision Res.* (2010) 50:72–87. doi: 10.1016/j.visres.2009.10.012
24. Adhikari P, Feigl B, Zele AJ. Rhodopsin and melanopsin contributions to the early redilation phase of the post-illumination pupil response (PIPR). *PLoS ONE* (2016) 11:e0161175. doi: 10.1371/journal.pone.0161175
25. Joyce DS, Feigl B, Cao D, Zele AJ. Temporal characteristics of melanopsin inputs to the human pupil light reflex. *Vision Res.* (2015) 107:58–66. doi: 10.1016/j.visres.2014.12.001
26. Neitz J, Neitz M. The genetics of normal and defective color vision. *Vision Res.* (2011) 51:633–51. doi: 10.1016/j.visres.2010.12.002
27. Provencio I, Rodriguez IR, Jiang G, Hayes WP, Moreira EF, Rollag MD. A novel human opsin in the inner retina. *J Neurosci.* (2000) 20:600–5. doi: 10.1523/JNEUROSCI.20-02-00600.2000
28. Gooley JJ, Mien IH, Hilaire MAS, Yeo S, Chua EC, van Reen E, et al. Melanopsin and rod – cone photoreceptors play different roles in mediating pupillary light responses during exposure to continuous light in humans. *J Neurosci.* (2012) 32:14242–53. doi: 10.1523/JNEUROSCI.1321-12.2012
29. Vartanian GV, Li BY, Chervenak AP, Walch OJ, Pack W, Ala-Laurila P, et al. Melatonin suppression by light in humans is more sensitive than previously reported. *J Biol Rhythms* (2015) 30:351–4. doi: 10.1177/0748730415585413
30. Koenig D, Hofer H. The absolute threshold of cone vision. *J Vis.* (2011) 11:21. doi: 10.1167/11.1.21
31. Mure LS, Rieux C, Hattar S, Cooper HM. Melanopsin-dependent nonvisual responses: evidence for photopigment bistability *in vivo*. *J Biol Rhythm* (2007) 22:411–24. doi: 10.1177/0748730407306043
32. Mure LS, Cornut P-L, Rieux C, Drouyer E, Denis P, Gronfier C, et al. Melanopsin bistability: a fly's eye technology in the human retina. *PLoS ONE* (2009) 4:e5991. doi: 10.1371/journal.pone.0005991
33. Emanuel AJ, Do MTH. Melanopsin tristability for sustained and broadband phototransduction. *Neuron* (2015) 85:1043–55. doi: 10.1016/j.neuron.2015.02.011
34. Mawad K, van Gelder RN. Absence of long-wavelength photic potentiation of murine intrinsically photosensitive retinal ganglion cell firing in vitro. *J Biol Rhythms* (2008) 23:387–91. doi: 10.1177/0748730408323063
35. Papamichael C, Skene DJ, Revell VL. Human nonvisual responses to simultaneous presentation of blue and red monochromatic light. *J Biol Rhythms* (2012) 27:70–8. doi: 10.1177/0748730411431447
36. Wong KY, Dunn FA, Berson DM. Photoreceptor adaptation in intrinsically photosensitive retinal ganglion cells. *Neuron* (2005) 48:1001–10. doi: 10.1016/J.NEURON.2005.11.016
37. Walker MT, Brown RL, Cronin TW, Robinson PR. Photochemistry of retinal chromophore in mouse melanopsin. *Proc Natl Acad Sci USA.* (2008) 105:8861–5. doi: 10.1073/pnas.0711397105
38. Sonoda T, Lee SK. A novel role for the visual retinoid cycle in melanopsin chromophore regeneration. *J Neurosci.* (2016) 36:9016–8. doi: 10.1523/JNEUROSCI.1883-16.2016
39. Buysse DJ, Reynolds CF III, Monk TH, Berman SR, Kupfer DJ. The Pittsburgh sleep quality index: a new instrument for psychiatric practice and research. *Psychiatry Res.* (1989) 28:193–213.
40. Horne JA, Östberg O. A self-assessment questionnaire to determine morningness-eveningness in human circadian rhythms. *Int J Chronobiol.* (1976) 4:97–110.
41. Revell VL, Skene DJ. Light-induced melatonin suppression in humans with polychromatic and monochromatic light. *Chronobiol Int.* (2007) 24:1125–37. doi: 10.1080/07420520701800652
42. Joyce DS, Feigl B, Zele AJ. The effects of short-term light adaptation on the human post-illumination pupil response. *Investig Opthalmology Vis Sci.* (2016) 57:5672. doi: 10.1167/iovs.16-19934
43. Dacey DM, Liao H-W, Peterson BB, Robinson FR, Smith VC, Pokorny J, et al. Melanopsin-expressing ganglion cells in primate retina signal colour and irradiance and project to the LGN. *Nature* (2005) 433:749–54. doi: 10.1038/nature03387
44. Lockley SW, Brainard GC, Czeisler CA. High sensitivity of the human circadian melatonin rhythm to resetting by short wavelength light. *J Clin Endocrinol Metab.* (2003) 88:4502–5. doi: 10.1210/jc.2003-030570
45. Zaidi FH, Hull JT, Peirson SN, Wulff K, Aeschbach D, Gooley JJ, et al. Short-wavelength light sensitivity of circadian, pupillary, and visual awareness in humans lacking an outer retina. *Curr Biol.* (2007) 17:2122–8. doi: 10.1016/j.cub.2007.11.034
46. Brainard GC, Sliney D, Hanifin JP, Glickman G, Byrne B, Greeson JM, et al. Sensitivity of the human circadian system to short-wavelength (420-nm) light. *J Biol Rhythms* (2008) 23:379–86. doi: 10.1177/07487304083 23089
47. Lucas RJ, Peirson SN, Berson DM, Brown TM, Cooper HM, Czeisler CA, et al. Measuring and using light in the melanopsin age. *Trends Neurosci.* (2014) 37:1–9. doi: 10.1016/j.tins.2013.10.004
48. Viénot F, Bailacq S, Rohellec JL. The effect of controlled photopigment excitations on pupil aperture. *Ophthalmic Physiol Opt.* (2010) 30:484–91. doi: 10.1111/j.1475-1313.2010.00754.x
49. Spitschan M, Jain S, Brainard DH, Aguirre GK. Opponent melanopsin and S-cone signals in the human pupillary light response. *Proc Natl Acad Sci USA.* (2014) 111:15568–72. doi: 10.1073/pnas.1400942111
50. Cao D, Nicandro N, Barrionuevo PA. A five-primary photostimulator suitable for studying intrinsically photosensitive retinal ganglion cell functions in humans. *J Vis.* (2015) 15:15.1.27. doi: 10.1167/15.1.27
51. Barrionuevo PA, Cao D. Luminance and chromatic signals interact differently with melanopsin activation to control the pupil light response. *J Vis.* (2016) 16:29. doi: 10.1167/16.11.29
52. Spitschan M, Bock AS, Ryan J, Frazzetta G, Brainard DH, Aguirre GK. The human visual cortex response to melanopsin-directed stimulation is accompanied by a distinct perceptual experience. *Proc Natl Acad Sci USA.* (2017) 114:12291–6. doi: 10.1073/pnas.1711522114
53. Murray IJ, Kremers J, McKeefry D, Parry NRA. Paradoxical pupil responses to isolated M-cone increments. *J Opt Soc Am A* (2018) 35:B66. doi: 10.1364/JOSAA.35.000B66
54. Woelders T, Leenheers T, Gordijn MCM, Hut RA, Beersma DGM, Wams EJ. Melanopsin- and L-cone-induced pupil constriction is inhibited by S- and M-cones in humans. *Proc Natl Acad Sci USA.* (2018) 115:792–7. doi: 10.1073/pnas.1716281115
55. Park JC, Moura AL, Raza AS, Rhee DW, Kardon RH, Hood DC. Toward a clinical protocol for assessing rod, cone, and melanopsin contributions to the human pupil response. *Invest Ophthalmol Vis Sci.* (2011) 52:6624–35. doi: 10.1167/iovs.11-7586
56. Melyan Z, Tarttelin EE, Bellingham J, Lucas RJ, Hankins MW. Addition of human melanopsin renders mammalian cells photoresponsive. *Nature* (2005) 433:741–5. doi: 10.1038/nature03344
57. Koyanagi M, Kubokawa K, Tsukamoto H, Shichida Y, Terakita A. Cephalochordate melanopsin: evolutionary linkage between invertebrate visual cells and vertebrate photosensitive retinal ganglion cells. *Curr Biol.* (2005) 15:1065–9. doi: 10.1016/j.cub.2005.04.063
58. Zhao X, Pack W, Khan NW, Wong KY. Prolonged inner retinal photoreception depends on the visual retinoid cycle. *J Neurosci.* (2016) 36:4209–17. doi: 10.1523/JNEUROSCI.2629-14.2016
59. Bailes HJ, Lucas RJ. Human melanopsin forms a pigment maximally sensitive to blue light (λmax ≈ 479 nm) supporting activation of G(q/11) and G(i/o) signalling cascades. *Proc Biol Sci.* (2013) 280:20122987. doi: 10.1098/rspb.2012.2987
60. Bowmaker JK, Dartnall HJ. Visual pigments of rods and cones in a human retina. *J Physiol.* (1980) 298:501–11.
61. Kardon R, Anderson SC, Damarjian TG, Grace EM, Stone E, Kawasaki A. Chromatic pupil responses: preferential activation of the melanopsin-mediated versus outer photoreceptor-mediated pupil light reflex. *Ophthalmology* (2009) 116:1564–73. doi: 10.1016/j.ophtha.2009.02.007
62. Herbst K, Sander B, Lund-Andersen H, Broendsted AE, Kessel L, Hansen MS, et al. Intrinsically photosensitive retinal ganglion cell function in relation to age: a pupillometric study in humans with special reference to the age-related optic properties of the lens. *BMC Ophthalmol.* (2012) 12:4. doi: 10.1186/1471-2415-12-4
63. Alpern M, Campbell FW. The spectral sensitivity of the consensual light reflex. *J Physiol.* (1962) 164:478–507. doi: 10.1113/jphysiol.1962.sp007033
64. Münch M, Léon L, Crippa SV, Kawasaki A. Circadian and wake-dependent effects on the pupil light reflex in response to narrow-bandwidth light pulses. *Invest Ophthalmol Vis Sci.* (2012) 53:4546–55. doi: 10.1167/iovs.12-9494

65. Bonmati-Carrion MA, Arguelles-Prieto R, Martinez-Madrid MJ, Reiter R, Hardeland R, Rol MA, et al. Protecting the melatonin rhythm through circadian healthy light exposure. *Int J Mol Sci.* (2014) 15:23448–500. doi: 10.3390/ijms151223448
66. Revell VL, Barrett DCG, Schlangen LJM, Skene DJ. Predicting human nocturnal nonvisual responses to monochromatic and polychromatic light with a melanopsin photosensitivity function. *Chronobiol Int.* (2010) 27:1762–77. doi: 10.3109/07420528.2010.516048
67. Bonmati-Carrion MA, Baño-Otalora B, Madrid JA, Rol MA. Light color importance for circadian entrainment in a diurnal (*Octodon degus*) and a nocturnal (*Rattus norvegicus*) rodent. *Sci Rep.* (2017) 7:8846. doi: 10.1038/s41598-017-08691-7

13

Arousal Effects on Pupil Size, Heart Rate and Skin Conductance in an Emotional Face Task

Chin-An Wang [1,2,3†], Talia Baird [1†], Jeff Huang [1], Jonathan D. Coutinho [1], Donald C. Brien [1] and Douglas P. Munoz [1]*

[1] Centre for Neuroscience Studies, Queen's University, Kingston, ON, Canada, [2] Graduate Institute of Humanities in Medicine, Taipei Medical University, Taipei, Taiwan, [3] Research Center of Brain and Consciousness, Taipei Medical University, Shuang Ho Hospital, New Taipei City, Taiwan

***Correspondence:**
Chin-An Wang
josh.wang@queensu.ca

† These authors have contributed equally to this work

Arousal level changes constantly and it has a profound influence on performance during everyday activities. Fluctuations in arousal are regulated by the autonomic nervous system, which is mainly controlled by the balanced activity of the parasympathetic and sympathetic systems, commonly indexed by heart rate (HR) and galvanic skin response (GSR), respectively. Although a growing number of studies have used pupil size to indicate the level of arousal, research that directly examines the relationship between pupil size and HR or GSR is limited. The goal of this study was to understand how pupil size is modulated by autonomic arousal. Human participants fixated various emotional face stimuli, of which low-level visual properties were carefully controlled, while their pupil size, HR, GSR, and eye position were recorded simultaneously. We hypothesized that a positive correlation between pupil size and HR or GSR would be observed both before and after face presentation. Trial-by-trial positive correlations between pupil diameter and HR and GSR were found before face presentation, with larger pupil diameter observed on trials with higher HR or GSR. However, task-evoked pupil responses after face presentation only correlated with HR. Overall, these results demonstrated a trial-by-trial relationship between pupil size and HR or GSR, suggesting that pupil size can be used as an index for arousal level involuntarily regulated by the autonomic nervous system.

Keywords: trial-by-trial, pupillometry, pupil dilation, parasympathetic and sympathetic system, locus ceruleus-norepinephrine

INTRODUCTION

Physiological arousal constantly changes throughout the day, and this fluctuation greatly influences behavior and performance. Fluctuations in arousal are commonly linked to changes of the sympathetic and parasympathetic activity in the autonomic nervous system. Galvanic skin response (GSR) is an independent index of sympathetic activity while heart rate (HR) is predominantly controlled by the parasympathetic nervous system (1–4). The sympathetic nervous system controls sweat gland activity, and increases in sympathetic activity produce corresponding increases in GSR (5). Although HR is predominantly linked to the parasympathetic system and parasympathetic activation decreases HR, it is antagonistically controlled by both sympathetic and parasympathetic activity which can produce increased or decreased HR, respectively (3, 4).

Pupil size is also modulated by the balanced activity of the parasympathetic and sympathetic nervous systems (6, 7). Although an increasing number of studies have used pupil size to index the level of arousal (8–15), limited research has focused on examining the relationships between pupil size, HR and GSR. Nevertheless, many studies have concurrently recorded these measures to mostly investigate the task-dependent modulation in these physiological indexes [e.g., (16–22)]. Moreover, pupil size is modulated by low-level visual properties such as luminance, color, visual contrast, and spatial frequencies (23–26). Furthermore, eye movements influence not only the accuracy of pupil size measurement in the video-based eye tracking system, but also the parasympathetic and sympathetic activity via the pathway through the midbrain superior colliculus (27–30). Therefore, distinct patterns of eye movements in different conditions could influence pupil size differently via this pathway. Notably, in previous research, factors such as visual contrast, spatial frequency, color, and eye movements are usually not adequately controlled for and may have confounded observed effects between pupil size and arousal level.

The goal of this study is to investigate trial-by-trial fluctuations in sympathetic and parasympathetic modulation of pupil size. To index sympathetic and parasympathetic activity, HR and GSR were recorded concurrently with pupil size. Emotional face stimuli were used to induce arousal fluctuation because they are often used to evoke emotional arousal [e.g., (31–33)]. Participants maintained central fixation during the trial, following the presentation of different emotional face stimuli with carefully controlled low-level visual properties (**Figure 1**). Considering the common sympathetic control of GSR and pupil size, and common parasympathetic control of HR and pupil size, we hypothesize that activation of the parasympathetic system should decrease HR and pupil size, and activation of the sympathetic system should increase GSR and pupil size, together predicting positive correlations between pupil size and HR or GSR. Moreover, because baseline pupil size and stimulus-evoked (referred to as task-evoked) pupil dilations are thought to reveal different neural processes [e.g., (8, 10, 12)], the epochs before and after face presentation were analyzed separately, to examine the correlations both in baseline and task-evoked responses.

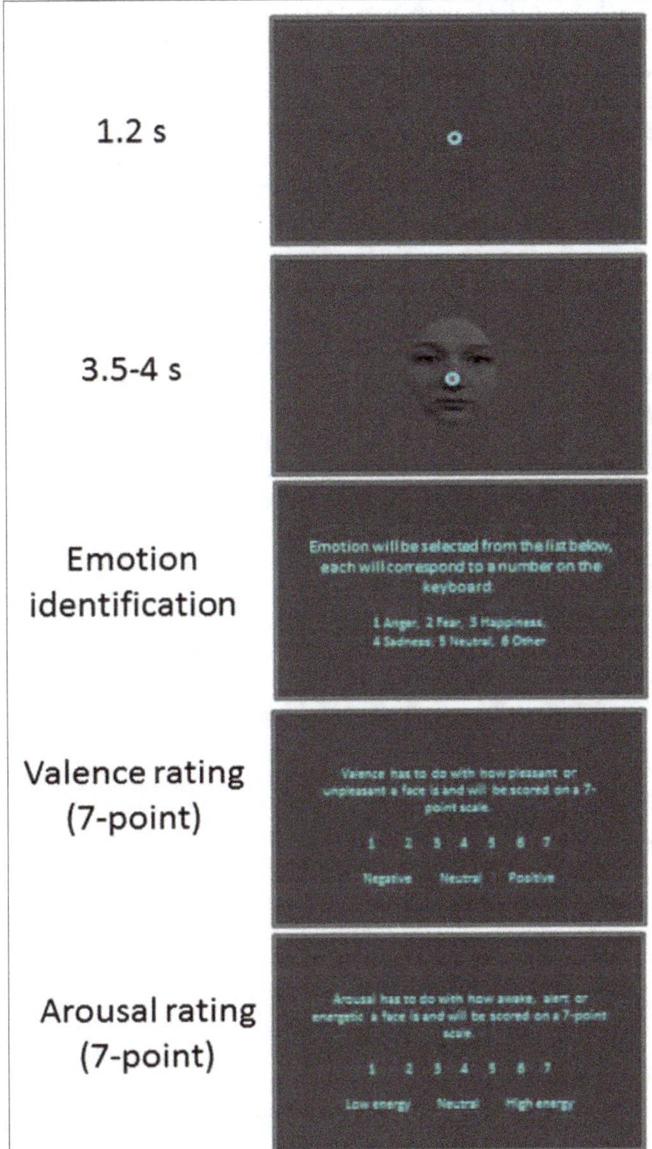

FIGURE 1 | Behavioral paradigm. Each trial began with a central fixation point on a gray background. After a delay, a face stimulus was presented and after a random delay the central fixation point and a face stimulus disappeared and participants were required to answer three questions about the face presented.

MATERIALS AND METHODS

Participants

All experimental procedures were reviewed and approved by the Human Research Ethics Board of Queen's University and were in accordance with the principles of the Canadian Tri-Council Policy Statement (TCPS-2 2014) on Ethical Conduct for Research Involving Humans, and the Declaration of Helsinki (34). Thirty participants (sixteen female) ranging between 18 and 24 years of age ($M = 21.76$, $SD = 1.56$) were recruited for this study. All participants had normal or corrected to normal vision, were naïve to the purpose of the experiment. Participants gave written informed consent and were compensated for their participation. Recruitment was limited to Caucasian participants because the face stimuli used in this experiment were all from Caucasian models.

Recording and Apparatus

Eye movements, pupil size, heart rate and skin conductance were recorded throughout the experiment. A video-based eye tracker (Eyelink-1000 binocular-arm, SR Research, Osgoode, ON, Canada), was used to measure eye position and pupil size with binocular recording at a sampling rate of 500 Hz (left eye was used). Eye position was tracked in order to ensure that participants maintained visual fixation on a point at the center of the screen throughout the trial. Heart rate was measured using a simple photo-sensor digital heart rate monitor that outputs a binary value based on blood flow through the ear (Grove Ear clip heart Beat Sensor). Skin conductance was measured using a galvanic skin conductance sensor (Q-S222

Galvanic Skin Response Sensor, Qubit Systems Inc., Kingston, ON, Canada), and the sensor monitored skin conductivity between two disposable tab electrodes attached to the index and middle fingers of the left hand. We used a 5 uSiemens range, which yielded a resolution of 0.0012 uS, and manually adjusted to an optimal range for each participant during the setup period, prior to the experiment. Both HR and GSR were recorded through an Arduino Uno digital acquisition board (https://www.arduino.cc) at a rate of 210 Hz with 10-bit resolution. Through a serial connection to the Arduino, the biometric recordings were controlled by the Experiment Builder program running the experiment. The biometric recordings could therefore be initiated and terminated by the same program controlling the display, and event marker codes could be placed in the biometric recordings at precise timings, allowing us to precisely align our trial stimulus events to the HR and GSR recordings. For convenience of comparison, all recordings were then interpolated to a 1 ms resolution using a spline interpolation for pupil area and GSR, and a linear interpolation for heart rate. Stimuli were presented on a 17-inch LCD monitor at a screen resolution of 1,280 × 1,024 pixels (60 Hz refresh rate), subtending a viewing angle of 32° × 26°, and the distance from the eyes to the monitor was set at 60 cm. Pupil area values recorded from the eye tracker were transformed to actual pupil size in diameter following previously described methods suggested by the Eyelink company (35, 36). Briefly, laser-printed dots between 2.0 and 6.0 mm in diameter were printed (false pupils), and placed at approximately the same position as the participants' pupil position during data recording. Eyelink pupil values from false pupils were used to transform Eyelink pupil values recorded from real participants to actual pupil diameter simply using a linear interpolation after taking the square root of all pupil area data. According to Eyelink, measurement error is below 1% with under 0.2% error for 3 mm or greater.

Behavioral Task

Participants were seated in a dark room and the experiment consisted of 6 practice trials followed by 100 trials. Each trial (**Figure 1**) began with the appearance of a central fixation point (FP) (0.6° diameter, 11 cd/m^2) on a gray background (11 cd/m^2). After 1,200 ms of central fixation, a centered facial stimulus (3° × 4°, 11 cd/m^2) with a central FP appeared for 3,500–4,000 ms. This was followed by three questions presented on the visual screen. First, the participants were asked to identify the emotion expressed by keying in a number on a keyboard attributed to one of six options: anger, happiness, fear, sadness, neutral, and other. Participants were then asked to rate the degree of arousal and valence of the stimuli using seven-point scales (17). When rating arousal, 1 indicated a low and 7 indicated a high degree of arousal. When rating valence, 1 indicated an unpleasant stimulus whereas, 7 indicated a pleasant stimulus, with 4 representing a neutral value. The next trial commenced after an inter-trial interval of 3–4 s.

Stimuli

Adult facial stimuli were selected from the Radboud Faces Database, which had been validated with respect to expression recognition, clarity, genuiness, attractiveness and valence (37) and used previously in our lab (38, 39). Images of 20 (10 male and 10 female) front facing, adult models expressing anger, happiness, fear, and sadness in addition to a neutral expression were incorporated into the fixation task. Images of separate models were used in the initial practice phase of the task. Oval face masks, previously used to isolate the face and eliminate distractions such as hair (40–42) were applied to all faces using Adobe Photoshop Creative Cloud 2015.5 (Adobe Systems Inc., San Jose, CA). Following our previous method (38, 39), after oval masking, Radboud face images were grayscale and adjusted to match the background luminance. They were aligned such that the nose of each image appeared at the FP location. Face stimuli were then filtered through the SHINE MATLAB toolbox to the normalize luminance, visual contrast and spatial frequency of facial images (43). Therefore, luminance, visual contrast and spatial frequency were controlled across all facial stimuli, and the overall luminance level remained unchanged during the trial.

Data Analysis

To maintain an accurate measure of pupil size, trials with an eye position deviation of more than 2° from the central FP or with detected saccades (>2°) during the required period of central fixation were excluded from analysis. Following the literature, a linear interpolation was performed using pre- and post-blink pupil values to replace pupil values during a detected blink (10, 44, 45). Trials were discarded when two eye blinks occurred within a time interval of 500 ms. The above criteria resulted in the removal of 11.0% of trials. Four participants were excluded from GSR analyses due to recording errors, and one participant was excluded from HR analyses due to recording errors. In addition, 48.7% of trials were removed from GSR analysis due to reading values beyond the range of the recording system (5 μsigmen). Note that, because there were at least 10 valid trials in a given condition for all included participants for each analysis (except for valence analysis, which only required 5 trials), the number of included participants was different among different analyses. Heart rate for each participant was analyzed by identifying the onset of each peak, representing a beat on our photo sensor. The timing of all beats for all trials were then overlaid to generate a raster plot of beats. This was then smoothed using a rectangular zero-phase (filtered both forward and reverse) filter of 100 ms to produce a continuous beat-per-minute trace for each trial type.

The raw values averaging from 1,000 ms before to the onset of the face presentation in pupil size, HR, and GSR were used to investigate the correlation among these measurements before the face presentation (referred to as pre-stimulus epoch). To investigate the task-evoked responses, baseline-correction procedure was used. For pupil size, a baseline pupil value for each trial was determined by averaging pupil size from 500 ms before to the onset of the face presentation, as used previously (36, 46). Pupil values were subtracted from this baseline value, and the mean change (from baseline) in an epoch from 500 to 3,000 ms after picture onset was used to indicate task-evoked pupil responses. Following previous research on heart rate and skin conductance analyses (47), baseline (averaging from 1,000 ms before to the face appearance) was subtracted from the GSR and HR values. For heart rate, the mean change (from baseline) in an epoch from 500 to 3,000 ms after stimulus onset was used. For skin conductance, the maximum change between 500 and 3,000 ms after face onset was computed with a log transform (log [GSR]). Note that outlier values beyond ±2.5 standard deviation were also excluded from analysis. To examine the hypothesis that pupil size should correlate with both HR and GSR with larger pupil size for higher HR or GSR, we performed correlational analyses and a one-tailed student *t*-test except where indicated. Bayesian *t*-test was also performed to inform statistical significance for pairwise comparisons, with a scale factor $r = 0.707$ (48). Moreover, Cohen's *d*, where appropriate, was calculated to estimate the effect size (49). One way repeated-measure ANOVA with Bonferroni-corrected *post hoc* comparisons was performed to assess the effect of emotion on behavioral responses, pupil size, heart rate, and skin conductance values.

To analyze, on a trial-by-trial basis, whether subjective arousal value for each face stimulus can be predicted by task-evoked responses of pupil size, HR, and GSR during face viewing, we employed a logistic regression approach. More specifically, we performed an individual logistic regression for each participant to estimate the predictive value of each task-evoked response to the arousal rating for each individual face stimulus presentation. The normalized beta-values (beta-values/standard errors of beta-values) from these individual logistic regressions were then subjected to two-tailed *t*-tests at the group-level to assess whether the beta-values were reliably different from zero.

Multiple regression analysis was used to determine if and how HR and GSR influenced pupil size. To estimate the contribution of HR and GSR on pupil size before and after face stimulus presentation on each trial, we performed the multiple regression analysis in the two epochs on a trial-by-trial basis separately for all participants using HR (Equation 1), GSR (Equation 2), or HR+GSR (Equation 3) as independent variables in the analysis. We then compared adjusted R-square values derived from the model in all participants using two-tailed student *t*-test to evaluate at the group-level whether combined HR+GSR explains significantly more variance of pupil size than the HR- or GSR-alone condition. If HR and GSR uniquely contribute to pupil size, adjusted R-square values of the combined conditions (HR+GSR) should be larger than the HR- or GSR- alone condition.

$$\text{Pupil size} = a^{*}\text{HR} + b$$

$$\text{Pupil size} = a^{*}\text{GSR} + b$$

$$\text{Pupil size} = a^{*}\text{HR} + b^{*}\text{GSR} + c$$

a, b, c were constant linear weights generated by the model.

RESULTS

Behavioral Performance in Recognizing Facial Emotions

Participants were engaged during the experiment because they performed the task accurately with correct responses made for 75, 90, 99, 90, and 85% of trials in the angry, fear, happy, sad, and neutral condition, respectively [**Figure 2A**, $F_{(4, 116)} = 27.33$, $p < 0.001$, $N = 30$]. Mean valence ratings (7-point scale) were 2.55, 2.92, 5.74, 2.73, and 3.65 in the angry, fear, happy, sad, and neutral condition, respectively [**Figure 2B**, $F_{(4, 116)} = 281.27$, $p < 0.001$, $N = 30$], and as expected, valence values were lower for negative emotions than positive or neutral emotions (all *p*s < 0.05). Mean arousal ratings (7-point scale) were 4.54, 5.53, 5.00, 3.25, and 3.14 in the angry, fear, happy, sad, and neutral condition, respectively [**Figure 2C**, $F_{(4, 116)} = 107.33$, $p < 0.001$, $N = 30$].

Dynamics of measured responses are shown in **Figure 3**. In general, pupil size decreased before face presentation and pupil dilation was observed after the face presentation (**Figure 3A**). Initial pupil constriction after central fixation, prior to stimulus presentation, has been observed in many studies, including those conducted in our lab. There is no good argument to explain this pupil constriction, but it is possible that this constriction may be associated with the beginning of central fixation or the engagement of attention. The observed pupil dilation was consistent with a recent study which presented affective stimuli centrally while controlling low-level visual properties of the stimuli (50). In addition, heart rate (HR) and GSR were simultaneously recorded (**Figures 3B,C**) to index activity of the parasympathetic and sympathetic system, respectively. We first examined the relationship between pupil diameter and HR or GSR before face presentation (pre-stimulus epoch), and then examined correlation of the task-evoked responses in pupil size, HR, and GSR after face presentation.

Pupil Diameter Correlated With Heart Rate and Skin Conductance Before Face Presentation

To investigate the influence of the parasympathetic system on pupil size before face presentation, we performed a correlation between pupil diameter (raw pupil size) and HR before the presentation of face stimuli (pre-stimulus epoch). Trials were divided into two groups according to HR in the pre-stimulus epoch (median-split), and pupil dynamics between higher and lower heart rate were different (**Figure 4A**), with larger pupil diameter when HR was higher [mean pupil size diameter of epoch from 500 ms to face onset: high: 4.89, low: 4.85, $t_{(23)} = 1.85$, $p = 0.035$, $\text{BF} = 0.93$, $d = 0.38$, $N = 24$, **Figure 4B**: high-low]. **Figure 4C** shows summary histogram of trial-by-trial correlation coefficients for all subjects, showing a positive correlation between HR and pupil diameter [median correlation coefficient: 0.06, $t_{(23)} = 2.3$, $p = 0.018$, $\text{BF} = 1.92$, $d = 0.64$, one-tailed paired *t*-test of R values against zeros], suggesting a correlation between heart rate and pupil diameter before face presentation. These results were consistent with the hypothesis that an increase in parasympathetic activity resulted in decreased heart rate and pupil size.

Correlation between GSR and pupil diameter was also observed before face presentation (**Figures 4D–F**). Trials were divided into two groups according to GSR during the pre-stimulus epoch, and pupil dynamics between higher and lower GSR (median-split) in the pre-stimulus epoch were different (**Figure 4D**), with significantly larger pupil diameter in the higher

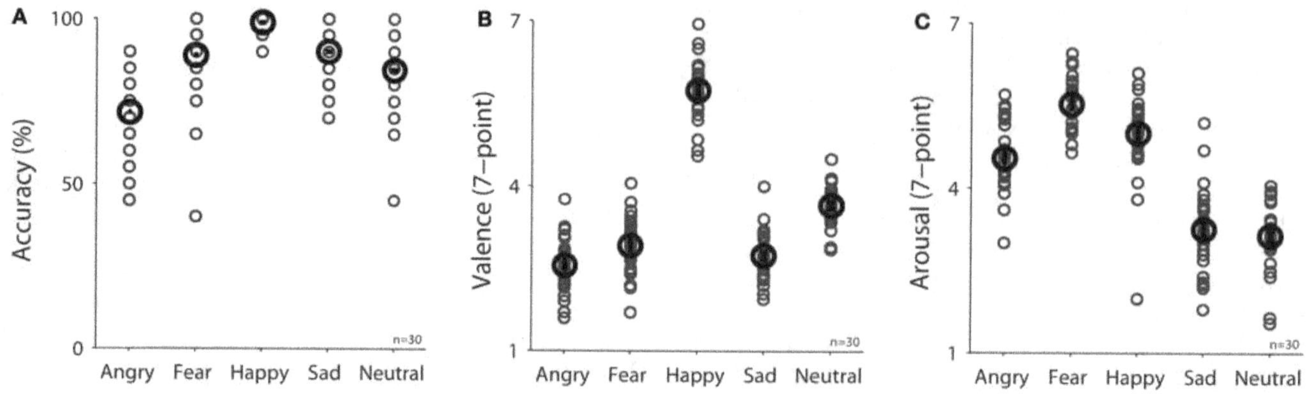

FIGURE 2 | Task performance in different emotional face conditions ($N = 30$) on **(A)** accuracy in emotion recognition, **(B)** valence rating, and **(C)** arousal rating. The black bold-circle represents the mean value across participants. The error-bar represents ±standard error across participants. The gray small-circle represents mean value for each participant. n, number of participants.

GSR condition, compared to the lower GSR condition [mean pupil size of epoch from 500 ms to face onset: high: 4.85, low: 4.76, $t_{(22)} = 2.26$, $p = 0.017$, BF = 1.79, $d = 0.47$, $N = 23$, **Figure 4E**: high-low]. **Figure 4F** shows summary histograms of trial-by-trial correlation coefficients for all subjects, showing a positive correlation between GSR and pupil diameter [median correlation coefficient: 0.05, $t_{(22)} = 1.8$, $p = 0.034$, BF = 0.87, $d = 0.53$]. Consistent with the hypothesis, these results suggest that activation of the sympathetic pathway caused an increase in GSR and pupil size. Overall, these results suggest a small but reliable correlation between pupil size and HR or GSR. Note that BF values were not decisive in these statistical tests, therefore the results should still be explained with caution.

No Modulation of Pupil Size, HR, GSR by Facial Emotional Stimuli

To investigate the modulation of task-evoked responses (see Methods) by emotional valence, we separated trials into three emotion categories (positive: 5–7 valence value; neutral: 4 valence value; negative: 1–3 valence value) according to the subjective valence ratings. Presentation of face stimuli evoked pupil dilation regardless of valence level (**Figure 5A**), which was similar to other studies (e.g., 50). However, in contrast to other studies using images (47, 51–53), emotional valence did not modulate evoked pupil responses, with mean pupil responses being 0.11, 0.14, and 0.12 in the positive, neutral, and negative conditions, respectively [$F_{(2,42)} = 2.22$, $p = 0.12$, all $ps > 0.23$, $N = 22$]. Although presentation of face stimuli generally decreased HR and increased GSR responses (**Figures 5B,C**), unlike other studies (17, 47, 54, 55), task-evoked responses in HR and GSR were not modulated by emotional valence, with mean HR change being −3.42, −2.5, and −3.19 in the positive, neutral, and negative conditions, respectively [**Figure 5B**, $F_{(2,42)} = 0.27$, $p = 0.76$, all $ps > 0.9$, $N = 22$], and mean GSR change was 0.049, 0.072, and 0.063 in the positive, neutral, and negative conditions, respectively [**Figure 5C**, $F_{(2,18)} = 0.43$, $p = 0.61$, all $ps > 0.9$, $N = 10$]. Note that there were only 10 participants included in GSR analysis, therefore the non-significant results could be due to a weak statistical power. Previous research has shown no differences in pupil responses evoked by emotional stimuli among positive, neutral, and negative emotions when the intensity of emotions is low (56) [similar results in GSR and HR (54)]. It is thus possible that the intensity of emotion in our stimuli was too low to produce a pronounced valence modulation because we specifically controlled low-level visual properties across all face stimuli. Notably, research has shown differences between explicit and implicit emotional processing (57–59), and weaker emotional modulation when the executive control is involved (60). Therefore, it is also possible that our explicit task requirement for emotion identification and valence and arousal rating automatically engaged the executive network, which greatly interrupted normal emotional face processing, resulting in weak emotional effects. Future research is required to address these possibilities.

Correlation Between Task-evoked Pupil Responses and Heart Rate and Skin Conductance

To examine the parasympathetic and sympathetic modulation on pupil size after face presentation, we performed correlations between task-evoked pupil responses and task-evoked HR or GSR (see Methods). Trials were divided into two groups according to task-evoked HR after face presentation (median-split), and pupil size between higher and lower HR were different (**Figure 6A**), with significantly larger pupil dilation when HR was higher [mean pupil size: high: 0.13, low: 0.098, $t_{(19)} = 2.47$, $p = 0.012$, $d = 0.55$, BF = 2.57, $N = 20$, **Figure 6B**: high-low]. **Figure 6C** shows summary histogram of trial-by-trial correlation coefficients for all subjects, showing a positive correlation between task-evoked pupil and HR responses [median correlation coefficient: 0.067, $t_{(23)} = 2.3$, $p = 0.017$, BF = 1.91, $d = 0.64$, $N = 24$], suggesting a correlation in task-evoked responses between heart rate and pupil size. In contrast, task-evoked pupil responses did not correlate with GSR after face presentation. Trials were divided into two groups

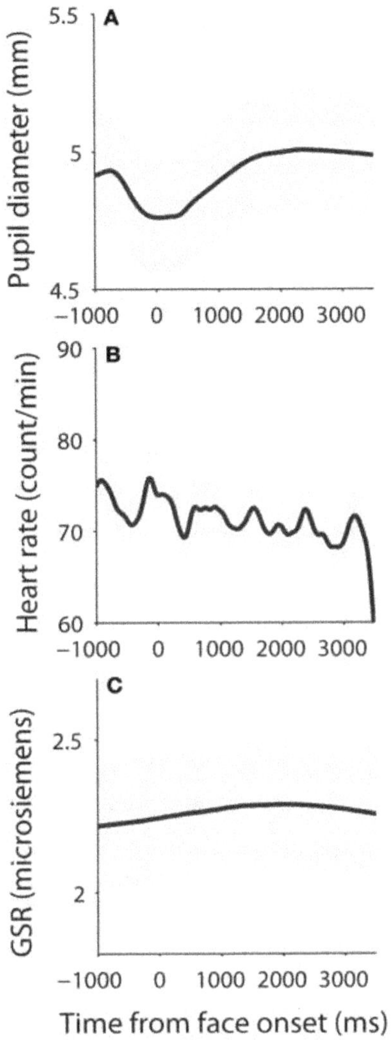

FIGURE 3 | Dynamics of pupil size, heart rate, and skin conductance responses. **(A)** Pupil diameter following the presentation of face stimuli. **(B)** Heart rate following the presentation of face stimuli. **(C)** Galvanic skin response following the presentation of face stimuli. The shaded gray regions surrounding the response represent ± standard error range (across participants). GSR, galvanic skin response.

according to task-evoked GSR after face presentation (median-split), and pupil dynamics between higher and lower GSR were not different (**Figure 6D**), with similar pupil dilations between two conditions [mean pupil size: high: 0.091, low: 0.092, $t_{(6)} = 0.07$, $p = 0.45$, BF = 0.35, $d = 0.03$, $N = 7$, **Figure 6E**: high-low]. **Figure 6F** shows summary histogram of trial-by-trial correlation coefficients for all subjects, showing again no correlations between task-evoked pupil and GSR responses [median correlation coefficient: 0.025, $t_{(22)} = 0.63$, $p = 0.27$, BF = 0.26, $d = 0.18$, $N = 23$]. Note that the number of subjects was different between these two analyses because median-split in the first analysis resulted in two conditions, and subjects required a sufficient number of trials in both conditions to be included in the analysis, resulting in fewer viable subjects.

GSR During Face Viewing Predicts Subsequent Arousal Rating

To examine trial-by-trial relationships between subjective arousal of emotional faces and task-evoked responses in pupil size, HR, or GSR, we performed logistic regression (see Methods). Task-evoked pupil responses during face viewing did not predict trial-by-trial variability of subjective arousal [**Figure 7**: mean beta-value: −0.24, $t_{(28)} = -1.14$, $p = 0.27$, BF = 0.36, $d = 0.29$, two-tailed paired t-test of ß values against zeros]. Responses in HR also failed to predict trial-by-trial variability of subjective arousal [**Figure 7**: two-tailed paired t-test: mean beta-value: −0.089, $t_{(27)} = -0.452$, $p = 0.65$, BF = 0.22, $d = 0.12$]. Yet, GSR responses during face viewing reliably predicted trial-by-trial variability of subjective arousal [**Figure 7**: two-tailed paired t-test: mean beta-value: 0.59, $t_{(22)} = 2.47$, $p = 0.022$, BF = 2.58, $d = 0.72$], suggesting that task-evoked GSR can predict subjective arousal in the context of emotional face viewing.

Modeling Pupil Size Using HR and GSR

Pupil size is controlled by the activity of the parasympathetic and sympathetic systems (7), therefore HR and GSR should influence a trial-by-trial fluctuation of pupil size differently. To test this hypothesis, we performed a multiple regression analysis, and used HR (Equation 1), GSR (Equation 2), or HR+GSR (Equation 3) on a trial-by-trial basis as independent variables to account for trial-by-trial pupil size fluctuation in both pre-stimulus and post-face (task-evoked responses) epochs ($N = 24$). Although trial-by-trial pupil size fluctuation in the pre-stimulus epoch explained by the model was generally small (**Figure 8A**), with the mean variance (adjusted R-squared) being 0.017, 0.086, and 0.092 in the HR, GSR, and HR+GSR condition in the pre-stimulus epoch, respectively, adjusted R-squared values were significantly higher in the HR+GSR condition than in the HR- or GSR-alone condition [two-tailed paired t-test: HR+GSR and HR: $t_{(23)} = 4.53$, $p = 0.00015$, BF = 188.00, $d = 0.92$; HR+GSR and GSR: $t_{(23)} = 4.18$, $p = 0.00036$, BF = 86.42, $d = 0.85$]. Similar, but not significant, patterns were observed in the post-face epoch (**Figure 8B**), with the mean variance (adjusted R-squared) being 0.034, 0.021, and 0.047 in the HR, GSR, HR+GSR condition, respectively [two-tailed paired t-test: HR+GSR and HR: $t_{(23)} = 1.34$, $p = 0.19$, BF = 0.47, $d = 0.35$; HR+GSR and GSR: $t_{(23)} = 1.38$, $p = 0.18$, BF = 0.50, $d = 0.34$]. These results suggest that both HR and GSR uniquely accounted for some fluctuations of pupil size on a trial-by-trial basis in the pre-stimulus epoch, arguably mediated by the parasympathetic and sympathetic system, respectively.

DISCUSSION

Pupil size is becoming an increasingly popular index of arousal and cognitive function, largely due to the popularity of the video-based eye-tracking system with automated pupillometry. Here, we directly examined the relationships between pupil size and parasympathetic and sympathetic activity, through simultaneous

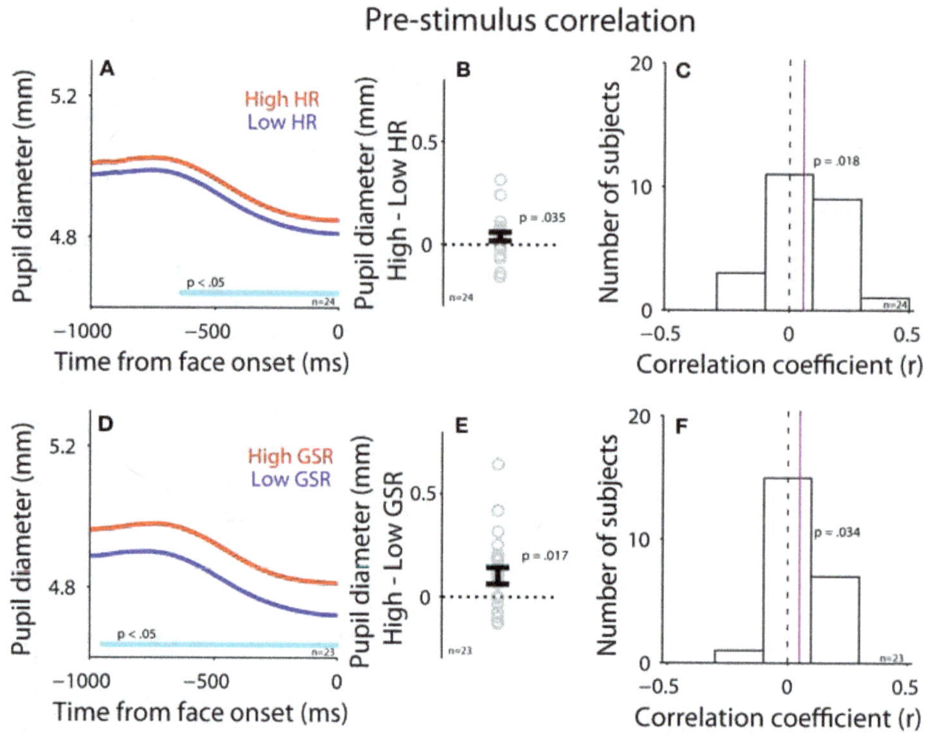

FIGURE 4 | Correlation between pupil diameter and HR or GSR before face presentation. **(A)** Pupil diameter following the presentation of face stimuli in higher or lower HR ($N = 24$). **(B)** Differences in pupil diameter between higher and lower HR conditions for each individual subject. **(C)** Distribution of correlation coefficients for the relationship between pupil diameter and HR for all subjects. **(D)** Pupil diameter following the presentation of face stimuli in higher or lower GSR ($N = 23$). **(E)** Differences in pupil diameter between higher and lower GSR conditions for each individual subject. **(F)** Distribution of correlation coefficients for the relationship between pupil diameter and GSR for all subjects. In **(A,D)**, the cyan bar on X-axis indicates the time line at which differences between the two conditions were statistically significant ($p < 0.05$). In **(B,E)**, the error-bar represents mean ± standard error across participants. In **(C,F)**, the vertical dotted line represents a zero value of the correlation coefficient ($r = 0$), and the vertical purple line represents the median value of the correlation coefficient. HR, heart rate; GSR, galvanic skin response; n, number of participants.

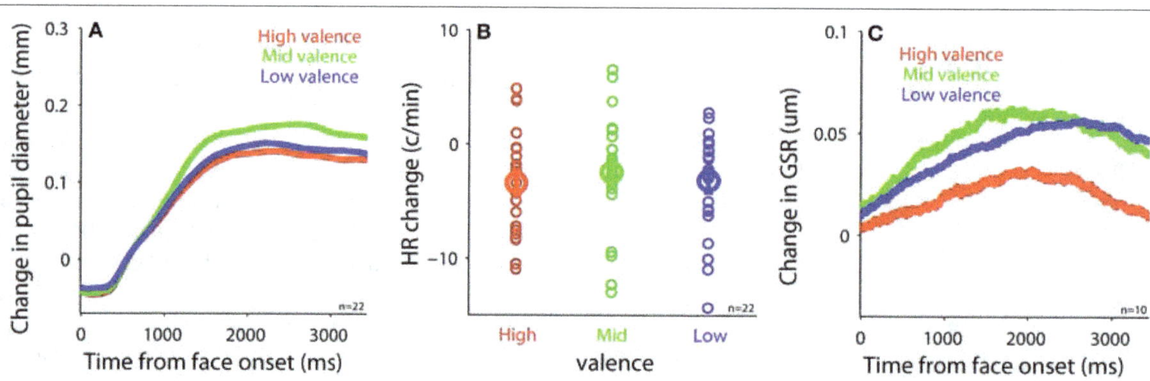

FIGURE 5 | Task-evoked responses after face presentation. **(A)** Change in pupil size following the presentation of face stimuli in different valence conditions ($N = 22$). **(B)** Heart rate change after face presentation in different valence conditions ($N = 22$). **(C)** Change in GSR after face presentation in different valence conditions ($N = 10$). In **(B)**, the bold-circle represents the mean value across participants. The error-bar represents ± standard error across participants. The colored small-circle represents mean value for each participant. HR, heart rate; GSR, galvanic skin response; n, number of participants.

recordings of pupil size, heart rate (HR), and galvanic skin response (GSR) during an emotional face recognition task. Pupil diameter on a trial-by-trial basis positively correlated with HR and GSR before face presentation: trials with larger pupil diameter prior to face presentation were accompanied by higher HR and GSR (**Figure 4**). Although trial-by-trial correlation between task-evoked pupil responses and GSR after face presentation was diminished (**Figure 6**), trial-by-trial variations

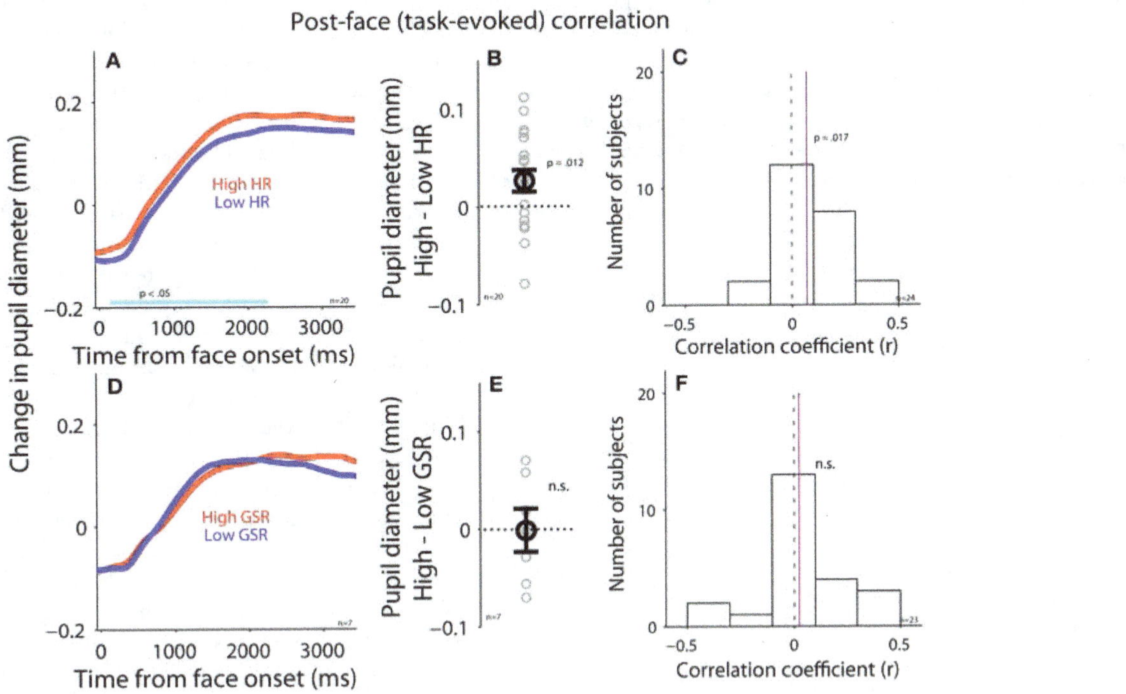

FIGURE 6 | Correlation between task-evoked pupil response and HR or GSR after face presentation. **(A)** Task-evoked pupil responses following the presentation of face stimuli in higher or lower HR ($N = 20$). **(B)** Differences in task-evoked pupil responses between higher and lower HR conditions for each individual subject. **(C)** Distribution of correlation coefficients for the relationship between task-evoked pupil responses and HR for all subjects ($N = 29$). **(D)** Task-evoked pupil responses following the presentation of face stimuli in higher or lower GSR ($N = 7$). **(E)** Differences in task-evoked pupil responses between higher and lower GSR conditions for each individual subject. **(F)** Distribution of correlation coefficients for the relationship between task-evoked pupil responses and GSR for all subjects ($N = 23$). In **(A,D)**, the cyan bar on X-axis indicates the time line at which differences between the two conditions were statistically significant ($p < 0.05$). In **(B,E)**, the bold-circle represents the mean value across participants. The error-bar represents ± standard error across participants. The colored small-circle represents mean value for each participant. In **(C,F)**, the vertical dotted line represents a zero value of the correlation coefficient ($r = 0$), and the vertical purple line represents the median value of the correlation coefficient. HR, heart rate; GSR, galvanic skin response; n.s., not statistically significant; n, number of participants.

in GSR after face presentation reliably predicted subsequent subjective arousal rating (**Figure 7**). Moreover, both HR and GSR, as an index of parasympathetic and sympathetic activity, uniquely accounted for the variance of pupil size fluctuation on a trial-by-trial basis (**Figure 8**). Together, our results suggest that pupil size correlated with measures of both the parasympathetic and sympathetic systems.

Autonomic Control of Pupil Size, Heart Rate, and Skin Conductance

Although HR, GSR and pupil size all associate with activity of the autonomic nervous system, the underlying neural substrate mediating each index is very different. Autonomic control of cardiac activity begins in the medulla. The nucleus of the solitary tract inhibits the sympathetic rostral ventrolateral medulla and activates the parasympathetic dorsal vagal nucleus (61) and nucleus ambiguus (62) which contribute to the vagal nerve. Neurons in the sympathetic rostral ventrolateral medulla project to preganglionic spinal cord neurons. Post-ganglionic sympathetic and parasympathetic neurons in the stellate (63) and cardiac ganglia (61), respectively, innervate the heart. Although predominantly controlled by the parasympathetic system, HR is also modulated by the sympathetic system. Sympathetic pre-ganglionic neurons in the spinal cord also innervate the adrenal medulla, a modified sympathetic prevertebral ganglion, stimulating the release of epinephrine and norepinephrine into the blood stream, which then travels to the heart (64). Sympathetic control of sweat gland activity begins in the preoptic sweat nucleus of the hypothalamus, which projects to preganglionic neurons in the intermediolateral spinal cord (65). These neurons travel through the ventral root of the spinal cord to innervate postganglionic sympathetic neurons in the paravertebral sympathetic chain ganglia. These neurons project to sympathetic terminals surrounding sweat glands (66). Therefore, increases in sympathetic activity produce corresponding increases in GSR (5).

Pupil size is controlled by the balanced activity of the sympathetic and parasympathetic nervous system, with parasympathetic and sympathetic innervation of the pupillae sphincter and dilator pupillae muscles of the iris, respectively (6, 7). Parasympathetic innervation of the pupillae sphincter comes from preganglionic neurons in the Edinger-Westphal nucleus in the midbrain [reviewed in (67)]. Preganglion neurons of the Edinger-Westphal nucleus project to postganglionic pupilloconstrictor neurons in the ciliary ganglion, which in turn control constrictor pupillae muscles directly through a short projection (68). In the sympathetic pathway, preganglionic sympathetic neurons located in the ciliospinal center of Budge, the C8-T2 segments of the spinal cord, project to sympathetic chain ganglia and travel to the superior cervical ganglia through the sympathetic trunk to the superior cervical ganglion (67). Here, post-ganglionic sympathetic neurons project to the dilatory pupillae via long and short ciliary nerves (69).

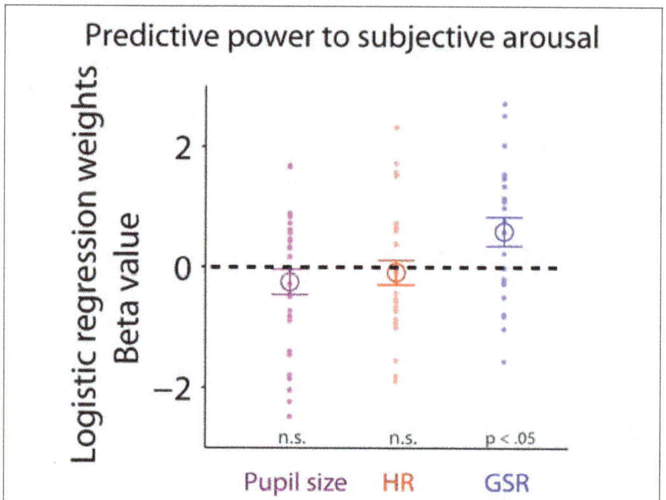

FIGURE 7 | Trial-by-trial relationship between subjective arousal and task-evoked pupil size, HR, and GSR. Individual normalized beta values from logistic regression analyses for pupil size, HR, and GSR on arousal rating ($N = 23$). The large-circle represents the mean value across participants. The error-bar represents ± standard error across participants. The colored small-dot represents mean value for each participant. HR, heart rate; GSR, galvanic skin response; n.s., not statistically significant.

Given the abovementioned pathways, pupil size should correlate with HR and GSR. Consistently, we found a positive trial-by-trial correlation between pupil diameter and HR or GSR before face presentation, with larger pupil diameter observed on trials with higher HR or larger GSR responses (**Figure 4**). Since HR is also modulated by the sympathetic pathway, the observed correlations between HR and pupil size can also be partly attributed by the sympathetic pathway. After face presentation, however, this correlation was diminished particularly between pupil size and GSR (**Figure 6**). The diminished correlation after face presentation could be due to low intensity of emotional face stimuli resulting from the control of low-level visual properties across stimuli including luminance, visual contrast, and spatial frequency. As a result, there were no differences in valence modulation of pupil size, HR, or GSR (**Figure 5**). The uncontrolled intensity of different emotions and different task requirements for emotional image stimuli may also explain a degree of inconsistency observed in the valence modulation of pupil size, HR, or GSR in the literature (17, 47, 52, 53, 55, 56, 70–73). Moreover, the inconsistency of the valence modulation with imaging viewing could also be attributed to inadequate control of low-level visual properties across stimuli and evoked eye movements across conditions. It is also interesting to note that this valence modulation of pupil dilation can be evoked with emotional written words, and previous studies have shown that larger pupil dilation is evoked by negative words than the neutral or positive words (71–75).

The regression model results suggested that HR and GSR accounted uniquely, arguably mediated separately by the parasympathetic and sympathetic systems, to trial-by-trial pupil size fluctuation because the combined HR and GSR conditions explained more pupil size variance than the HR- or GSR- alone condition (**Figure 8**). Notably, ~10% of variance in pupil size

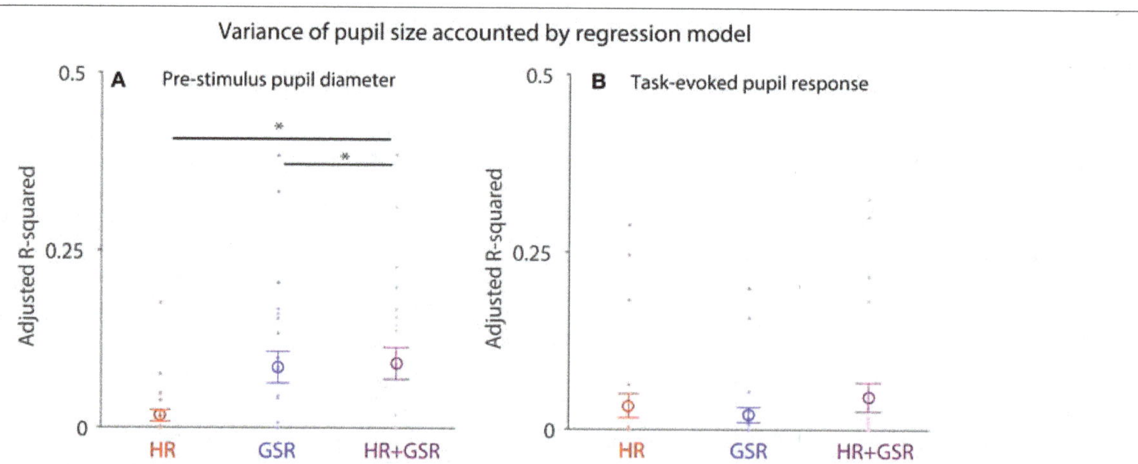

FIGURE 8 | Contribution of HR and GSR on trial-by-trial variation in pupil size before (pre-stimulus) and after (task-evoked) face presentation. **(A)** Adjusted R-square values derived from the regression model using baseline HR+GSR, HR, or GSR as independent variables to explain trial-by-trial variation in pupil diameter before face presentation (baseline). **(B)** Adjusted R-square values derived from the regression model using task-evoked HR+GSR, HR, or GSR as independent variables to explain trial-by-trial variation in task-evoked pupil size after face presentation. The large-circle represents the mean value across participants. The error-bar represents ± standard error across participants. The colored small-dot represents mean value for each participant. HR, heart rate; GSR, galvanic skin response. *indicates differences are statistically significant.

was explained by HR and GSR in the model. These results could imply that pupil size is more sensitive to autonomic arousal than HR and GSR, because, as described previously, it more directly links to the autonomic nervous system than other indices. It is also possible that pupil size is influenced by other factors which have not been identified. Together, it is important to investigate the influence of the emotional intensity on different autonomic indexes to study the emotional arousal in the future.

Locus Ceruleus-Norepinephrine (LC-NE) Account for Pupil Size Fluctuation

The LC-NE system has been associated with many functions arguably via arousal mechanisms (76–80), and pupil size variation is regularly linked to the LC-NE system (8). Relationship between pupil size and LC activity has been demonstrated in studies recording neuronal activity in behaving animals (81–85). In humans, drugs assumed to alter LC activity also change pupil size (86), and pupil diameter correlates with LC activation in fMRI study (87, 88). Moreover, drugs that alter arousal state interrupt functional connectivity of the arousal circuit mediated through the LC (89). Notably, there are two modes of LC activity that have been described: tonic and phasic mode, both of which have important behavioral relevance (8) and are thought to affect baseline pupil size and task-evoked pupil dilations, respectively (10, 12). Our results showing a stronger correlation between pupil diameter and HR or GSR before face presentation (baseline pupil size) suggest that tonic LC activity is particularly correlated with the sympathetic and parasympathetic activity observed in the current study. Notably, some other areas such as amygdala and limbic structures may also play an important role in the relation between emotional processing and pupil size [e.g., (90–92)] and therefore possibly contributed to the correlation observed in the current study.

Other Influence of Pupil Size by Low-level Visual Properties and Oculomotor Pathway

To fully understand the modulation of pupil size, it is also important to consider other influences on the pupil. Pupil size is also modulated by low-level visual properties in addition to the well-described luminance modulation, and pupil responses to different colors, visual contrast, and spatial frequencies have been observed both in humans and animals (23–26). However, research examining the relationship between pupil size and emotional arousal has mostly only focused on the control of the luminance modulation. Furthermore, eye movements can influence not only the accuracy of pupil size measurement in any video-based camera, but also pupil size itself even if the recording accuracy is maintained through some sorts of calibration. This is because the superior colliculus, a subcortical center for saccadic eye movements (93–95), links to not only shifts of attention and gaze, but also pupil size (30, 96, 97). Weak microstimulation of the SCi (or frontal eye field) evokes pupil dilation without evoking saccadic eye movements (27–29). The superior colliculus-to-pupil control pathway suggests that distinct patterns of eye movements could modulate pupil size differently through the mediated activity in the superior colliculus. In summary, the influences of these factors on pupil size should be carefully considered in the interpretation of any pupil results.

CONCLUSION

Pupil size can change independently of changes in luminance, and this trial-by-trial fluctuation in pupil size has largely been attributed to changes in the autonomic arousal level. Here, we showed that pupil size on a trial-by-trial basis particularly before face presentation correlated with both HR and GSR, respectively, indexing activity of parasympathetic and sympathetic branches of the autonomic nervous system. These results suggest that pupil size can be used as an index for the parasympathetic and sympathetic activity on a trial-by-trial basis. Many other factors are also associated with or related to the autonomic system such as blood pressure and glucose level. It is therefore important to record other autonomic indices in addition to pupil size to better understand the modulation of pupil size by the autonomic function.

AUTHOR CONTRIBUTIONS

C-AW and DM designed research. TB performed research. C-AW and DB contributed unpublished reagents, analytic tools. C-AW and TB analyzed data. C-AW, TB, JH, JC, and DM wrote the paper.

ACKNOWLEDGMENTS

We thank Ann Lablans, Brittney Armitage-Brown, and Mike Lewis for outstanding technical assistance as well as members of the Munoz lab for comments on an earlier version of the manuscript. This work was supported by Canadian Institutes of Health Research Grant (MOP-FDN-148418) and the Canada Research Chair Program to DM.

REFERENCES

1. Akselrod S, Gordon D, Ubel FA, Shannon DC, Berger AC, Cohen RJ. Power spectrum analysis of heart rate fluctuation: a quantitative probe of beat-to-beat cardiovascular control. *Science* (1981) 213:220–2.
2. Boucsein W. *Electrodermal Activity*. New York, NY; Dordrecht; Heidelberg; London: Springer Science+Business Media, LLC (2012).
3. Craft N, Schwartz JB. Effects of age on intrinsic heart rate, heart rate variability, and AV conduction in healthy humans. *Am J Physiol.* (1995) 268:H1441–52. doi: 10.1152/ajpheart.1995.268.4.H1441
4. Mendelowitz D. Advances in parasympathetic control of heart rate and cardiac function. *News Physiol Sci.* (1999) 14: 155–161.
5. Sugenoya J, Iwase S, Mano T, Ogawa T. Identification of sudomotor activity in cutaneous sympathetic nerves using sweat expulsion as the effector response. *Eur J Appl Physiol Occup Physiol.* (1990) 61:302–8.
6. Fotiou F, Fountoulakis KN, Goulas A, Alexopoulos L, Palikaras A. Automated standardized pupillometry with optical method for purposes of clinical practice and research. *Clin Physiol.* (2000) 20:336–47. doi: 10.1046/j.1365-2281.2000.00259.x

7. Loewenfeld IE. *The Pupil: Anatomy, Physiology, and Clinical Applications.* Boston, MA: Butterworth-Heinemann (1999).
8. Aston-Jones G, Cohen JD. An integrative theory of locus coeruleus-norepinephrine function: adaptive gain and optimal performance. *Annu Rev Neurosci.* (2005) 28:403–50. doi: 10.1146/annurev.neuro.28.061604.135709
9. Ebitz RB, Platt ML. Neuronal activity in primate dorsal anterior cingulate cortex signals task conflict and predicts adjustments in pupil-linked arousal. *Neuron* (2015) 85:628–40. doi: 10.1016/j.neuron.2014.12.053
10. Nassar MR, Rumsey KM, Wilson RC, Parikh K, Heasly B, Gold JI. Rational regulation of learning dynamics by pupil-linked arousal systems. *Nat Neurosci.* (2012) 15:1040–46. doi: 10.1038/nn.3130
11. Eldar E, Cohen JD, Niv Y. The effects of neural gain on attention and learning. *Nat Neurosci.* (2013) 16:1146–53. doi: 10.1038/nn.3428
12. de Gee JW, Knapen T, Donner TH. Decision-related pupil dilation reflects upcoming choice and individual bias. *Proc Natl Acad Sci USA.* (2014) 111:E618–25. doi: 10.1073/pnas.1317557111
13. Murphy PR, Vandekerckhove J, Nieuwenhuis S. Pupil-linked arousal determines variability in perceptual decision making. *PLoS Comput Biol.* (2014) 10:e1003854. doi: 10.1371/journal.pcbi.1003854
14. Urai AE, Braun A, Donner TH. Pupil-linked arousal is driven by decision uncertainty and alters serial choice bias. *Nat Commun.* (2017) 8:14637. doi: 10.1038/ncomms14637
15. de Gee JW, Colizoli O, Kloosterman NA, Knapen T, Nieuwenhuis S, Donner TH. Dynamic modulation of decision biases by brainstem arousal systems. *Elife* (2017) 6:e23232. doi: 10.7554/eLife.23232
16. Tursky B, Shapiro D, Crider A, Kahneman D. Pupillary, heart rate, and skin resistance changes during a mental task. *J Exp Psychol.* (1969) 79:164–7.
17. Libby WL, Lacey BC, Lacey JI. Pupillary and cardiac activity during visual attention. *Psychophysiology* (1973) 10:270–94.
18. Morrow LA, Steinhauer SR. Alterations in heart rate and pupillary response in persons with organic solvent exposure. *Biol Psychiatry* (1995) 37:721–30. doi: 10.1016/0006-3223(94)00204-G
19. Jennings JR, van der Molen MW, Steinhauer SR. Preparing the heart, eye, and brain: foreperiod length effects in a nonaging paradigm. *Psychophysiology* (1998) 35:90–8.
20. Scott TR, Wells WH, Wood DZ, Morgan DI. Pupillary response and sexual interest reexamined. *J Clin Psychol.* (1967) 23:433–8. doi: 10.1002/1097-4679(196710)23:4<433::AID-JCLP2270230408>3.0.CO;2-2
21. Colman FD, Paivio A. Pupillary response and galvanic skin response during an imagery task. *Psychon Sci.* (1969) 16:296–7. doi: 10.3758/BF03332696
22. Bond AJ, James DC, Lader MH. Physiological and psychological measures in anxious patients. *Psychol Med.* (1974) 4:364. doi: 10.1017/S00332917000 45803
23. Barbur J. "Learning from the pupil-studies of basic mechanisms and clinical applications," in *The Visual Neurosciences*, eds L. M. Chalupa, and J. S. Werner (Cambridge, MA: MIT Press), 641–56.
24. Gamlin PD, Zhang H, Harlow A, Barbur JL. Pupil responses to stimulus color, structure and light flux increments in the rhesus monkey . *Vision Res.* (1998) 38:3353–8.
25. Barbur JL, Prescott NB, Douglas RH, Jarvis JR, Wathes CM. A comparative study of stimulus-specific pupil responses in the domestic fowl (Gallus gallus domesticus) and the human. *Vision Res.* (2002) 42:249–55. doi: 10.1016/S0042-6989(01)00279-6
26. Barbur JL, Harlow AJ, Sahraie A. Pupillary responses to stimulus structure, colour and movement. *Ophthalmic Physiol Opt.* (1992) 12:137–41.
27. Wang C-A, Boehnke SE, White BJ, Munoz DP. Microstimulation of the monkey superior colliculus induces pupil dilation without evoking saccades. *J Neurosci.* (2012) 32:3629–36. doi: 10.1523/JNEUROSCI.5512-11.2012
28. Ebitz RB, Moore T. Selective modulation of the pupil light reflex by microstimulation of prefrontal cortex. *J Neurosci.* (2017) 37:5008–18. doi: 10.1523/JNEUROSCI.2433-16.2017
29. Lehmann SJ, Corneil BD. Transient pupil dilation after subsaccadic microstimulation of primate frontal eye fields. *J Neurosci.* (2016) 36:3765–76. doi: 10.1523/JNEUROSCI.4264-15.2016
30. Wang C-A, Munoz DP. A circuit for pupil orienting responses: implications for cognitive modulation of pupil size. *Curr Opin Neurobiol.* (2015) 33:134–40. doi: 10.1016/j.conb.2015.03.018
31. Vuilleumier P, Richardson MP, Armony JL, Driver J, Dolan RJ. Distant influences of amygdala lesion on visual cortical activation during emotional face processing. *Nat Neurosci.* (2004) 7:1271–8. doi: 10.1038/nn1341
32. Balconi M, Lucchiari C. Consciousness and arousal effects on emotional face processing as revealed by brain oscillations. A gamma band analysis. *Int J Psychophysiol.* (2008) 67:41–6. doi: 10.1016/J.IJPSYCHO.2007.10.002
33. Adolphs R, Russell JA, Tranel D. A role for the human amygdala in recognizing emotional arousal from unpleasant stimuli. *Psychol Sci.* (1999) 10:167–71. doi: 10.1111/1467-9280.00126
34. World Medical Association. *Bull World Health Organ.* World Medical Association Declaration of Helsinki. Ethical principles for medical research involving human subjects. (2001) 79:373–4. Available online at: http://www.ncbi.nlm.nih.gov/pubmed/11357217 (Accessed May 16, 2018).
35. Steiner GZ, Barry RJ. Pupillary responses and event-related potentials as indices of the orienting reflex. *Psychophysiology* (2011) 48:1648–55. doi: 10.1111/j.1469-8986.2011.01271.x
36. Wang C-A, Munoz DP. Modulation of stimulus contrast on the human pupil orienting response. *Eur J Neurosci.* (2014) 40:2822–32. doi: 10.1111/ejn.12641
37. Langner O, Dotsch R, Bijlstra G, Wigboldus DHJ, Hawk ST, van Knippenberg A. Presentation and validation of the radboud faces database. *Cogn Emot.* (2010) 24:1377–88. doi: 10.1080/02699930903485076
38. Soncin S, Brien DC, Coe BC, Marin A, Munoz DP. Contrasting emotion processing and executive functioning in attention-deficit/hyperactivity disorder and bipolar disorder. *Behav Neurosci.* (2016) 130:531–43. doi: 10.1037/bne0000158
39. Yep R, Soncin S, Brien DC, Coe BC, Marin A, Munoz DP. Using an emotional saccade task to characterize executive functioning and emotion processing in attention-deficit hyperactivity disorder and bipolar disorder. *Brain Cogn.* (2018) 124:1–13. doi: 10.1016/j.bandc.2018.04.002
40. Bokde ALW, Dong W, Born C, Leinsinger G, Meindl T, Teipel SJ, et al. Task difficulty in a simultaneous face matching task modulates activity in face fusiform area. *Brain Res Cogn Brain Res.* (2005) 25:701–10. doi: 10.1016/j.cogbrainres.2005.09.016
41. Leinsinger G, Born C, Meindl T, Bokde ALW, Britsch S, Lopez-Bayo P, et al. Age-dependent differences in human brain activity using a face- and location-matching task: an FMRI study. *Dement Geriatr Cogn Disord.* (2007) 24:235–46. doi: 10.1159/000107098
42. White M, Li J. Matching faces and expressions in pixelated and blurred photos. *Am J Psychol.* (2006) 119:21–8. doi: 10.2307/20445316
43. Willenbockel V, Sadr J, Fiset D, Horne GO, Gosselin F, Tanaka JW. Controlling low-level image properties: the SHINE toolbox. *Behav Res Methods* (2010) 42:671–84. doi: 10.3758/BRM.42.3.671
44. Karatekin C, Bingham C, White T. Oculomotor and pupillometric indices of pro- and antisaccade performance in youth-onset psychosis and attention deficit/hyperactivity disorder. *Schizophr Bull.* (2010) 36:1167–86. doi: 10.1093/schbul/sbp035
45. Wang C-A, Huang J, Yep R, Munoz DP. Comparing pupil light response modulation between saccade planning and working memory. *J Cogn.* (2018) 1:33. doi: 10.5334/joc.33
46. Wang C-A, Blohm G, Huang J, Boehnke SE, Munoz DP. Multisensory integration in orienting behavior: pupil size, microsaccades, and saccades. *Biol Psychol.* (2017) 129:36–44. doi: 10.1016/j.biopsycho.2017.07.024
47. Bradley MM, Miccoli L, Escrig MA, Lang PJ. The pupil as a measure of emotional arousal and autonomic activation. *Psychophysiology* (2008) 45:602–7. doi: 10.1111/j.1469-8986.2008.00654.x
48. Rouder JN, Speckman PL, Sun D, Morey RD, Iverson G. Bayesian t tests for accepting and rejecting the null hypothesis. *Psychon Bull Rev.* (2009) 16:225–37. doi: 10.3758/PBR.16.2.225
49. Hentschke H, Stüttgen MC. Computation of measures of effect size for neuroscience data sets. *Eur J Neurosci.* (2011) 34:1887–94. doi: 10.1111/j.1460-9568.2011.07902.x
50. Finke JB, Deuter CE, Hengesch X, Schächinger H. The time course of pupil dilation evoked by visual sexual stimuli: exploring the underlying ANS mechanisms. *Psychophysiology* (2017) 54:1444–58. doi: 10.1111/psyp.12901
51. Kashihara K, Okanoya K, Kawai N. Emotional attention modulates microsaccadic rate and direction. *Psychol Res.* (2014) 78:166–79. doi: 10.1007/s00426-013-0490-z

52. Kuzinas A, Noiret N, Bianchi R, Laurent É. The effects of image hue and semantic content on viewer's emotional self-reports, pupil size, eye movements, and skin conductance response. *Psychol Aesthetics Creat Arts* (2016) 10:360–71. doi: 10.1037/a0040274
53. Schirillo JA. Pupil dilations reflect why rembrandt biased female portraits leftward and males rightward. *Front Hum Neurosci.* (2014) 7:938. doi: 10.3389/fnhum.2013.00938
54. Bradley MM, Codispoti M, Cuthbert BN, Lang PJ. Emotion and motivation I: defensive and appetitive reactions in picture processing. *Emotion* (2001) 1:276–98. doi: 10.1037/1528-3542.1.3.276
55. Gomez P, von Gunten A, Danuser B. Autonomic nervous system reactivity within the valence-arousal affective space: modulation by sex and age. *Int J Psychophysiol.* (2016) 109:51–62. doi: 10.1016/j.ijpsycho.2016.10.002
56. Oliva M, Anikin A. Pupil dilation reflects the time course of emotion recognition in human vocalizations. *Sci Rep.* (2018) 8:4871. doi: 10.1038/s41598-018-23265-x
57. Winston JS, O'Doherty J, Dolan RJ. Common and distinct neural responses during direct and incidental processing of multiple facial emotions. *Neuroimage* (2003) 20:84–97. doi: 10.1016/S1053-8119(03)00303-3
58. D'Hondt F, Szaffarczyk S, Sequeira H, Boucart M. Explicit and implicit emotional processing in peripheral vision: a saccadic choice paradigm. *Biol Psychol.* (2016) 119:91–100. doi: 10.1016/j.biopsycho.2016.07.014
59. Critchley H, Daly E, Phillips M, Brammer M, Bullmore E, Williams S, et al. Explicit and implicit neural mechanisms for processing of social information from facial expressions: a functional magnetic resonance imaging study. *Hum Brain Mapp.* (2000) 9:93–105. doi: 10.1002/(SICI)1097-0193(200002)9:2<93::AID-HBM4>3.0.CO;2-Z
60. Cohen N, Moyal N, Lichtenstein-Vidne L, Henik A. Explicit vs. implicit emotional processing: the interaction between processing type and executive control. *Cogn Emot.* (2016) 30:325–39. doi: 10.1080/02699931.2014.1000830
61. Klabunde RE. *Cardiovascular Physiology Concepts.* Lippincott Williams & Wilkins/Wolters Kluwer (2011). Available online at: https://books.google.ca/books?hl=zh-TW&lr=&id=27ExgvGnOagC&oi=fnd&pg=PP2&dq=Cardiovascular+Physiology+Concepts&ots=_i9x1hf5gv&sig=qv8yNqFSEMLOTbEVcSAORhBc8FY#v=onepage&q=CardiovascularPhysiologyConcepts&f=false (Accessed July 9, 2018).
62. Agarwal SK, Calaresu FR. Electrical stimulation of nucleus tractus solitarius excites vagal preganglionic cardiomotor neurons of the nucleus ambiguus in rats. *Brain Res.* (1992) 574:320–4. doi: 10.1016/0006-8993(92)90833-U
63. Pardini BJ, Lund DD, Schmid PG. Innervation patterns of the middle cervical–stellate ganglion complex in the rat. *Neurosci Lett.* (1990) 117:300–6.
64. Feher J. The adrenal medulla and integration of metabolic control. In: *Quantitative Human Physiology* (Cambridge, MA:Elsevier; Academic Press). p. 820–7. doi: 10.1016/B978-0-12-382163-8.00089-X
65. Smith CJ, Johnson JM. Responses to hyperthermia. Optimizing heat dissipation by convection and evaporation: neural control of skin blood flow and sweating in humans. *Auton Neurosci.* (2016) 196:25–36. doi: 10.1016/j.autneu.2016.01.002
66. Sato K, Kang WH, Saga K, Sato KT. Biology of sweat glands and their disorders. I. normal sweat gland function. *J Am Acad Dermatol.* (1989) 20:537–63.
67. McDougal DH, Gamlin PD. Autonomic control of the eye. *Compr Physiol.* (2015) 5:439–73. doi: 10.1002/cphy.c140014
68. Lowenstein O, Loewenfeld IE. Mutual role of sympathetic and parasympathetic in shaping of the pupillary reflex to light; pupillographic studies. *Arch Neurol Psychiatry* (1950) 64:341–77.
69. Ruskell GL. Access of autonomic nerves through the optic canal, and their orbital distribution in man. *Anat Rec A Discov Mol Cell Evol Biol.* (2003) 275:973–8. doi: 10.1002/ar.a.10108
70. Paivio A, Simpson HM. The effect of word abstractness and pleasantness on pupil size during an imagery task. *Psychon Sci.* (1966) 5:55–6. doi: 10.3758/BF03328277
71. Silk JS, Dahl RE, Ryan ND, Forbes EE, Axelson DA, Birmaher B, et al. Pupillary reactivity to emotional information in child and adolescent depression: links to clinical and ecological measures. *Am J Psychiatry* (2007) 164:1873–80.doi: 10.1176/appi.ajp.2007.06111816
72. Siegle GJ, Granholm E, Ingram RE, Matt GE. Pupillary and reaction time measures of sustained processing of negative information in depression. *Biol Psychiatry* (2001) 49:624–36. doi: 10.1016/S0006-3223(00)01024-6
73. Siegle GJ, Steinhauer SR, Carter CS, Ramel W, Thase ME. Do the seconds turn into hours? Relationships between sustained pupil dilation in response to emotional information and self-reported rumination. *Cognit Ther Res.* (2003) 27:365–82. doi: 10.1023/A:1023974602357
74. Silk JS, Siegle GJ, Whalen DJ, Ostapenko LJ, Ladouceur CD, Dahl RE. Pubertal changes in emotional information processing: pupillary, behavioral, and subjective evidence during emotional word identification. *Dev Psychopathol.* (2009) 21:7–26. doi: 10.1017/S0954579409000029
75. Siegle GJ, Steinhauer SR, Friedman ES, Thompson WS, Thase ME. Remission prognosis for cognitive therapy for recurrent depression using the pupil: utility and neural correlates. *Biol Psychiatry* (2011) 69:726–33. doi: 10.1016/j.biopsych.2010.12.041
76. Sara SJ. The locus coeruleus and noradrenergic modulation of cognition. *Nat Rev Neurosci.* (2009) 10:211–23. doi: 10.1038/nrn2573
77. Sara SJ, Bouret S. Orienting and reorienting: the locus coeruleus mediates cognition through arousal. *Neuron* (2012) 76:130–41. doi: 10.1016/j.neuron.2012.09.011
78. Benarroch EE. The locus ceruleus norepinephrine system: functional organization and potential clinical significance. *Neurology* (2009) 73:1699–704. doi: 10.1212/WNL.0b013e3181c2937c
79. Carter ME, Yizhar O, Chikahisa S, Nguyen H, Adamantidis A, Nishino S, et al. Tuning arousal with optogenetic modulation of locus coeruleus neurons. *Nat Neurosci.* (2010) 13:1526–33. doi: 10.1038/nn.2682
80. McCall JG, Al-Hasani R, Siuda ER, Hong DY, Norris AJ, Ford CP, et al. CRH engagement of the locus coeruleus noradrenergic system mediates stress-induced anxiety. *Neuron* (2015) 87:605–20. doi: 10.1016/j.neuron.2015.07.002
81. Varazzani C, San-Galli A, Gilardeau S, Bouret S. Noradrenaline and dopamine neurons in the reward/effort trade-off: a direct electrophysiological comparison in behaving monkeys. *J Neurosci.* (2015) 35:7866–77. doi: 10.1523/JNEUROSCI.0454-15.2015
82. Joshi S, Li Y, Kalwani RM, Gold JI. Relationships between pupil diameter and neuronal activity in the locus coeruleus, colliculi, and cingulate cortex. *Neuron* (2016) 89:221–34. doi: 10.1016/j.neuron.2015.11.028
83. Reimer J, Froudarakis E, Cadwell CR, Yatsenko D, Denfield GH, Tolias AS. Pupil fluctuations track fast switching of cortical states during quiet wakefulness. *Neuron* (2014) 84:355–62. doi: 10.1016/j.neuron.2014.09.033
84. Reimer J, McGinley MJ, Liu Y, Rodenkirch C, Wang Q, McCormick DA, et al. Pupil fluctuations track rapid changes in adrenergic and cholinergic activity in cortex. *Nat Commun.* (2016) 7:13289. doi: 10.1038/ncomms13289
85. McGinley MJ, Vinck M, Reimer J, Batista-Brito R, Zagha E, Cadwell CR, et al. Waking state: rapid variations modulate neural and behavioral responses. *Neuron* (2015) 87:1143–61. doi: 10.1016/j.neuron.2015.09.012
86. Hou RH, Freeman C, Langley RW, Szabadi E, Bradshaw CM. Does modafinil activate the locus coeruleus in man? Comparison of modafinil and clonidine on arousal and autonomic functions in human volunteers. *Psychopharmacology* (2005) 181:537–49. doi: 10.1007/s00213-005-0013-8
87. Murphy PR, O'Connell RG, O'Sullivan M, Robertson IH, Balsters JH. Pupil diameter covaries with BOLD activity in human locus coeruleus. *Hum Brain Mapp.* (2014) 35:4140–54. doi: 10.1002/hbm.22466
88. Clewett DV, Huang R, Velasco R, Lee T-H, Mather M. Locus coeruleus activity strengthens prioritized memories under arousal. *J Neurosci.* (2018) 38:1558–74. doi: 10.1523/JNEUROSCI.2097-17.2017
89. Song AH, Kucyi A, Napadow V, Brown EN, Loggia ML, Akeju O. Pharmacological modulation of noradrenergic arousal circuitry disrupts functional connectivity of the locus ceruleus in humans. *J Neurosci.* (2017) 37:6938–45. doi: 10.1523/JNEUROSCI.0446-17.2017
90. Demos KE, Kelley WM, Ryan SL, Davis FC, Whalen PJ. Human amygdala sensitivity to the pupil size of others. *Cereb Cortex* (2008) 18:2729–34. doi: 10.1093/cercor/bhn034

91. Harrison NA, Wilson CE, Critchley HD. Processing of observed pupil size modulates perception of sadness and predicts empathy. *Emotion* (2007) 7:724–9. doi: 10.1037/1528-3542.7.4.724
92. Lee KH, Siegle GJ. Different brain activity in response to emotional faces alone and augmented by contextual information. *Psychophysiology* (2014) 51:1147–57. doi: 10.1111/psyp.12254
93. Katnani HA, Gandhi NJ. Order of operations for decoding superior colliculus activity for saccade generation. *J Neurophysiol.* (2011) 106:1250–9. doi: 10.1152/jn.00265.2011
94. Hall WC, Moschovakis A. *The Superior Colliculus: New Approaches for Studying Sensorimotor Integration. Methods & New Frontiers in Neuroscience.* Boca Raton, FL; London; New York, NY; Washington, DC: CRC Press (2003).
95. White BJ, Munoz DP. The superior colliculus. In: Liversedge S, Gilchrist I, Everling S, editors. *Oxford Handbook of Eye Movements.* Oxford, UK: Oxford University Press. p. 195–213.
96. Corneil BD, Munoz DP. Overt responses during covert orienting. *Neuron* (2014) 82:1230–43. doi: 10.1016/j.neuron.2014.05.040
97. Krauzlis RJ, Lovejoy LP, Zenon A. Superior colliculus and visual spatial attention. *Annu Rev Neurosci.* (2013) 36:165–82. doi: 10.1146/annurev-neuro-062012-170249

14

Patterns of Pupillary Activity During Binocular Disparity Resolution

Carey D. Balaban [1], Alex Kiderman [2], Mikhaylo Szczupak [3], Robin C. Ashmore [2] and Michael E. Hoffer [3,4,5]*

[1] Departments of Otolaryngology, Neurobiology, Communication Sciences and Disorders, and Bioengineering, University of Pittsburgh, Pittsburgh, PA, United States, [2] Neuro Kinetics, Inc., Pittsburgh, PA, United States, [3] Department of Otolaryngology, University of Miami Hospital, Miami, FL, United States, [4] Neurological Surgery, University of Miami Hospital, Miami, FL, United States, [5] Sports Performance and Wellness Institute, University of Miami Hospital, Miami, FL, United States

***Correspondence:**
Carey D. Balaban
cbalaban@pitt.edu

This study examined the dynamic coordination between disconjugate, vergence eye movements, and pupil size in 52 normal subjects during binocular disparity stimulation in a virtual reality display. Eye movements and pupil area were sampled with a video-oculographic system at 100 Hz during performance of two tasks, (1) fusion of a binocular disparity step (±1.5° of visual angle in the horizontal plane) and (2) pursuit of a sinusoidally varying binocular disparity stimulus (0.1 Hz, ±2.6° of visual angle in the horizontal plane). Pupil size data were normalized on the basis of responses to homogeneous illumination increments ranging from 0.42 to 65.4 cd/m^2. The subjects produced robust vergence eye movements in response to disparity step shifts and high fidelity sinusoidal vergence responses (R^2 relative to stimulus profile: 0.933 ± 0.088), accompanied by changes in pupil area. Trajectory plots of pupil area as a function of vergence angle showed that the pupil area at zero vergence is altered between epochs of linear vergence angle—pupil area relations. Analysis with a modified Gath-Geva clustering algorithm revealed that the dynamic relationship between the ocular vergence angle and pupil size includes two different transient, synkinetic response patterns. The near response pattern, pupil constriction during convergence and pupil dilation during divergence, occurred ~80% of the time across subjects. An opposite, previously undescribed synkinetic pattern was pupil constriction during divergence and pupil dilatation during convergence; it occurred ~15% of the time across subjects. The remainder of the data were epochs of uncorrelated activity. The pupil size intercepts of the synkinetic segments, representing pupil size at initial tropia, had different relationships to vergence angle for the two main coordinated movement types. Hippus-like movements of the pupil could also be accompanied by vergence movements. No pupil coordination was observed during a conjugate pursuit task. In terms of the current dual interaction control model (1), findings suggest that the synkinetic eye and pupillary movements are produced by a dynamic switch of the influence of vergence related information to pupil control, accompanied by a resetting of the pupil aperture size at zero-vergence.

Keywords: convergent eye movements, virtual environment, pupil responses, synkinesias, human

INTRODUCTION

Visual cues for locating three-dimensional objects include binocular disparity, blur, and size change. These cues are used to control disconjugate (convergence and divergence) eye movements that track objects as they vary in depth. Binocular disparity drives an extraocular control process named fusional convergence, while blur-driven eye movements are termed accommodative convergence. These disconjugate eye movements are accompanied by pupil size changes and lens accommodation. For example, when tracking an approaching object, the "near triad" synkinesis (2) is a coordinated execution of convergent eye movements, pupillary constriction (miosis), and increased lens curvature. The opposite response occurs when one tracks a receding object; the eyes will diverge, pupil dilate, and the lens curvature decreases. The dynamic interactions between accommodation and accommodative vergence eye movements have been studied extensively and modeled quantitatively (3–5). This study examines dynamic coupling between vergence eye movements and pupil control during binocular disparity vergence tasks.

Instantaneous pupil size reflects several control signals to sympathetic and parasympathetic preganglionic neurons. The most extensively studied dynamic pupillary control system is the consensual pupillary light response, the adjustments of pupil size for ambient illumination (6–12). The pupillary component of accommodative responses has been termed the "pupillary near reflex" (13, 14). Physiological hippus, a spontaneous fluctuation in pupil diameter at a dominant frequency of ~0.5–0.7 Hz, is produced by variations in central parasympathetic drive (15). Slower pupillary fluctuations related to respiratory cycle control and/or respiratory sinus arrhythmia also appear to be modulated by variations in parasympathetic outflow (16). Finally, factors such as attentional load and task experience can influence pupil size during performance of cognitive tasks (17). These cognitive influences appear to be mediated by a central network that includes descending cortical pathways to the supraoculomotor area and surrounding reticular formation (1, 18, 19).

Concepts of control of the pupillary component of the near response were summarized recently in a modified dual interaction model by McDougal and Gamlin (1), which posits a central interaction between blur and binocular disparity controllers (3) that is upstream to their individual contributions to pupillary size control. Their model includes a pupillary light reflex pathway, influenced by global luminance pathways through the pretectum (**Figure 1**). Independent assessment of these subsystems is clearly possible and it would both test and refine these operating models of coordinated extraocular muscle and pupil motor activities.

This study uses a virtual reality display system to introduce binocular disparity alone, with neither blur of the image nor changes in ambient illumination. This selective stimulus allows a comparison of eye movement and pupillary size control during a binocular disparity step task, a binocular disparity pursuit task, and a versional pursuit task at the same frequency. The model predictions are then analyzed on two scales. A macroscale analysis examines vergence eye movement response as the product of a simple transfer function model for the binocular disparity resolution controller. The coupled component of the pupil response is represented by a transfer function from the literature (9), which assumes that pupil size at zero vergence remains invariant. A microscale analysis, on the other hand, uses time series approaches to identify epochs of synkinetic relationships between vergence eye movements and pupil area, which include gain differences and changes in both the range and the center of the range for pupil area regulation. These latter analyses demonstrate that the coordination of extraocular muscle-driven vergence and pupillary area during dynamic vergence pursuit differ from the features revealed by the traditional step testing (steady state measurements at two fixation points or binocular disparities). More significantly, the disparity-induced convergence pursuit task revealed previously undescribed, synkinetic patterns of dynamic coordination of pupillary and extraocular muscle responses.

MATERIALS AND METHODS

Control subjects were recruited at Madigan Army Medical Center (35 subjects: 26 males, 9 females) and the University of Miami (17 subjects: 10 males, 7 females). Subjects ranged in age from 21 to 45 years [mean 28.7 ± 6.3 (S.D.) years]. Informed consent was obtained. Control subjects were selected who had no history of otologic or ophthalmologic disorders, and no history of traumatic brain injury or neurologic disorders. In addition, these control subjects were not taking any prescription or over the counter medicines that would impair or affect vestibular function or performance on the test battery. The project was approved by the IRBs at the University of Miami, Madigan Army Medical Center, and the University of Pittsburgh.

The experimental apparatus used in this study was a portable 3D head mounted display (HMD) system with integrated clinical eye tracking technology (I—PAS ™; I-Portal® Portable Assessment System, Neuro Kinetics, Inc., Pittsburgh, PA, USA). Within this device, each eye views an independent circular segment of a 1,920 × 1,080 pixel stimulus display that subtends a 60° diagonal field of view. The device has integral video-based eye tracking, performed under continuous 940 nm infrared illumination at a sampling rate of 100 Hz. Pupils are detected by identification of luminance boundaries. The pupil area is measured for each image, and eye position is calculated from the centroid of the identified pupil. Horizontal (±30° range) and vertical (±20° range) eye tracking spatial resolution is on the order of 0.02°, while spatial resolution for torsional eye movement (±10° range) is < 0.1°. Subjects can also adjust the focus of the video image across a 6 diopter range.

Neuro Kinetics VEST™ software was used to run the battery of tests and for data collection. All stimuli were rendered in the virtual environment that was created by the enclosed video display, and stimulus refresh rates were synchronized with the eye tracking sampling rate. Eye movement recordings were calibrated for a series of conjugate horizontal and vertical gaze shifts, using spot targets subtending ~0.1° of visual angle. For calibrating the pupillary light reflex, the subjects viewed a 5°

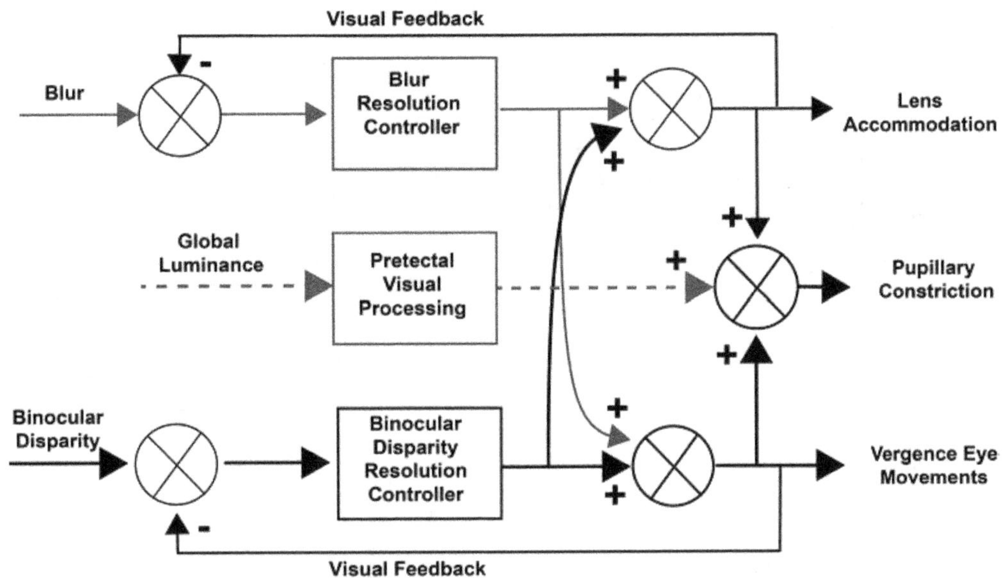

FIGURE 1 | Dual interaction model for coordinated control of vergence eye movements and pupil size. This basic dual interaction model (1) includes separate paths for the influence of blur, binocular disparity, and global illumination on lens curvature, pupil size, and ocular convergence. Blur provides primary control for lens adjustments, binocular disparity drives convergence (to prevent diplopia), and global illumination drives the pupillary light reflex.

(visual angle) disc centered on the visible area of each screen half, illuminated at intensities ranging from 0.42 to 65.4 cd/m^2. For analysis of responses during vergence tasks, the pupil area (A_{raw}) was normalized for each subject based on pupillary light reflex responses. The maximum (A_{max}) and minimum (A_{min}) pupil areas were determined separately for left and right eyes for responses to low (0.42 cd/m^2) and high (65.4 cd/m^2) brightness stimulus. The normalized values were calculated for each eye as $A_{norm} = 100^*(A_{raw}-A_{min})/(A_{max}-A_{min})$; the instantaneous mean of the left and right pupil values was used for identification of synkinetic oculomotor and pupil response components.

Targets for the disparity fusion ("vergence tracking") task were a white square with red center that covered $\sim 0.1^\circ$ visual angle of each eye. The total field luminance during presentation of the square, measured with a spot luminance detector incorporating a LDM-9901 sensor (Gigahertz-Optik, Germany), ranged from 0.05 to 0.06 cd/ m^2. The vergence disparity step task began with the illuminated targets at a central fixation position for each eye. The targets were then shifted at 4 s intervals between a disparity requiring a 1.5° convergence and a disparity requiring a 1.5° divergence in order to achieve binocular fusion. Five cycles of alternating convergence and divergence were presented over a 40 s duration (**Figure 2A**). For the vergence pursuit (tracking) task, the trial began with illumination of the two monocular targets at the initial focal point phoria (equivalent to ~1 m in virtual depth). The target then moved smoothly through 3 cycles of a sinusoidal profile, such that the monocular targets moved simultaneously laterally and then medially to produce binocular disparity (i.e., the left eye target moved leftward while the right eye target moved rightward, then the left eye target moved rightward while the right eye target moved leftward) with a cycle duration of 10 s. During this sinusoidal movement, the maximum deviation of the response from the initial position was ±2.6° of visual angle in the horizontal plane. Since there is no stimulus blur introduced, the accommodation produced by this vergence angle is expected to be on the order of 0.5 diopter and to be linear with visual angle (20). For the versional smooth pursuit task, the stimuli monocular spots were moved sinusoidally to the left and then to the right (±10° excursion) with a cycle duration of 10 s.

The calibrated data were exported as Excel files and analyzed with MATLAB (MathWorks, Natick, MA) and SPSS Statistics 24 (IBM). The eye movements in the disparity step task were modeled as the weighted sum of first order high and low pass representations of the vergence target position with a processing delay. Nonlinear least squares regression ("lsqnonlin.m" function in MATLAB) was used to estimate parameters for the vergence disparity response as a weighted sum of phasic ($\frac{K_{vh}se^{-t_v s}}{s+1}$) and tonic ($\frac{K_{vl}e^{-t_v s}}{0.25s+1}$) processes, with delay t_v and gains K_{vh} (phasic process) and K_{vl}, (tonic process), respectively. The delay parameter accounts for the reaction time to the binocular disparity step stimulus; it was set at zero for the binocular disparity pursuit task. Based upon Sun et al. (9), the pupil dynamics were fitted from the vergence data by a transfer function for pupil motion, $\frac{K_p e^{-t_p s}}{0.28s+1}$, with delay t_p and gain K_p, which estimates the near response sensitivity directly. Symmetry was tested by fitting separate gains for half-cycles of convergence vs. divergence and for half-cycles of pupil constriction versus dilatation.

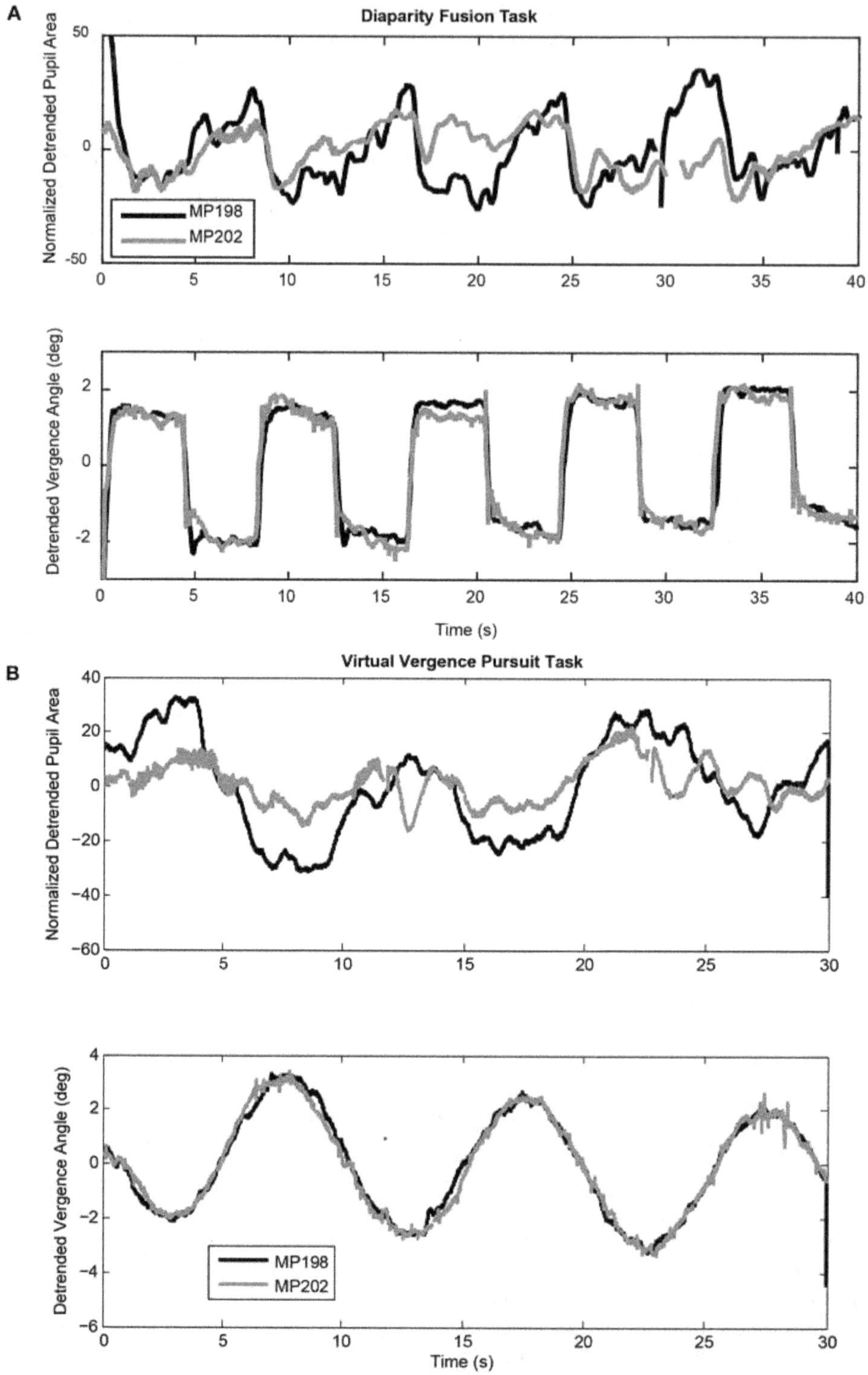

FIGURE 2 | Examples of coordinated pupil and eye movements during the virtual binocular disparity vergence task. **(A)** Detrended data from two subjects (MP198 and MP202) during a step binocular disparity fusion task. The upper panel shows the normalized pupil area traces and the lower panel shows the ocular vergence angle relative to the tropia at calibration. **(B)** Detrended data from the same subjects for a binocular disparity tracking task at 0.1 Hz. Note the highly consistent vergence eye movements for both the binocular disparity step tasks and the disparity tracking tasks of both subjects. Data from MP198 before detrending are shown in the supplemental data section (**Figure S1**).

RESULTS

General Observations

Both binocular fusion stimuli produced robust, high fidelity convergent, and divergent eye movements. The binocular disparity step stimuli produced an alternating sequence of rapid converging and diverging movements to fuse the disparate targets (**Figure 2A**, lower trace). The binocular disparity pursuit stimulus (**Figure 2B**) also produced a robust tracking sequence of divergent and convergent eye movements. These eye movements are a primary response to binocular disparity. They are accompanied by pupillary responses that vary during eye movements and between subjects. The deterministic properties and variability in the relationship between the pupillary responses and eye movements will now be examined for each disparity task.

The findings are described sequentially from the perspectives of macroscale and microscale behavior. Metrics of macroscale behavior were derived by (1) analysis of responses relative to the stimulus profile, and (2) analyses based upon a lumped parameter linear systems approach for eye and pupil movements from an entire trial. These approaches are presented initially for the binocular disparity step and binocular disparity pursuit tasks. These macroscale approaches assume that both the range and the center of the range for pupil area regulation are stationary during a measurement trial. The ensuing microscale perspective uses bivariate analyses of the coordinated trajectories of eye and pupil movements to characterize independent and synkinetic control epochs. This microscale analysis explicitly characterizes time-dependent behavior of the pupil regulatory range and its relationship to vergence angle regulation.

Macroscale Analysis Approach

Binocular Disparity Step

The binocular disparity step stimulus sequence produced alternating convergent and divergent eye movements, accompanied by a more variable modulation of pupil area (**Figure 2A**). **Table 1A** shows average measurements of the pupil area and the vergence angle of the eyes during the steady state of the convergence and divergence fusion responses; the ratio of these measures has been used in the literature to provide an estimate of the static (or steady-state) sensitivity of the pupil "near response." The oculomotor vergence responses were symmetric for converging and diverging disparity fusion movements. In contrast to the symmetric oculomotor vergence behavior, the average magnitude of pupillary area changes was significantly greater in the diverging direction than the converging direction (**Table 1A**, paired *t*-test, $t_{(49)} = 6.25$, $p < 0.01$). The near response magnitudes, estimated for constriction in the converged, and dilation during diverged eye movements, were also significantly greater in the diverged direction ($p < 0.01$). The lumped peak-to-peak estimate of the near response magnitude was 6.21 ± 0.60 % area (relative to light reflex range)/degree for constriction during convergence (relative to resting tropia) or dilation during divergence.

The impression that the converging eye movement responses were brisker than the diverging responses (**Figure 2A**, lower traces) was tested by linear systems modeling of the eye movement responses as the sum of high and low pass representations of the vergence target position (see Methods). The goodness of fit of the model to the vergence eye movements was very robust, with average coefficients of determination (R^2) of 0.84 ± 0.03. The estimated processing delays (t_v) were 0.26 ± 0.02 s and the estimated gains are listed in **Table 1B**. The high pass gain values were rectified, but of the same magnitude for shifts of the stimuli in either nasal or temporal directions; hence, there was a phasic convergence when disparity changed abruptly. The low pass magnitudes for the convergent and divergent eye movements were symmetric and did not differ from the static responses estimates in **Table 1A**.

The contribution of pupillary motion dynamics to this directional asymmetry was tested by modeling pupil motion as a function of the drive that produces the vergence eye movements (9). The gain estimate from this model represents the responsiveness of normalized pupil diameter per degree of vergence (gain of the pupil "near response"). The model

TABLE 1 | Disparity step task responses.

Component	Direction	Average magnitude or *Gain* (±SE)	Near response sensitivity
A. MEASUREMENTS FROM STEADY-STATE EPOCHS (n = 52 SUBJECTS)			
Vergence	Toward midline (convergent disparity)	1.40 ± 0.07° *0.93 ± 0.05*	
	Away (divergent disparity)	1.44 ± 0.07° *0.96 ± 0.05*	
Pupil	Toward midline	7.60 ± 0.89%** (Normalized re: light response)	−5.39 ± 0.52 %/° convergence**
	Away	10.00 ± 0.88% (Normalized re: light response)	−7.13 ± 0.60 %/° convergence

***p < 0.01 relative to opposite direction.*

Component	Direction	Magnitude or *Gain* ± S.E.	Comment
B. MODEL PARAMETERS (n = 52 SUBJECTS)			
High pass vergence magnitude	Converge	0.173 ± 0.045 *0.108 ± 0.017*	*Fully Rectified and Symmetric*
	Diverge	−0.169 ± 0.035 *−0.105 ± 0.013*	
Low pass vergence magnitude	Converge	1.409 ± 0.069 *0.88 ± 0.04*	*Symmetric*
	Diverge	1.485 ± 0.071 *0.93 ± 0.04*	
Pupil (re: vergence; "near response gain")	Constrict	−5.032 ± 0.610 % / °convergence	*Asymmetric ($p < 0.001$)*
	Dilate	−7.983 ± 0.595 %/ °convergence	

Gains, shown in italic font below the response magnitudes, were obtained by dividing magnitudes by the virtual stimulus magnitude in that direction, 2.6°.

TABLE 2 | Sinusoidal vergence pursuit modulation parameters for eye movements and pupil size.

Component	Direction	Magnitude or *Gain* [±SE]	Phase angle re: Stimulus (±SE)	R^2 (±SE)
A. SINUSOIDAL ANALYSIS				
Vergence	Toward midline	2.54 ± 0.11° *0.98 ± 0.04*	172.75 ± 1.26° (3.015 ± 0.022 rad)	0.933 ± 0.088
	Away	2.26 ± 0.10° *0.87 ± 0.04*		
Pupil	Toward midline	23.54 ± 1.57% (Normalized re: light response)	−8.37 ± 4.87° (−0.146 ± 0.085 rad)	0.563 ± 0.198
	Away	13.43 ± 1.96% (Normalized re: light response)		

Component	Direction	Magnitude or *Gain* [± SE]	Comment
B. MODEL PARAMETERS			
High pass vergence magnitude	Both (rectified)	0.255 ± 0.084 *0.098 ± 0.032*	
Low pass vergence magnitude	Converge	2.422 ± 0.128 *0.93 ± 0.05*	*Symmetric*
	Diverge	2.246 ± 0.127 *0.86 ± 0.05*	
Pupil (re: vergence; "near response gain")	Constrict	−7.841 ± 0.727 %/° convergence	*Asymmetric (paired t, t = 2.8, p < 0.01)*
	Dilate	−8.413 ± 0.646 %/° convergence**	

Gains, shown in italic font below the response magnitudes, were obtained by dividing magnitudes by the virtual stimulus magnitude in that direction, 2.6°.
***p < 0.01, paired t-test.*

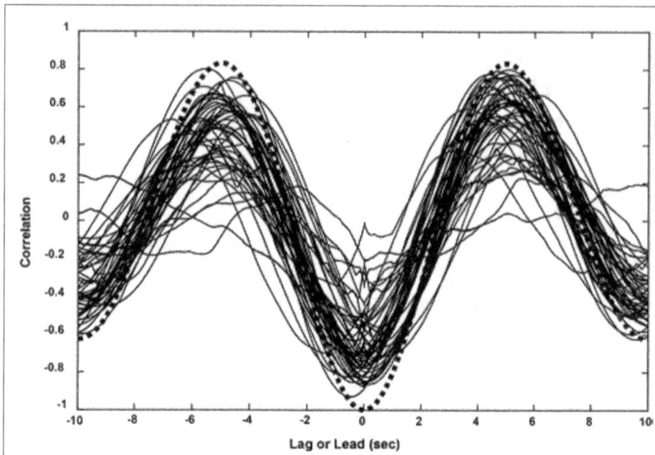

FIGURE 3 | Cross-correlation functions for eye movement and pupil responses (sinusoidal pursuit task) from all 52 subjects. The functions corresponded closely to the theoretical result for two cosines at the stimulus frequency of 0.1 Hz (black dashed line).

from the literature explained roughly 30% of the variance in the pupil traces as a function of only the vergence behavior ($R^2 = 0.28 \pm 0.03$) and the estimate of the delay parameter (0.19 ± 0.02 s) did not differ significantly from the 0.2 s delay estimate for the pupillary motor reaction during the light response (9). Consistent with the outcome of the steady state analysis (**Table 1A**), the average sensitivity (% area/degree convergence) when diverging was significantly greater than the sensitivity converging [paired $t_{(49)} = 6.97, p < 0.001$].

Sinusoidal Tracking Task

The subjects' tracking of the virtual stimuli (disparity simulation varying sinusoidally from 2.6° divergence to 2.6° convergence at 0.1 Hz) produced symmetric smooth convergence eye movements, accompanied by consensual pupillary area changes. Examples of the average vergence angle and average pupillary area (normalized to the light reflex response) are shown in **Figure 2B**. The initial divergent eye movement tracking was accompanied by pupillary dilation, followed by convergent eye tracking movements that were accompanied primarily by pupillary constriction. The modulation amplitudes of the eye movement [paired $t_{(51)} = 4.37, p < 0.001$] and of the pupil area [paired $t_{(51)} = 5.19, p < 0.001$] were both greater pursuing virtual targets toward the midline, which is a convergence response, than during a divergence response (**Table 2A**). The eye movements displayed extremely high fidelity to a sinusoidal tracking profile. The modulation in the convergence direction did not differ significantly from the intended ± 2.6° vergence modulation, but the divergence response was smaller. There was a small linear drift of −0.011± 0.002 (SE) deg/s in the center of modulation toward divergence, which is equivalent to a gradual divergence (relative to initial tropia) by ∼ 0.33° over the 30 s task [$t_{(51)} = -4.64, p < 0.01$]. The pupil size was modulated out of phase with the vergence angle (average difference: 167.6 ± 2.5° or 2.925 ± 0.043 rad), but there was no significant linear drift in pupil size during the 30 s task [$t_{(51)} = -0.671, p > 0.5$]. Cross-correlation functions for the detrended subject data (**Figure 3**) showed the configuration for the correlation of two out-of-phase sine waves (dashed black line) confirming that the virtual stimulus elicited coordinated performance of oculomotor and pupillary components of the near triad.

Linear systems modeling of the binocular disparity pursuit eye movement responses as the sum of high and low pass representations of the vergence target position was conducted to test the hypothesis that the same basic model can characterize the response dynamics for both binocular disparity step and pursuit responses. Based upon the results for the binocular disparity step response (**Table 1B**), a single sensitivity parameter was used to characterize a fully rectified high pass component (**Table 2B**). Repeated measures ANOVA indicated no significant differences in gain estimates for either high or low pass components of the vergence eye movements from the step versus pursuit tasks. In contrast to the results of the binocular disparity step task (which has higher frequency components), the estimates of the pupil near response sensitivity (%/° convergence) for this single, low frequency pursuit task did not differ for converging and diverging movements during the pursuit task. The steady-state sensitivity of the pupillary near response during sinusoidal vergence tracking was estimated directly from the data by (a) the lagged slope (from autoregression analysis) of the bivariate relationship for pupil area as a function of vergence angle (-7.97 ± 0.62 % area/° vergence) and (b) the ratio of the average peak modulations of the pupil area and vergence movements (-8.22 ± 0.62 % area/° vergence). The linear modeling approach was also used to estimate the dynamic near response sensitivity from the vergence pursuit response, using the transfer function $\frac{K_p e^{-t_p s}}{0.28s+1}$. The delay parameter t_p was set at 0.19 s, the average value from the binocular disparity step response analysis (above). The model could account for approximately half of the variance in the pupil traces ($R^2 = 0.51 \pm 0.03$ S.E.). The near response sensitivity, estimated for the converging (-7.84 ± 0.73 % area/° convergence) and diverging (-8.41 ± 0.65 % area/° convergence) directions, were significantly greater in the diverged direction (paired t-test, $p < 0.01$). The model-based, average near response sensitivity estimate for the pursuit task (-8.13 ± 0.75 % area/° convergence) was greater (paired t-test, $p < 0.05$) than for the step task (-6.51 ± 0.56 % area/° convergence).

These findings are consistent with the prevailing concept (1, 3) that there is a central coupling between binocular disparity processing and pupillary control. However, the variations in the estimates of the magnitude of this "near response" component in pupillary control provided motivation for a more detailed analysis of the dynamic coordination of pupil and vergence eye movement control during the disparity tracking task.

Microscale Analysis Approach

Binocular Disparity Step Eye-Pupil Trajectories

The magnitude of the pupillary responses varied on a movement-by-movement basis during reproducible vergence eye movements (e.g., **Figure 2A**). The variability between epochs of dynamic pupillary area changes across a consistent pattern of vergence eye movements is shown in trajectory plots of normalized pupil size as a function of vergence angle (**Figure 4**). Successive sample points (100 Hz sample rate) are shown for convergent (red dots) and divergent (black dots) disparity-driven responses. Relationships during steady-state fusion are represented by green dots; cyan lines show the connected trajectory. The representative cases have several noteworthy features. Firstly, a wide range of instantaneous pupillary areas were observed at the convergent and divergent fusion targets during the task. Secondly, the pupillary areas at the initial tropia (represented as zero detrended vergence) tended to differ during the convergent versus the divergent eye movements [Repeated Measures ANOVA, main effect of direction, $F_{(1, 36)} = 82.45$, $p < 0.001$], which indicates that the set point for pupillary control relative to vergence angle is changing on a movement-by-movement basis during the fixation/fusion periods of the task (green dots). Finally, the pupillary component of individual disparity responses shows three patterns relative to the consistent pattern of vergence eye movements (**Figure 4**): epochs of (1) almost exclusively eye movement ("horizontal segments") or pupil area changes ("vertical segments"), (2) combinations that reflect a near response pattern (pupil constriction with convergence and dilation with divergence, larger gray arrows) and (3) a pattern that is opposite the near response (e.g., some MP198 data segments in **Figure 4** show dilation with convergence, small gray arrows).

Sinusoidal Pursuit Task Eye-Pupil Trajectories

Bivariate plots of detrended pupil areas as a function of the detrended disjunctive eye movement measurements showed extensive epochs of linear coupling during the virtual vergence tracking task. Data from a representative subject is shown in **Figure 5** (left panel). Like the disparity fusion task plots in **Figure 4,** each subject showed epochs with different quasilinear associations between concurrent pupil areas and vergence angles, including segments with a near response pattern (pupil constriction with convergence and dilation with divergence, larger gray arrows) and segments with an opposite movement pattern, dilation while converging (smaller gray arrows). Each bivariate plot is dominated typically by a series of parallel segments reflecting the pupillary constriction during convergence (near response pattern), offset by differences in a pupil size set-point. Because the sampled detrended normalized pupil area and detrended vergence angles from each session are a bivariate time series, an analysis technique was applied to objectively identify segments with a homogeneous linear slope. This slope provides an empirical estimate of the influence of the hypothetical disparity control mechanism [McDoughal and Gamlin (1)] on pupillary size. A modified Gath-Geva clustering algorithm (21) was used for objective fuzzy segmentation of the time series into 15 segments with homogeneous properties, based upon preliminary analyses indicating that results were unaffected by more granular divisions of the data into more segments. This published algorithm first applies a principal component decomposition to identify a component that represents the instantaneous pupillary area relative to instantaneous vergence angle. It then applies a clustering algorithm to decompose the data into linear segments, based upon measured homogeneity of the segments, and the fuzzy sets that are used to represent the segments in time.

The distribution of the slopes of linear segments had relative peaks in both the negative and positive slope directions (**Figure 5**, right panel). A fuzzy c-means clustering algorithm [(22), MATLAB routine "fcm.m"] indicated that the boundary between two clusters, with at least 0.65 fuzzy class membership, was demarcated by cutoffs of ≤ -2% pupil area range /deg vergence ("near response" pattern) and ≥ 2% pupil area range /deg vergence (opposite pattern). The remaining segments with >0.35 to < 0.65 membership in either class were considered to have a "flat" slope (yellow in **Figure 6,** right panel). Applying these boundaries across all subjects, 67% of the segments (range: 7–15 segments/subject, average: 10) showed the near response type (slope ≤ -2% pupil area range /deg vergence, average $R^2 = 0.670 \pm 0.015$) and 27% (range:

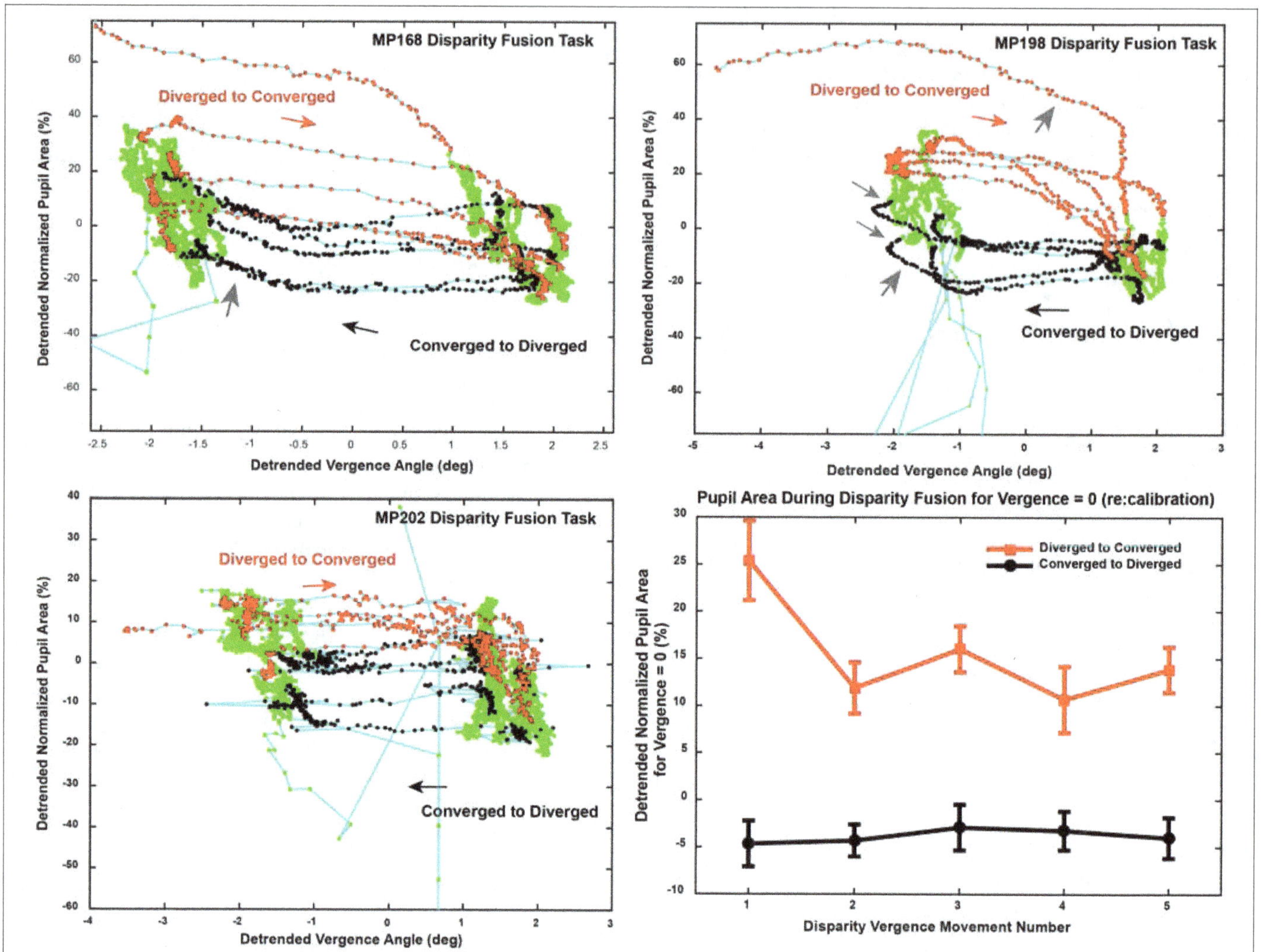

FIGURE 4 | Trajectory of the vergence angle and pupil area during the binocular fusion step task is shown in the upper and lower left panels. The upper right (MP198) and lower left (MP202) panels area are plotted from data shown in in **Figure 2A**. Successive sample points (100 Hz sample rate) are plotted in green, with the dots indicating the convergent (red dots) and divergent (black dots) disparity-driven responses. The directions of the trajectories between fixations is indicated with arrows. Note that response patterns include periods when there are (1) almost exclusively vergence eye movements (horizontally oriented segments), (2) almost exclusively pupil area changes (vertically oriented segments), (3) combinations that reflect a near response pattern (pupil constriction with convergence and dilation with divergence, larger gray arrows) and (3) a pattern that is opposite the near response (smaller gray arrows). The lower right panel shows the average pupil area (normalized to light reflex range) at zero vergence for successive increments) to show the stability across repeated binocular disparity steps.

0–8 segments/subject, average: 4) of the segments showed the opposite relationship (slope $\geq$ 2% pupil area range /deg vergence, average $R^2 = 0.651 \pm 0.024$). The flat segments [6% of segments across subjects (range: 0–4 segments/subject), yellow in **Figure 5**, right panel] had a significantly lower, but still reasonably strong R^2 value (0.421 ± 0.052). The near response-type segments were of significantly longer duration (2.39 ± 0.06 s, Tukey HSD tests, $p < 0.01$) than either the segments with opposite polarity (1.17 ± 0.09 s) or the flat (absolute slope <2% pupil area range/deg vergence) slope segments (1.38 ± 0.19 s), which did not differ from each other. Slope and duration of segments were uncorrelated. Hence, the near response pattern was present 82.8 ± 1.5% (mean ± SE) of the time during vergence trials for individual subjects, while the opposite pattern was present ~16% of the time.

The dominant "near response" pattern, a negative linear relationship between the vergence angle and pupil diameter (slope ≤ -2 % of pupil area range per degree of vergence) consisted of segments with an average slope of 13.3 ± 0.6 % of pupil area range per degree of vergence (mean ± SE).The high coefficient of determination ($R^2 = 0.670 \pm 0.015$) suggests that binocular disparity is a prominent drive during these segments for pupillary constriction during convergence and pupillary dilation during divergence. The magnitudes of the slopes of these segments were significantly greater than the steady state estimates of near response sensitivity and the near response sensitivity estimate from the disparity fusion task in each subject, as shown

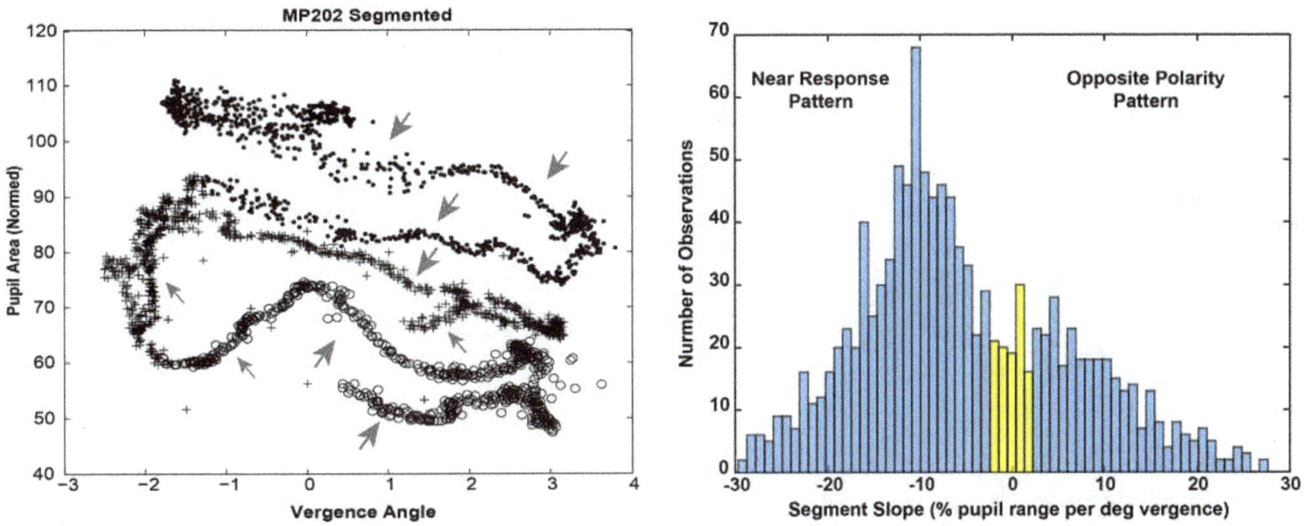

FIGURE 5 | The left panel shows the trajectory of the vergence angle and pupil area for one of the traces shown during the binocular disparity pursuit task in **Figure 2B**. Note that the graph appears as a series of parallel quasi-linear segments, offset by differences in a pupil size set-point. The right panel shows the bimodal distribution of linear segment slopes. A fuzzy c-means clustering algorithm [(22), MATLAB routine "fcm.m"] indicated that the boundary between two clusters, with at least 0.65 fuzzy class membership (shown in blue), was demarcated by cutoffs of $\leq -2\%$ pupil area range /deg vergence ("near response" pattern) and $\geq 2\%$ pupil area range /deg vergence (opposite pattern). The intermediate observations (flat slope) are shown in yellow.

by repeated measures analysis of variance [$F_{(3, 147)} = 38.71, p < 0.001$] followed by pairwise comparisons ($p < 0.001$ for each case).

The zero vergence intercept of the pupil-area for these linear segments estimates the set point of pupil area for each segment, relative to the initial tropia during calibration (defined arbitrarily as 0°). This new set point is likely to reflect other signals for the pupil control, including "aftereffects" of disparity that alter vergence phoria (3) and effects related to cognitive processing load. The intercepts varied with the binocular disparity at the start of the segment for both the near response (negative slope) and positive slope segments (**Figure 6**). Nonlinear regression was used to model the pupil set points (zero-vergence angle intercepts) as the sum of a constant offset, a linear trend with time and an asymmetric sinusoidal modulation (**Table 2**). For near response segments, the set point tended to dilate while the target disparity is converged, and to constrict while the target disparity is diverged. Approximately 24% of the variance in the set point of the near response linear segments reflects a constant dilation of almost 4% of light response range and symmetric modulation of about 14.6% of light response range. The pupil size and vergence angle traces from these "near response segments" are extracted and superimposed on the left side of **Figure 7**. Although the pupil set point changes produce variability, these pupil response segments show smooth, continuous modulation during vergence eye movements.

The consistency and dominance of the inverse linear relationship between pupillary area and vergence angle ("near response pattern") is obvious after alignment of the segments by subtraction of the pupil-size intercept from each segment (**Figure 8**). The near response segments form a tight, overlapping cloud of points with a negative correlation, supporting the hypothesis that the parallel, negative slope segments in the raw data (**Figure 4**) are the products of a coordinated near response motor program with different pupil size set points. However, there were short periods when pupil area increased with ocular convergence (**Figure 8**, small arrows) and periods showing either vergence movements without pupil area changes or pupil area changes without eye movement (**Figure 8**, large arrows).

The linear segments that did not show the near response pattern were divided by the c-means cluster analysis (above) into segments with a positive slope (slope ≥ 2 % of pupil area per degree vergence, membership of at least 0.65 in the positive histogram mode in **Figure 5**) and flat response segments (absolute slope <2 % of pupil area per degree vergence, membership <0.65 in both modes). During the latter segments, the pupillary responses and eye movements are uncorrelated. During the former period, the positively sloped segments (213 total in 52 subjects; 4 segments per subject) averaged a slope of 15.5 ± 0.8 % of pupil area range per degree of vergence (mean $\pm$ SE), which was of similar magnitude, but of the opposite polarity to the near response, and a similarly robust within-segment R^2 for the linear relationship (0.65 ± 0.02). Because the coefficient of determination was very strong during these epochs, it appears that binocular disparity is a prominent drive for pupillary dilation during convergence or pupillary constriction during divergence, which is opposite in polarity to the "near response." However, the durations of these positive slope responses (1.17 ± 0.08 s, mean $\pm$ SE) were significantly shorter than the near response (negative slope) segments (Tukey HSD test, $p < 0.01$).

For the segments with a positive vergence angle-pupil size relationship, the vergence angle at the start of the

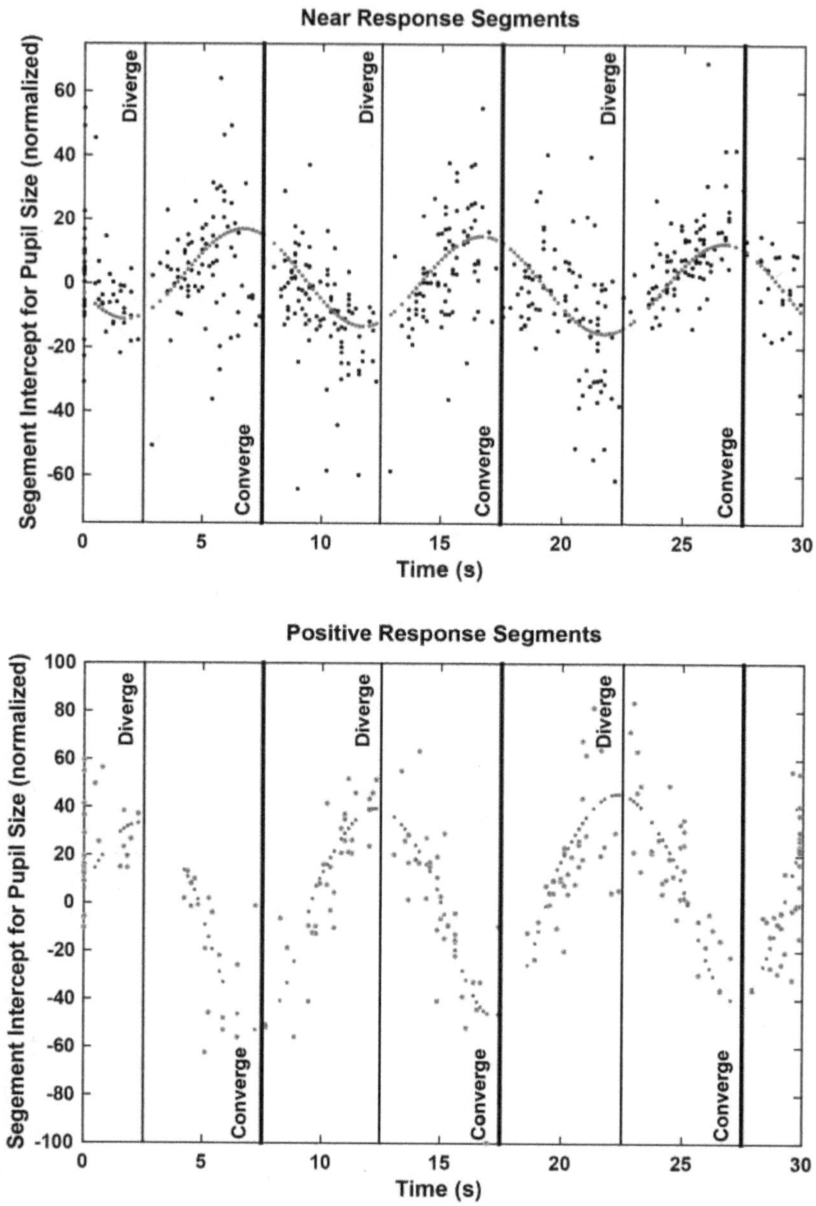

FIGURE 6 | Plots of the pupil size intercepts across all subjects for linear segments of coordinated eye movement and pupil vergence accommodation patterns. The segment intercept is plotted at the onset of the segment; the stimulus times for maximum divergence and convergence are shown by vertical lines.

segment accounted for ~54% of the variance in the (new) pupil size set point (**Figure 6**, lower panel and **Table 3**). The constant component was a dilation of only about 1% and the modulation was asymmetric. The set point for the pupil was more constricted during convergence with a peak modulation of 58% of normalized pupil size. The pupil set point was more dilated during divergence with a modulation of 38% of normalized pupillary range. When the pupil size and vergence angle traces from these "positive slope segments" are extracted and superimposed (right side of **Figure 7**), these asymmetric set point adjustments are reflected in discontinuities in the pupil response segments during convergence vs. divergence. Hence, these epochs seem to be a second motor program for pupillary regulation during binocular disparity-driven oculomotor responses.

The flat response segments were infrequent observations (44/780 total segments in 52 subjects, ~1 segment per subject). Their slope was nearly zero (0.1 ± 1.8 % of pupil area range per degree of vergence), their durations (1.38 ± 0.19 s, mean ± SE) were comparable to the positive slope segments, and their within-segment R^2 for the linear relationship (0.42 ± 0.05) was significantly lower than for the positive or negative slope segments (Tukey HSD tests, $p < 0.01$). These findings indicate that pupillary activity is uncorrelated with vergence during a

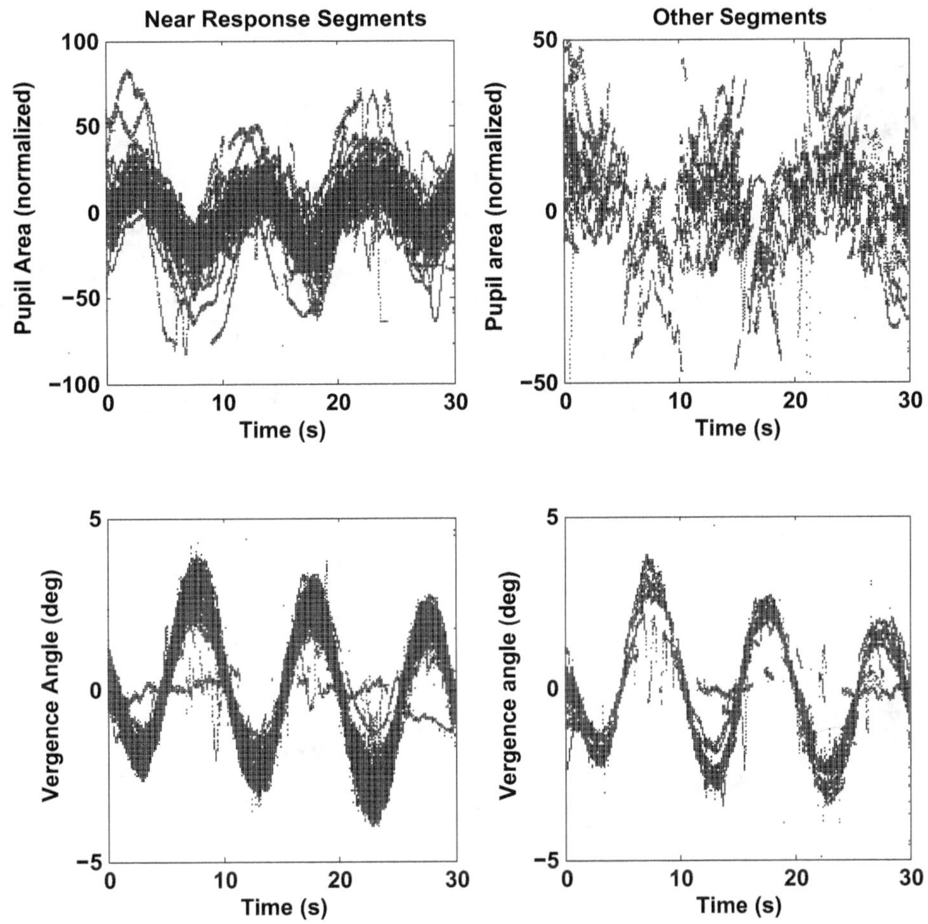

FIGURE 7 | Pupil size recordings (upper graphs) and vergence angle recordings (lower graph) are shown for data segments showing a negative linear relationship between pupil area and vergence angle ("Near Response Segments," left side) and for segments showing either a positive linear relationship between pupil area and vergence angle or a flat relationship ("Other Response Segments," left side). Segments of detrended data from all subjects are superimposed, including one outlier subject with little vergence tracking. Note the out-of-phase modulation of the pupil and vergence traces for the "Near Response Segments".

small period of time during the binocular disparity tracking task.

The relative prevalence of linear segments showing a near response pattern and other pupil-oculomotor (flat or positive correlation) patterns during disparity vergence tracking are shown at each time point in **Figure 9**. Data from the single subject with low fidelity disparity vergence tracking are included. The vergence eye movements did not vary during the segments showing pupillary near responses or other responses; rather the differences in slopes can be attributed to the pupillary size responses alone (**Figure 7**). The near response pattern was most prevalent when the eye positions were converged (i.e., binocular disparity closer) relative to the initial tropia. The response segments showing the opposite relationship (e.g., constriction with divergence) were most common with divergence from the initial tropia point. The flat segments were uncommon and showed no preference for binocular disparity.

The linear segment analysis can also be used to decompose the pupil data into two components, a purely vergence eye movement related component (product of slope of linear segment and detrended vergence eye movement data) and the residual pupillary activity representing a component unrelated to vergence. The decompositions from two representative data sets are shown in **Figure 10** (left panels). A frequency domain assessment of the relative contributions of these mechanisms to periodic changes in pupil area is shown in the right panels of **Figure 10**. Several features are notable from this analysis. First, activity coordinated with the 0.1 Hz disparity-driven vergence eye tracking is dominant at low frequencies (below ~0.25 Hz). Second, power spectral density was prominent in the hippus-like frequency range (0.5–0.7 Hz) in the residual data trace. Third, the appreciable power in the hippus frequency range (0.5–0.7 Hz range) of the vergence-associated pupil activity represents coordinated disparity-driven vergence-pupil responses.

Conjugate (Versional) Smooth Pursuit Task

In contrast to the dynamic binocular disparity pursuit task, there was no evidence of coordination of eye movements (conjugate

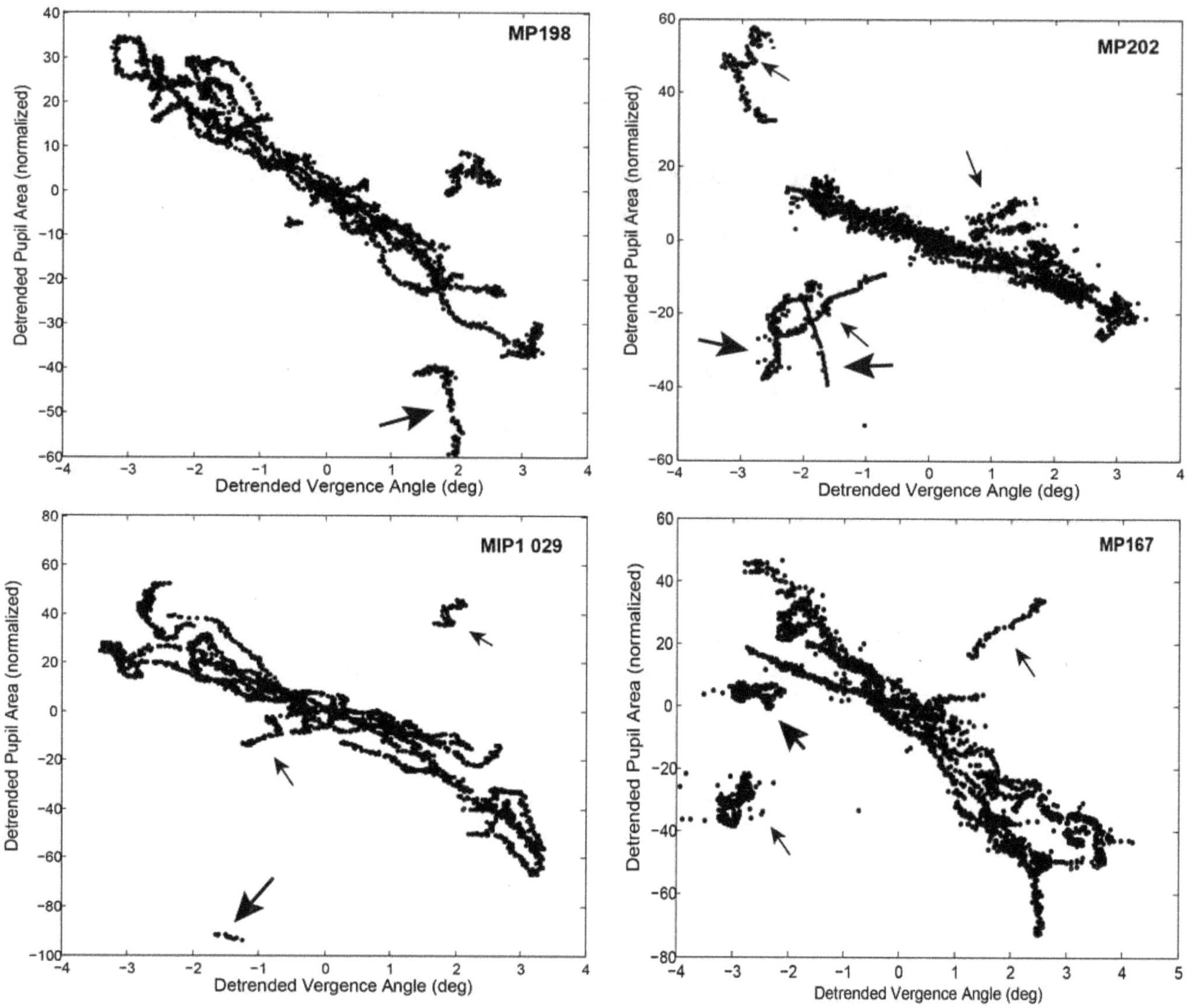

FIGURE 8 | Time-implicit plots of detrended pupil area as function of detrended vergence angle, after subtraction of the pupil area intercept from each linear segment. Note the overlap between the segments representing a coordinated near response pattern. Thin arrows indicate segments with a positively correlated relationship between vergence angle and pupil area. Thick arrows indicate segments with little covariation (uncorrelated eye movement and pupil movement).

or disconjugate components) and pupil size regulation during performance of horizontal or vertical conjugate smooth pursuit tasks ($\pm 10°$) at 0.1 Hz. The versional movements were accompanied by variable, small vergence movements that were accompanied by pupil size changes. The macroscale analysis model had a relatively poor fit to the pupil data as a function of vergence movements, accounting for <25% of the variance in the pupil size shifts [$R^2 = 0.232 \pm 0.023$ (S.E.,) compared to $R^2 = 0.51 \pm 0.03$ (S.E.) for the disparity pursuit task]. Application of the Gath-Geva algorithm identified linear segments of ocular vergence-pupil coordination with a lower R^2 value (0.400 ± 0.012 S.E.) than the vergence pursuit task (0.655 ± 0.027 S.E.), which can be seen in the "noisy" trajectory of the pupil as a function of vergence eye position in **Figure 11** (left panel, compare with **Figure 5**, left pane). The distribution of the slopes of the segments had a single peak (**Figure 11**, right panel). In terms of the divisions for the relationships during binocular fusion, 55.9% of the segments had negative slope (< −2% pupil area range per degree vergence), with a mean slope of -13.63 ± 0.65 (S.E.) pupil area range per degree vergence, an average duration of 1.86 ± 0.09 (S.E.) seconds and an average R^2 value of 0.414 ± 0.016 (S.E.). The positive slope segments (>2% pupil area range per degree vergence) constituted 27.1% of the sample, had a mean slope of 17.68 ± 1.32 (S.E.) % pupil area range per degree vergence, an average duration of 1.71 ± 0.17 (S.E.) seconds and an average R^2 value of 0.427 ± 0.023 (S.E.). Finally, the flat slope segments (between −2 and 2% pupil area range per degree vergence) constituted 17.0% of the sample, had a mean slope of

TABLE 3 | Estimated parameters for model components reflected in pupil intercept estimates for piecewise linear coordination patterns.

	Offset	Linear slope	Modulation diverging (%)	Modulation converging (%)	Phase re: stimulus (dilation re: convergence)
Near response pattern ($R^2 = 0.241$)	3.96	−0.21 /s	14.51	14.75	0.50 rad lead (796 ms lead)
Positive-slope pattern ($R^2 = 0.543$)	0.9	0.62 /s	30.88	58.18	2.98 rad lag

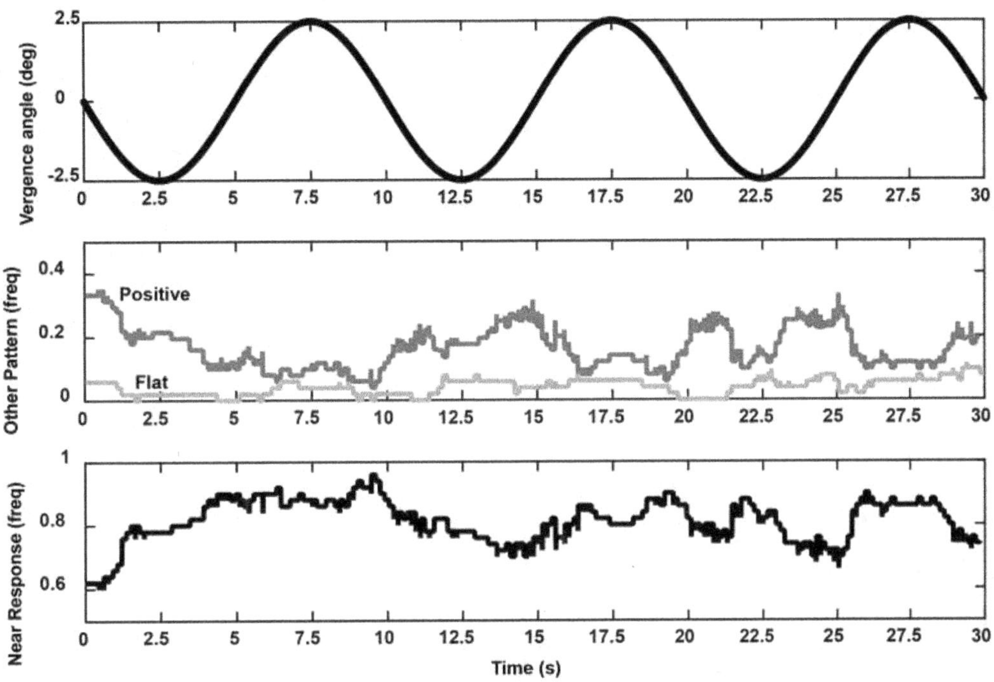

FIGURE 9 | Frequency of occurrence of a coordinated near response segment (i.e., pupil constriction-convergence/pupil dilation-divergence linear relationship, lower panel), positive slope segment (i.e., pupil dilation-convergence/pupil constriction-divergence linear relationship), or flat relationship (middle panel) during the vergence task. These summaries are taken from pooled data from all 52 subjects. The upper trace shows the stimulus pattern (divergence negative re: baseline tropia).

$-0.07\pm$ 0.10 (S.E.) % pupil area range per degree vergence, an average duration of $2.81\pm$ 0.19 (S.E.) seconds and an average R^2 value of 0.353 ± 0.027 (S.E.).

DISCUSSION

This study utilized a head-mounted virtual reality display with integrated clinical eye tracking capabilities to characterize the association between pupil activity and vergence eye movements that are generated in response to a rapid (binocular disparity step) or a gradual (sinusoidal disparity pursuit) shift in binocular disparity of small targets. Because target luminance, sharpness and size were maintained, responses were purely to binocular disparity. They did not appear during conjugate pursuit on the same device. Robust vergence eye movements were elicited by convergent and divergent motion of fixation points presented to each eye. For a disparity fusion task, the disparity between target displays to each eye shifted abruptly to require movements (convergence or divergence) to resolve diplopia. For a disparity vergence pursuit task, disparity followed a sinusoidal profile with a period of 10 s. This approach is analogous to Rashbass and Westheimer's classic studies of disjunctive eye movements (23), which used cathode ray tubes for simultaneous monocular stimuli. As in the earlier studies for higher disparity frequencies, the gradual binocular disparity was sufficient to elicit sinusoidal tracking and concurrent pupil size changes, without changing either global luminance or apparent size of the fixation points.

In terms of the model in **Figure 1**, the stimulus-related eye and pupil movements during binocular disparity stimulation are a function of (a) the eye movement vergence response to resolve the disparity and (b) the response dynamics of the pupil to the internal signal driving the vergence eye movements. The coordination between vergence eye movements and pupil area was analyzed from two perspectives, which we can term macroscale and microscale. The macroscale analysis analyzed the responses as a single continuous process, which estimates parameters for vergence eye movements, pupil area changes, and coordination of the eye and pupil movements with an implicit

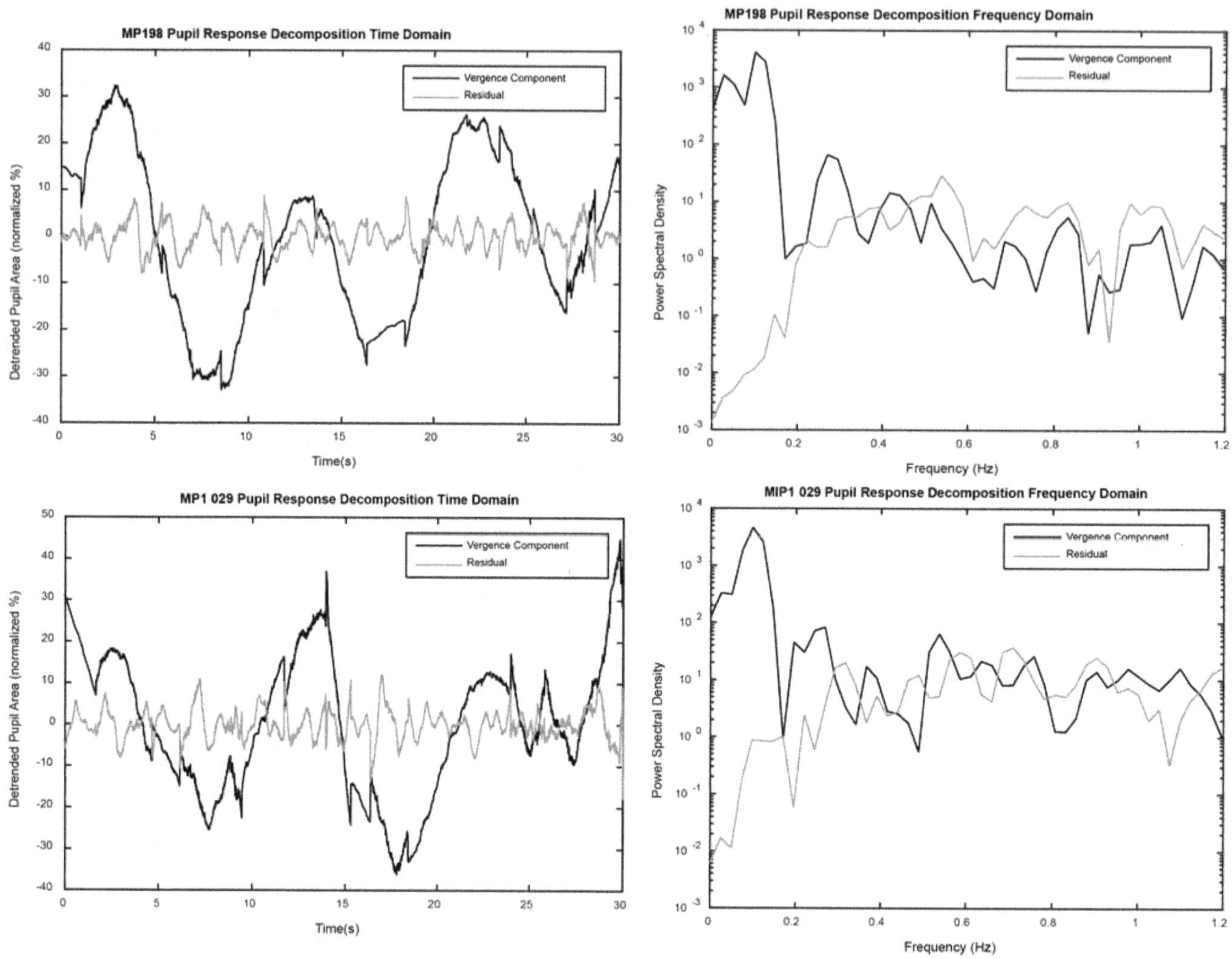

FIGURE 10 | The left panels show a decomposition of the detrended pupil data into components predicted by (1) the relationship with detrended vergence eye movements alone (black) and (2) the residual (gray). The power spectral densities for each component (right panels) were calculated with the "periodogram.m" function in MATLAB (MathWorks, Inc., Natick, MA), using a full length Hamming window and a 4,096 point fast Fourier transform.

assumption that pupil size at zero vergence remains invariant. The microscale analysis assesses the movements as a sequence of discrete epochs of coordinated activity, which includes explicit identification of (a) recalibrations of the pupil area at zero vergence and (b) epochs of synkinetic activity with different operating characteristics for pupil area adjustments in relation to vergence eye movements.

The combination of a disparity step test and a disparity smooth pursuit task at a single, low frequency permit an examination of synkinetic control in a ballistic (step) versus a pursuit task. For the ballistic movement task, the model analysis suggested that 28 ± 3% of the variance of the pupil response could be explained by modeled coordination with the vergence eye movements alone. For the pursuit task, a larger proportion (51 ± 3%) of the variance of the pupil response was explained by the pupil movements modeled from the vergence behavior. Further, the pupil sensitivity for the pursuit task (−8.13 ± 0.75 % area/° convergence) was significantly greater than for the step task (−6.51 ± 0.56 % area/° convergence). The residual activity (unrelated to dynamic ocular convergence) includes physiological hippus (15), slower pupillary fluctuations related to respiratory cycle control and/or respiratory sinus arrhythmia (16), attentional load and task experience (17). These findings motivate a more detailed study of the frequency dependence of contributions by disparity resolution control to pupil movement.

Analyses indicated that there is an active recalibration process for baseline pupil area during both binocular disparity tasks, which sets a control point for pupil aperture (area). This is obvious from stimulus cycle-to-cycle shifts of the pupil size at zero vergence in bivariate plots of pupil area as a function of the vergence angle (**Figures 4, 5**). For the disparity pursuit task, they varied weakly with eye position (**Figure 6**). The relationship between pupil area and vergence angle during a binocular disparity pursuit task also displayed epochs with two different

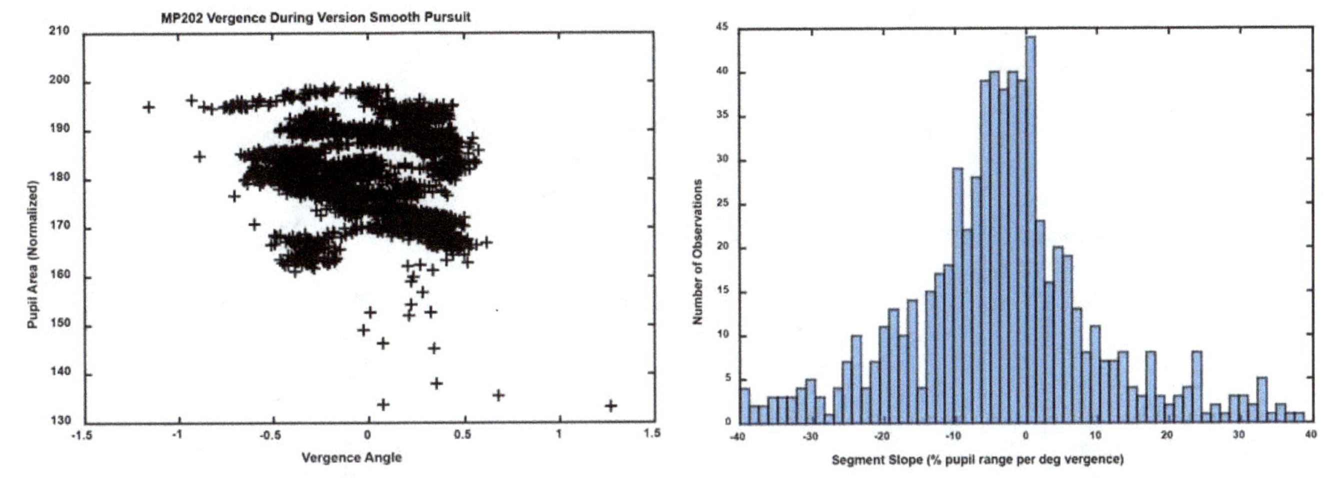

FIGURE 11 | The left panel shows the trajectory of the vergence angle and pupil area for the same unit shown in **Figure 5** (left panel). Note that the graph appears as a series of noisy quasi-linear segments, offset by differences in a pupil size set-point. The right panel shows the unimodal distribution of linear segment slopes.

patterns for coordinated pupil and vergence eye movement control, as well as infrequent epochs of independent regulation of eye movements and pupil area. The eye movement and pupil area measurements were coordinated closely more than 90% of the time during this binocular disparity-induced tracking task. These movements could be divided analytically into epochs of (1) "near response" (linear negative relationship between pupil area and vergence angle [convergence positive]), (2) positively correlated response (linear positive relationship between pupil area and vergence angle), and (3) uncorrelated response epochs. These relationships dominate bivariate plots of the instantaneous pupil size as a function of instantaneous vergence angle (e.g., **Figures 5, 8**). The tight linear correlation (average R^2 of at least 0.65) for the two former response epochs suggest that they represent distinct control modes for pupillary control during visual tracking of approaching and receding targets, governed by opposite polarities of drive from the binocular disparity control mechanism postulated in the literature (1). There are also different behavior patterns governing the pupil set-points for the linear trajectories for both the "near response" segments and the positive correlation segments, suggesting that they represent different polarity pupil area control programs during vergence tracking. Epochs of these pupillary control modes are also recognizable in the binocular disparity fusion task responses (**Figure 4**). Because the vergence eye movement responses followed stimuli with extremely high fidelity, we suggest that the apparent coordination between disparity-driven ocular and pupillary responses is produced by a real-time selection of different modes of disparity controller drives for pupillary control. This effect is unrelated to hippus, which remains when the vergence eye movement-dependent activity is subtracted from the pupil data (**Figure 10**, left panels).

The consistency and fidelity of the vergence eye movements support the view from previous studies that they reflect the output of a binocular disparity controller, which eliminates diplopia by moving the eyes to fuse the disparate stimulus features (1, 3). Previous studies have then viewed the pupillary, vergence, and lens accommodation during near responses as the result of interactions between binocular disparity and blur controllers that produce a continuous, coordinated pupillary constriction with ocular convergence and pupillary dilation with ocular divergence (1, 3). The results of this study suggest the former approach is inadequate for explaining dynamic properties of responses driven by binocular disparity in isolation. Rather, the eye movement and pupillary responses during resolution of either a step or a sinusoidal binocular disparity stimulus appear to consist of successive epochs of uncorrelated activity, coordinated near response activity (pupil constriction with convergence/dilation with divergence) and a coordinated opposite response pattern (pupillary dilation with convergence/constriction with divergence). The piecewise linearity of pupil area regulation with respect to vergence angle suggests that the controller co-regulates iris dilator and sphincter muscle activity. It seems premature to propose an alternate model from these unexpected findings. However, one may speculate (**Figure 12**) that program selection may be mediated by cerebro-ponto-cerebellar networks influencing premotor mechanisms in the supraoculomotor area (1, 18).

In a study of workers with prolonged near vision work at video displays, Ukai et al. (24) reported an adaptive increase in pupillary constriction at 0D accommodation relative to the prolonged near vision work period. Because the depth of field of the human eye varies as the reciprocal of pupil diameter (25), the modulation in the set points for pupil area regulation may be setting tolerances for blur during disparity-driven tracking. If we assume an average pupil diameter dynamic range of 2.5–8.5 mm, then the pupil area dynamic range will vary between 4.9 and 56.7 mm^2 and the midpoint of the area range (zero on the detrended normalized plots) will be 30.8 mm^2 (diameter of 6.3 mm). Hence, 10% of the range would be 5.2 mm^2. For the near response pupillary control epochs, the modulation of the pupil area operating point for each segment relative to

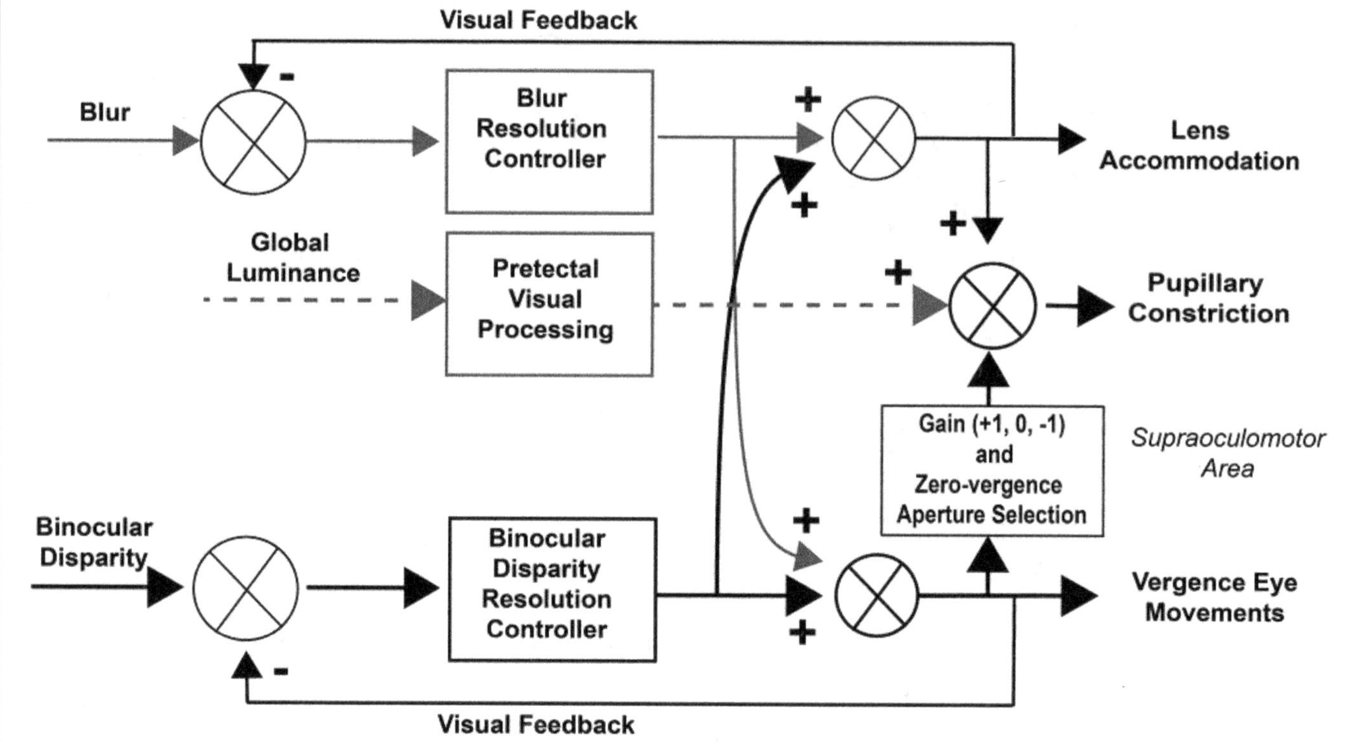

FIGURE 12 | Modified dual interaction model. This model adds a three-state gain selection switch and zero-vergence aperture reset for the influence of disparity signals on pupillary control to the basic McDoughal and Gamlin model (1), which accounts for the epochs of pupil-vergence synkinesia that are observed during 0.1 Hz binocular disparity tracking. The binocular disparity pathways are highlighted in black to mirror the selective stimulation used in this study.

initial (calibration baseline) tropia (defined as zero vergence) is relatively small (±15% pupil constriction re: 50% area during divergence) and noisy ($R^2 = 0.24$). By contrast, after the selection of a positive relationship between pupil area and vergence angle, the set points for pupil size regulation are more tightly correlated, with vergence angle relative to the initial tropia ($R^2 = 0.54$), and the magnitudes are greater. The modulation magnitudes are equivalent to $\sim\!-5.2$ mm^2 (constriction re: 50% area) during convergence and $+1.7$ mm^2 (dilation re: 50% area) during divergence. These findings suggest collectively that the near response segments and the positively correlated segments are pupillary motor programs to produce different depth of field attributes during the performance of vergence eye movements. The different epochs of correlated eye movement and pupil size activity were associated preferentially with convergent vs. divergent eye alignment. The near response segments were most prevalent when the eye alignment was convergent (relative to initial or baseline tropia), while the converse was true for the segments showing a positive correlation between pupil area and vergence angle. The segments showing flat (no correlated) relationship were infrequent and showed no clear preference for eye alignment.

The effects of variable iris diaphragm apertures on image properties are well known to expert photographers. Techniques for image *bokeh* provide insight into the utility of different motor programs for regulating both the set point and dynamic control of pupil area during disconjugate eye movements. In photography, bokeh is achieved by opening the iris diaphragm to reduce the depth of field, which produces a subtle blur of objects that are not precisely within the focal plane. This strategy establishes a subtle demarcation of figure (target) from background relationships (26). From this aperture control perspective, two features are apparent from the piecewise linear relationships between pupil area and ocular vergence. Firstly, the resetting of the "baseline" pupil size at zero vergence for each segment may set a static baseline blur of the background relative to the target for a linear variation of pupil area with vergence angle. Secondly, we observed two different scenarios for dynamic aperture effects during disparity-driven vergence. A first scenario is dilation of the pupil during divergence (a component of the "near response"). The second scenario is dilation during convergence, which is a component of the coordinated response with opposite polarity, that occurs preferentially at diverged disparity targets (about 30% of the time). Ueda et al. (27) reported that the threshold velocity for dynamic visual acuity (Landot C orientation at constant distance from subject) increased significantly in subjects after mydriasis induction with Mydrin-P (phenylephrine) eye drops. Because topical phenylephrine does not affect lens accommodation (28), the change in dynamic acuity suggests that the dilating aperture effects may increase the dynamic visual acuity range for tracking target motion when binocular disparity fusion requires divergence of the eyes.

Conversely, the dominant pattern of dynamic pupillary constriction during convergence (near response) increases depth of field and decreases blur as the eyes converge. An opposite scenario was episodic pupillary constriction with divergence, particularly when the targets were diverged from the center (positive slope pattern). From a perceptual perspective, this strategy would decrease blur and facilitate target identification. In addition, the increased depth of field would facilitate alignment of the right and left disparate targets in the face of a background. In summary, co-regulation of convergence and pupil area can be considered as control system that is useful in setting figure (target) to background relationships during dynamic tracking, with concomitant generation of blur to affect control of lens accommodation (**Figure 1**). Rather than a simple reflex, the multiple patterns of coordination suggest that we view this circuit as an interactive controller that sets an aperture effect characteristic for epochs of visual information sampling. Hence, it will be of considerable interest to investigate the occurrence of the repertoire of dynamic pupillary control patterns under viewing conditions that include blur and relative size changes of the targets.

ETHICS STATEMENT

This study was carried out in compliance with human subject ethical guidelines and regulations of United States government agencies, including Departments of Health and Human Services and the Food and Drug Administration. The protocol was approved by the Institutional Review Boards of the University of Miami (Protocol #20150286), Madigan Army Medical Center (#214005, IRBNet #393240-1) and Naval Medical Center, San Diego (#NMCSD.2013.060). All subjects gave written informed consent in accordance with the Declaration of Helsinki.

AUTHOR CONTRIBUTIONS

CB and MH contributed to design, data analysis, and writing the manuscript. MS contributed to study coordination, data collection, and writing the manuscript. AK and RA contributed to technical aspect of hardware and device software design, both for implementation and in the methods section of the manuscript.

FUNDING

This work was supported by a Head Health Challenge II Award (National Football League, UnderArmor, and General Electric).

ACKNOWLEDGMENTS

The authors gratefully acknowledge the expert assistance of Jim Buskirk, Sara Murphy, Constanza Pelusso, MD, Kathryn Marshall, PhD, Sean Wise, MD, and James Crawford, MD in subject recruitment and the conduct of the study.

SUPPLEMENTARY MATERIAL

Figure S1 | These graphs show the appearance of eye tracking data for subject MP198 during the binocular disparity pursuit task. The detrended data are shown in **Figure 2B**.

REFERENCES

1. McDougal DH, Gamlin PDR. Autonomic control of the eye. *Compr Physiol* (2015) 5:439–73. doi: 10.1002/cphy.c140014
2. Leigh RJ, Zee DS. *The Neurology of Eye Movements, 4th Edn.* New York, NY: Oxford University Press (2006).
3. Schor CM. A dynamic model of cross-coupling between accommodation and convergence: simulations of step and frequency responses. *Optomet Visual Sci.* (1992) 69:258–69. doi: 10.1097/00006324-199204000-00002
4. Fincham EF, Walton J. The reciprocal actions of accommodation and convergence. *J Physiol.* (1957) 137:488–508. doi: 10.1113/jphysiol.1957.sp005829
5. Kent PR. Convergence accommodation. *Am J Optomet Arch Am Acad Optomet.* (1958) 35:393–406. doi: 10.1097/00006324-195808000-00001
6. Krenz WC, Stark L. Systems model for pupil size effect. II. Feedback model. *Biol Cybern* (1985) 51:391–7.
7. Privitera CM, Stark LW. A binocular pupil model for simulation of relative afferent pupil defects and the swinging flashlight test. *Biol Cybern* (2006) 94:215–24. doi: 10.1007/s00422-005-0042-8
8. Stark L, Sherman PM. A servoanalytic study of the consensual pupil reflex to light. *J Neurophysiol.* (1957) 20:17–26. doi: 10.1152/jn.1957.20.1.17
9. Sun F, Krenz WC, Stark LW. A systems model for pupil size effect. I. Transient data. *Biol Cybern* (1983) 48:101–8. doi: 10.1007/BF00344393
10. Sun F, Tauchi P, Stark L. Dynamic pupillary response controlled by the pupil size effect. *Exp Neurol.* (1983) 82:313–24. doi: 10.1016/0014-4886(83)90404-1
11. Sun W, Sun F, Hung G. Neural network mosaic model for pupillary responses to spatial stimuli. *Biol Cybern* (1998) 79:131–8. doi: 10.1007/s004220050465
12. Watson AB, Yellott JI. A unified formula for light adapted pupil size. *J Vision* (2012) 12:1–16. doi: 10.1167/12.10.12
13. Marg E, Morgan MW. The pupillary near reflex: the relation of pupillary diameter to accommodation and the various components of convergence. *Am J Optomet Arch Am Acad Optomet.* (1949) 26:183–98. doi: 10.1097/00006324-194905000-00001
14. Marg E, Morgan MW. Further investigation of the pupillary near reflex. *Am J Optomet Arch Am Acad Optomet.* (1950) 27:217–25. doi: 10.1097/00006324-195005000-00001
15. Turnbull PPK, Irani N, Lim N, Phillips JR. Origins of pupillary hippus in the autonomic nervous system. *Invest Ophthalmol Visual Sci.* (2017) 58:197–203. doi: 10.1167/iovs.16-20785
16. Borgdorff P. Respiratory fluctuations in pupil size. *Am J Physiol.* (1975) 228:1094–102. doi: 10.1152/ajplegacy.1975.228.4.1094
17. Wahn B, Ferris DP, Hairston WD, König P. Pupil sizes scale with attentional load and task experience in a multiple object tracking task. *PLoS ONE* (2016) 11:e0168087. doi: 10.1371/journal.pone.0168087
18. Gamlin PDR. Neural mechanisms for the control of vergence eye movements. *Ann NY Acad Sci.* (2002) 956:264–72. doi: 10.1111/j.1749-6632.2002.tb02825.x
19. May PJ, Porter JD, Gamlin PDR. Interconnections between the primate cerebellum and midbrain near-response regions. *J Comp Neurol.* (1992) 315:98–116. doi: 10.1002/cne.903150108

20. Kersten D, Legge GE. Convergence accommodation. *J Opt Soc Am.* (1983) 73:332–8. doi: 10.1364/JOSA.73.000332
21. Abonyi J, Feil B, Nemeth S, Arva P. Modified Gath-Geva clustering for fuzzy segmentationof multivariate time series. *Fuzzy Sets Syst.* (2005) 149:39–56. doi: 10.1016/j.fss.2004.07.008
22. Bezdek JC. *Pattern Recognition with Fuzzy Objective Function Algorithms.* Nadler M, editor. New York, NY: Plenum Press (1981). doi: 10.1007/978-1-4757-0450-1
23. Rashbass C, Westheimer G. Disjunctive eye movements. *J Physiol.* (1961) 159:339–60. doi: 10.1113/jphysiol.1961.sp006812
24. Ukai K, Tsuchiya K, Ishikawa S. Induced pupillary hippus following near vision: increased occurrence in visual display unit workers. *Ergonomics* (1997) 40:1201–11. doi: 10.1080/001401397187441
25. Ogle KN, Schwartz JT. Depth of focus of the human eye. *J Opt Soc Am.* (1959) 49:273–80. doi: 10.1364/JOSA.49.000273
26. Lanman D, Raskar R, Taubin G. Modeling and synthesis of aperture effects in cameras. In: Brown P, Cunningham DW, Interrante V, McCormack J, editors. *Computational Aesthetics in Graphics, Visualization, and Imaging.* Aire-la-Ville: The Eurographics Association (2008). p. 81–8.
27. Ueda T, Nawa Y, Yukawa E, Taketani F, Hara Y. Change in dynamic visual acuity (DVA) by pupil dilation. *J Hum Fact Ergonom Soc.* (2006) 48:651–5. doi: 10.1518/001872006779166299
28. Ostrin AL, Glasser A. The effects of phenylephrine on pupil diameter and accommodation in rhesus monkeys. *Invest Ophthalmol Visual Sci.* (2004) 451:215–22. doi: 10.1167/iovs.03-0704

15

Non-Linearities in the Rod and Cone Photoreceptor Inputs to the Afferent Pupil Light Response

Pablo Alejandro Barrionuevo[1*], *J. Jason McAnany*[2], *Andrew J. Zele*[3] *and Dingcai Cao*[2*]

[1] Instituto de Investigación en Luz, Ambiente y Visión, Consejo Nacional de Investigaciones Científicas y Técnicas–Universidad Nacional de Tucumán, San Miguel de Tucumán, Argentina, [2] Department of Ophthalmology and Visual Sciences, University of Illinois at Chicago, Chicago, IL, United States, [3] Visual Science Laboratory, School of Optometry and Vision Science & Institute of Health and Biomedical Innovation, Queensland University of Technology, Brisbane, QLD, Australia

Correspondence:
Pablo Alejandro Barrionuevo
pbarrionuevo@herrera.unt.edu.ar
Dingcai Cao
dcao98@uic.edu

Purpose: To assess the nature and extent of non-linear processes in pupil responses using rod- and cone-isolating visual beat stimuli.

Methods: A four-primary photostimulating method based on the principle of silent substitution was implemented to generate rod or cone isolating and combined sinusoidal stimuli at a single component frequency (1, 4, 5, 8, or 9 Hz) or a 1 Hz beat frequency (frequency pairs: 4 + 5, 8 + 9 Hz). The component frequencies were chosen to minimize the melanopsin photoresponse of intrinsically photosensitive retinal ganglion cells (ipRGCs) such that the pupil response was primarily driven by outer retinal photoreceptor inputs. Full-field (Ganzfeld) pupil responses and electroretinograms (ERGs) were recorded to the same stimuli at two mesopic light levels (−0.9 and 0 log cd/m^2). Fourier analysis was used to derive the amplitudes and phases of the pupil and ERG responses.

Results: For the beat frequency condition, when modulation was restricted to the same photoreceptor type at the higher mesopic level (0 log cd/m^2), there was a pronounced pupil response to the 1 Hz beat frequency with the 4 + 5 Hz frequency pair and rare beat responses for the 8 + 9 Hz frequency pair. At the lower mesopic level there were few and inconsistent beat responses. When one component modulated the rod excitation and the other component modulated the cone excitation, responses to the beat frequency were rare and lower than the 1 Hz component frequency condition responses. These results were confirmed by ERG recordings.

Conclusions: There is non-linearity in both the pupil response and electroretinogram to rod and cone inputs at mesopic light levels. The presence of a beat response for modulation components restricted to a single photoreceptor type, but not for components with cross-photoreceptor types, indicates that the location of a non-linear process in the pupil pathway occurs at a retinal site earlier than where the rod and cone signals are combined, that is, at the photoreceptor level.

Keywords: retina, ERG analysis, pupil, photoreceptors cells, beats, mesopic light level, non-linearity

INTRODUCTION

The response of the pupil to radiance information, the "pupil light reflex" (PLR), is mediated by phototransduction in rods, cones and by the photopigment melanopsin that is expressed in intrinsically photosensitive retinal ganglion cells (ipRGCs) (1–4). The olivary pretectal nucleus (OPN) commands pupillary movements, and it receives afferent signals from ipRGCs (2, 5, 6). Classical PLR studies used two types of stimulation paradigms, including pulsed and flickering stimulation. The best known is the PLR to a pulse of light, in which, roughly, two main stages in the temporal domain can be identified: the transient (or phasic) stage and the tonic (or sustained) stage. This pulsed PLR paradigm has revealed that cones are prevalent in the phasic stage, while rods and melanopsin are mostly conducting the tonic response (7–9). Another approach includes analyzing pupillary responses to flickering stimulation in the frequency domain through Fourier transformation (10–12). With this approach, it is determined that melanopsin, rods, L- and M-cones provide excitatory input to the pupil pathway, whereas S-cones provide inhibitory inputs (10, 12, 13). This is consistent with the spectral characteristics of primate ipRGCs receptive fields (14), although recent studies reported inhibitory responses for M-cones inputs (15, 16). Cone contributions to the flicker pupil response summate linearly with rod and/or melanopsin contributions (11), and melanopsin is combined linearly with luminance information (L + M + S) and [(L + M) – S] chromatic signals (10). However, a non-linear "winner takes all" mechanism has been identified with predominant participation of rods and melanopsin (8, 17), and this type of mechanism seems to account for the combination of melanopsin and (L – M) chromatic signals (10). Besides this evidence, the non-linear properties of rod and cone inputs to the pupil response were rarely investigated.

A tool to study non-linear mechanisms in the afferent pupillary pathway is through beat responses, which are a signature of non-linear processing (18). When two sinusoidal stimuli of different frequencies are processed by a non-linear system a response appears with a frequency corresponding to the difference of those frequencies; this phenomenon is called a beat. Oscillations at the beat frequency therefore reveal that the system is responding non-linearly to the stimulation. Beat responses have been used to study non-linearities in the auditory system (19) and in vision for example, to study binocular interactions (20, 21).

Non-linearities in the pupil pathway have been suggested in the retina or iris muscle (22, 23). Howarth and colleagues (22) used a beat paradigm with monocular and dichoptic stimulation and inferred that the site of the non-linearity preceded the locus where signals from the two eyes are integrated. Retinal non-linearities can account for the effects of saturation and rectification in cell responses (24). Saturation is caused by the limited dynamic range of retinal cells whereas rectification causes a cell response to sinusoidal stimulation (positive or negative) to be excluded or inverted (25, 26). The presence of beats in electroretinogram (ERG) recordings, has been attributed to rectification within the outer retina (18).

The purpose of this study was to isolate non-linear processes in the afferent pupil responses to rod and cone inputs using visual beat stimuli. If a beat response is observed in both the pupil light response and electroretinogram, the origin of the non-linearities will likely be in the retina.

METHODS

Observers

Three male observers (age 24–43 years) participated in the study. All have normal color vision (assessed by the Neitz OT anomaloscope and the Farnsworth-Munsell 100-hue test). Ophthalmological examinations excluded any retinal or optic nerve condition that could affect the results. The study protocols were approved by the Institutional Review Board at University of Illinois at Chicago and adhered to the tenets of the Declaration of Helsinki.

Apparatus

A ColorDome Ganzfeld in an Espion^3 electrophysiology system (Diagnosys LLC, Lowell, MA, USA) was used for stimulus presentation. We used the "dim ring" of LEDs in the ColorDome Ganzfeld to produce light levels within mesopic range. The "dim ring" had 4 LEDs with dominant wavelengths as 470 nm ("blue"), 524 nm ("green"), 588 nm ("amber"), and 636 nm ("red") nm. The ColorDome Ganzfeld was programmed to serve as a four-primary photostimulator that could control the excitations of rods and three types of cones (S-, M-, and L-cones) independently using silent substitution (27). The cone excitations were computed based on the Smith-Pokorny cone fundamentals for the CIE 1964 10° Standard Observer (26). The cone chromaticities were described in a relative cone-troland space, which plots S/(L + M) vs. L/(L + M) (28). For an equal-energy-spectrum (*EES*) light, the L/(L + M) value is 0.667 and the S/(L + M) value is 1.0. The cone luminance is the sum of the L and M cone excitations and is specified in photopic cd/m^2. Rod excitation was computed based on the scotopic luminous efficiency function, $V'(\lambda)$, with normalization such that 1 photopic cd/m^2 of *EES* light defines rod excitation of 1 rod cd/m^2.

Since the built-in calibration provided by the Diagnosys system was based on the CIE 1931 2° standard observer, we calibrated the light outputs from the ColorDome LEDs so that we could specify stimuli in the CIE 1964 10° colorimetric system. The spectral distribution of each LED was measured with a PhotoResearch PR-670 spectroradiometer. The CIE 10° luminance of each LED at its maximum were calculated from the spectral measurements.

Pupil responses were recorded by an EyeLink II eyetracker (SR Research) at a 250 Hz sampling rate. The Espion^3 electrophysiology system controlling the ColorDome triggered the eyetracker to synchronize the stimulation presentation and recording. Full-field electroretinograms (ERGs) were recorded in the Espion^3 electrophysiology system with bandwidths of 0.3 and 300 Hz at a 2,000 Hz sampling rate using *DTL Plus* corneal electrodes, which were referred to ear clip electrodes and a wrist

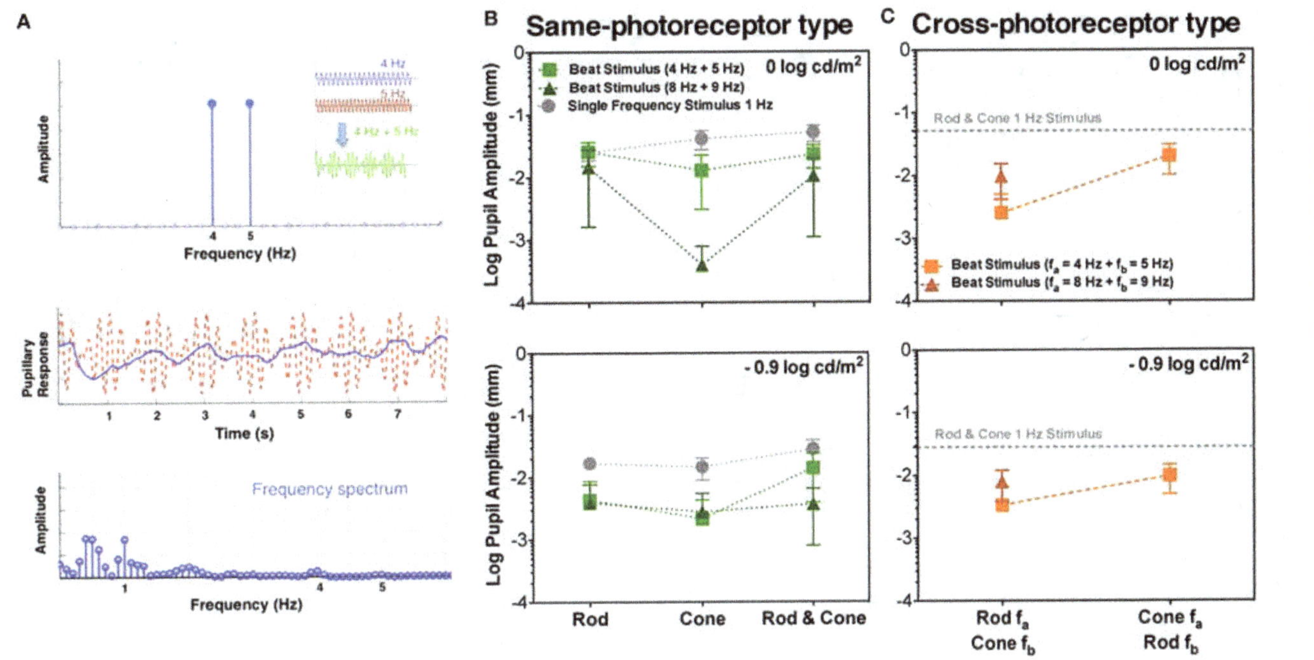

FIGURE 1 | Beats in the pupillary responses. **(A)** Linear system frequency response for combined sinusoidal stimulations at 4 and 5 Hz (top panel; temporal profile in the inset). Middle and bottom panels contain responses of S1 to Rod & Cone 4 Hz + Rod & Cone 5 Hz in the temporal and frequency domains, respectively. Averaged beat responses across participants are shown for combined 4 and 5 Hz (squares), and combined 8 and 9 Hz (triangles) in comparison with pupil responses for 1 Hz stimulation (circles) for same-photoreceptor type condition **(B)**, and Cross-photoreceptor type condition **(C)**. Error bars represent SEM.

electrode ground. Head position was maintained using a chin rest in front of the ColorDome stimulator.

Stimuli

We generated three types of photoreceptor-isolated sinusoidal stimuli at two mesopic light levels: (1) isolated rod stimuli ("Rod," only rod excitation was modulated while maintaining constant cone excitations), (2) isolated cone luminance stimuli ("Cone," only cone luminance, L + M, was modulated while maintaining constant rod excitation), and (3) combined rod and cone stimuli ("Rod & Cone," both rod and cone luminance signals were modulated in phase). To achieve a large contrast range for both the rod or cone modulations, the time-averaged chromaticity was set to $L/(L + M) = 0.77$ and $S/(L + M) = 0.20$ in a relative cone troland space (27). The time-averaged photopic luminances were -0.9 log cd/m^2 (0.13 photopic cd/m^2 or 0.10 scotopic cd/m^2 or 11 log quanta/cm^2/s) or 0 log cd/m^2 (1.0 photopic cd/m^2 or 0.82 scotopic cd/m^2 or 11.9 log quanta/cm^2/s), in order to minimize the melanopsin contribution. The low adaptation luminance was achieved by covering the ColorDome with a calibrated 0.9 log unit neutral density filter. The rod and/or cone excitations were sinusoidally modulated at 25% Michelson contrast. For pupil measurements, the stimuli were modulated at one frequency at 1, 4, 5, 8, or 9 Hz alone (i.e., component frequency condition), or at two frequencies with the same phase (i.e., beat frequency condition). The frequency pairs (4 + 5 Hz, or 8 + 9 Hz) generated a 1 Hz beat frequency, the optimal beat frequency for the pupil light response (22). A beat stimulus in the temporal domain is shown in **Figure 1A** (top panel). The component frequencies were chosen because at these frequencies, melanopsin sensitivity is minimal (29). Although the pupil response was weak, the photoreceptor response was still measureable (11). The beat stimuli could be the combination of the same photoreceptor types or different photoreceptor types (**Table 1**).

TABLE 1 | Beat conditions tested.

	Rod 4 Hz	Cone 4 Hz	Rod and Cone 4 Hz
Rod 5 Hz	Same-	Cross-	
Cone 5 Hz	Cross-	Same-	
Rod and Cone 5 Hz			Same-
	Rod 8 Hz	**Cone 8 Hz**	**Rod & Cone 8 Hz**
Rod 9 Hz	Same-	Cross-	
Cone 9 Hz	Cross-	Same-	
Rod and Cone 9 Hz			Same-

Photoreceptor type combinations assessed for 4 + 5 Hz pairs (top) and 8 + 9 Hz pairs (bottom).

Procedure: Pupil Response and ERG Recording

The pupil response and ERGs were recorded binocularly in separate sessions. Each pupil recording session started with

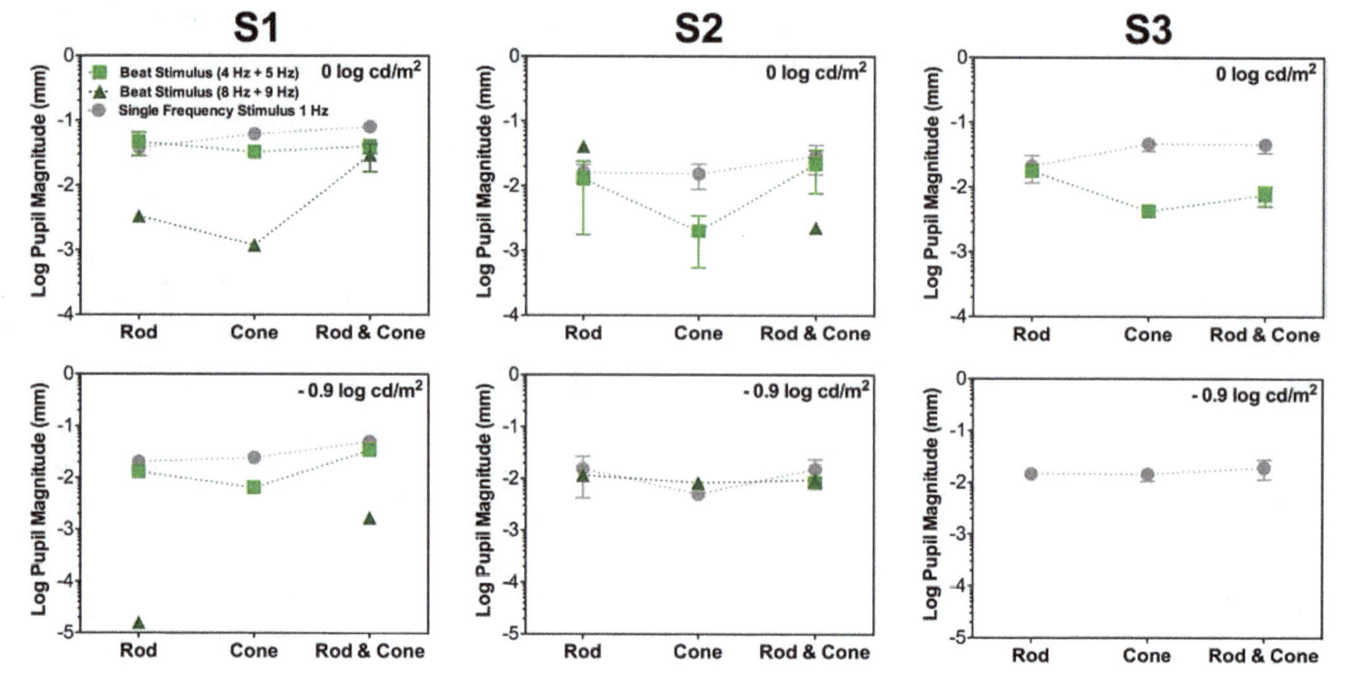

FIGURE 2 | Data for the same photoreceptor type condition for individual participants; S1 (left column), S2 (middle column), and S3 (right column). Upper panels contains data for 0 log cd/m^2, lower panels for −0.9 log cd/m^2. Error bars represents SEM. For this condition thee three participants elicited beat responses. S1's beat responses were elicited in all cases except for Cone 8 Hz + Cone 9 Hz at −0.9 log cd/m^2. For S2 (middle column), beat responses were elicited in all conditions for 4 + 5 Hz pair at 0 log cd/m^2 and only for Rod & Cone condition at −0.9 log cd/m^2. For 8 + 9 Hz pair no beat responses were obtained for Cone condition at 0 log cd/m^2. For S3 (right column), no beat responses were elicited at −0.9 log cd/m^2 or for 8 + 9 Hz stimuli at 0 log cd/m^2.

30 min of dark adaptation and included two mesopic light levels (0.9 log cd/m^2 followed by 0 log cd/m^2). For each light level, the observers adapted to a steady background for 2 min before recording. Data were collected over 10 s period for a trial with a 10 s interval between trials. Each session lasted ~1.5 h. Sufficient rest was given between conditions.

For the binocular ERG recording, both eyes were dilated with 1% tropicamide drops and dark-adapted for 15 min before ERG measurements. The same photoreceptor isolating stimuli used with the pupil recordings were used for the ERG measurements with the combination of 4 and 5 Hz frequencies. The recording procedure was similar to the pupil recordings. Individual trials that included an eye movement or blink artifact (i.e., maximum amplitude $\geq$ 200 μV) were removed automatically by the Diagnosys Espion[3] electrophysiology system or manually by the ERG technician during the recordings. Fifteen sweeps were recorded for each condition. One session lasted ~1.5 h. Each session was repeated three times on different days.

Data Analysis

For all stimulus conditions, the pupil or ERG responses from the two eyes of each observer were similar and the data from the two eyes were averaged. The averaged waveform for each condition at a light level was subjected to a discrete Fourier transformation (2,500 samples) to extract the amplitude and phase of the first harmonic. Noise for the pupil responses was estimated in the frequency domain from the component frequency conditions: 4, 5, 8, and 9 Hz, averaging the component amplitude obtained at 1 Hz in each case. For the ERG experiment, noise was estimated based on the amplitudes of a test frequency with a steady background light. The difference in the extracted amplitude and noise amplitude for each condition was computed for each observer. If the amplitude was smaller than the noise level for a condition, the amplitude for that condition was set as zero for further statistical analysis. The data were summarized as mean and standard error (SEM). Then the amplitudes with noise removed were compared using repeated measures ANOVA or paired *T*-test.

RESULTS

Pupillary Recordings

A typical pupil response of one participant obtained for the beat frequency condition with the combined Rod & Cone 4 Hz + Rod & Cone 5 Hz at 0 log cd/m^2 is shown in **Figure 1A** (middle panel for the temporal domain and bottom panel for the frequency domain). A pupillary response at the 1 Hz beat frequency is apparent when the stimulation is a combination of signals at 4 and 5 Hz; a linear system cannot produce a response at this beat frequency, indicating a non-linear process in the afferent pupil response. Average pupil amplitude responses of the 1 Hz component for the three participants at two mesopic light levels are shown in **Figures 1B,C**. Beat pupil responses were evident with the 4 + 5 Hz stimulus pairs for all photoreceptor types (Rod,

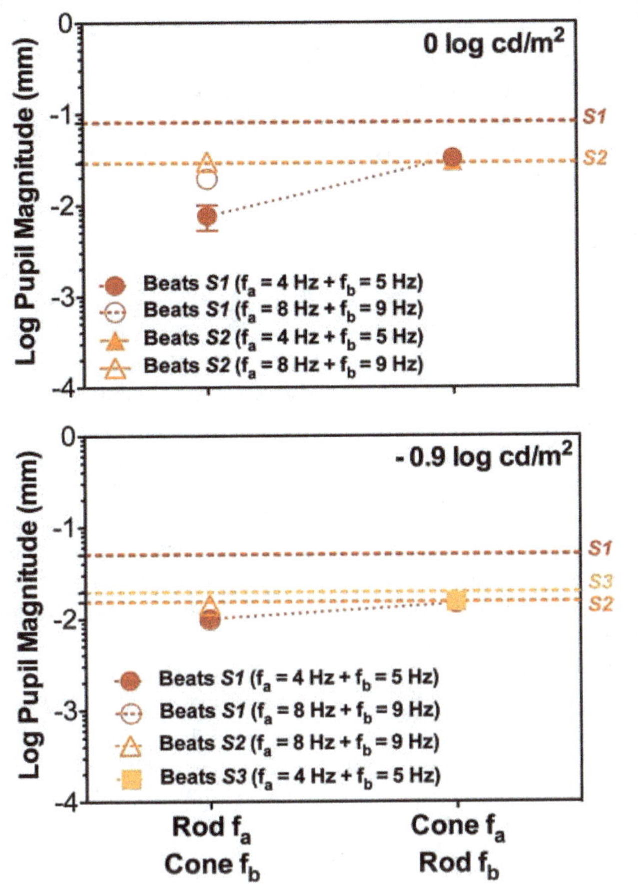

FIGURE 3 | Data for the cross photoreceptor type condition for individual participants; S1 (red circles), S2 (orange triangles), and S3 (light orange squares). Dashed lines represents the Rod & Cone 1 Hz single frequency data for each subject. Upper panel contains data for 0 log cd/m^2, lower panel for −0.9 log cd/m^2. Error bars represents SEM. Cross-photoreceptor type results were rare and reduced with respect to Rod & Cone 1 Hz data. S1's pupillary recordings showed cross beat responses for both light levels. For S2 beat responses were obtained for Rod 8 Hz combined with Cone 9 Hz at both light levels, and for combination of Cone 4 Hz and Rod 5 Hz at 0 log cd/m^2. For S3, beat responses were obtained when Cone 4 Hz was combined with Rod 5 Hz at the lower light level. Beat amplitudes for S2 and S3 were comparable to results for Rod & Cone 1 Hz stimulus.

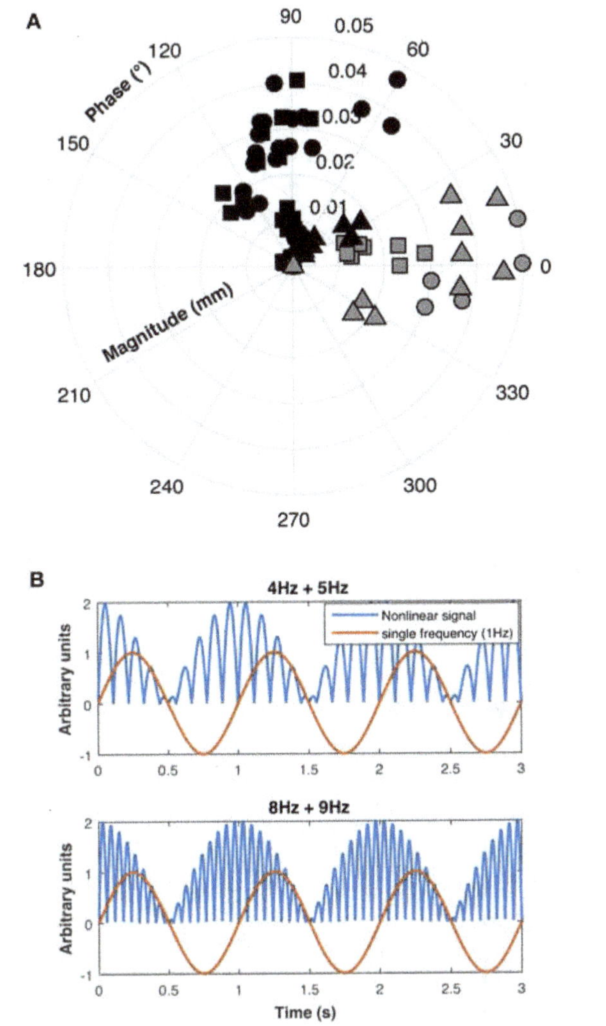

FIGURE 4 | (A) Polar plot of individual results for the three participants (S1: circles, S2: squares, and S3: triangles) for beat responses (black symbols) and single 1 Hz responses (gray symbols), **(B)** This panel shows that beat phase caused by rectification is shifted 90° with respect to single frequency phase.

Cone, or Rod & Cone) in the three participants at 0 log cd/m^2, and only for S1 at −0.9 log cd/m^2 (square symbols, **Figure 2**). Rod-Cone phase differences were similar for the beat frequency condition (15.74 ± 7.03°) and component frequency condition [10.94 ± 3.66°, $t_{(4)} = 0.605$, $p = 0.58$].

Considering the different photoreceptor combinations at 8 and 9 Hz at 0 log cd/m^2 (**Figure 1B**, upper panel), the averaged beat responses were present for participants S1 and S2 only (**Figure 2**). At lower light level, the amplitude of the responses were reduced and the differences between beat responses and single frequency responses were not significant for the three photoreceptor combinations, $F_{(2,12)} = 2.95$, $p = 0.128$ (**Figure 1B**, lower panel). Individual results showed very small or null responses with the three combinations for participant S1 and null responses for S3 (**Figure 2**).

Finally, beat stimuli modulating the cross photoreceptor types elicited beat responses in few cases (**Figures 1C, 3**). Participant S1's pupillary recordings showed beat responses for both light levels, however, for S2, beat responses were obtained for the Rod 8 Hz combined with Cone 9 Hz at both light levels, and for combination of Cone 4 Hz and Rod 5 Hz at 0 log cd/m^2, whereas, S3's beat responses were obtained when Cone 4 Hz was combined with Rod 5 Hz at the lower light level (**Figure 3**). No response were obtained for Cone 8 Hz + Rod 9 Hz at both light levels for any participant (**Figures 1C, 3**).

A polar plot of the pupillary responses of the three participants are shown in **Figure 4A**. The phase of the beat responses are shifted 90° with respect to the single frequency response phases, which is evidence for a non-linearity in the pupillary signal processing, possibly due to rectification which introduces a similar phase shift between the beat and component frequencies (**Figure 4B**).

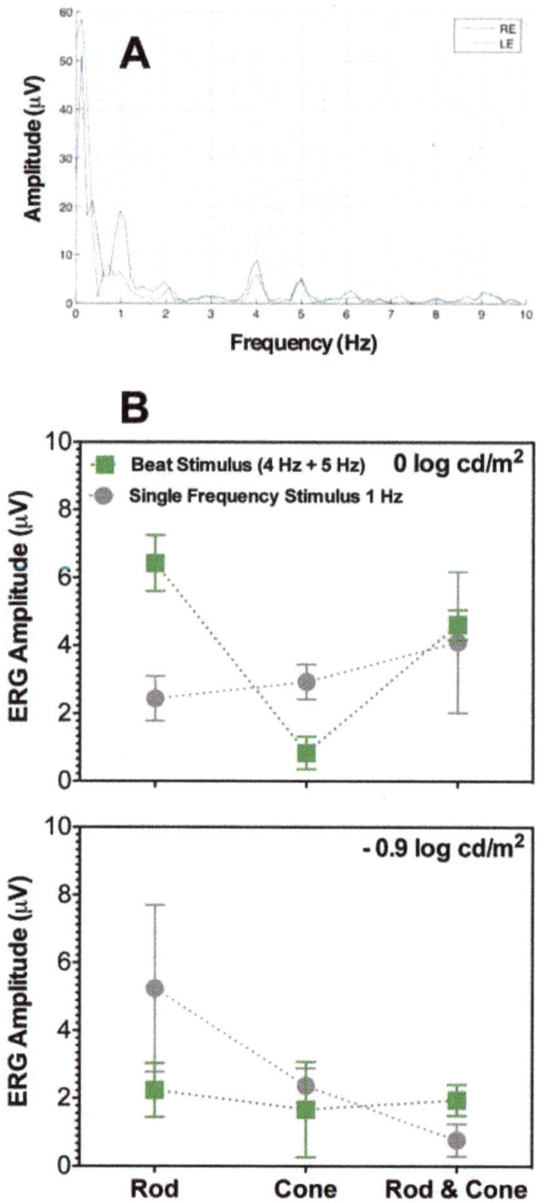

FIGURE 5 | Beats in ERG recordings. **(A)** Frequency beat response of S1 to Rod & Cone 4 Hz + Rod & Cone 5 Hz condition. **(B)** Averaged beat responses for combined 4 and 5 Hz (squares) in comparison with results for single 1 Hz stimulation. Error bars represent SEM.

ERG Recordings

To determine if beat responses observed in pupillary measurements occurred at the retinal level, a second experiment was conducted by obtaining the ERG recordings of the three participants using similar stimuli modulations (4 Hz + 5 Hz) for the same-photoreceptor types.

The frequency profile of the ERG amplitudes for participant S1 at 0 log cd/m^2 for the combined Rod & Cone 4 Hz + Rod & Cone 5 Hz condition (**Figure 5A**) shows clear peaks appear at 1, 4, and 5 Hz. Beat ERG responses were obtained for most cases.

Figure 5B shows the averaged results for the three participants. At both 0 log cd/m^2 (**Figure 5B**, upper panel) and −0.9 log cd/m^2 (**Figure 5B**, lower panel), the beat responses were similar to the single frequency responses [$F_{(1,8)} = 0.85$, $p = 0.4$; $F_{(1,8)} = 0.5$, $p = 0.52$; respectively]. The pattern of the ERG data was generally consistent with the pupillary responses.

DISCUSSION

Substantial pupillary beat responses were obtained for combined sinusoidal stimulations at 4 Hz and 5 Hz of the same-photoreceptor type (Rod 4 Hz + Rod 5 Hz, Cone 4 Hz + Cone 5 Hz, and Rod & Cone 4 Hz + Rod & Cone 5 Hz) at the higher mesopic light level (0 log cd/m^2), and were consistent across participants. Beat responses observed in the 4 + 5 Hz pupil response were similarly obtained in ERG recordings, confirming that non-linearities are present at the retinal level. According the analysis of the phase difference between beat data and single 1 Hz data (**Figure 4**), a rectification process may be involved. At the lower mesopic light level, the beat responses were inconsistent, likely because at this illumination level the signal-to-noise ratios are decreased and the cones are at the lower end of their operating range. This was also evident for the same-photoreceptor combination type with the 8 and 9 Hz stimulation (at both light levels). A similar outcome was observed for the cross-photoreceptor type condition. However, for participant S1 beat responses were obtained in most cases, meaning that individual differences are important in retinal non-linearities to elicit beat responses. Individual differences as those found in our study can emerge from many sources, such as fatigue, emotional states, other sensory inputs and refractive errors (30, 31). It will be interesting to investigate this issue in the future.

A previous study evaluating pupillary beat responses used higher frequency stimuli in the range of 10–25 Hz (22). These authors claimed this frequency range is optimal for binocular conditions, however we found strong beats in the 4–5 Hz range and weaker beat responses in the range of 8–9 Hz. It is known that the flicker pupil light response has a cut-off resolution frequency in the order of ~8–9 Hz (11, 32–34), but other factors, such as the conditions in which the experiments were carried out could explain this difference. They used a brighter photopic background (~15,000 photopic td) compared to our dimmer mesopic lighting (~10 photopic td), had a higher modulation depth (~80 vs. 25% for this study), and used broadband lights. As such, we observed beat responses for same-photoreceptor type condition, and the amplitude of the beat response could be larger with higher light levels for cones activation. We did not run experiments for source frequencies higher than 9 Hz, so we cannot rule out the appearance of beats at higher frequencies as those used by Howarth and colleagues (22). More research is needed to understand the relationship between light level and the optimal frequency range to modulate non-linear responses.

Since the discovery of intrinsically photosensitive retinal ganglion cells (ipRGCs) in mammals (5, 14, 35), understanding of the retinal circuit to control pupillary response to light has been advanced. From the five types of ipRGCs detected in the rodent retina (36, 37), M1 cells disproportionally innervate the OPN (5, 38). In primate retinas, outer cells are the counterparts of the rodent M1 cells (39). Outer cells have their dendrites in the OFF sublamina of the interplexiform layer near the inner nuclear layer and are innervated by bipolar and amacrine cells (40, 41). It was suggested that diffuse bipolars DB6 convey excitatory inputs to L and M cones, while dopaminergic amacrines convey major inhibitory signals (10, 40, 42). Considering the pathways conveying rods signals, it was shown that there is no direct innervation of rod bipolar cell to ipRGCs (39). In primates rod and cone signals are combined at the outer retina through the rod-cone gap junction pathway, at the inner retina through the rod->rod bipolar->AII amacrine->cone bipolar pathway, and potentially through horizontal cells feedback between photoreceptors (43, 44). For pupillary responses it was suggested that the most probable pathway to activate phasic pupillary movements is via rod-cone gap junctions->DB6 bipolar cells (10).

Our results showed weaker and more sparse beats in the cross-photoreceptor type condition than in the same-photoreceptor type condition. Therefore, same-photoreceptor non-linear processing produced stronger signals (able to evoke pupillary movements) than cross-photoreceptor non-linear processing, which in turn means that the non-linearities occur before rod and cone signals interact. Since beat responses were also obtained in the ERG measurements, which are predominantly mediated by photoreceptors and bipolar cells, the candidate locus of the non-linearity is in the photoreceptoral (rod and cone) level or bipolar cell level.

Since we did not find consistent beat responses in the cross photoreceptor type condition, we cannot make further inferences about the presence of non-linear rod-cone interactions. In this work we examined beats for sinusoidal stimuli with same phase. A possible way to analyze rod-cone interactions is by systematically changing the phase difference between the rod and cone photoreceptor modulations, in conditions where beat responses are elicited. The presence of non-linear pupil responses in the outer retina may have applications in the study of retinal degenerations involving rods and/or cones, with different diseases (e.g., Retinitis pigmentosa, age-related macular degeneration) expected to have different signature beats depending on the degree of photoreceptor degeneration.

AUTHOR CONTRIBUTIONS

PB and DC conceived, designed and performed the experiments, and wrote the manuscript. JM and AZ critically revised the manuscript. All authors approved the final manuscript version.

ACKNOWLEDGMENTS

Agencia Nacional de Promoción Científica y Tecnológica PICT 2016-3312 (PB). Consejo Nacional de Investigaciones Cientificas y Técnicas P-UE 0114 ILAV (PB). Australian Research Council Discovery Projects ARC-DP170100274 (AZ and DC) and Australian Research Council Future Fellowship ARC-FT180100458 (AZ). National Institutes of Health research grant R01EY026004 (JM), UIC core grant for vision research P30-EY001792, Unrestricted Departmental Grant (DC, JM), and a Dolly Green Scholar award (JM) from the Research to Prevent Blindness.

REFERENCES

1. Gamlin PD, McDougal DH, Pokorny J, Smith VC, Yau K-W, Dacey DM. Human and macaque pupil responses driven by melanopsin-containing retinal ganglion cells. *Vision Res.* (2007) 47:946–54. doi: 10.1016/j.visres.2006.12.015
2. Guler AD, Ecker JL, Lall GS, Haq S, Altimus CM, Liao H-W, et al. Melanopsin cells are the principal conduits for rod/cone input to non-image forming vision. *Nature* (2008) 453:102–5. doi: 10.1038/nature06829
3. Hattar S, Lucas RJ, Mrosovsky N, Thompson S, Douglas RH, Hankins MW, et al. Melanopsin and rod–cone photoreceptive systems account for all major accessory visual functions in mice. *Nature* (2003) 424:75–81. doi: 10.1038/nature01761
4. Panda S, Provencio I, Tu DC, Pires SS, Rollag MD, Castrucci AM, et al. Melanopsin is required for non-image-forming photic responses in blind mice. *Science* (2003) 301:525–7. doi: 10.1126/science.1086179
5. Hattar S, Liao H-W, Takao M, Berson DM, Yau K-W. Melanopsin-containing retinal ganglion cells: architecture, projections, and intrinsic photosensitivity. *Science* (2002) 295:1065–70. doi: 10.1126/science.1069609
6. Viney TJ, Balint K, Hillier D, Siegert S, Boldogkoi Z, Enquist LW, et al. Local retinal circuits of melanopsin-containing ganglion cells identified by transsynaptic viral tracing. *Curr Biol.* (2007) 17:981–8. doi: 10.1016/j.cub.2007.04.058
7. Adhikari P, Zele AJ, Feigl B. The Post-Illumination Pupil Response (PIPR). *Invest Opthalmol Vis Sci.* (2015) 56:3838–49. doi: 10.1167/iovs.14-16233
8. McDougal DH, Gamlin PD. The influence of intrinsically photosensitive retinal ganglion cells on the spectral sensitivity and response dynamics of the human pupillary light reflex. *Vision Res.* (2010) 50:72–87. doi: 10.1016/j.visres.2009.10.012
9. Park JC, Moura AL, Raza AS, Rhee DW, Kardon RH, Hood DC. Toward a clinical protocol for assessing rod, cone, and melanopsin contributions to the human pupil response. *Invest Ophthalmol Vis Sci.* (2011) 52:6624–35. doi: 10.1167/iovs.11-7586
10. Barrionuevo PA, Cao D. Luminance and chromatic signals interact differently with melanopsin activation to control the pupil light response. *J Vis.* (2016) 16:29. doi: 10.1167/16.11.29
11. Barrionuevo PA, Nicandro N, McAnany JJ, Zele AJ, Gamlin P, Cao D. Assessing rod, cone, and melanopsin contributions to human pupil flicker responses. *Invest Ophthalmol Vis Sci.* (2014) 55:719–27. doi: 10.1167/iovs.13-13252
12. Spitschan M, Jain S, Brainard DH, Aguirre GK. Opponent melanopsin and S-cone signals in the human pupillary light response. *Proc Natl Acad Sci USA.* (2014) 111:15568–72. doi: 10.1073/pnas.1400942111
13. Cao D, Nicandro N, Barrionuevo PA. A five-primary photostimulator suitable for studying intrinsically photosensitive retinal ganglion cell functions in humans. *J Vis.* (2015) 15:27. doi: 10.1167/15.1.27
14. Dacey DM, Liao H-W, Peterson BB, Robinson FR, Smith VC, Pokorny J, et al. Melanopsin-expressing ganglion cells in primate retina signal colour and irradiance and project to the LGN. *Nature* (2005) 433:749–754. doi: 10.1038/nature03387
15. Woelders T, Leenheers T, Gordijn MCM, Hut RA, Beersma DGM, Wams EJ. Melanopsin- and L-cone–induced pupil constriction is inhibited by S- and M-cones in humans. *Proc Natl Acad Sci USA.* (2018) 115:792–7. doi: 10.1073/pnas.1716281115

16. Murray IJ, Kremers J, McKeefry D, Parry NRA. Paradoxical pupil responses to isolated M-cone increments. *JOSA A* (2018) 35:B66–71. doi: 10.1364/JOSAA.35.000B66
17. Lall GS, Revell VL, Momiji H, Al Enezi J, Altimus CM, Güler AD, et al. Distinct contributions of rod, cone, and melanopsin photoreceptors to encoding irradiance. *Neuron* (2010) 66:417–28. doi: 10.1016/j.neuron.2010.04.037
18. Burns SA, Elsner AE, Kreitz MR. Analysis of nonlinearities in the flicker ERG. *Optom Vis Sci.* (1992) 69:95–105. doi: 10.1097/00006324-199202000-00002
19. Wever EG. Beats and related phenomena resulting from the simultaneous sounding of two tones: I. *Psychol Rev.* (1929) 36:402–18. doi: 10.1037/h0072876
20. Baitch LW, Levi DM. Evidence for nonlinear binocular interactions in human visual cortex. *Vision Res.* (1988) 28:1139–43. doi: 10.1016/0042-6989(88)90140-X
21. Baitch LW, Levi DM. Binocular beats: psychophysical studies of binocular interaction in normal and stereoblind humans. *Vision Res.* (1989) 29:27–35. doi: 10.1016/0042-6989(89)90171-5
22. Howarth PA, Bailey IL, Berman SM, Heron G, Greenhouse DS. Location of nonlinear processes within the pupillary pathway. *Appl Opt.* (1991) 30:2100–5. doi: 10.1364/AO.30.002100
23. Milton J. Pupil light reflex: delays and oscillations. In: *Nonlinear Dynamics in Physiology and Medicine Interdisciplinary Applied Mathematics.* New York, NY: Springer (2003). p. 271–301.
24. Demb JB. Functional circuitry of visual adaptation in the retina. *J Physiol.* (2008) 586:4377. doi: 10.1113/jphysiol.2008.156638
25. Demb JB, Zaghloul K, Haarsma L, Sterling P. Bipolar cells contribute to nonlinear spatial summation in the brisk-transient (Y) ganglion cell in mammalian retina. *J Neurosci.* (2001) 21:7447–54. doi: 10.1523/JNEUROSCI.21-19-07447.2001
26. Spekreijse H. Rectification in the goldfish retina: analysis by sinusoidal and auxiliary stimulation. *Vision Res.* (1969) 9:1461–72. doi: 10.1016/0042-6989(69)90062-5
27. Shapiro AG, Pokorny J, Smith VC. Cone-rod receptor spaces with illustrations that use CRT phosphor and light-emitting-diode spectra. *J Opt Soc Am A Opt Image Sci Vis.* (1996) 13:2319–28. doi: 10.1364/JOSAA.13.002319
28. Smith VC, Pokorny J. The design and use of a cone chromaticity space: a tutorial. *Color Res Appl.* (1996) 21:375–83. doi: 10.1002/(SICI)1520-6378(199610)21:5<375::AID-COL6>3.0.CO;2-V
29. Zele AJ, Feigl B, Adhikari P, Maynard ML, Cao D. Melanopsin photoreception contributes to human visual detection, temporal and colour processing. *Sci Rep.* (2018) 8:3842. doi: 10.1038/s41598-018-22197-w
30. Loewenfeld IE, Lowenstein O. *The Pupil: Anatomy, Physiology, and Clinical Applications.* Detroit: Iowa State University Press (1993).
31. Winn B, Whitaker D, Elliott DB, Phillips NJ. Factors affecting light-adapted pupil size in normal human subjects. *Invest Ophthalmol Vis Sci.* (1994) 35:1132–7.
32. Webster JG, Heller SL. Modeling the pupillary light reflex at higher frequencies. In *Proc. Annu. Conf. Engineering in Medicine and Biology.* Vol. 10 (1968).
33. Clarke RJ, Zhang H, Gamlin PDR. Characteristics of the pupillary light reflex in the alert rhesus monkey. *J Neurophysiol.* (2003) 89:3179–89. doi: 10.1152/jn.01131.2002
34. Joyce DS, Feigl B, Cao D, Zele AJ. Temporal characteristics of melanopsin inputs to the human pupil light reflex. *Vision Res.* (2015) 107:58–66. doi: 10.1016/j.visres.2014.12.001
35. Berson DM, Dunn FA, Takao M. Phototransduction by retinal ganglion cells that set the circadian clock. *Science* (2002) 295:1070–3. doi: 10.1126/science.1067262
36. Berson DM. Intrinsically photosensitive retinal ganglion cells. In: Werner JS, Chalupa LM, editors. *The New Visual Neurosciences.* Cambridge, MA: The MIT Press (2014). p. 183–96.
37. Feigl B, Zele AJ. Melanopsin-expressing intrinsically photosensitive retinal ganglion cells in retinal disease: *Optom Vis Sci.* (2014) 91:894–903. doi: 10.1097/OPX.0000000000000284
38. Hattar S, Kumar M, Park A, Tong P, Tung J, Yau K-W, et al. Central projections of melanopsin-expressing retinal ganglion cells in the mouse. *J Comp Neurol.* (2006) 497:326–49. doi: 10.1002/cne.20970
39. Liao H-W, Ren X, Peterson BB, Marshak DW, Yau K-W, Gamlin PD, et al. Melanopsin-expressing ganglion cells on macaque and human retinas form two morphologically distinct populations. *J Comp Neurol.* (2016) 524:2845–72. doi: 10.1002/cne.23995
40. Grünert U, Jusuf PR, Lee SC, Nguyen DT. Bipolar input to melanopsin containing ganglion cells in primate retina. *Vis Neurosci.* (2011) 28:39–50. doi: 10.1017/S095252381000026X
41. Jusuf PR, Lee SCS, Hannibal J, Grünert U. Characterization and synaptic connectivity of melanopsin-containing ganglion cells in the primate retina. *Eur J Neurosci.* (2007) 26:2906–21. doi: 10.1111/j.1460-9568.2007.05924.x
42. Neumann S, Haverkamp S, Auferkorte ON. Intrinsically photosensitive ganglion cells of the primate retina express distinct combinations of inhibitory neurotransmitter receptors. *Neuroscience* (2011) 199:24–31. doi: 10.1016/j.neuroscience.2011.10.027
43. Grimes WN, Songco-Aguas A, Rieke F. Parallel processing of rod and cone signals: retinal function and human perception. *Annu Rev Vis Sci.* (2018) 4:123–41. doi: 10.1146/annurev-vision-091517-034055
44. Zele AJ, Cao D. Vision under mesopic and scotopic illumination. *Front Psychol.* (2015) 5:1594. doi: 10.3389/fpsyg.2014.01594

16

Melanopsin Retinal Ganglion Cells and Pupil: Clinical Implications for Neuro-Ophthalmology

Chiara La Morgia[1,2]*, *Valerio Carelli*[1,2] *and Michele Carbonelli*[1]

[1] *Unità Operativa Complessa Clinica Neurologica, IRCCS Istituto delle Scienze Neurologiche di Bologna, Ospedale Bellaria, Bologna, Italy,* [2] *Dipartimento di Scienze Biomediche e Neuromotorie, Università di Bologna, Bologna, Italy*

Correspondence:
Chiara La Morgia
chiara.lamorgia@unibo.it

Melanopsin retinal ganglion cells (mRGCs) are intrinsically photosensitive RGCs that mediate many relevant non-image forming functions of the eye, including the pupillary light reflex, through the projections to the olivary pretectal nucleus. In particular, the post-illumination pupil response (PIPR), as evaluated by chromatic pupillometry, can be used as a reliable marker of mRGC function *in vivo*. In the last years, pupillometry has become a promising tool to assess mRGC dysfunction in various neurological and neuro-ophthalmological conditions. In this review we will present the most relevant findings of pupillometric studies in glaucoma, hereditary optic neuropathies, ischemic optic neuropathies, idiopathic intracranial hypertension, multiple sclerosis, Parkinson's disease, and mood disorders. The use of PIPR as a marker for mRGC function is also proposed for other neurodegenerative disorders in which circadian dysfunction is documented.

Keywords: melanopsin retinal ganglion cells, light, pupil, neurodegeneration, optic nerve, optic neuropathies, Alzheimer, Parkinson

INTRODUCTION

Melanopsin retinal ganglion cells (mRGCs) are intrinsically photosensitive RGCs expressing the photopigment melanopsin (1, 2). They constitute about 0.2–1% of total RGCs and contribute to the photoentrainment of circadian rhythms, through their projections to the suprachiasmatic nucleus (SCN), but also to other anatomical structures devoted to non-image forming functions of the eye. These include pupil regulation through their projections to the olivary pretectal nucleus (OPN) in the midbrain (3–5) and brain structures relevant for emotional processing (6). Recent data support the notion that distinct subpopulations of mRGCs mediate different functions in the central nervous system, including circadian rhythm regulation and pupil light reflex (PLR) through their projections to the OPN (5, 7).

The mRGC contribution to the pupil function has been extensively investigated over the recent years and it is now clear that rods mediate mainly the transient pupil contraction, whereas mRGCs contribute to the steady-state pupil constriction (8–11). In fact, mRGCs are characterized by a unique property, which is the capability of firing without fatigue in response to continuous stimulation, consistent with the intrinsic activation of these cells (12). In particular, post-illumination pupil response (PIPR), measured after 1.7 s from onset of the light stimulus, and its magnitude can be considered as specific measures of mRGC function (13). Different protocols, using different light paradigms and experimental setting of stimulation, have been tested and now established to assess *in vivo* PLR mediated by mRGCs (13, 14). Specifically, the contribution of mRGCs to pupil response has been evaluated using blue (470 nm) and red (640 nm) light, being the blue light able to maximally stimulating mRGCs (13–15).

The PLR mediated by mRGCs has been investigated in different ophthalmological conditions including glaucoma (16–18), retinitis pigmentosa (19), diabetes (20), Leber's congenital amaurosis (14), age-related macular degeneration (21), and ischemic optic neuropathies (22, 23). Moreover, various neurological and psychiatric disorders have been evaluated, including hereditary optic neuropathies (24–29), seasonal affective disorder (SAD) (30), idiopathic intracranial hypertension (IIH) (31, 32), multiple sclerosis (MS) (33), and Parkinson's disease (PD) (34).

In this review we will focus on pupillometry findings in neuro-ophthalmological disorders in which pupil and circadian functions have been investigated. In particular, we include disorders affecting the optic nerve such as glaucoma and hereditary optic neuropathies, neurodegenerative disorders with optic nerve involvement and circadian dysfunction and affective disorders for which a relevant role of mRGCs has been postulated. We will highlight the potential role of mRGC-mediated pupil function as an *in vivo* objective tool and possible biomarker for evaluating mRGC function in different neurodegenerative disorders.

MELANOPSIN RGCs AND PUPIL IN GLAUCOMA AND ANTERIOR ISCHEMIC OPTIC NEUROPATHY

Glaucoma is a chronic optic neuropathy characterized by loss of peripheral visual field secondary to a progressive and extensive loss of RGCs and their optic nerve fibers (35). The pathophysiology of glaucoma is not yet completely understood, even though two common and pivotal events are the increase in intraocular pressure and impaired microcirculation (vascular deregulation), both preceding the RGC death (36). Previous studies in monkey models of glaucoma reported that all classes of RGCs are susceptible to injury or damage since the early stages of the disease including the sub-population of mRGCs (37). Concordantly, recent clinical studies have shown high prevalence of sleep and circadian disorders, as well as depression in glaucoma patients, implying that the mRGC-driven photoentrainment of circadian rhythms may be affected in patients with glaucoma (38–41).

In the last years, several studies were published aimed at measuring *in vivo* the integrity of mRGC system in glaucoma by assessing the PLR (16–18). Overall, the results and the conclusions of these studies have been frequently inconsistent because of the different protocols and methodology adopted for chromatic pupillography. In fact, many variables may affect the results, such as time of dark adaptation, light stimulus (duration, intensity, and wavelength), time to measure the intrinsic melanopsin-mediated PIPR, direct or consensual pupil stimulation, and so on (see **Table 1**).

Nonetheless, it is now clearly proven that the PLR, and particularly the PIPR, is altered in moderate and advanced stages of glaucoma, despite the use of different chromatic illumination paradigms (16–18, 27, 42, 43). These findings are also correlated with functional and structural features of the glaucomatous pathology, as demonstrated by the fact that PIPR is inversely correlated with the mean deviation in the visual fields (17, 42, 43). Moreover, an inverse correlation between PLR to high-irradiance blue light and optic disc cupping measured by Heidelberg Retinal Tomography was found (42), and the reduction of PLR to blue and red light correlates with retinal nerve fiber layer (RNFL) thinning (44, 45). These results are in line with a study demonstrating that there is a correlation between the severity of the glaucoma and the reduction of the PIPR (16). This is concordant with the knowledge that in glaucoma the central 10 degrees of the retina, where the mRGCs are more concentrated, are affected only in the last stages of the disease. However, in the last 2 years, a new method of light delivery (quadrant field pupillometry) (44), and a new light stimulation protocol (increasing light regimens) (45) were used to better investigate the pre-perimetric and early-stage glaucoma. By stimulating only the portion of the retina most precociously affected in glaucoma it was shown that the superonasal quadrant PIPR differentiates patients suspected of having glaucoma and with early glaucoma from healthy controls, and this finding correlated with RNFL thinning measured by OCT (44). Furthermore, by increasing logarithmically the light stimuli intensity, PLR is reduced in patients with early-stage glaucoma compared with controls at moderate to high irradiances with both blue and red light, and the maximal pupillary constriction amplitude is correlated to the RNFL thickness (45). To highlight the possible correlation of different measurements of mRGC functions, it is also worth mentioning that in advanced glaucoma, individuals with greater light-induced melatonin suppression (a measure of the retino-hypothalamic tract function) have also a smaller PIPR (27).

Finally, a functional damage of the mRGC-mediated PLR has been reported in the affected eyes of patients with unilateral or bilateral anterior ischemic optic neuropathy (AION), specifically 10 patients with unilateral non-arteritic ischemic optic neuropathy (NAION), 1 bilateral NAION, and 7 patients with bilateral AION associated with optic disc drusen, compared to the unaffected and control eyes (22). Differently, previous studies failed to demonstrate differences in the PLR between NAION and control eyes (23). Furthermore, if the bright blue stimuli were presented bilaterally and simultaneously to both eyes, bilateral AION patients showed, through binocular summation, the same post-stimulus pupil size of patients with unilateral AION and controls (22).

MELANOPSIN RGCs AND PUPIL IN HEREDITARY MITOCHONDRIAL OPTIC NEUROPATHIES

Mitochondrial optic neuropathies are inherited disorders of the optic nerve due to mitochondrial DNA (mtDNA) mutations affecting the mitochondrial-encoded subunits of complex I of the respiratory chain complex, pathogenic for Leber's hereditary Optic Neuropathy (LHON) or to mutations of the nuclear gene *OPA1* causing Dominant Optic Atrophy (DOA) (46, 47). These inherited mitochondrial disorders are characterized by the selective loss of RGCs, in particular those originating the

TABLE 1 | Pupillometry findings in glaucoma and in anterior ischemic optic neuropathy.

	Population	PLR Methods	Main findings
Kankipati et al. (17)	16 glaucoma patients 19 healthy controls	10 s light stimulus of blue (470 nm) or red (623 nm) to one eye after dilation (60°). Consensual PIPR: average pupil diameter over a period of 30 s, starting 10 s after light offset minus baseline pupil diameter	Patients net PIPR (blue PIPR minus red PIPR) was significantly smaller than in controls and inversely correlated with the MD in visual field of the tested eye
Feigl et al. (16)	25 glaucoma patients 16 healthy controls	10 s blue (488 nm) and red (610 nm) stimuli presented to the right eye, and the consensual pupil response of the left eye was measured (7°) PIPR: average pupil diameter 20–50 s after light offset	The blue PIPR was significantly smaller between controls and patients with advanced glaucoma, as well as between early and advanced glaucoma patients
Nissen et al. (18)	11 unilateral glaucoma patients 11 healthy controls	10 s of darkness (baseline pupil), 20 s of exposure stimulus (red-660 nm and blue-470 nm) and 50 s of darkness (post-exposure). The area under the curve (AUC) of consensual pupil was calculated for: (1) during the 20 s of light-on, (2) during the first 10 s after light was turned off and (3) from 10 to 30 s after light was turned off (AUC30–50 s)	The pupillary response to blue light was decreased in the glaucomatous eyes of unilateral glaucoma. In the unaffected eyes, the pupillary response to blue light did not differ from that of healthy controls
Rukmini et al. (42)	40 glaucoma patients 161 healthy controls	Narrowband blue (469 nm) or red (631 nm) (After 1 min dark adaptation). Pupillary constriction amplitude (%) after 2-min irradiance of gradually increasing light stimuli (ranging from 6.8 to 13.8 Log photons/cm^2/s)	In glaucomatous eyes, reduced pupillary responses to high-irradiance blue light were associated with greater visual field loss (MD) and optic disc cupping
Kelbsch et al. (43)	25 glaucoma patients 16 Ocular Hypertension (OH) patients 16 healthy controls	28 lx, red (605 nm) or blue (420 nm) light with a duration of either 1 or 4 s. The consensual PIPR was recorded	PIPR blue-red was reduced in glaucoma patients compared to normals ($p < 0.001$) and OH ($p < 0.01$). There was no significant difference between OH and controls. PIPR was inversely correlated with MD in the tested eye
Münch et al. (27)	11 LHON patients 11 glaucoma patients 22 healthy controls	Post-stimulus pupil size at 6 s from light offset (1 s stimulus red and blue) was recorded before, and immediately after light exposure (2 h of bright light exposure)	Only glaucoma patients demonstrated a relative attenuation PRL and at advanced stages of disease also melatonin suppression abnormal response
Adhikari et al. (44)	12 glaucoma suspects 22 early glaucoma patients 12 late glaucoma patients 21 healthy controls	(After 10 min dark adaptation) Post-stimulus pupil size at 6 s from light offset (1 s, blue-464 nm, 15.5 log quanta.cm^{-2} s^{-1} blue light presented in the supero-nasal quadrant field)	Supero-nasal field melanopsin PIPR measurements differentiated mRGC dysfunction in glaucoma suspects and early glaucoma from healthy controls and showed a linear correlation with RNFL thickness
Najjar et al. (45)	46 early stage glaucoma patients 90 controls	Pupillary constriction amplitude (%) after 2-min irradiance of gradually increasing light stimuli (ranging from 8.5 to 14.5 Log photons/cm^2/s) for blue light (462 nm) and (from 8.5 to 14 Log photons/cm^2/s) for red light (638 nm)	Maximum amplitude of pupil constriction was reduced in patients with early-stage glaucoma compared with controls for blue and red stimuli. This reduction was dependent on the irradiance of the light exposure, and showed a linear correlation with RNFL thickness
Herbst et al. (23)	10 unilateral NAION patients 11 controls	Consensual pupil responses during and after exposure to continuous 20 s blue (470 nm) or red (660 nm) light of high intensity (300 cd/m^2) were recorded in each eye	Compared with the responses of the controls, the blue light post-illumination pupil responses were similar in the affected eyes and increased in the fellow non-affected eyes. This suggests a possible adaptive phenomenon, of ipRGCs in both eyes
Tsika et al. (22)	10 unilateral NAION patients 8 bilateral AION patients (1 NAION and 7 AION associated with optic disc drusen) 29 controls	Post-stimulus pupil size (PSPS) at 6 s following monocular as well as binocular light stimulation of 1 s (red-635 nm, blue-464 nm) at different intensities (1.0, 1.5, and 2.0 log cd/m^2)	PSPS to all monocularly-presented light stimuli were impaired in AION eyes. To binocular light stimulation, the PSPS of AION patients was similar to controls

papillo-macular bundle, thus leading to optic atrophy secondary to mitochondrial dysfunctions with the invariable outcome of severe visual loss (46). In both disorders, previous data suggested the maintenance of the PLR even in the chronic stage of the disease, pointing to a pupil-visual dissociation (48, 49). In fact, in these disorders recent histological studies demonstrated a relative preservation of mRGCs compared to the massive loss of regular RGCs in both LHON and DOA, which supports the maintenance of the PLR in these patients (50). At this regard, interestingly, a previous post mortem study demonstrated the relative sparing of the retinofugal fibers to the pretectum in a LHON case, supporting the maintenance of the mRGC projections to the pretectum, which constitute the afferent pathway of the PLR (51). The reasons for the robustness of mRGCs in mitochondrial optic neuropathies are still unknown and under investigation, even though the possible role of peculiar metabolic properties, including the size of the soma, has been proposed (50, 52, 53). More recently, pupillometric studies showed a relative maintenance of the mRGC-mediated pupil response in LHON and DOA patients (24–29) (**Table 2**). Similarly to the maintenance of the PLR a preserved light-induced melatonin suppression has been demonstrated in LHON and DOA patients supporting a relative preservation of these cells in hereditary mitochondrial optic neuropathies (50). Interestingly, the preservation of mRGCs and PLR has also been demonstrated in an OPA1-mouse model (54).

MELANOPSIN RGCs AND PUPIL IN OTHER NEUROLOGICAL DISORDERS

In the last years the mRGC-mediated pupil light response has been investigated in various neurological disorders, including IIH, MS, and PD (31–34).

In a cohort of 13 IIH patients compared to 13 controls it was reported a significant reduction of PLR under melanopsin and rod paradigms in IIH subjects, suggesting the potential use of these parameters as an objective measure of RGC dysfunction in IIH (31). However, the abnormal mRGC-driven PLR has not been reported in a cohort of drug naïve IIH patients (32).

A significant reduction of the sustained pupil response to blue light in the eyes with thinner ganglion cell layer (GCL) + inner plexiform layer (IPL) was demonstrated in a group of 24 MS patients, in particular in those with a previous history of optic neuritis, compared to 15 controls (33). The authors proposed the use of the sustained pupil response to light mediated by mRGCs as a surrogate biomarker for neurodegeneration, including the retinohypothalamic tract, in MS patients (33). In consideration that mRGCs are a fundamental conduit for circadian photoentrainment, the sustained PLR to light may be used as a surrogate marker for RHT integrity and consequently for circadian measurements including melatonin rhythm. This may be relevant for potential light therapeutic interventions in these patients (33). Congruently, previous studies demonstrated an abnormal melatonin rhythm in MS patients (55).

An attenuated PIPR for short wavelength and reduced pupil constriction amplitude for long wavelength stimulation was described in a group of 17 early PD patients compared to a control group (34). Pupil metrics in this group were not influenced by disease severity, sleep quality, medications, or OCT measurements and were controlled for unrest pupil conditions. The authors proposed the pupil response mediated by mRGCs as potential biomarker for non-motor symptoms in PD, such as sleep and circadian dysfunction (34). In fact, there is a large body of evidence supporting the occurrence of circadian dysfunction in PD (56).

Finally, a recent study reported the occurrence of PLR dysfunction in R6/2 and Q175 Huntington's disease (HD) mouse models, with a prevalent contribution of cone dysfunction in young-middle-aged mice and of mRGCs in old mice (57). HD is a neurodegenerative disorder in which circadian dysfunction is a prominent and early disease trait pointing again to a possible mRGC dysfunction (56, 58).

Based on these recent findings, it seems reasonable that other neurological disorders, for which there is evidence of circadian dysfunction and mRGC pathology, such as Alzheimer's disease (AD) (59, 60), HD (56–58), and possibly others, may present an abnormal mRGC-driven PLR.

MELANOPSIN RGCs AND PUPIL IN AFFECTIVE DISORDERS

SAD is a psychiatric condition characterized by the recurrence of depression in winter, in relation to low levels of ambient light in this season (61). Even if the etiology of this disorder is still elusive, the possible role of individual seasonal variation in retinal sensitivity, and in particular of retinal subsensitivity in SAD has been proposed (62–64). Moreover, a polymorphism in the melanopsin (*OPN4*) gene (P10L) has been associated with SAD, suggesting that mRGCs and sensitivity to light may play a relevant role in the pathogenesis of SAD (65). Based on these premises, Roecklein and coauthors investigated the PIPR in 15 individuals with SAD compared to 15 controls. They found a reduced PIPR and a lower PIPR percent change in response to blue light in SAD subjects compared to controls, implying an abnormal mRGC-mediated response to light, as measured by PLR in SAD (30). Moreover, the PIPR response after blue light varied in relation to the OPN4 I394T genotype, another polymorphic variant, suggesting again a possible influence of genetic predisposition in modulating the sensitivity to light in SAD (30). Interestingly, this polymorphic variant has also been found to influence the steady-state pupil diameter in controls (66).

Differently, the melanopsin-mediated PIPR measurements were not significantly different between eight patients with non-seasonal depression and 13 age-matched healthy controls matched for day-light exposure (67). This finding possibly implies a different pathophysiological mechanism in SAD and non-seasonal depression. However, another study using a different light stimulation protocol, showed an abnormal PIPR in both seasonal-depressed and non-seasonal depressed patients (68).

DISCUSSION

Intrinsically photosensitive retinal ganglion cells, the mRGCs, are unique photoreceptors located in the inner retina, which

TABLE 2 | Pupillometry findings in neurological disorders.

	Population	PLR Methods	Main findings
Moura et al. (24)	10 LHON patients 16 controls	1 s red (640 nm) and blue (470 nm) light flashes at 1, 10, 100, and 250 cd/m² luminance Monocular undilated stimulation, patch of the other eye	Overall maintenance of PLR in LHON patients despite the severity of optic atrophy
Kawasaki et al. (25)	1 LHON patient (14448/ND6) one eye affected	20 s red (660 nm) and blue (470 nm) light at 100 and 300 cd/m^2 in affected and unaffected eye	Similar sustained PLR in the affected and unaffected eye suggesting preservation of mRGCs in the affected eye
Kawasaki et al. (26)	8 HON patients 8 controls	1 or 30 s red (635 ± 20 nm) (1 cd/m^2) and blue (463 ± 26 nm) (−4 to 2.5 log cd/m^2) light Simultaneous stimulation of both undilated eyes	No significant difference between HON and controls in terms of PLR parameters
Münch et al. (27)	11 HON patients 11 glaucoma 22 controls	1 s or 30 s light stimulus at 635 ± 20 nm (red light) and 464 ± 26 nm (blue light) Simultaneous stimulation of both undilated eyes	Similar sustained response after blue light in HON patients compared to controls
Nissen et al. (28)	29 OPA1 mutation patients carrying the c.983A > G (n = 14) or c.2708_ 2711delTTAG mutation (n = 15) 40 controls	Isoluminant (300 cd/m^2) red (660 nm) or blue (470 nm) light flash (20 s) Monocular stimulation and recording of the controlateral eye	No differences between OPA1 patients and controls in terms of PIPR
Loo et al. (29)	5 OPA1 patients 54 controls	Red (631 nm) and blue (469 nm) light stimulation (order of light exposure random) gradually increasing intensity from 6.8 to 13.8 log photons/cm^2/s1 over 2 min (preceded and followed by 1 min of darkness)	Dose-response curve (mean constriction amplitude) for blue and red light similar between OPA1 patients and controls
Roecklein et al. (30)	15 SAD patients 15 controls	Red (632.9 nm) and blue (467.7 nm) 30 s light stimuli presented to both eyes and pupil recorded in LE	Reduced PIPR and lower PIPR percent change to blue light in SAD compared to controls
Park et al. (31)	13 IIH patients 13 controls	1 s blue and light flashes (rod, melanopsin and rod conditions) Monocular undilated stimulation, patch of the other eye	Smaller PLRs (transient and sustaineide response) under melanopsin and rod paradigms in IIH patients compared to controls
Ba-Ali et al. (32)	13 drug-naïve IIH patients 13 controls		No difference in melanopsin-driven PLR
Meltzer et al. (33)	24 MS patients 15 controls	1 s red (622 nm) and blue (463 nm) administered alternatively to each eye (max 2.6 log lux)	Reduced PIPR (melanopsin-driven PLR) to blue light in MS eyes with thinner GCL + IPL and with previous optic neuritis
Joyce et al. (34)	17 PD patients 12 controls	Pulsed (8 s) or phasic (12 s) blue (465 nm) or red (638 nm) light stimulation Recording of the consensual response with the stimulated eye dilated	Reduced PIPR and pupil constriction amplitude in PD patients compared to controls

express the photopigment melanopsin (1, 2, 7). The presence of melanopsin makes these cells maximally sensitive to blue light at 470–480 nm and able to spontaneously spike for a long period, even when isolated from the surrounding retinal structures (7, 12). The mRGCs are crucial for non-image forming functions of the eye including circadian photoentrainment, sleep and melatonin synthesis, and PLR. Of particular importance, in this context, is the possibility of using some pupil metrics, such as the PIPR, as a specific signature of mRGC function *in vivo* (8, 13, 56) for ophthalmological and neurodegenerative disorders, which may present circadian dysfunction. In fact, mRGCs contribute mainly to the sustained component of the PLR and, using blue wavelength light, it is possible to isolate the melanopsin contribution to the PLR.

The availability of the mRGC-mediated PLR as a tool to indirectly test the circadian system status, as recently proposed (69), opens new avenues in the analysis of circadian, sleep, and non-motor features in many neurodegenerative disorders. Interestingly, it has been demonstrated in 15 healthy subjects, using combined evaluations including pupillometry, actigraphy, light sensors and body temperature, a close inverse relationship between pupil light response metrics and circadian status (70). In particular, for the pupil recordings it was used a protocol in which the right eye was dilated and different light stimuli including different light wavelength were tested (5 min stimuli) with 40 min of darkness between the light stimulations. Pupil parameters were analyzed using *ad-hoc* software. For the actigraphic recordings the subjects wore an actigraph with light sensor and non-parametric circadian measures, such as intradaily variability, interdaily stability, relative amplitude, L5 and M5, were obtained (70). The authors proposed the Circadian Status Index as an integrative measure to unify three aspects (robustness, timing, and level) of the three circadian rhythm measures (temperature, activity, and light), as well as a global parameter for pupil metrics (circadian photoreception PLR). However, the authors found an inverse relationship between the pupil and circadian metrics. These contradictory findings between circadian status robustness and the PLR might be referred to individual differences in the M1 cell population of mRGCs. Larger studies, more uniform light stimulation protocols and the inclusion of more circadian and pupil metrics are warranted to analyze the possible correlations between pupil metrics and circadian status. In fact, the current available pupillometric studies all suffer the limitation of great heterogeneity of stimulation protocols and consequent lack of reproducibility of their results. Similarly, all these studies are generally underpowered by the limited number of subjects analyzed.

Finally, since mRGCs are contributing to other non-visual functions of the eye, and different class of mRGCs have different projections to the CNS contributing to different functions (5), it must be emphasized that the finding of an abnormal mRGC-mediated PLR does not mean necessarily a global dysfunction of these cells. Overall, the availability of an easily accessible metric for mRGC function, in conjunction with other tests, such as melatonin suppression test, actigraphic recordings, and functional MRI, may represent a comprehensive strategy to further exploring the function of these cells in patients with different neuro-ophthalmological conditions.

CONCLUSIONS AND FUTURE DIRECTIONS

In conclusion, the use of PLR mediated by mRGCs, as a measure of mRGC function, is of particular relevance for neurodegenerative disorders for which there is already evidence of circadian and sleep dysfunction, such as PD, AD, and HD. Similarly, it might be also relevant for other neurological disorders with evidence of circadian dysfunction such as frontotemporal dementia (71), Lewy-Body dementia (72), Progressive Supranuclear Palsy (73, 74), and possibly prion diseases, in particular fatal familial insomnia (75). Moreover, the study of PLR mediated by mRGCs might be particularly intriguing for conditions, in which light sensitivity is a predominant feature, such as photophobia (76, 77) and photosensitivity in epilepsy (78). At this regard, an abnormal PLR has been recently documented in migraineous photophobic subjects, even though it was not specifically assessed the mRGC contribution to PLR (79, 80).

Overall, after adequate standardization of light protocols, the availability of an easy accessible tool to assess mRGC function, as a surrogate marker for more general non-image forming functions of the eye, including circadian rhythms and sleep, is a particularly promising biomarker for neurodegenerative disorders.

AUTHOR CONTRIBUTIONS

CLM and MC were responsible for conception, design, drafting, and revision of the manuscript. VC was responsible for conception and revision of the manuscript.

FUNDING

This work was supported by the Ministry of Health Young Researcher project (GR-2013-02358026) (to CLM) and by the Italian Ministry of Health and of Research and the Gino Galletti Foundation (to VC).

REFERENCES

1. Berson DM, Dunn FA, Takao M. Phototransduction by retinal ganglion cells that set the circadian clock. *Science* (2002) 295:1070–3. doi: 10.1126/science.1067262
2. Hattar S, Liao HW, Takao M, Berson DM, Yau KW. Melanopsin-containing retinal ganglion cells: architecture, projections, and intrinsic photosensitivity. *Science* (2002) 295:1065–70. doi: 10.1126/science.1069609
3. Hannibal J, Hindersson P, Ostergaard J, Georg B, Heegaard S, Larsen PJ, et al. Melanopsin is expressed in PACAP-containing retinal ganglion cells of the human retinohypothalamic tract. *Invest Ophthalmol Vis Sci.* (2004) 45:4202–9. doi: 10.1167/iovs.04-0313
4. Hannibal J, Christiansen AT, Heegaard S, Fahrenkrug J, Kiilgaard JF. Melanopsin expressing human retinal ganglion cells: subtypes, distribution, and intraretinal connectivity. *J Comp Neurol.* (2017) 525:1934–61. doi: 10.1002/cne.24181
5. Chen SK, Badea TC, Hattar S. Photoentrainment and pupillary light reflex are mediated by distinct populations of ipRGCs. *Nature* (2011) 476:92–5. doi: 10.1038/nature10206
6. LeGates TA, Altimus CM, Wang H, Lee HK, Yang S, Zhao H, et al. Aberrant light directly impairs mood and learning through melanopsin-expressing neurons. *Nature* (2012) 491:594–8. doi: 10.1038/nature11673
7. Sand A, Schmidt TM, Kofuji P. Diverse types of ganglion cell photoreceptors in the mammalian retina. *Prog Retin Eye Res.* (2012) 31:287–302. doi: 10.1016/j.preteyeres.2012.03.003
8. Gamlin PD, McDougal DH, Pokorny J, Smith VC, Yau KW, Dacey DM. Human and macaque pupil responses driven by melanopsin-containing retinal ganglion cells. *Vision Res.* (2007) 47:946–54. doi: 10.1016/j.visres.2006.12.015
9. Kawasaki A, Kardon RH. Intrinsically photosensitive retinal ganglion cells. *J Neuroophthalmol.* (2007) 27:195–204. doi: 10.1097/WNO.0b013e31814b1df9
10. Young RS, Kimura E. Pupillary correlates of light-evoked melanopsin activity in humans. *Vision Res.* (2008) 48:862–71. doi: 10.1016/j.visres.2007.12.016

11. Keenan WT, Rupp AC, Ross RA, Somasundaram P, Hiriyanna S, Wu Z, et al. A visual circuit uses complementary mechanisms to support transient and sustained pupil constriction. *Elife* (2016) 5:e15392. doi: 10.7554/eLife.15392
12. Wong KY. A retinal ganglion cell that can signal irradiance continuously for 10 hours. *J Neurosci.* (2012) 32:11478–85. doi: 10.1523/JNEUROSCI.1423-12.2012
13. Adhikari P, Zele AJ, Feigl B. The post-illumination pupil response (PIPR). *Invest Ophthalmol Vis Sci.* (2015) 56:3838–49. doi: 10.1167/iovs.14-16233
14. Park JC, Moura AL, Raza AS, Rhee DW, Kardon RH, Hood DC. Toward a clinical protocol for assessing rod, cone, and melanopsin contributions to the human pupil response. *Invest Ophthalmol Vis Sci.* (2011) 52:6624–35. doi: 10.1167/iovs.11-7586
15. Kardon R, Anderson SC, Damarjian TG, Grace EM, Stone E, Kawasaki A. Chromatic pupil responses: preferential activation of the melanopsin-mediated versus outer photoreceptor-mediated pupil light reflex. *Ophthalmology* (2009) 116:1564–73. doi: 10.1016/j.ophtha.2009.02.007
16. Feigl B, Mattes D, Thomas R, Zele AJ. Intrinsically photosensitive (melanopsin) retinal ganglion cell function in glaucoma. *Invest Ophthalmol Vis Sci.* (2011) 52:4362–7. doi: 10.1167/iovs.10-7069
17. Kankipati L, Girkin CA, Gamlin PD. The post-illumination pupil response is reduced in glaucoma patients. *Invest Ophthalmol Vis Sci.* (2011) 52:2287–92. doi: 10.1167/iovs.10-6023
18. Nissen C, Sander B, Milea D, Kolko M, Herbst K, Hamard P, et al. Monochromatic pupillometry in unilateral glaucoma discloses no adaptive changes subserved by the ipRGCs. *Front Neurol.* (2014) 5:15. doi: 10.3389/fneur.2014.00015
19. Kardon R, Anderson SC, Damarjian TG, Grace EM, Stone E, Kawasaki A. Chromatic pupillometry in patients with retinitis pigmentosa. *Ophthalmology* (2011) 118:376–81. doi: 10.1016/j.ophtha.2010.06.033
20. Feigl B, Zele AJ, Fader SM, Howes AN, Hughes CE, Jones KA, et al. The post-illumination pupil response of melanopsin-expressing intrinsically photosensitive retinal ganglion cells in diabetes. *Acta Ophthalmol.* (2012) 90:e230–4. doi: 10.1111/j.1755-3768.2011.02226.x
21. Feigl B, Zele AJ. Melanopsin-expressing intrinsically photosensitive retinal ganglion cells in retinal disease. *Optom Vis Sci.* (2014) 91:894–903. doi: 10.1097/OPX.0000000000000284
22. Tsika C, Crippa SV, Kawasaki A. Differential monocular vs. binocular pupil responses from melanopsin-based photoreception in patients with anterior ischemic optic neuropathy. *Sci Rep.* (2015) 5:10780. doi: 10.1038/srep10780
23. Herbst K, Sander B, Lund-Andersen H, Wegener M, Hannibal J, Milea D. Unilateral anterior ischemic optic neuropathy: chromatic pupillometry in affected, fellow non-affected and healthy control eyes. *Front Neurol.* (2013) 4:52. doi: 10.3389/fneur.2013.00052
24. Moura AL, Nagy BV, La Morgia C, Barboni P, Oliveira AG, Salomão SR, et al. The pupil light reflex in Leber's hereditary optic neuropathy: evidence for preservation of melanopsin-expressing retinal ganglion cells. *Invest Ophthalmol Vis Sci.* (2013) 54:4471–7. doi: 10.1167/iovs.12-11137
25. Kawasaki A, Herbst K, Sander B, Milea D. Selective wavelength pupillometry in Leber hereditary optic neuropathy. *Clin Exp Ophthalmol.* (2010) 38:322–4. doi: 10.1111/j.1442-9071.2010.02212.x
26. Kawasaki A, Collomb S, Léon L, Münch M. Pupil responses derived from outer and inner retinal photoreception are normal in patients with hereditary optic neuropathy. *Exp Eye Res.* (2014) 120:161–6. doi: 10.1016/j.exer.2013.11.005
27. Münch M, Léon L, Collomb S, Kawasaki A. Comparison of acute non-visual bright light responses in patients with optic nerve disease, glaucoma and healthy controls. *Sci Rep.* (2015) 5:15185. doi: 10.1038/srep15185
28. Nissen C, Rönnbäck C, Sander B, Herbst K, Milea D, Larsen M, et al. Dissociation of pupillary post-illumination responses from visual function in confirmed OPA1 c.983A > G and c.2708_2711delTTAG autosomal dominant optic atrophy. *Front Neurol.* (2015) 6:5. doi: 10.3389/fneur.2015.00005
29. Loo JL, Singhal S, Rukmini AV, Tow S, Amati-Bonneau P, Procaccio V, et al. Multiethnic involvement in autosomal-dominant optic atrophy in Singapore. *Eye* (2017) 31:475–80. doi: 10.1038/eye.2016.255
30. Roecklein K, Wong P, Ernecoff N, Miller M, Donofry S, Kamarck M, et al. The post illumination pupil response is reduced in seasonal affective disorder. *Psychiatr Res.* (2013) 210:150–8. doi: 10.1016/j.psychres.2013.05.023
31. Park JC, Moss HE, McAnany JJ. The pupillary light reflex in idiopathic intracranial hypertension. *Invest Ophthalmol Vis Sci.* (2016) 57:23–9. doi: 10.1167/iovs.15-18181
32. Ba-Ali S, Jensen RH, Larsen LS, Lund-Andersen H, Hamann S. The melanopsin-mediated pupillary light response is not changed in patients with newly diagnosed idiopathic intracranial hypertension. *Neuroophthalmology* (2017) 42:65–72. doi: 10.1080/01658107.2017.1344251
33. Meltzer E, Sguigna PV, Subei A, Beh S, Kildebeck E, Conger D, et al. Retinal architecture and melanopsin-mediated pupillary response characteristics: a putative pathophysiologic signature for the retino-hypothalamic tract in multiple sclerosis. *JAMA Neurol.* (2017) 74:574–82. doi: 10.1001/jamaneurol.2016.5131
34. Joyce DS, Feigl B, Kerr G, Roeder L, Zele AJ. Melanopsin-mediated pupil function is impaired in Parkinson's disease. *Sci Rep.* (2018) 8:7796. doi: 10.1038/s41598-018-26078-0
35. Weinreb RN, Aung T, Medeiros FA. The pathophysiology and treatment of glaucoma: a review. *JAMA* (2014) 311:1901–11. doi: 10.1001/jama.2014.3192
36. Nickells RW, Howell GR, Soto I, John SW. Under pressure: cellular and molecular responses during glaucoma, a common neurodegeneration with axonopathy. *Annu Rev Neurosci.* (2012) 35:153–79. doi: 10.1146/annurev.neuro.051508.135728
37. Jakobs TC, Libby RT, Ben Y, John SW, Masland RH. Retinal ganglion cell degeneration is topological but not cell type specific in DBA/2J mice. *J Cell Biol.* (2005) 171:313–25. doi: 10.1083/jcb.200506099
38. Onen SH, Mouriaux F, Berramdane L, Dascotte JC, Kulik JF, Rouland JF. High prevalence of sleep-disordered breathing in patients with primary open-angle glaucoma. *Acta Ophthalmol Scand.* (2000) 78:638–41. doi: 10.1034/j.1600-0420.2000.078006638.x
39. Drouyer E, Dkhissi-Benyahya O, Chiquet C, WoldeMussie E, Ruiz G, Wheeler LA, et al. Glaucoma alters the circadian timing system. *PLoS ONE* (2008) 3:e3931. doi: 10.1371/journal.pone.0003931
40. Lanzani MF, de Zavalía N, Fontana H, Sarmiento MI, Golombek D, Rosenstein RE. Alterations of locomotor activity rhythm and sleep parameters in patients with advanced glaucoma. *Chronobiol Int.* (2012) 29:911–9. doi: 10.3109/07420528.2012.691146
41. Wang H, Zhang Y, Ding J, Wang N. Changes in the circadian rhythm in patients with primary glaucoma. *PLoS ONE* (2013) 29:e62841. doi: 10.1371/journal.pone.0062841
42. Rukmini AV, Milea D, Baskaran M, How AC, Perera SA, Aung T, et al. Pupillary responses to high-irradiance blue light correlate with glaucoma severity. *Ophthalmology* (2015) 122:1777–85. doi: 10.1016/j.ophtha.2015.06.002
43. Kelbsch C, Maeda F, Strasser T, Blumenstock G, Wilhelm B, Wilhelm H, et al. Pupillary responses driven by ipRGCs and classical photoreceptors are impaired in glaucoma. *Graefes Arch Clin Exp Ophthalmol.* (2016) 254: 1361–70. doi: 10.1007/s00417-016-3351-9
44. Adhikari P, Zele AJ, Thomas R, Feigl B. Quadrant field pupillometry detects melanopsin dysfunction in glaucoma suspects and early glaucoma. *Sci Rep.* (2016) 6:33373. doi: 10.1038/srep33373
45. Najjar RP, Sharma S, Atalay E, Rukmini AV, Sun C, Lock JZ, et al. Pupillary responses to full-field chromatic stimuli are reduced in patients with early-stage primary open-angle glaucoma. *Ophthalmology* (2018) 125:1362–71. doi: 10.1016/j.ophtha.2018.02.024
46. Carelli V, Ross-Cisneros FN, Sadun AA. Mitochondrial dysfunction as a cause of optic neuropathies. *Prog Retin Eye Res.* (2004) 23:53–89. doi: 10.1016/j.preteyeres.2003.10.003
47. Yu-Wai-Man P, Griffiths PG, Chinnery PF. Mitochondrial optic neuropathies-disease mechanisms and therapeutic strategies. *Prog Retin Eye Res.* (2011) 30:81–114. doi: 10.1016/j.preteyeres.2010.11.002
48. Bremner FD, Tomlin EA, Shallo-Hoffmann J, Votruba M, Smith SE. The pupil in dominant optic atrophy. *Invest Ophthalmol Vis Sci.* (2001) 42:675–8.
49. Wakakura M, Yokoe J. Evidence for preserved direct pupillary light response in Leber's hereditary optic neuropathy. *Br J Ophthalmol.* (1995) 79:442–6.
50. La Morgia C, Ross-Cisneros FN, Sadun AA, Hannibal J, Munarini A, Mantovani V, et al. Melanopsin retinal ganglion cells are resistant to neurodegeneration in mitochondrial optic neuropathies. *Brain* (2010) 133:2426–38. doi: 10.1093/brain/awq155

51. Bose S, Dhillon N, Ross-Cisneros FN, Carelli V. Relative post-mortem sparing of afferent pupil fibers in a patient with 3460 Leber's hereditary optic neuropathy. *Graefes Arch Clin Exp Ophthalmol.* (2005) 243:1175–9. doi: 10.1007/s00417-005-0023-6
52. La Morgia C, Ross-Cisneros FN, Hannibal J, Montagna P, Sadun AA, Carelli V. Melanopsin-expressing retinal ganglion cells: implications for human diseases. *Vision Res.* (2011) 51:296–302. doi: 10.1016/j.visres.2010.07.023
53. Georg B, Ghelli A, Giordano C, Ross-Cisneros FN, Sadun AA, Carelli V, et al. Melanopsin-expressing retinal ganglion cells are resistant to cell injury, but not always. *Mitochondrion* (2017) 36:77–84. doi: 10.1016/j.mito.2017.04.003
54. Perganta G, Barnard AR, Katti C, Vachtsevanos A, Douglas RH, MacLaren RE, et al. Non-image-forming light driven functions are preserved in a mouse model of autosomal dominant optic atrophy. *PLoS ONE* (2013) 8:e56350. doi: 10.1371/journal.pone.0056350
55. Damasceno A, Moraes AS, Farias A, Damasceno BP, dos Santos LM, Cendes F. Disruption of melatonin circadian rhythm production is related to multiple sclerosis severity: a preliminary study. *J Neurol Sci.* (2015) 353:166–8. doi: 10.1016/j.jns.2015.03.040
56. La Morgia C, Ross-Cisneros FN, Sadun AA, Carelli V. Retinal ganglion cells and circadian rhythms in Alzheimer's disease, Parkinson's disease, and beyond. *Front Neurol.* (2017) 8:162. doi: 10.3389/fneur.2017.00162
57. Ouk K, Hughes S, Pothecary CA, Peirson SN, Jennifer Morton A. Attenuated pupillary light responses and downregulation of opsin expression parallel decline in circadian disruption in two different mouse models of Huntington's disease. *Hum Mol Genet.* (2016) 25:5418–32. doi: 10.1093/hmg/ddw359
58. Morton AJ. Circadian and sleep disorder in Huntington's disease. *Exp Neurol.* (2013) 243:34–44. doi: 10.1016/j.expneurol.2012.10.014
59. La Morgia C, Ross-Cisneros FN, Koronyo Y, Hannibal J, Gallassi R, Cantalupo G, et al. Melanopsin retinal ganglion cell loss in Alzheimer disease. *Ann Neurol.* (2016) 79:90–109. doi: 10.1002/ana.24548
60. Feng R, Li L, Yu H, Liu M, Zhao W. Melanopsin retinal ganglion cell loss and circadian dysfunction in Alzheimer's disease. *Mol Med Rep.* (2016) 13:3397–400. doi: 10.3892/mmr.2016.4966
61. Magnusson A, Partonen T. The diagnosis, symptomatology, and epidemiology of seasonal affective disorder. *CNS Spectr.* (2005) 10:625–34; quiz 1–14. doi: 10.1017/s1092852900019593
62. Wehr TA, Duncan WC Jr, Sher L, Aeschbach D, Schwartz PJ, Turner EH, et al. A circadian signal of change of season in patients with seasonal affective disorder. *Arch Gen Psychiatr.* (2001) 58:1108–14. doi: 10.1001/archpsyc.58.12.1108
63. Hébert M, Dumont M, Lachapelle P. Electrophysiological evidence suggesting a seasonal modulation of retinal sensitivity in subsyndromal winter depression. *J Affect Disord.* (2002) 68:191–202. doi: 10.1016/s0165-0327(00)00192-0
64. Rohan KJ, Roecklein KA, Lacy TJ, Vacek PM. Winter depression recurrence one year after cognitive-behavioral therapy, light therapy, or combination treatment. *Behav Ther.* (2009) 40:225–38. doi: 10.1016/j.beth.2008.06.004
65. Roecklein KA, Rohan KJ, Duncan WC, Rollag MD, Rosenthal NE, Lipsky RH, et al. A missense variant (P10L) of the melanopsin (OPN4) gene in seasonal affective disorder. *J Affect Disord.* (2009) 114:279–85. doi: 10.1016/j.jad.2008.08.005
66. Higuchi S, Hida A, Tsujimura S, Mishima K, Yasukouchi A, Lee SI, et al. Melanopsin gene polymorphism I394T is associated with pupillary light responses in a dose-dependent manner. *PLoS ONE* (2013) 8:e60310. doi: 10.1371/journal.pone.0060310
67. Feigl B, Ojha G, Hides L, Zele AJ. Melanopsin-driven pupil response and light exposure in non-seasonal major depressive disorder. *Front Neurol.* (2018) 9:764. doi: 10.3389/fneur.2018.00764
68. Berman G, Muttuvelu D, Berman D, Larsen JI, Licht RW, Ledolter J, Kardon et al. Decreased retinal sensitivity in depressive disorder: a controlled study. *Acta Psychiatr Scand.* (2018) 137:231–40. doi: 10.1111/acps.12851
69. Markwell EL, Feigl B, Zele AJ. Intrinsically photosensitive melanopsin retinal ganglion cell contributions to the pupillary light reflex and circadian rhythm. *Clin Exp Optom.* (2010) 93:137–49. doi: 10.1111/j.1444-0938.2010.00479
70. Bonmati-Carrion MA, Hild K, Isherwood C, Sweeney SJ, Revell VL, Skene DJ, et al. Relationship between human pupillary light reflex and circadian system status. *PLoS ONE* (2016) 11:e0162476. doi: 10.1371/journal.pone.0162476
71. Merrilees J, Hubbard E, Mastick J, Miller BL, Dowling GA. Rest-activity and behavioral disruption in a patient with frontotemporal dementia. *Neurocase* (2009) 15:515–26. doi: 10.1080/13554790903061371
72. Harper DG, Stopa EG, McKee AC, Satlin A, Fish D, Volicer L. Dementia severity and Lewy bodies affect circadian rhythms in Alzheimer disease. *Neurobiol Aging* (2004) 25:771–81. doi: 10.1016/j.neurobiolaging.2003.04.009
73. De Pablo-Fernández E, Courtney R, Warner TT, Holton JL. A histologic study of the circadian system in Parkinson disease, multiple system atrophy, and progressive supranuclear palsy. *JAMA Neurol.* (2018) 75:1008–12. doi: 10.1001/jamaneurol.2018.0640
74. Suzuki K, Miyamoto T, Miyamoto M, Hirata K. The core body temperature rhythm is altered in progressive supranuclear palsy. *Clin Auton Res.* (2009) 19:65–8. doi: 10.1007/s10286-009-0510-7
75. Roguski A, Gill AC. The role of the mammalian prion protein in the control of sleep. *Pathogens* (2017) 6:E58. doi: 10.3390/pathogens6040058
76. Noseda R, Copenhagen D, Burstein R. Current understanding of photophobia, visual networks and headaches. *Cephalalgia* (2018) 1:333102418784750. doi: 10.1177/0333102418784750
77. Noseda R, Kainz V, Jakubowski M, Gooley JJ, Saper CB, Digre K, Burstein R. A neural mechanism for exacerbation of headache by light. *Nat Neurosci.* (2010) 13:239–45. doi: 10.1038/nn.2475
78. Martins da Silva A, Leal B. Photosensitivity and epilepsy: current concepts and perspectives—A narrative review. *Seizure* (2017) 50:209–18. doi: 10.1016/j.seizure.2017.04.001
79. Cortez MM, Rea NA, Hunter LA, Digre KB, Brennan KC. Altered pupillary light response scales with disease severity in migrainous photophobia. *Cephalalgia* (2017) 37:801–11. doi: 10.1177/03331024166 73205
80. Mylius V, Braune HJ, Schepelmann K. Dysfunction of the pupillary light reflex following migraine headache. *Clin Auton Res.* (2003) 13:16–21. doi: 10.1007/s10286-003-0065-y

17

Melanopsin and Cone Photoreceptor Inputs to the Afferent Pupil Light Response

Andrew J. Zele[1,2*], *Prakash Adhikari*[1,2], *Dingcai Cao*[3] *and Beatrix Feigl*[1,4,5]

[1] *Institute of Health and Biomedical Innovation, Queensland University of Technology (QUT), Brisbane, QLD, Australia,*
[2] *School of Optometry and Vision Science, Queensland University of Technology (QUT), Brisbane, QLD, Australia,*
[3] *Department of Ophthalmology and Visual Sciences, University of Illinois at Chicago, Chicago, IL, United States,* [4] *School of Biomedical Sciences, Queensland University of Technology (QUT), Brisbane, QLD, Australia,* [5] *Queensland Eye Institute, Brisbane, QLD, Australia*

***Correspondence:**
Andrew J. Zele
andrew.zele@qut.edu.au

Background: Retinal photoreceptors provide the main stage in the mammalian eye for regulating the retinal illumination through changes in pupil diameter, with a small population of melanopsin-expressing intrinsically photosensitive retinal ganglion cells (ipRGCs) forming the primary afferent pathway for this response. The purpose of this study is to determine how melanopsin interacts with the three cone photoreceptor classes in the human eye to modulate the light-adapted pupil response.

Methods: We investigated the independent and combined contributions of the inner and outer retinal photoreceptor inputs to the afferent pupil pathway in participants with trichromatic color vision using a method to independently control the excitations of ipRGCs, cones and rods in the retina.

Results: We show that melanopsin-directed stimuli cause a transient pupil constriction generated by cones in the shadow of retinal blood vessels; desensitizing these penumbral cone signals uncovers a signature melanopsin pupil response that includes a longer latency (292 ms) and slower time (4.1x) and velocity (7.7x) to constriction than for cone-directed stimuli, and which remains sustained post-stimulus offset. Compared to melanopsin-mediated pupil responses, the cone photoreceptor-initiated pupil responses are more transient with faster constriction latencies, higher velocities and a secondary constriction at light offset. The combined pupil responses reveal that melanopsin signals are additive with the cone signals.

Conclusions: The visual system uses the L–, M–, and S–cone photoreceptor inputs to the afferent pupil pathway to accomplish the tonic modulations of pupil size to changes in image contrast. The inner retinal melanopsin-expressing ipRGCs mediate the longer-term, sustained pupil constriction to set the light-adapted pupil diameter during extended light exposures.

Keywords: pupil light reflex, melanopsin, cone, photoreceptor, intrinsically photosensitive retinal ganglion cells

INTRODUCTION

In humans and non-human primates, melanopsin-expressing ipRGCs have an intrinsic photoresponse (1, 2), receive extrinsic rod and cone inputs and project to the olivary pretectal nucleus (OPN) (1, 3) to form the primary afferent pupil pathway and regulate the pupil aperture (2, 4–12). Pupil diameter is critical for modulating retinal illumination, enhancing visual performance by varying ocular aberrations and depth of focus (13) and is a clinically significant biomarker in neuro-ophthalmology (14, 15). The relative rod, cone and melanopsin-expressing intrinsically photosensitive retinal ganglion cell (ipRGC) contributions to the pupil light response (PLR) have been explored in both animals and humans having different photoreceptor spectral responses and post-receptoral pathways, using different methodological approaches. When all ocular photoreceptors (rods, cones, and ipRGCs) are knocked-out in transgenic mice, there is no PLR (16). In transgenic mice with ipRGCs that do not express the melanopsin photopigment, the PLR is normal at low irradiances and reduced at high irradiances, indicating that rods and cones can contribute to the PLR without activating melanopsin (17, 18). In rod-cone knock-out mice, the PLR is present, but with reduced response amplitude, indicating that melanopsin-expressing ipRGCs alone can mediate the pupil response (17). Similarly, in non-human primates (macaque) following pharmacological blockade of rod and cone signals, the PLR is present with lower amplitude, slower dynamics, and persists after light offset (2); immunotoxin ablation of the OPN4 melanopsin gene in rhesus monkeys results in a reduction in the maximum pupil constriction amplitude and elimination of the post-illumination pupil response (19). When mouse ipRGCs are selectively ablated however, the PLR is absent, indicating the rod-cone pathway does require ipRGCs for a functional pupil response (20). The animal models therefore show that ipRGCs, rods and cones are complementary in their signaling to the pupil control pathway (18, 21–23). However, transgenic animal models that by design, knock-out photoreceptors, cannot be used to independently control the level of activation and interaction between the different photoreceptor inputs to the PLR and so alternate methods are required.

The relative photoreceptor contributions to human PLR can be studied using psychophysical methodologies that independently control the photoreceptor excitations. Outer retinal receptors drive the transient pupil constriction (2, 4, 7, 24–29), but the melanopsin, L–, M–, and S-cone inputs have not been separated in normally-sighted people to identify their independent and combined contributions. After light offset, the redilation of the post-illumination pupil response (PIPR) in the dark is modulated by both rhodopsin and melanopsin during its early-redilation phase (4) and then entirely by melanopsin (2, 30); there has been no direct measurement of the melanopsin control of the PIPR under light-adapted photopic conditions, nor the melanopsin interaction with cone signals. Extrinsic cone inputs to the OPN are mediated via ipRGCs through retinal interneurons (19, 31, 32) and there is evidence for an independent post-retinal pathway for chromatically opponent inputs to the afferent pupil response (26, 33). To determine the melanopsin contribution to the light-adapted PLR, the intrinsic melanopsin response must be separated from the outer retinal (rod and cone) photoreceptor responses. Here we isolate the melanopsin and cone contributions to the PLR for photoreceptor-directed incremental light pulses using a method of silent-substitution (6, 34) that independently controls their relative activity under conditions that provide constant rod photoreceptor excitation. The outcomes of this study reveal the separate and combined contributions of melanopsin and cones to light-adapted, photopic pupil responses in humans with trichromatic color vision.

MATERIALS AND METHODS

Participants and Ethics Statement

All experimental protocols were approved by the Queensland University of Technology (QUT) Human Research Ethics Committee (approval no: 1700000510) and conducted in accordance with their guidelines. Test protocols were completed in compliance with the tenets of the Declaration of Helsinki and all participants provided informed and written consent after the nature and possible consequences of the experiments were explained. Four healthy participants with trichromatic color vision (2 females, 2 males, 23–41 years; one observer was an Author) and no systemic disease took part in this study in accordance with the human research ethics approval. All observers underwent a comprehensive ophthalmic examination, including fundus examination, ocular coherence tomography, color vision (D-15 and Rayleigh color match), visual acuity, contrast sensitivity (Pelli-Robson) and intra-ocular pressure to exclude any retinal or optic nerve disease.

Apparatus and Calibrations

A calibrated five-primary Maxwellian-view photostimulator with 12-bit resolution and a ~488 Hz upper frequency limit (6) was used to generate all test stimuli. This photostimulator includes five narrowband primary lights comprising light emitting diodes (LED) and interference filters with peak wavelengths (full widths at half maximum) at 456 nm (10 nm), 488 nm (11 nm), 540 nm (10 nm), 594 nm (14 nm), and 633 nm (15 nm) that were combined using fiber optic cables and a homogenizer and focused by an achromatic doublet field lens in the plane of a 2 mm artificial pupil in Maxwellian view. The outputs of the primary lights were controlled by an Arduino based stimulation system, a LED driver (TLC5940), a microcontroller (Arduino Uno SMDR3, Model A000073) and calibrated neutral density filters (Ealing, Natick, MA, USA) using custom engineered software (Xcode 3.2.3, 64-bit, Apple, Inc., Cupertino, CA, USA). The spectral outputs of five primary lights were measured with a spectroradiometer (StellarNet, Tampa, FL, USA); luminance outputs measured with an ILT1700 Research Radiometer (International Light Technologies, Inc., Peabody, MA, USA) as a function of the duty cycle of the LED driver were used to compute the linearization coefficients (6).

The excitations of melanopsin, rhodopsin and the three cone opsins were independently controlled using the principle of silent substitution (6, 34). The L– M– and S-cone, rod (R) and ipRGC (i) excitations were calculated based on CIE 1964 10° standard observer cone fundamentals (35), the CIE 1951 scotopic luminosity function, and melanopsin spectral sensitivity function (30, 36), respectively. For a 1 photopic Troland (Td) light metameric to an equal energy spectrum, the photoreceptor excitation relative to photopic luminance with a 2:1 L:M cone ratio is l = L/(L+M) = 0.6667, m = M/(L+M) = 0.3333, s = S/(L+M) = 1, r = R/(L+M) = 1 and intrinsic melanopsin i = I/(L + M) = 1. Measurements were performed with a 2000 photopic Td adapting stimulus field chromaticity that had an orange appearance (l = 0.752, s = 0.105, r = 0.319, and i = 0.235). Using the principle of silent substitution to selectively modulate one photoreceptor class, or a combination of up to four photoreceptor classes, unique scaling coefficients for the each of the 5-primary lights are calculated using linear algebra (6, 37, 38) for the nominated Weber contrast [C = $(Td_{max}-Td_{min})/Td_{min}*100\%$] of the photoreceptor excitation(s). For example, a 6% Weber contrast +L–M stimulus increases the L-cone excitation by 6% contrast relative to the photoreceptor excitation at the adapting background level, and decreases the M-cone excitation by −6% contrast; the result of this +L–M photoreceptor excitation is a chromaticity change (i.e., a magenta appearing light modulation) without altering the mean retinal illumination or the intrinsic melanopsin-ipRGC, rod and S-cone photoreceptor excitations relative to the adapting background level.

To nullify individual differences in pre-receptoral filtering and photoreceptor spectral sensitivities between the observer and the CIE 1964 10° standard observer, participants performed heterochromatic flicker photometry (HFP) settings between a reference primary (cyan; 100 Td mean illuminance, 15 Hz square wave counterphase flicker) and each of the test primaries (red, green, blue and amber) (38). The 15 Hz modulation frequency is beyond the temporal resolution of the chromatic mechanisms (39, 40), of melanopsin photoreception (10) and therefore likely mediated by the inferred luminance pathway (35, 41). During each HFP setting, the observer minimized the appearance of flicker by controlling the radiance of the test primary using a method of adjustment. For each test-reference wavelength combination, the final setting was the average of 15 repeats; the theoretical 10° standard observer data was then scaled by the observer's average HFP settings.

Experimental Design: Pupil Light Responses

The stimulus was a 30° diameter circular field with the central 10.5° blocked to eliminate the effect of macular pigment. A small hole (<1 min arc) in the center of this macular blocker was used for fixation. Prior to all experimental sessions, the observers were adapted to the dark-room illumination (< 0.0003 lux) for 15 min followed by a 2 min adaptation to the 2000 Td orange field. In order to maintain a constant retinal illumination during the stimulus presentation (42), consensual pupil responses in the un-stimulated eye were infrared LED illuminated (λmax = 851 nm) and imaged with a camera (640 X 480 pixels; 60 Hz; Point Gray FMVU-03MTM-CS; Richmond, BC, Canada; Computar TEC55 55 mm telecentric lens; Computar, Cary, NC, USA) following our established procedures (30, 43). The consensual pupil responses were measured using 5,000 and 1,000 ms incremental pulses of five photoreceptor excitation combinations: [1] melanopsin-directed stimuli (17% Weber contrast) with no change in the excitation of the rods and three cone types, [2] L– and M–cones modulated in-phase to produce a cone luminance increment (+L+M; 10% Weber contrast) with no change in the excitation of S–cones, rods or melanopsin, [3] S–cone increments (+S; 10% Weber contrast) with no change in the excitation of melanopsin, rods, L– and M–cones, [4] a counterphase equiluminant L– and M–cone modulation (+L–M; 6% Weber contrast) with no change in L+M cone luminance or the excitation of S–cones, rods or melanopsin, and [5] the additive mixture of melanopsin (17% Weber contrast) with each of the photoreceptor combinations specified in [2–4].

The inter-stimulus interval included temporal white noise that randomly modulated the S-cone, M-cone, L-cone, and rod photoreceptor excitations (40% Michelson contrast) (44, 45) without changing the melanopsin photoreceptor excitation (10). The purpose of the temporal white noise is to limit the effect of any non-melanopsin photoreceptor absorptions on the melanopsin-directed pupil responses by desensitizing penumbral cones in the shadow of the retinal vasculature; for the 17% Weber contrast, melanopsin-directed pulse on the 2000 Td adaptation field, the penumbral L–, M–, and S–cone contrasts were 0.2, 0.5, and 0.6%, respectively and the rod contrast was 0.2%. The physically measured open-field cone contrast, which is the difference between the theoretical and measured irradiances of the five primary lights for the S M L R i photoreceptor excitations for the melanopsin-directed stimulus, was 0.0, 0.1, and 1.3% for the L–, M–, and S–cone contrasts, respectively, and 0.3% for the rod contrast. The rod contrast in all cone isolating conditions was ≤0.3%.

For the pupil measurements, each trial was separated by a 1 ms blank interval (46) and the trial repeated 10 times during a single recording sequence that was repeated at least 10 times (~100 trials per observer per stimulus condition; 8 conditions X 2 stimulus durations = ~1,600 total trials per observer). Testing sessions were <1.5 h to avoid the effect of observer fatigue and sleepiness on pupil responses. Data were measured during the day to minimize the influence of circadian variation on melanopsin-mediated pupil responses (9); each participant was scheduled at the same test time for their test sessions on different days.

Analysis Metrics for the Pupil Light Responses

The PLR was quantified with reference to a baseline pupil diameter defined as the average of the 100 ms pre-stimulus data immediately before onset of the stimulus pulse. The PLR latency (in milliseconds) is the time to 1% pupil constriction after pulse onset; the peak constriction amplitude (% baseline diameter) is the smallest pupil diameter in response to stimulus onset, and the time at this maximum constriction is defined as the time to peak (in seconds). The pupil constriction velocity from stimulus pulse onset is the peak constriction amplitude divided by the time to peak (%.s^{-1}). The light-adapted pupil diameter following stimulus offset (% baseline) was quantified at 1.8 s post-stimulus; although this metric is sometimes referred to as the post-stimulus pupil response (PSPR) when measured under light-adapted conditions (47), we adopted the more common notation, post-illumination pupil response (1.8 s PIPR). The pupil traces represent the global average of all repeats from all observers (~100 trials per observer per condition); the ±95% confidence limits were estimated from all stimulus trials for all observers for the respective stimulus conditions.

Confirmation of Photoreceptor Isolation

We performed multiple control measurements to confirm the observer calibration and photoreceptor isolation. Firstly, a 500 ms, 18% Weber contrast rod incremental pulse with no change in melanopsin or cone excitations at a 5 Troland adaptation level was invisible after photopigment bleach and highly conspicuous after dark adaptation. Secondly, the cone excitations perceptually matching a 500 ms, 18% contrast rod incremental pedestal at a 5 Td background were equivalent to a decrease in L/[L+M], an increase in S/[L+M] and an increase in [L+M] (48). Finally, a 500 ms rod incremental pulse was invisible when presented at the maximum achievable contrast (18.5%) at a 5000 photopic Td adaptation level. The data clearly show that different photoreceptor-directed conditions produce pupil responses with different amplitude and timings. Individual differences in luminous efficiency, including any effect from photoreceptor polymorphisms, were corrected for during the HFP, as were individual differences in lens density (6, 10).

RESULTS

We first established that continuous presentation of the temporal white noise (i.e., no stimulus) that randomly modulates the S-cone, M-cone, L-cone, and rod photoreceptor excitations (without changing the melanopsin photoreceptor excitation) does not produce a pupil constriction (**Figure 1A**). The hippus evident in the pupil traces may be due to parasympathetic nervous system activity (49). Similarly, turning the noise off for a period equal to a 1,000 ms stimulus pulse and during which time this blank is equal to the time average illuminance of the adapting field, there is also no change in the pupil response (**Figure 1B**).

Pupil responses to melanopsin-directed stimuli measured with and without temporal white noise reveal the independent contribution of melanopsin (**Figure 2A**); the pupil responses for the 5,000 ms pulses are shown in the left panels, and for the 1,000 ms pulses in the right panels. The transient pupil constriction to the onset of a melanopsin-directed stimulus pulse is generated by penumbral cone signals (**Figure 2A**, cyan line); desensitizing penumbral cones and any residual high and low frequency cone responses using the temporal white noise (10) uncovers the signature melanopsin pupil response which includes a latency to constriction (5,000 ms pulse: 633.3 ± 43.3 ms; 1,000 ms pulse: 612.5 ± 42.7 ms) that is longer than for cones, with a slower velocity to constriction (5,000 ms pulse: 0.8 ± 0.02 %.s^{-1}; 1,000 ms pulse: 2.3 ± 0.4 %.s^{-1}) that remains sustained post-stimulus offset (**Figure 2A**, green lines; **Table 1**). For melanopsin-directed stimuli, the pupil responses to 5,000 ms pulses have a slower velocity to constriction than to 1,000 ms pulses (**Table 1**) because the velocity of the sustained melanopsin-mediated pupil constriction during light stimulation decreases over time. The time to peak constriction is 4.1x slower than for the average cone-directed PLR (5,000 ms; **Table 1**).

The cone photoreceptor-initiated pupil responses (**Figures 2B–D**) include higher transience (+L–M > +L+M > S-cone) than for melanopsin, with faster constriction latencies (range for 1,000 and 5,000 ms pulses: 325 to 491 ms), higher velocities (range for 1,000 and 5,000 ms pulses: 2.6 to 11.1%.s^{-1}), and larger peak amplitudes to light onset (**Table 1**). That the stimulus contrast was ~30x higher than the +L–M visual detection threshold and ~2x higher than the +L+M detection threshold (10) resulted in the +L–M directed stimuli producing larger constriction amplitudes and higher constriction velocities than did +L+M directed stimuli. For cone-directed pulses (no change in the melanopsin excitation), the pupil rapidly redilates to baseline after stimulus offset whereas melanopsin-directed

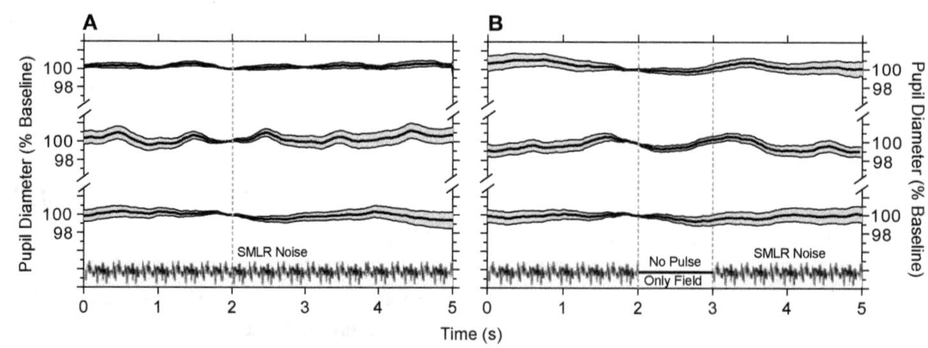

FIGURE 1 | Pupil responses to temporal white noise. **(A)** Temporal white noise is presented for 5,000 ms then repeated; pupil diameter is steady during continuous presentation of the temporal white noise. **(B)** A 1,000 ms blank equal to the time average chromaticity and retinal illuminance of the orange field (no pulse, only field) is inserted within the temporal white noise; this blank field does not cause a pupil constriction. Panels show the average ±95% confidence limits for each of three observers (traces vertically offset; ~100 trials per observer). Pupil responses are normalized to the diameter at 2 s (vertical line) during each 5,000 ms repeat.

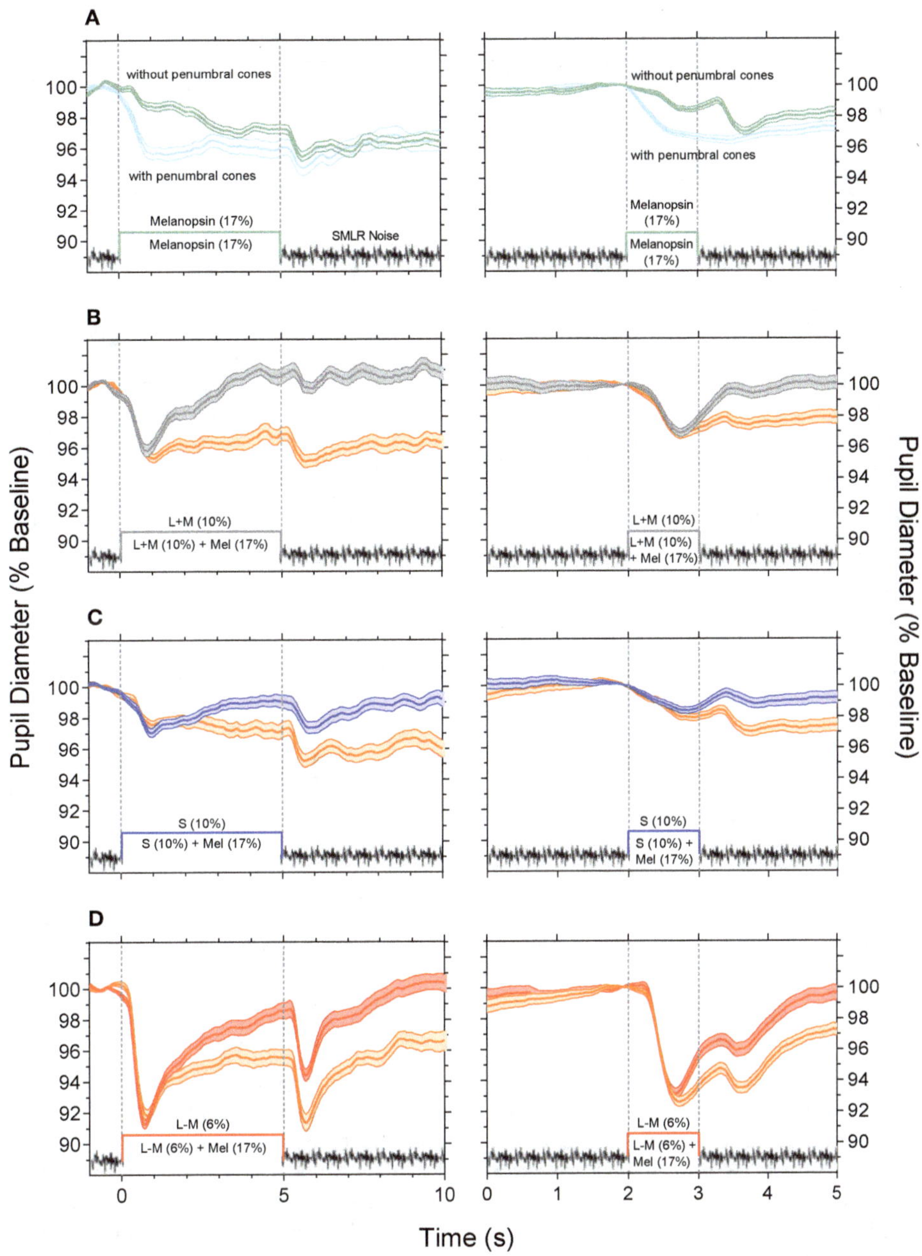

FIGURE 2 | Light-adapted pupil responses measured under photoreceptor isolating conditions and with combined cone- and melanopsin-directed stimuli. **(A)** Melanopsin-directed pupil responses (17% Weber contrast in all measurements) measured with temporal white noise (without penumbral cones; green lines) and without temporal white noise (with penumbral cones; cyan lines). **(B)** +L+M cone luminance directed pupil responses (10% Weber contrast; grey lines) and the combined+ L+M cones and melanopsin responses (orange lines). **(C)** S-cone directed pupil responses (10% Weber contrast; blue lines) and the combined S-cone and melanopsin responses (orange lines). **(D)** +L–M directed pupil responses (6% Weber contrast; red lines) and the combined +L–M and melanopsin responses (orange lines). In all panels the data show the average ±95% confidence limits of 4 observers (~100 trials per observer). Dotted vertical lines indicate the onset and offset of the incremental pulses. Left column shows the PLR with 5,000 ms incremental pulses; right column shows the PLR with 1,000 ms incremental pulses. The average light-adapted baseline pupil diameter for all observers across all conditions was 4.43 mm ± 0.21 (mean ± SEM).

pulses produce sustained post-stimulus constrictions (1.8 s PIPR range for 1,000 ms cone-directed pulses: 0.3 to 1.1% vs. 1.9% for melanopsin-directed pulses; 5,000 ms cone-directed pulses: 0.1 to 2.1% vs. 3.9% for melanopsin-directed pulses) (**Figures 2B–D**; **Table 1**). The redilation component in response to luminance (+L+M) directed stimuli (**Figure 2B**, gray lines) is faster than that for S-cone (**Figure 2C**, blue lines) and +L-M directed stimuli (**Figure 2D**, red lines) and all show a second constriction between 291 and 425 ms after stimulus offset. We note that the observers verbally reported the presence of a prominent

TABLE 1 | The pupil light reflex (PLR) metrics (mean ± SEM) with 5,000 ms pulses and 1,000 ms pulses for different photoreceptor isolating conditions.

	Photoreceptor directed stimulation						
Pupil metrics 5,000 ms pulse	**Mel (17%)***	**L+M (10%)**	**S (10%)**	**L−M (6%)**	**L+M + Mel**	**S + Mel**	**L−M + Mel**
PLR Latency (ms)	633.3 ± 43.3	341.7 ± 49.3	491.7 ± 64.4	325.0 ± 4.8	412.5 ± 45.8	579.2 ± 81.5	354.2 ± 12.5
Peak Constriction Amplitude (%)	3.2 ± 0.2	4.5 ± 0.6	3.1 ± 0.2	8.9 ± 0.4	4.8 ± 0.3	3.8 ± 0.4	8.5 ± 0.7
Time to Peak (s)	4.0 ± 0.3	0.9 ± 0.1	1.2 ± 0.2	0.8 ± 0.04	1.7 ± 0.6	2.8 ± 0.8	0.9 ± 0.1
Constriction Velocity (%.s^{-1})	0.8 ± 0.02	5.0 ± 1.0	2.6 ± 0.3	11.1 ± 1.0	3.6 ± 0.8	1.7 ± 0.4	9.8 ± 1.2
1.8 s PIPR (%)	3.9 ± 0.7	0.1 ± 0.1	2.1 ± 0.5	2.1 ± 1.0	3.9 ± 0.7	4.1 ± 0.6	5.4 ± 0.6
Pupil metrics 5,000 ms pulse	**Mel (17%)***	**L+M (10%)**	**S (10%)**	**L−M (6%)**	**L+M + Mel**	**S + Mel**	**L−M + Mel**
PLR Latency (ms)	612.5 ± 42.7	395.8 ± 46.3	445.8 ± 114.3	366.7 ± 9.6	379.2 ± 48.8	425.0 ± 62.9	341.7 ± 22.1
Peak Constriction Amplitude (%)	2.1 ± 0.2	3.1 ± 0.2	2.1 ± 0.3	7.0 ± 1.0	3.4 ± 0.2	2.5 ± 0.4	7.6 ± 0.7
Time to Peak (s)	0.9 ± 0.1	0.8 ± 0.03	0.9 ± 0.1	0.7 ± 0.01	0.9 ± 0.1	0.8 ± 0.1	0.8 ± 0.03
Constriction Velocity (%.s^{-1})	2.3 ± 0.4	4.1 ± 0.3	2.6 ± 0.6	9.9 ± 1.6	4.1 ± 0.5	3.0 ± 0.3	10.0 ± 1.3
1.8 s PIPR (%)	1.9 ± 0.1	0.3 ± 0.2	1.1 ± 0.3	0.6 ± 0.1	2.1 ± 0.1	2.4 ± 0.4	3.0 ± 0.3

*The units for the metrics and Weber contrasts of the photoreceptor isolating conditions are given in the parentheses. Mel, melanopsin; PIPR, post-illumination pupil response. *Measured with temporal white noise (without penumbral cones).*

afterimage following offset of the +L−M and S−cone stimuli, and a faint afterimage following offset of the +L+M stimuli. When melanopsin combines with cone signals (**Figures 2B–D**, orange lines), the faster temporal response of cones mediates the transient pupil constrictions to stimulus onset and the slower melanopsin signal maintains the pupil constriction during continuous light stimulation and after stimulus offset, with a larger amplitude sustained constriction during the longer (5,000 ms) stimulus exposure. Together, these interactions reveal melanopsin- and cone-directed pupil responses at photopic illuminations under light-adapted conditions that provide no change in rod photoreceptor contrast.

Overlaying all the photoreceptor-directed pupil light responses highlights the transient constriction generated by the cone signals, and the slower, sustained response generated by melanopsin (**Figure 3A**). The combined melanopsin- and cone-directed pupil responses (**Figure 3B**) show an initial transient constriction followed by a sustained constriction that is absent from the cone-directed pupil responses; the secondary constriction after stimulus offset is present in all conditions (**Figures 3A,B**). In **Figure 3C**, the difference between the photoreceptor-directed (**Figure 3A**) and the combined pupil responses (**Figure 3B**) reveals that melanopsin contributions to each of the cone-directed pupil responses manifests as a slow constriction to stimulus onset that remains sustained following stimulus offset, and which is equivalent to the melanopsin-directed pupil response (without penumbral cone intrusion; **Figure 2A**). For the combined pupil responses, the melanopsin contribution appears to be additive to the cone-directed inputs, with similar patterns for both the longer (5,000 ms) and shorter (1,000 ms) duration pulses.

DISCUSSION

We observe that the pupil light response is modulated by interactions between all three cone photoreceptor signals and melanopsin, with clear differences in their relative contributions. The constriction response mediated intrinsically via melanopsin includes a longer latency and slower velocity than for cones (**Figures 2A, 3A**); the melanopsin-mediated sustained pupil constriction continues post-stimulus (**Figures 2A, 3C**). Importantly, this shows that under light-adapted conditions, the putative melanopsin contribution to the pupil after

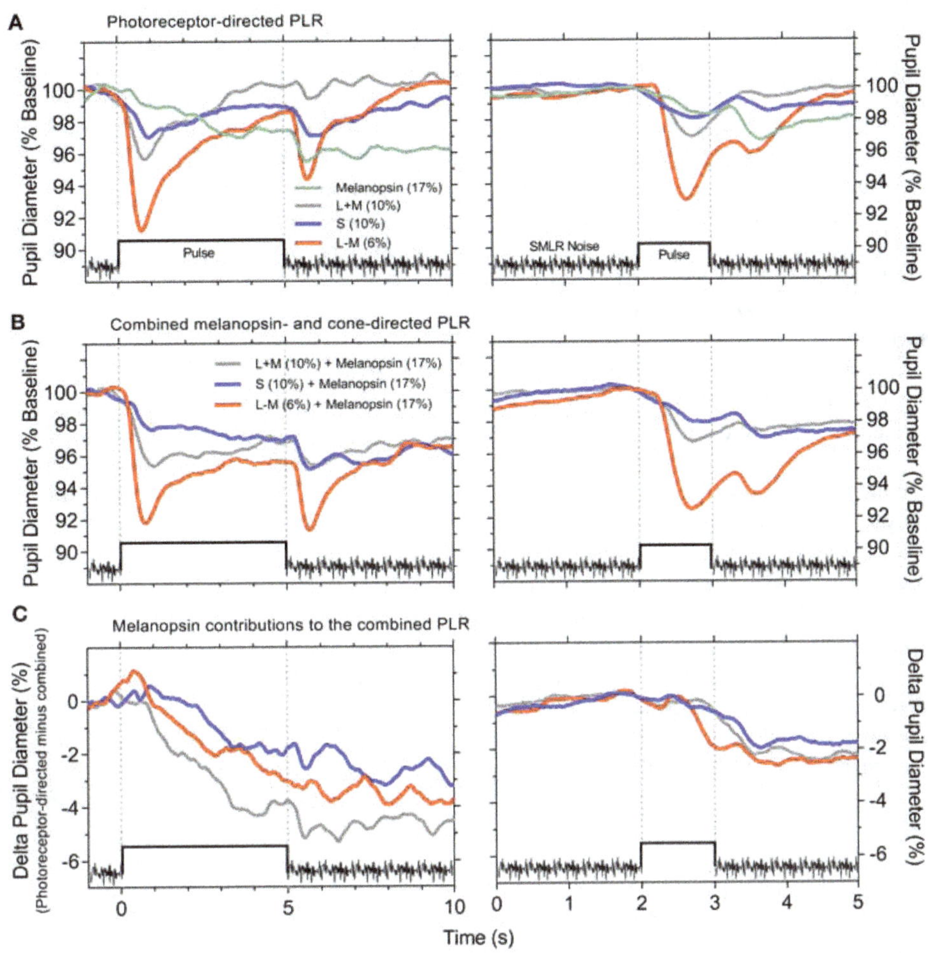

FIGURE 3 | Photoreceptor-directed and combined pupil light responses (PLR). **(A)** Photoreceptor-directed PLR. **(B)** Combined melanopsin- and cone-directed PLR. **(C)** Melanopsin contributions to the combined PLR [difference between the data in **(A,B)**]. The PLR traces are an overlay of the average pupil responses from **Figure 2** ($n = 4$ observers) on the same timescale for the 5,000 ms stimulus pulse (left panels) and 1,000 ms stimulus pulse (right panels). Stimulus contrasts are specified within the panels.

stimulus offset (i.e., post-stimulus) mirrors the sustained post-illumination pupil response observed in the dark. Therefore, irrespective of adaptation condition, the implication is that the sustained activity of inner retinal melanopsin-expressing ipRGCs in response to the lighting conditions (i.e., stimulus and/or mean adaptation level) will set the light-adapted pupil diameter, as it does after stimulus offset in the dark, analogs to the post-illumination pupil response (2, 30). In comparison, cone-mediated pupil responses to changes in image contrast are transient with a rapid redilation to the light-adapted baseline pupil diameter.

For cone isolated tonic pupil responses (i.e., no change in melanopsin excitation), the S-cone directed stimuli (~1.4x visual threshold) produce a robust second pupil constriction at stimulus offset that is, relative to the respective peak pupil constriction, larger than for the chromatic +L−M stimuli (~30x visual threshold and which produce color opponent after-images) and luminance +L+M stimuli (~2x visual threshold) (**Figure 3A** and **Table 1**); these findings indicate that pupil responses to S-cone directed incremental lights (27, 28) reveal inhibitory inputs to the pupil pathway, as observed for phasic pupil responses to periodic modulation (6, 8, 10, 12). Such inhibitory responses are also present with the chromatic +L−M directed incremental pulses, that with flicker stimuli may indicate antagonism between the opponent cone inputs (50, 51). Residual-cone input is not likely to drive this second constriction in the melanopsin-directed pupil responses because the noise does not produce a transient pupil constriction (**Figure 1**). Recordings from ipRGCs in primate retina do however, reveal a transient hyperpolarization at light offset (2) and so the secondary constriction may therefore originate in ipRGCs, as the major pathway of outer retinal signals to the OPN. Another possibility is that this secondary constriction is related to the colored afterimage (28, 52, 53). Illusory changes in brightness can also induce a pupil constriction (54). That this secondary constriction is more prominent with both the longer duration (5,000 ms) melanopsin-directed pulses (with penumbral cone intrusion) and the cone-directed pulses (**Figure 3A**; left vs. right panels), indicates that temporal adaptation differentially alters the strength of afterimage (consistent with the observer reports) and therefore the amplitude of the second constriction.

As for mice, stimulus duration is an important determinant of the photoreceptor inputs to the afferent pupil response in humans. Transgenic mouse models however, show weak cone contributions to the pupil; transient pupil responses in mice are driven predominantly through the relay of rod signals to ipRGCs, through persistent, sustained pupil responses from ipRGCs during continuous light stimulation (22) and additive cone and melanopsin inputs that contribute to constriction (55). Here we show that cone signals drive human tonic pupil responses (**Figure 1**), in addition to rods (5, 7, 25). With melanopsin-directed stimuli, the latency to constriction is 292 ms longer than to a +L+M-cone luminance directed stimulus (5,000 ms pulse; **Table 1** and **Figure 3**), strikingly similar to the ~280 ms difference in constriction latency between melanopsin only (rod-cone knockout) and wild-type mice (17). Such similarities serve to highlight the precision of the silent-substitution methodology for isolating melanopsin-mediated photoreceptor responses.

For the tonic pupil constriction to narrowband, aperiodic pulsed stimuli, the primary view is that the most sensitive outer or inner retinal process will mediate the constriction (i.e., winner take all) (25); stimulus irradiances that are suprathreshold for a melanopsin photoresponse increase channel membrane openings and decrease input impedance to shunt outer retinal signals extrinsically to ipRGCs (25). This study shows that when illumination conditions drive both, melanopsin and cones, the tonic pupil constrictions are always dominated by cones because of the slower constriction velocity of melanopsin, whereas during prolonged light exposure, melanopsin combines with cones to maintain constriction, then after stimulus offset the light-adapted pupil diameter is controlled by melanopsin.

AUTHOR CONTRIBUTIONS

AZ, BF, and DC conceived, designed, and supervised the project. PA and AZ performed the experiments. All Authors participated in the analysis and interpretation of the experiments. AZ and BF wrote the manuscript. All Authors critically revised and approved the final manuscript version.

ACKNOWLEDGMENTS

Supported by the Australian Research Council Discovery Projects ARC-DP170100274 (AZ, BF, and DC) and Australian Research Council Future Fellowship ARC-FT180100458 (AZ).

REFERENCES

1. Dacey DM, Liao HW, Peterson BB, Robinson FR, Smith VC, Pokorny J, et al. Melanopsin-expressing ganglion cells in primate retina signal colour and irradiance and project to the LGN. *Nature.* (2005) 433:749–54. doi: 10.1038/nature03387
2. Gamlin PD, McDougal DH, Pokorny J, Smith VC, Yau KW, Dacey DM. Human and macaque pupil responses driven by melanopsin-containing retinal ganglion cells. *Vis Res.* (2007) 47:946–54. doi: 10.1016/j.visres.2006.12.015
3. Hannibal J, Kankipati L, Strang CE, Peterson BB, Dacey D, Gamlin PD. Central projections of intrinsically photosensitive retinal ganglion cells in the macaque monkey. *J Comp Neurol.* (2014) 522:2231–48. doi: 10.1002/cne.23588
4. Adhikari P, Feigl B, Zele AJ. Rhodopsin and melanopsin contributions to the early redilation phase of the post-illumination pupil response (PIPR). *PLoS ONE.* (2016) 11:e0161175. doi: 10.1371/journal.pone.0161175
5. Barrionuevo PA, Nicandro N, McAnany JJ, Zele AJ, Gamlin P, Cao D. Assessing rod, cone, and melanopsin contributions to human pupil flicker responses. *Invest Ophthalmol Vis Sci.* (2014) 55:719–27. doi: 10.1167/iovs.13-13252
6. Cao D, Nicandro N, Barrionuevo PA. A five-primary photostimulator suitable for studying intrinsically photosensitive retinal ganglion cell functions in humans. *J Vis.* (2015) 15:15.1.27. doi: 10.1167/15.1.27
7. Gooley JJ, Ho Mien I, St. Hilaire MA, Yeo SC, Chua EC, van Reen E, et al. Melanopsin and rod-cone photoreceptors play different roles in mediating pupillary light responses during exposure to continuous light in humans. *J Neurosci.* (2012) 32:14242–53. doi: 10.1523/JNEUROSCI.1321-12.2012
8. Spitschan M, Jain S, Brainard DH, Aguirre GK. Opponent melanopsin and S-cone signals in the human pupillary light response. *Proc Natl Acad Sci USA.* (2014) 111:15568–72. doi: 10.1073/pnas.1400942111
9. Zele AJ, Feigl B, Smith SS, Markwell EL. The circadian response of intrinsically photosensitive retinal ganglion cells. *PLoS ONE.* (2011) 6:e17860. doi: 10.1371/journal.pone.0017860
10. Zele AJ, Feigl B, Adhikari P, Maynard ML, Cao D. Melanopsin photoreception contributes to human visual detection, temporal and colour processing. *Sci Rep.* (2018) 8:3842. doi: 10.1038/s41598-018-22197-w
11. Barbur JL, Harlow AJ, Sahraie A. Pupillary responses to stimulus structure, colour and movement. *Ophthalmic Physiol Opt.* (1992) 12:137–41.
12. Barrionuevo PA, McAnany JJ, Zele AJ, Cao D. Non-linearities in the rod and cone photoreceptor inputs to the afferent pupil light response. *Front Neurol.* (2018) 9:1140. doi: 10.3389/fneur.2018.01140
13. McDougal DH, Gamlin PD. Autonomic control of the eye. *Compr Physiol.* (2015) 5:439–73. doi: 10.1002/cphy.c140014
14. Kawasaki A, Kardon RH. Intrinsically photosensitive retinal ganglion cells. *J Neuroophthalmol.* (2007) 27:195–204. doi: 10.1097/WNO.0b013e31814b1df9
15. Feigl B, Zele AJ. Melanopsin-expressing intrinsically photosensitive retinal ganglion cells in retinal disease. *Optom Vis Sci.* (2014) 91:894–903. doi: 10.1097/OPX.0000000000000284
16. Hattar S, Lucas RJ, Mrosovsky N, Thompson S, Douglas RH, Hankins MW, et al. Melanopsin and rod-cone photoreceptive systems account for all major accessory visual functions in mice. *Nature.* (2003) 424:76–81. doi: 10.1038/nature01761
17. Lucas RJ, Douglas RH, Foster RG. Characterization of an ocular photopigment capable of driving pupillary constriction in mice. *Nat Neurosci.* (2001) 4:621–6. doi: 10.1038/88443
18. Lucas RJ, Hattar S, Takao M, Berson DM, Foster RG, Yau KW. Diminished pupillary light reflex at high irradiances in melanopsin-knockout mice. *Science.* (2003) 299:245–7. doi: 10.1126/science.1077293
19. Ostrin LA, Strang CE, Chang K, Jnawali A, Hung LF, Arumugam B, et al. Immunotoxin-induced ablation of the intrinsically photosensitive retinal ganglion cells in rhesus monkeys. *Front Neurol.* (2018) 9:1000. doi: 10.3389/fneur.2018.01000

20. Guler AD, Ecker JL, Lall GS, Haq S, Altimus CM, Liao HW, et al. Melanopsin cells are the principal conduits for rod-cone input to non-image-forming vision. *Nature.* (2008) 453:102–5. doi: 10.1038/nature06829
21. Hattar S, Liao HW, Takao M, Berson DM, Yau KW. Melanopsin-containing retinal ganglion cells: architecture, projections, and intrinsic photosensitivity. *Science.* (2002) 295:1065–70. doi: 10.1126/science.1069609
22. Keenan WT, Rupp AC, Ross RA, Somasundaram P, Hiriyanna S, Wu Z, et al. A visual circuit uses complementary mechanisms to support transient and sustained pupil constriction. *Elife.* (2016) 5:e15392. doi: 10.7554/eLife.15392
23. Kostic C, Crippa SV, Martin C, Kardon RH, Biel M, Arsenijevic Y, et al. Determination of rod and cone influence to the early and late dynamic of the pupillary light response. *Invest Ophthalmol Vis Sci.* (2016) 57:2501–8. doi: 10.1167/iovs.16-19150
24. Alpern M, Campbell FW. The spectral sensitivity of the consensual light reflex. *J Physiol.* (1962) 164:478–507.
25. McDougal DH, Gamlin PD. The influence of intrinsically-photosensitive retinal ganglion cells on the spectral sensitivity and response dynamics of the human pupillary light reflex. *Vis Res.* (2010) 50:72–87. doi: 10.1016/j.visres.2009.10.012
26. Young RS, Kimura E. Pupillary correlates of light-evoked melanopsin activity in humans. *Vis Res.* (2008) 48:862–71. doi: 10.1016/j.visres.2007.12.016
27. Barbur JL, Sahraie A, Simmons A, Weiskrantz L, Williams SC. Residual processing of chromatic signals in the absence of a geniculostriate projection. *Vis Res.* (1998) 38:3447–53.
28. Kimura E, Young RS. S-cone contribution to pupillary responses evoked by chromatic flash offset. *Vis Res.* (1999) 39:1189–97.
29. Vienot F, Brettel H, Dang TV, Le Rohellec J. Domain of metamers exciting intrinsically photosensitive retinal ganglion cells (ipRGCs) and rods. *J Opt Soc Am A.* (2012) 29:A366–76. doi: 10.1364/JOSAA.29.00A366
30. Adhikari P, Zele AJ, Feigl B. The Post-Illumination Pupil Response (PIPR). *Invest Ophthalmol Vis Sci.* (2015) 56:3838–49. doi: 10.1167/iovs.14-16233
31. Grünert U, Jusuf PR, Lee SC, Nguyen DT. Bipolar input to melanopsin containing ganglion cells in primate retina. *Vis Neurosci.* (2011) 28:39–50. doi: 10.1017/S095252381000026X
32. Nasir-Ahmad S, Lee SC, Martin PR, Grünert U. Melanopsin-expressing ganglion cells in human retina: morphology, distribution, and synaptic connections. *J Comp Neurol.* (2017) 527:312–27. doi: 10.1002/cne.24176
33. Gamlin PD, Zhang H, Harlow A, Barbur JL. Pupil responses to stimulus color, structure and light flux increments in the rhesus monkey. *Vis Res.* (1998) 38:3353–8.
34. Estévez O, Spekreijse H. The "silent substitution" method in visual research. *Vis Res.* (1982) 22:681–91.
35. Smith VC, Pokorny J. Spectral sensitivity of the foveal cone photopigments between 400 and 500 nm. *Vis Res.* (1975) 15:161–71.
36. Enezi J, Revell V, Brown T, Wynne J, Schlangen L, Lucas R. A "melanopic" spectral efficiency function predicts the sensitivity of melanopsin photoreceptors to polychromatic lights. *J Biol Rhythms.* (2011) 26:314–23. doi: 10.1177/0748730411409719
37. Shapiro AG, Pokorny J, Smith VC. Cone-rod receptor spaces with illustrations that use CRT phosphor and light-emitting-diode spectra. *J Opt Soc Am A.* (1996) 13:2319–28.
38. Zele AJ, Adhikari P, Cao D, Feigl B. Melanopsin driven enhancement of cone-mediated visual processing. *Vis Res.* (2019). doi: 10.1016/j.visres.2019.04.009
39. Brindley GS, Du Croz JJ, Rushton WA. The flicker fusion frequency of the blue-sensitive mechanism of colour vision. *J Physiol.* (1966) 183:497–500.
40. Swanson WH, Ueno T, Smith VC, Pokorny J. Temporal modulation sensitivity and pulse detection thresholds for chromatic and luminance perturbations. *J Opt Soc Am A.* (1987) 4:1992–2005.
41. Guth SL, Lodge HR. Heterochromatic additivity, foveal spectral sensitivity, and a new color model. *J Opt Soc Am.* (1973) 63:450–62.
42. Kelbsch C, Strasser T, Chen Y, Feigl B, Gamlin PD, Kardon R, et al. Standards in Pupillography. *Front Neurol.* (2019) 10:129. doi: 10.3389/fneur.2019.00129
43. Feigl B, Ojha G, Hides L, Zele AJ. Melanopsin-driven pupil response and light exposure in non-seasonal major depressive disorder. *Front Neurol.* (2018) 9:764. doi: 10.3389/fneur.2018.00764
44. Hathibelagal AR, Feigl B, Kremers J, Zele AJ. Correlated and uncorrelated invisible temporal white noise alters mesopic rod signaling. *J Opt Soc Am A.* (2016) 33:A93–103. doi: 10.1364/JOSAA.33.000A93
45. Zele AJ, Feigl B, Kambhampati PK, Aher A, McKeefry D, Parry N, et al. A temporal white noise analysis for extracting the impulse response function of the human electroretinogram. *Transl Vis Sci Technol.* (2017) 6:1. doi: 10.1167/tvst.6.6.1
46. Zele AJ, Feigl B, Kambhampati PK, Hathibelagal AR, Kremers J. A method for estimating intrinsic noise in electroretinographic (ERG) signals. *Doc Ophthalmol.* (2015) 131:85–94. doi: 10.1007/s10633-015-9510-1
47. Joyce DS, Feigl B, Zele AJ. The effects of short-term light adaptation on the human post-illumination pupil response. *Invest Ophthalmol Vis Sci.* (2016) 57:5672–80. doi: 10.1167/iovs.16-19934
48. Cao D, Pokorny J, Smith VC, Zele AJ. Rod contributions to color perception: linear with rod contrast. *Vis Res.* (2008) 48:2586–92. doi: 10.1016/j.visres.2008.05.001
49. Turnbull PR, Irani N, Lim N, Phillips JR. Origins of pupillary hippus in the autonomic nervous system. *Invest Ophthalmol Vis Sci.* (2017) 58:197–203. doi: 10.1167/iovs.16-20785
50. Murray IJ, Kremers J, McKeefry D, Parry NRA. Paradoxical pupil responses to isolated M-cone increments. *J Opt Soc Am A.* (2018) 35:B66–71. doi: 10.1364/JOSAA.35.000B66
51. Woelders T, Leenheers T, Gordijn MCM, Hut RA, Beersma DGM, Wams EJ. Melanopsin- and L-cone-induced pupil constriction is inhibited by S- and M-cones in humans. *Proc Natl Acad Sci USA.* (2018) 115:792–7. doi: 10.1073/pnas.1716281115
52. Newsome DA. Afterimage and pupillary activity following strong light exposure. *Vis Res.* (1971) 11:275–88.
53. Tsujimura S, Wolffsohn JS, Gilmartin B. Pupil responses associated with coloured afterimages are mediated by the magno-cellular pathway. *Vis Res.* (2003) 43:1423–32. doi: 10.1016/S0042-6989(03)00145-7
54. Laeng B, Endestad T. Bright illusions reduce the eye's pupil. *Proc Natl Acad Sci USA.* (2012) 109:2162–7. doi: 10.1073/pnas.1118298109
55. Hayter EA, Brown TM. Additive contributions of melanopsin and both cone types provide broadband sensitivity to mouse pupil control. *BMC Biol.* (2018) 16:83. doi: 10.1186/s12915-018-0552-1

18

The Method of Silent Substitution for Examining Melanopsin Contributions to Pupil Control

Manuel Spitschan[1*] *and Tom Woelders*[2]

[1] *Department of Experimental Psychology, University of Oxford, Oxford, United Kingdom,* [2] *Chronobiology Unit, Groningen Institute for Evolutionary Life Sciences, University of Groningen, Groningen, Netherlands*

Correspondence:
Manuel Spitschan
manuel.spitschan@psy.ox.ac.uk

The human pupillary light response is driven by all classes of photoreceptors in the human eye—the three classes of cones, the rods, and the intrinsically photosensitive retinal ganglion cells (ipRGCs) expressing the photopigment melanopsin. These photoreceptor classes have distinct but overlapping spectral tuning, and even a monochromatic light with a wavelength matched to the peak spectral sensitivity of a given photoreceptor will stimulate all photoreceptors. The method of silent substitution uses pairs of lights ("metamers") to selectively stimulate a given class of photoreceptors while keeping the activation of all others constant. In this primer, we describe the method of silent substitution and provide an overview of studies that have used it to examine inputs to the human pupillary light response.

Keywords: pupil, melanopsin, silent substitution, color vision, pupillometry, ipRGC (intrinsically photosensitive retinal ganglion cell), metamers

INTRODUCTION

At the input level, the size of the pupil is controlled by the activity of the different photoreceptors in the human eye (1). These different photoreceptors differ in many respects: their wavelength tuning (spectral sensitivity), their temporal properties, their operating range and their distribution across the retina. The goal of this primer is to describe the method of silent substitution for examining photoreceptor-specific pupil responses. We start with the fundamentals underlying the method of silent substitution, provide an overview of studies that have used this method, provide a practical guide and *R* code to implement silent substitution and highlight a few challenges to the method of silent substitution.

FUNDAMENTALS

Overlapping Spectral Sensitivities of the Human Photoreceptors

Photoreception in the human retina is based on the signals produced by the three types of cones—the long[L]-wavelength-sensitive cones, the medium[M]-wavelength-sensitive cones, and the short[S]-wavelength-sensitive cones—, the rods, and the intrinsically photosensitive retinal ganglion cells (ipRGCs), which contain the photopigment melanopsin (2–6). ipRGCs receive synaptic input from cones and rods but, in the absence of those inputs, these cells themselves are photosensitive due to the expression of the melanopsin photopigment in the cell membrane. The peak spectral sensitivities (λ_{max}) of the human photoreceptors are distinct. The photopigments (cone opsins) in the L, M, and S cones peak around 420, 530, and 558 nm, respectively; rhodopsin, the pigment in rods, has a peak at around 495 nm. Finally, the melanopsin photopigment has a peak spectral sensitivity at around 480 nm. Even though these peaks are spectrally distinct and distant, the spectral sensitivities overlap quite extensively due to the relative broadband tuning of photopigments (**Figure 1A**). One challenge in targeting the operation of a single class of photoreceptor is that the spectral sensitivities of the photoreceptors *in vivo* does not necessarily correspond to the spectral sensitivity of a pigment. All light that reaches the retina is filtered by the lens and ocular media (7), thereby shifting the effective spectral sensitivity. Typically, this pre-receptoral filtering is accounted for in the spectral sensitivities for cones, rods, and melanopsin-containing ipRGCs.

Non-specificity of Single-Wavelength Lights

An important desideratum for examining how the different photoreceptors contribute to the human pupillary light response is that stimuli produce responses specific to a given photoreceptor class. One consequence of the extensive spectral overlap of the photoreceptors is that most light sources activate all photoreceptors, and therefore, the responses elicited are largely nonspecific. For example, monochromatic light with a peak spectral output of 490 nm will activate melanopsin maximally relative to the other photoreceptors, but it will also lead to substantial activation of rods and the cones (**Figure 1B**). The relative amounts by which a monochromatic light of a given wavelength activates all photoreceptors is directly predicted from the relative spectral sensitivity of the photoreceptors at that wavelength. Monochromatic lights have been of great use in determining the spectral sensitivity of the sustained pupil constrictions that match that of melanopsin (8–11). This specific type of measurement is called the "post-illumination pupil response," abbreviated PIPR, in which the pupil response is typically measured in response to a non-specific short-wavelength light flash and a non-specific long-wavelength light flash against a dim or no background.

Principle of Univariance

One property of photoreceptors is the *principle of univariance* (12), which states that a given photoreceptor has only scalar output, namely its photocurrent: It cannot distinguish between changes in intensity and changes in wavelength. This is shown in **Figure 1C** using theoretical lights containing power at only a single wavelength (monochromatic light): Lights E_1, E_2, and E_3 all nominally elicit the same photoreceptor excitation. Lights E_1 and E_3 have their peak emission at the 50% point of spectral sensitivity on either side of the peak; light E_2 is scaled to be 50% of the emission of lights E_1 and E_3. To the photoreceptor (in this case melanopsin), which weights the input light by its spectral sensitivity, the lights are equally effective. The key insight is that photoreceptors integrate light of different wavelengths, weighting the input spectrum by their spectral sensitivity and summing it up. A consequence of the principle of univariance is that single photoreceptors are color-blind: Whether two lights differ in wavelength or intensity cannot be determined from the photoreceptor output alone.

Wavelength Exchange

Because photoreceptors weight input light by their spectral sensitivity function, in the case of two photoreceptors, it is possible to find two lights and scale them such that the excitation of one of the photoreceptors remains constant in this wavelength exchange, while the other one "sees" a difference. This is shown in **Figure 1D**: The peak emissions of lights E_1 and E_2 have been chosen to match the two 50% points of the S-cone spectral sensitivity, thereby eliciting the same responses. This is called *silencing* the S cones. Because the spectral sensitivity of melanopsin is different from that of the S cones, our two lights E_1 and E_2 necessarily produce a different response, and in this case we call melanopsin the *stimulated* photoreceptor. Wavelength exchange for two photopigments is the most simple case of silent substitution. But, with the exception of certain classes of color-blindness such as rod monochromacy, the human retina contains five photoreceptors. Fortunately, the same principle can be extended to more than two photoreceptors.

THE METHOD OF SILENT SUBSTITUTION

In the method of silent substitution, pairs of light are found that have the property that they stimulate the targeted photoreceptor class (or classes) whilst not changing the excitation of the other photoreceptors, the silenced ones. The method has a long history for determining the properties of the mechanisms of human color vision (13, 14).

Fundamentals

To introduce the method of silent substitution we begin with an example from human color vision. Human color vision is trichromatic under daylight conditions, i.e., when rods do not participate: A color-normal observer can match the color appearance of any light using a combination of three primary lights (15). Under these conditions, it is assumed that only the three classes of cones participate in the color match; it follows that because three photoreceptors participate, three independent primary lights need to be used. It is impossible to match the activation of three photoreceptors in one condition using just two primary lights.

In general, to stimulate one class of photoreceptor classes out of N_R photoreceptor classes while leaving the activation of the other $N_R - 1$ unchanged, at least N_R primary lights (N_p) are necessary. When $N_R = N_P$ (i. e. there are as many primary lights as photoreceptor classes under consideration), there is only one algebraic solution to match the activation of the $N_R - 1$ photoreceptors under one set of settings for the N_P lights to another other setting that will only stimulate the remaining photoreceptor class.

For the case of four photoreceptor classes in the human retina (three classes of cones and melanopsin), four lights are necessary to match the activation of cones and stimulate melanopsin. When including the rods, five lights are necessary to match the activation of cones and rods and stimulate melanopsin.

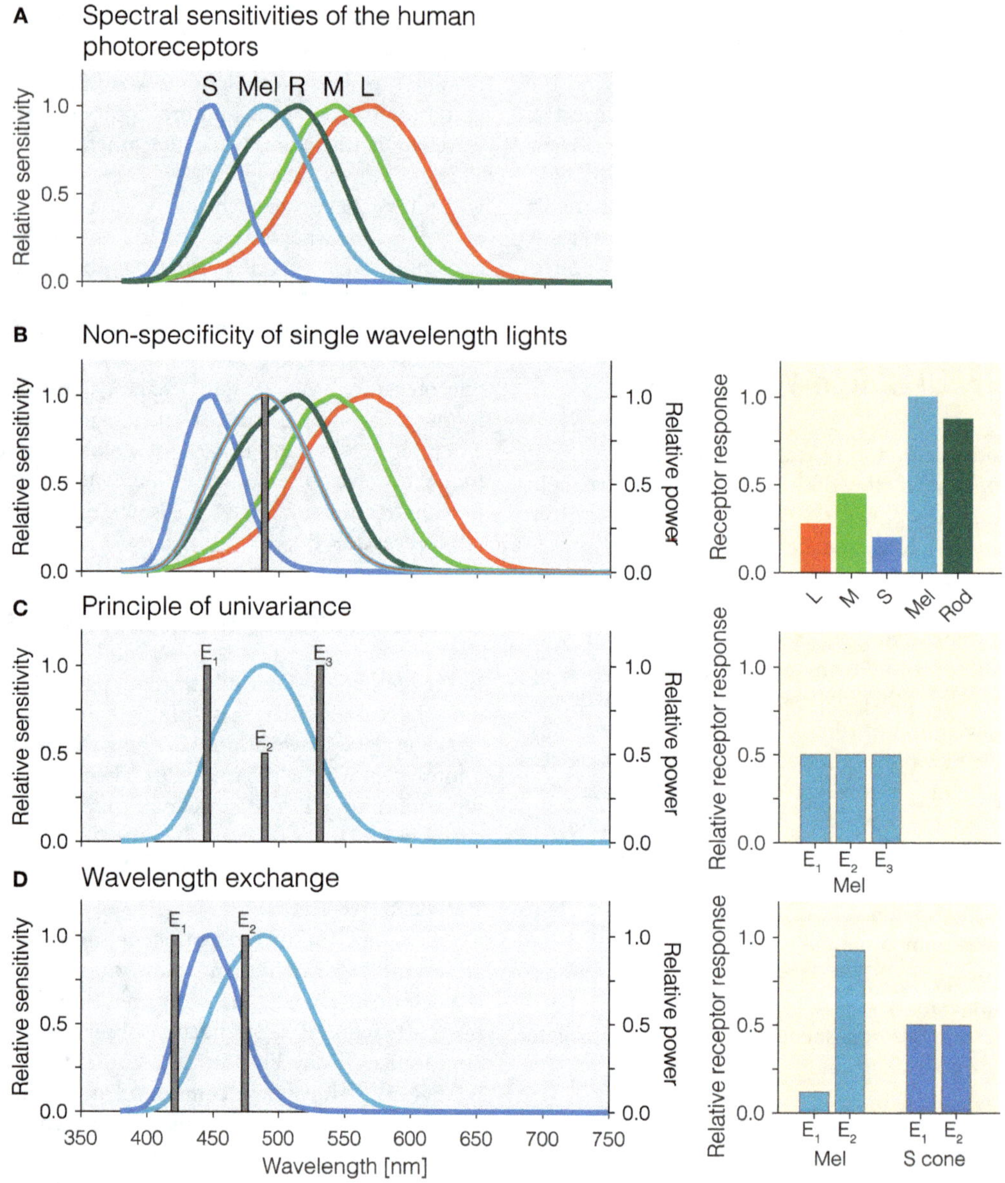

FIGURE 1 | (A) Overlapping spectral sensitivities of the human photoreceptors. **(B)** Non-specificity of single-wavelength lights. Right panel: Pattern of photoreceptor responses to the single-wavelength light at 490 nm. **(C)** Principle of univariance. Right panel: Pattern of photoreceptor responses to the single-wavelength lights E_1, E_2, and E_3 designed to elicit the same response in melanopsin. **(D)** Wavelength exchange between two short-wavelength lights E_1 and E_2 which stimulate S cones at the same level but yield different photoreceptor responses for melanopsin. Right panel: Pattern of excitations for lights E_1 and E_2.

It is possible to have more primary lights than photoreceptors under consideration, i.e., $N_R < N_P$. This would for example be the case when there were, e.g., eight independent primaries and the retina to be studied was a human one. In that case, there are infinitely many solutions to match the activation of the N_R-1 photoreceptors under one set of settings for the N_P lights to any other setting that will only stimulate the remaining photoreceptor class. In practice, this is typically solved by implementing a numerical optimization which maximizes the contrast seen by the stimulated photoreceptor while setting a constraint to have no contrast on the unstimulated ones, and enforcing additional constraints on the optimisation.

Contrast

The term contrast refers to a specific quantity, which is the fractional difference of activation of a photopigment around a background:

$$I = \frac{I_{modulation} - I_{background}}{I_{background}}$$

Intuitively, when the light-adapted background activates a given photoreceptor by some amount, e.g., 100 (arbitrary units), and the modulation activates it by a higher amount, e.g., 120 (arbitrary units), the contrast in that case would be 0.2 or 20%. Contrast can be specified either as fractions or as percentages.

An Intuitive Example

We now describe an example case for the method of silent substitution corresponding to the stimuli used in Spitschan, Jain, Brainard and Aguirre (16). These authors used a calibrated spectrally tuneable light source that modified the output of a broadband Xenon arc lamp using a digital micromirror device (DMD) to produce, effectively, arbitrary spectral power distributions. While this is a special case of light sources, most experimenters have used a set of discrete lights, the intensities of which are controlled to produce silent substitution stimuli. *The goal is to produce two lights with spectral power distributions that do not differ in the amount they activate the cones, and only yield a change in the amount they activate melanopsin.* Such pairs of stimuli are also called metamers–they are indistinguishable to the cones, despite having different spectral power distributions. In this example, we ignore the rods.

1. Background spectrum: In the first instance, we begin with a background spectrum of known spectral power distribution (**Figure 2A**). We call this the background spectrum because the observer is typically light-adapted to this spectrum, and the silent-substitution stimuli are shown to the observer "around" this background in the form of pulses or temporal modulations. This background spectrum elicits a pattern of photoreceptors responses (**Figure 2B**, right panel). The activation of photoreceptors is calculated by weighting the spectrum by the spectral sensitivities and summing it up for each photoreceptor class.
2. Increasing melanopsin activation: Pragmatically, we can increase the amount of light seen by melanopsin by simply increasing the amount of light emitted near the melanopsin peak. This is shown in **Figure 2B**. However, this is only partly successful: Because of the overlapping peak spectral sensitivities of the human photoreceptors, such an increase in emitted light leads to an increase in activation of all photoreceptors (**Figure 2B**, middle panel). Rather than considering the absolute amount of activation of the photoreceptors (which is also dependent on the exact light level), it is customary to speak of contrast (**Figure 2B**, right panel). Contrast here refers to the percentage difference in activation of photoreceptors between the modulation spectrum (red line in **Figure 2B**) and the background spectrum (**Figure 2A** and dashed line in **Figures 2B–F**). As can be seen in the right panel in **Figure 2B**, the increase in light near the melanopsin peak leads to an increase in contrast to all photoreceptors. To reiterate, the desideratum here is to have no contrast seen by L, M and S cones, and positive contrast seen by melanopsin.
3. Silencing S cones: To zero, or silence, the S cones, we decrease the amount of short-wavelength light, to which the S cones are most sensitive (**Figure 2C**). This indeed leads to a silencing of S cones (**Figure 2C**, middle panel). There is no difference in the absolute activation of S cones, and consequently, the S cone contrast is zero–they are silent.
4. Silencing L and M cones: To silence the L and M cones, a similar trick is applied: Light near the peak spectral sensitivity of L and M cones is decreased to reduce the overall absolute activation of L and M cones (**Figure 2D**). However, we note that there has been an "overshoot" in the decrease in L and M cones activation (**Figure 2D**, middle panel): The modulation spectrum is now producing *less* activation in the L and M cones than the background spectrum. This translates into a small amount of negative contrast seen by the L and M cones (**Figure 2D**, right panel). This can be overcome by again increasing the amount of long-wavelength light in the modulation spectrum (**Figure 2E**), thereby equalizing the activation of L and M cones relative to the background spectrum (**Figure 2D**, middle panel). The L, M and S cones are now silent (**Figure 2E**, right panel), and melanopsin is stimulated at 50%. Because no attempt was taken to silence the rods, they are also stimulated by this spectral exchange.
5. Inverting the melanopsin activation: The modulation spectrum shown in **Figure 2E** (red line) produces a significant increase in melanopsin excitation. By "mirroring" the modulation spectrum around the background spectrum (i.e., an increase in emitted light in the positive modulation spectrum becomes a decrease by the same amount in emitted light in the negative modulation spectrum), we can also generate a negative (rather than a positive) melanopsin stimulus (**Figure 2F**, blue line), thereby producing negative, or decremental, contrast on melanopsin (**Figure 2F**, right panel). In practice, negative and positive modulation spectra are alternated to yield the highest differential activation possible.

A Quantitative Example

We provide a quantitative example along with code in **Appendices A1, A2**, respectively. We use the stimuli from Woelders et al. (17) for this example.

History of Silent Substitution

The method of silent substitution has enjoyed use in empirical work well before the discovery of melanopsin and the ipRGCs. We point the reader to Estévez and Spekreijse (13) for an exposé of the early history of the method, which indeed dates back to experiments involving wavelength exchanges performed in 1906 (18) (see above section "Wavelength exchange"). From the insight that metameric lights such as those obtained in color matching experiments are silent substitution stimuli (i.e., matching the activation of the three cone types), the extension to experimentally control more photoreceptors is conceptually straightforward. In the 1990s, methods to manipulate four photoreceptors independently (three cone classes and rods) using mixtures of four primary lights were developed (18, 19). These methods were then expanded to examining melanopsin function either by

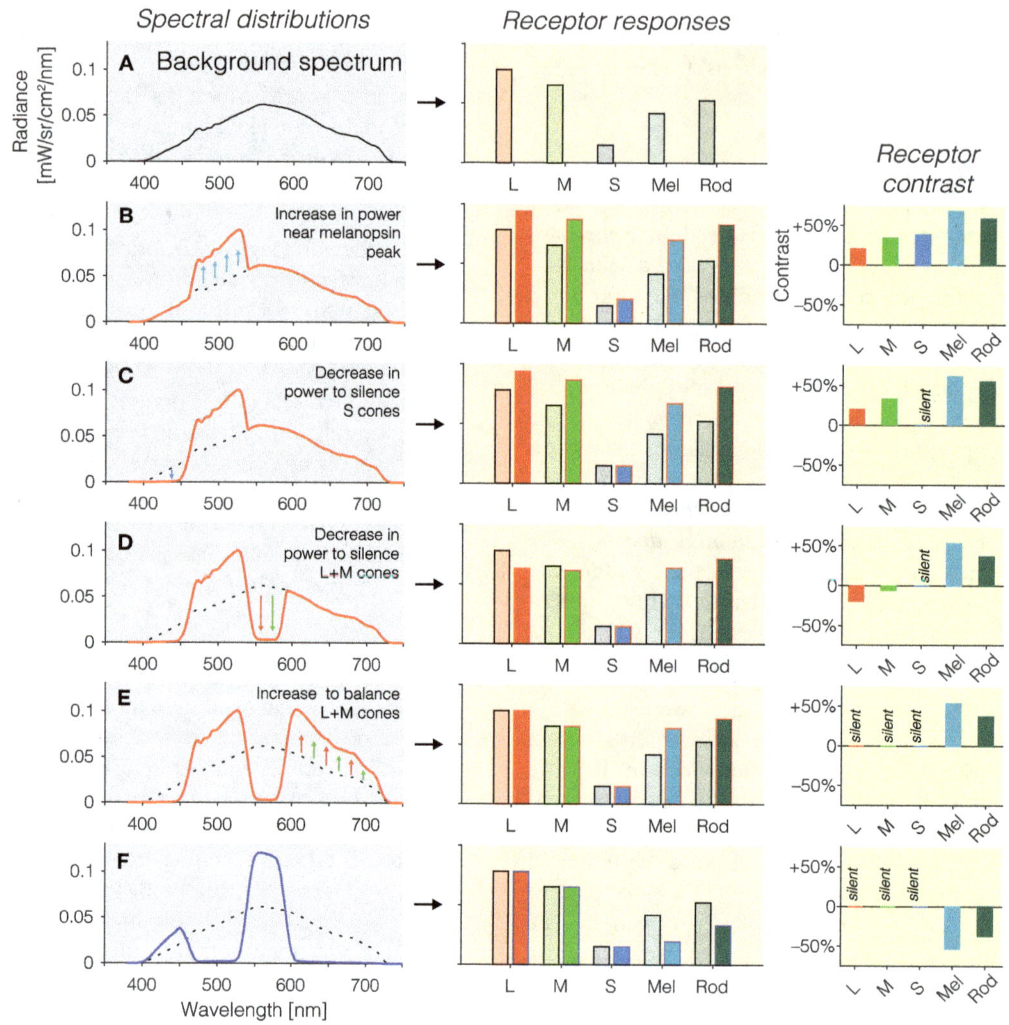

FIGURE 2 | (A) Background spectrum (left panel) to which the observer is light-adapted, eliciting a pattern of responses in the photoreceptors (right panel). **(B)** Increase in emitted light near the melanopsin peak relative to the background spectrum (left panel; dashed line = background spectrum, red line = modulation spectrum) leads to an increase in the excitation of all photoreceptors (middle panel), or equivalently, positive contrast on the photoreceptors (right panel). **(C)** To balance the excitation of the S cones, a decrease in emitted short-wavelength light (left panel) leads to silencing of the S cones (middle panel), or equivalently, zero contrast on the S cones (right panel). **(D)** To balance the excitation of the L and M cones, a decrease in emitted medium-wavelength light (left panel) leads to a reduction in L and M cone activity (middle panel) but not yet zero contrast on the L and M cones (right panel); indeed, the contrast seen by the L and M cones is now negative. **(E)** To silence the excitation of the L and M cones, a decrease in emitted long-wavelength light (left panel) leads to balancing of the L and M cones (middle panel), or equivalently, zero contrast on the L and M cones (right panel). The contrast seen by melanopsin is 50%. **(F)** The modulation spectrum shown in **(E)** yields positive contrast relative to the background spectrum but the spectrum can also be "mirrored" around the background spectrum, thereby leading to a negative modulation of melanopsin (and rods).

assuming rod saturation at high light levels (20), or using five primaries (21).

OVERVIEW OF SILENT SUBSTITUTION STUDIES CONCERNING THE PUPIL

We provide an overview of extant studies examining specifically melanopsin photoreception using the method of silent substitution in **Table 1** and hope that it serves to the reader as an orientation to the literature. This overview includes literature available in early September 2018. We note that both authors of this article have published papers using the method of silent substitution which are included in the table [M.S.: (16, 28), T.W.: (17)]. The table shows that there is a set of experimental parameters that are subject to the experimenters' discretion. We summarise these here.

Number of Primaries

As described above (*The method of silent substitution–Fundamentals*), when stimulating melanopsin, at least four (for matching the cones) or five (for matching both cones and rods) independent primary lights are necessary. Most silent

TABLE 1 | Studies examining human pupil responses with silent substitution.

References	Number of primaries	Primary wavelengths [nm]	Viewing geometry	Field size	Modulations [max. contrast]	Background light level	N observers	Temporal properties	Spectral sensitivities assumed
Tsujimura et al. (20)	4	470, 500, 525, 615 nm ± 20–36 nm	Diffusing screen in front of integrating sphere	20° field size	Melanopsin [−53%] Luminance [−53%] Isochromatic [−53%]	301 cd/m^2 to 642 cd/m^2 to 982 cd/m^2	6	10 min stimuli 5 min background	Cones: CIEPO2006 Melanopsin: Dartnall nomogram at 482 nm Assumes macular and lens filtering from CIEPO2006 Optical density 0.5
Viénot et al. (21)	5	473 ± 25 nm 511 ± 33 nm 530 ± 36 nm 595 ± 15 nm 627 ± 20 nm	Light booth with white paint	Ganzfeld	Melanopsin-only (cone and rod silent) [3.4%] Multiple mixed modulations	35 cd/m^2	10	Measurement after 1 min of continuous exposure	Cones: CIEPO2006 Rods: V'(λ) Melanopsin: Stockman-Sharpe shifted to peak at 482 nm; optical density 0.1; lens from Stockman & Sharpe
Tsijumura and Tokuda, (22)	4	468, 524, 599, and 633 nm (test) 466 nm, 500 nm, 517 nm, 596 nm (background) ±15–38 nm	Diffusing screen in front of integrating sphere	Annulus id 5 od 18° Total field 23°	8%	612 cd/m^2 background 1,109 cd/m^2 test field	6	Sinusoidal & square wave stimuli	Cones: CIEPO2006, 10° Melanopsin: Dartnall nomogram at 480 nm Assumes macular and lens filtering from CIEPO2006 Optical density 0.4
Spitschan et al. (16)	128	n/a	Viewing of surface through lens	27.5° circular, central 5° blocked	S, (L+M), melanopsin, (L+M+melanopsin) [50%]	382–1,033 cd/m^2	16	Sinusoidal, 0.01 – 2 Hz	10° Stockman–Sharpe/CIE cone fundamentals, melanopsin estimated by shifting Stockman-Sharpe nomogram to λ_{max} = 480 nm, corrected for prereceptoral filtering (same as cones, optical density 0.3).
Barrionuevo et al. (23)	4	442, 516, 594, and 634 nm (one set) 466, 514, 590, and 634 nm (second set)	Ganzfeld	54° field	Mixed joint modulations, no melanopsin-isolaing modulation	0.002–100 cd/m^2	3 (authors)	Sinusoidal, 0.5–8 Hz	Smith–Pokorny cone fundamentals Enezi et al. melanopsin function

(Continued)

TABLE 1 | Continued

References	Number of primaries	Primary wavelengths [nm]	Viewing geometry	Field size	Modulations [max. contrast]	Background light level	*N* observers		Spectral sensitivities assumed
Cao et al. (25)	5	456, 488, 540, 592, 633	Maxwellian view	30° circular, central 10.5° blocked	Experiment 1: S, M, L, Rod, Melanopsin [16%] Experiment 2: CSF	Experiment 1: 200 Photopic Td Experiment 2: 2,000 Photopic Td	3	Sinusoidal, 1 Hz	Smith–Pokorny cone fundamentals applied for the CIE 1964 10° Standard Observer CIE 1951 scotopic luminosity function Enezi et al. melanopsin function
Barrionuevo and Cao, (24)	5	456, 488, 540, 592, 633	Maxwellian view	30° circular, central 10.5° blocked	Experiment 1: S, M, L, Rods, Melanopsin, (L+M+S) [17%], red-green [4% M, −4% L] Experiment 2: LMS [17% each], L+M [17% each], LMS + melanopsin [16% each], Rods + melanopsin [9% each], S + melanopsin [16% each], red-green + melanopsin [2% M, −2% L, 8% melanopsin]	2–20,000 Photopic Td	3 (2 authors)	Sinusoidal, 1 Hz	Smith–Pokorny cone fundamentals applied for the CIE 1964 10° Standard Observer CIE 1951 scotopic luminosity function Enezi et al. melanopsin function
Spitschan et al. (28)	56	n/a	Viewing of surface through lens	64° circular, central 5° blocked	25–400%	100–200 cd/m^2	4	Tapered pulses (3 s, 14–16 s ISI)	CIE 2006 parametric model
Woelders et al. (17)	5	465, 500, 515, 595	Diffusing screen in front of LEDs	24.68° horizontal, 12.13° vertical	S, M, L, Melanopsin [23%]	Background or average of 8.5 melanopic lux	16	Square-wave (0.25–4 Hz)	α-opic lux (Lucas et al.): Govardovski nomograms, λ_{max} from Dartnall, optical densities 0.3, 0.38, 0.38 (S, M, L)
Murray et al. (27)	4	460, 524, 590, 635	Ganzfeld	Central 7° of surface covered with disk of no reflective black material.	L, M, (L+M+S) [11% Weber]	17 cd/m^2	5	Square-wave (1 s increment/ decrement followed by ISI of 2 s)	Stockman Sharpe cone fundamentals
Zele et al. (26)	5	456, 488, 540, 592, 633	Maxwellian view	30° circular, central 10.5° blocked	Color:[7%, 22% or 24% Weber] CFF and pupil: (L+M), S, melanopsin [17% Michelson]	2,000 photopic Td (detection thresholds and pupil) 200–5,000 Td (CFF)	4 (2 authors)	Pupil: 1 Hz sinusoidal	Smith–Pokorny cone fundamentals applied for the CIE 1964 108 Standard Observer CIE 1951 scotopic luminosity function Enezi et al. melanopsin function

substitution studies that have examined pupil responses to photoreceptor-specific modulations have employed a finite set of LEDs (four or five), though using spectrally tuneable light sources, more effective primaries are possible.

Peak Wavelength and Width of the Primary Lights

In the case where the primary lights are discrete (such as LEDs), the peak emission wavelengths are subject to design considerations when building the apparatus. Both the choice of peak wavelengths and primary widths affects the contrast available for the silent substitution modulations. The contrast available is also called the *gamut*. In principle, choosing broader primaries will reduce also the amount of susceptibility to individual differences in the cone spectral sensitivities (29). In practice, unless a spectrally tuneable light source is used allowing to create arbitrary spectral power distributions, the choices of primary wavelengths and widths is limited by what is commercially available. When building a system, we recommend first estimating the gamut for a given configuration of peak wavelengths and widths.

Viewing Geometry

Typical viewing geometries include Ganzfeld viewing conditions (in which the stimulus is a homogenous field in an integrating sphere) or Maxwellian view (in which an image is focused on the entrance pupil of the observer). These again depend on the type of design used when building the stimulation system.

Field Size

As can be seen in the table, the field sizes used in the field vary somewhat, and will again depend on constraints set by the optical apparatus used to deliver the stimuli, as well as theoretical considerations such as the distribution of the photoreceptor types across the retina.

Modulations and Contrast

Depending on the spectra of the primary lights, different amounts of contrast are available to stimulate melanopsin. Typically, the highest contrast can be achieved when LEDs are chosen of which the distribution of peak wavelengths is as broad as possible.

Background Light

The choice of background light level is again somewhat arbitrary in many situations, though experimenters typically strive to be well in photopic conditions, where rods are assumed to be saturated, and can therefore be ignored (but see *Rod intrusion* below).

Spectral Sensitivities Assumed

The extent to which a given melanopsin-stimulating modulation silences the cones depends on the spectral sensitivities assumed. Various spectral sensitivities are available (30). Choosing the wrong spectral sensitivities can lead to artefactual results, unless care is taken to correct the modulations. We recommend the use of the CIE 2006 "physiologically relevant" cone fundamentals (31) as it allows for flexible extensions to simulate individual differences parametrically (32). For melanopsin, there is currently no standard(ised) spectral sensitivity, though by using a template (also called nomogram) centered at 480 nm and assuming a low peak optical density, such a spectral sensitivity can easily be derived (33, 34).

CHALLENGES TO SILENT SUBSTITUTION

There are various sources of uncertainty when using silent substitution stimuli. We highlight a few of these here.

Retinal Inhomogenities

The human retina is inhomogeneous. One obvious feature of the retina making it inhomogeneous is the spatial location of the macular pigment around the fovea, with a drop-off toward the periphery. A consequence of macular pigment is that all light seen by the fovea is filtered through the pigment, thereby shifting the effective peak spectral sensitivity of the foveal cones vs. the peripheral cones. In addition, there are also differences in how much photopigment is expressed in foveal vs. peripheral cones—the optical densities are different. Another source of retinal inhomogeneity is that cones that are in the partial shadow of retinal blood vessels—penumbral cones—have a different spectral sensitivity than the open-field cones (35). Effectively, for the method of silent substitution, this means that that there are three additional photoreceptor classes that need to be silenced, and therefore, more primaries are necessary. Practically, penumbral cones can be desensitized using a white-noise stimulus (26), or silenced, though with a significant drop in contrast (36).

Individual Differences in the Cone Spectral Sensitivities

There are individual differences in the spectral sensitivities of the cones and this biological variability will affect the degree to which the cones are truly silenced in a melanopsin-directed modulation. Inter-observer differences have been a concern in the accurate specification of cone signals well before the discovery of melanopsin (37–39). Biological variability arises from inter-observer variability in lens density, macular pigment density, taxial density of the pigment (32, 37–39); and the peak spectral sensitivity due to polymorphisms in the opsin genes (40–43). A given set of cone fundamentals only describes the average spectral sensitivities within a population and ignoring biological variability will introduce error. In the field of melanopsin-mediated pupillometry, some experimenters correct the stimuli by having the observers perform a color matching procedure (25, 26), while others (16, 17, 28) simulate the variability of the stimuli using simulations based on estimates of the biological variability of parameters of the cones (32).

Melanopsin Bistability and Tristability

The method of silent substitution assumes that melanopsin the spectral sensitivity of melanopsin can be described by a single function. There is ample evidence that melanopsin is a bistable (44–49) or tristable photopigment (50). While the cone and rod photopigment is regenerated in the retinal pigment epithelium (RPE), melanopsin, being expressed in ipRGCs in the inner retina, and therefore removed from the RPE is thought to rely on a different mechanism for pigment regeneration. A bistable (or tristable) photopigment relies on light itself to regenerate the pigment, and that this regeneration process again is wavelength-dependent and therefore has a separate spectral sensitivity. It is controversial whether the multistable photochemistry of melanopsin has physiological consequences (51–53). Under conditions of adaptating to a constant background light as employed in silent substitution, melanopsin will be in photoequlibrium, i.e., the different states of the pigment will exist in fixed (though possibly unknown) proportions.

Rod Intrusion

Under daylight conditions, rods are typically thought to be saturated (54, 55), though the range of light levels in which both rods and cones are known to be active is substantial (56, 57). Using a five-primary stimulator [e.g., (25, 26)], it is possible to generate melanopsin-directed stimuli which not only silence the cones but also silence rods. Typically, when rods are silenced, the contrast available to melanopsin is typically only around 1/3 relative to a stimulus in which rods are ignored, though this will depend on the choice of background.

Scatter

The human eye is an imperfect optical system. In cases where the stimulus is a spatially extended light source and there is light outside the primary stimulation area (both centrally, if the macular region is blocked, and in the far periphery), there will be undesired stimulation of potentially unadapted photoreceptors (such as the rods). This can be addressed by adding a light outside the primary stimulation area that light-adapts the photoreceptors outside of the primary stimulation area.

Device Uncertainty

The light source used may not be stable over time and change spectral output between operations, or throughout the sessions. These drifts in device output need to be either calibrated, or at least characterized.

EXPLOITING PROPERTIES OTHER THAN SPECTRAL SENSITIVITY

We have noted in the introduction that the photoreceptors contributing to pupillary control differ not only in their spectral sensitivity (as is exploited in the method of silent substitution) but also in their temporal properties, their operating range and their distribution across the retina. These properties might also be exploited to selectively stimulate melanopsin. For example, the retinal location corresponding to the blind spot does not contain rods and cones, but light might stimulate melanopsin in the axons of ipRGCs. Delivering a stimulus only in the blind spot would therefore ensure that only melanopsin would be activated (58–60), but there could be scatter on rod and cone photoreceptors near the blind spot, and accidental displacement of a small circumscribed stimulus field would need to be controlled for. In the temporal domain, melanopsin photoreception is much slower than cone- and rod-mediated photoreception, and thus, the temporal properties of a stimulus can be optimized to bias the measured response toward melanopsin-mediated properties, e.g., the steady-state pupil size under continuous light (61).

CONCLUSION

The method of silent substitution is a powerful technique to stimulate a specific photoreceptor class or specific photoreceptor classes in the living human retina while leaving other classes un-stimulated. The method has been used successfully to examine the photoreceptor contributions to the human pupillary light responses. The method is not failsafe as several factors need to be considered (retinal inhomogeneities, individual differences, rod intrusion, scatter, and device uncertainty), but these can be addressed experimentally or in simulation. We hope that the method of silent substitution will gain traction to tease apart the contributions of different photoreceptors to human vision and to elucidate their role in the non-invasive assessment of the human visual system using pupillometry.

AUTHOR CONTRIBUTIONS

All authors listed have made a substantial, direct and intellectual contribution to the work, and approved it for publication.

FUNDING

MS is supported by a Sir Henry Wellcome Trust Fellowship (Wellcome Trust 204686/Z/16/Z).

ACKNOWLEDGMENTS

We thank Prof. Hannah Smithson for comments on the manuscript.

REFERENCES

1. McDougal DH, Gamlin PD. Autonomic control of the eye. *Compr Physiol.* (2015) 5:439–73. doi: 10.1002/cphy.c140014
2. Provencio I, Rodriguez IR, Jiang G, Hayes WP, Moreira EF, Rollag MD. A novel human opsin in the inner retina. *J Neurosci.* (2000) 20:600–5. doi: 10.1523/JNEUROSCI.20-02-00600.2000

3. Hattar S, Liao HW, Takao M, Berson DM, Yau KW. Melanopsin-containing retinal ganglion cells: architecture, projections, and intrinsic photosensitivity. *Science* (2002) 295:1065–70. doi: 10.1126/science.1069609
4. Berson DM, Dunn FA, Takao M. Phototransduction by retinal ganglion cells that set the circadian clock. *Science* (2002) 295:1070–3. doi: 10.1126/science.1067262
5. Dacey DM, Liao HW, Peterson BB, Robinson FR, Smith VC, Pokorny J, et al. Melanopsin-expressing ganglion cells in primate retina signal colour and irradiance and project to the LGN. *Nature* (2005) 433:749–54. doi: 10.1038/nature03387
6. Lucas RJ, Hattar S, Takao M, Berson DM, Foster RG, Yau KW. Diminished pupillary light reflex at high irradiances in melanopsin-knockout mice. *Science* (2003) 299:245–7. doi: 10.1126/science.1077293
7. Norren DV, Vos JJ. Spectral transmission of the human ocular media. *Vision Res.* (1974) 14:1237–44. doi: 10.1016/0042-6989(74)90222-3
8. Gamlin PD, McDougal DH, Pokorny J, Smith VC, Yau KW, Dacey DM. Human and macaque pupil responses driven by melanopsin-containing retinal ganglion cells. *Vision Res.* (2007) 47:946–54. doi: 10.1016/j.visres.2006.12.015
9. McDougal DH, Gamlin PD. The influence of intrinsically-photosensitive retinal ganglion cells on the spectral sensitivity and response dynamics of the human pupillary light reflex. *Vision Res.* (2010) 50:72–87. doi: 10.1016/j.visres.2009.10.012
10. Adhikari P, Zele AJ, Feigl B. The post-illumination pupil response (PIPR). *Invest Ophthalmol Vis Sci.* (2015) 56:3838–49. doi: 10.1167/iovs.14-16233
11. Kankipati L, Girkin CA, Gamlin PD. Post-illumination pupil response in subjects without ocular disease. *Invest Ophthalmol Vis Sci.* (2010) 51:2764–9. doi: 10.1167/iovs.09-4717
12. Rushton WA. Pigments and signals in colour vision. *J Physiol.* (1972) 220:1P-P.
13. Estévez O, Spekreijse H. The "silent substitution" method in visual research. *Vision Res.* (1982) 22:681–91. doi: 10.1016/0042-6989(82)90104-3
14. Estévez O, Spekrijse H. A spectral compensation method for determining the flicker characteristics of the human colour mechanisms. *Vision Res.* (1974) 14:823–30. doi: 10.1016/0042-6989(74)90147-3
15. Brainard DH, and Stockman A. Colorimetry. In: Bass M editor. *OSA Handbook of Optics*, 3rd Edn. New York, NY: McGraw-Hill (2010). pp. 10.11–10.56.
16. Spitschan M, Jain S, Brainard DH, Aguirre GK. Opponent melanopsin and S-cone signals in the human pupillary light response. *Proc Natl Acad Sci USA.* (2014) 111:15568–72. doi: 10.1073/pnas.1400942111
17. Woelders T, Leenheers T, Gordijn MCM, Hut RA, Beersma DGM, Wams EJ. Melanopsin- and L-cone-induced pupil constriction is inhibited by S- and M-cones in humans. *Proc Natl Acad Sci USA.* (2018) 115:792–7. doi: 10.1073/pnas.1716281115
18. Shapiro AG, Pokorny J, Smith VC. Cone-rod receptor spaces with illustrations that use CRT phosphor and light-emitting-diode spectra. *J Opt Soc Am A Opt Image Sci Vis.* (1996) 13:2319–28. doi: 10.1364/JOSAA.13.002319
19. Pokorny J, Smithson H, Quinlan J. Photostimulator allowing independent control of rods and the three cone types. *Vis Neurosci.* (2004) 21:263–7. doi: 10.1017/S0952523804213207
20. Tsujimura S, Ukai K, Ohama D, Nuruki A, Yunokuchi K. Contribution of human melanopsin retinal ganglion cells to steady-state pupil responses. *Proc Biol Sci.* (2010) 277:2485–92. doi: 10.1098/rspb.2010.0330
21. Viénot F, Bailacq S, Rohellec JL. The effect of controlled photopigment excitations on pupil aperture. *Ophthalmic Physiol Opt.* (2010) 30:484–91. doi: 10.1111/j.1475-1313.2010.00754.x
22. Tsujimura S, Tokuda Y. Delayed response of human melanopsin retinal ganglion cells on the pupillary light reflex. *Ophthalmic Physiol Opt.* (2011) 31:469–79. doi: 10.1111/j.1475-1313.2011.00846.x
23. Barrionuevo PA, Nicandro N, McAnany JJ, Zele AJ, Gamlin P, Cao D. Assessing rod, cone, and melanopsin contributions to human pupil flicker responses. *Invest Ophthalmol Vis Sci.* (2014) 55:719–27. doi: 10.1167/iovs.13-13252
24. Barrionuevo PA, Cao D. Luminance and chromatic signals interact differently with melanopsin activation to control the pupil light response. *J Vis.* (2016) 16:29. doi: 10.1167/16.11.29
25. Cao D, Nicandro N, Barrionuevo PA. A five-primary photostimulator suitable for studying intrinsically photosensitive retinal ganglion cell functions in humans. *J Vis*. (2015) 15:15.1.27. doi: 10.1167/15.1.27
26. Zele AJ, Feigl B, Adhikari P, Maynard ML, Cao D. Melanopsin photoreception contributes to human visual detection, temporal and colour processing. *Sci Rep.* (2018) 8:3842. doi: 10.1038/s41598-018-22197-w
27. Murray IJ, Kremers J, McKeefry D, Parry NRA. Paradoxical pupil responses to isolated M-cone increments. *J Opt Soc Am A Opt Image Sci Vis.* (2018) 35:B66–B71. doi: 10.1364/JOSAA.35.000B66
28. Spitschan M, Bock AS, Ryan J, Frazzetta G, Brainard DH, Aguirre GK. The human visual cortex response to melanopsin-directed stimulation is accompanied by a distinct perceptual experience. *Proc Natl Acad Sci USA.* (2017) 114:12291–6. doi: 10.1073/pnas.1711522114
29. Ramanath R. Minimizing observer metamerism in display systems. *Color Res Appl.* (2009) 34:391–8. doi: 10.1002/col.20523
30. Stockman A, Brainard DH. Color vision mechanisms. In: Bass M editor. *OSA Handbook of Optics*, 3rd Edn. New York, NY: McGraw-Hill (2010). pp. 11.11–11.104.
31. CIE. *Fundamental Chromaticity Diagram With Physiological Axes–Part 1.*Technical Report 170-1, Central Bureau of the Commission Internationale de l' Éclairage, (Vienna) (2006).
32. Asano Y, Fairchild MD, Blondé L. Individual colorimetric observer model. *PLoS ONE* (2016) 11:e0145671. doi: 10.1371/journal.pone.0145671
33. Enezi JA, Revell V, Brown T, Wynne J, Schlangen L, Lucas R. A "melanopic" spectral efficiency function predicts the sensitivity of melanopsin photoreceptors to polychromatic lights. *J Biol Rhythms* (2011) 26:314–23. doi: 10.1177/0748730411409719
34. Lucas RJ, Peirson SN, Berson DM, Brown TM, Cooper HM, Czeisler CA, et al. Measuring and using light in the melanopsin age. *Trends Neurosci.* (2014) 37:1–9. doi: 10.1016/j.tins.2013.10.004
35. Spitschan M, Aguirre GK, Brainard DH. Selective stimulation of penumbral cones reveals perception in the shadow of retinal blood vessels. *PLoS ONE* (2015) 10:e0124328. doi: 10.1371/journal.pone.0124328
36. Spitschan M, Datta R, Stern AM, Brainard DH, Aguirre GK. Human visual cortex responses to rapid cone and melanopsin-directed flicker. *J Neurosci.* (2016) 36:1471–82. doi: 10.1523/JNEUROSCI.1932-15.2016
37. Smith VC, Pokorny J. Chromatic-discrimination axes, CRT phosphor spectra, and individual variation in color vision. *J Opt Soc Am A Opt Image Sci Vis.* (1995) 12:27–35. doi: 10.1364/JOSAA.12.000027
38. Golz J, MacLeod DI. Colorimetry for CRT displays. *J Opt Soc Am A Opt Image Sci Vis.* (2003) 20:769–81. doi: 10.1364/JOSAA.20.000769
39. Webster MA, MacLeod DI. Factors underlying individual differences in the color matches of normal observers. *J Opt Soc Am A* (1988) 5:1722–35. doi: 10.1364/JOSAA.5.001722
40. Neitz J, Jacobs GH. Polymorphism of the long-wavelength cone in normal human colour vision. *Nature* (1986) 323:623–5. doi: 10.1038/323623a0
41. Neitz J, Jacobs GH. Polymorphism in normal human color vision and its mechanism. *Vision Res.* (1990) 30:621–36. doi: 10.1016/0042-6989(90)90073-T
42. Merbs SL, Nathans J. Absorption spectra of the hybrid pigments responsible for anomalous color vision. *Science* (1992) 258:464–6. doi: 10.1126/science.1411542
43. Sanocki E, Lindsey DT, Winderickx J, Teller DY, Deeb SS, Motulsky AG. Serine/alanine amino acid polymorphism of the L and M cone pigments: effects on Rayleigh matches among deuteranopes, protanopes and color normal observers. *Vision Res.* (1993) 33:2139–52. doi: 10.1016/0042-6989(93)90012-L
44. Sexton TJ, Golczak M, Palczewski K, Van Gelder RN. Melanopsin is highly resistant to light and chemical bleaching *in vivo*. *J Biol Chem.* (2012) 287:20888–97. doi: 10.1074/jbc.M111.325969
45. Matsuyama T, Yamashita T, Imamoto Y, Shichida Y. Photochemical properties of mammalian melanopsin. *Biochemistry* (2012) 51:5454–62. doi: 10.1021/bi3004999
46. Mure LS, Cornut PL, Rieux C, Drouyer E, Denis P, Gronfier C, et al. Melanopsin bistability: a fly's eye technology in the human retina. *PLoS ONE* (2009) 4:e5991. doi: 10.1371/journal.pone.0005991

47. Mure LS, Rieux C, Hattar S, Cooper HM. Melanopsin-dependent nonvisual responses: evidence for photopigment bistability *in vivo*. *J Biol Rhythms* (2007) 22:411–24. doi: 10.1177/0748730407306043
48. Melyan Z, Tarttelin EE, Bellingham J, Lucas RJ, Hankins MW. Addition of human melanopsin renders mammalian cells photoresponsive. *Nature* (2005) 433:741–5. doi: 10.1038/nature03344
49. Panda S, Nayak SK, Campo B, Walker JR, Hogenesch JB, Jegla T. Illumination of the melanopsin signaling pathway. *Science* (2005) 307:600–4. doi: 10.1126/science.1105121
50. Emanuel AJ, Do MT. Melanopsin tristability for sustained and broadband phototransduction. *Neuron* (2015) 85:1043–55. doi: 10.1016/j.neuron.2015.02.011
51. Mawad K, Van Gelder RN. Absence of long-wavelength photic potentiation of murine intrinsically photosensitive retinal ganglion cell firing *in vitro*. *J Biol Rhythms* (2008) 23:387–91. doi: 10.1177/0748730408323063
52. Rollag MD. Does melanopsin bistability have physiological consequences? *J Biol Rhythms* (2008) 23:396–9. doi: 10.1177/0748730408323067
53. Brown TM, Allen AE, al-Enezi J, Wynne J, Schlangen L, Hommes V, et al. The melanopic sensitivity function accounts for melanopsin-driven responses in mice under diverse lighting conditions. *PLoS ONE* (2013) 8:e53583. doi: 10.1371/journal.pone.0053583
54. Aguilar M, Stiles WS. Saturation of the rod mechanism of the retina at high levels of stimulation. *Opt Acta* (1954) 1:59–65. doi: 10.1080/713818657
55. Adelson EH. Saturation and adaptation in the rod system. *Vision Res.* (1982) 22:1299–312. doi: 10.1016/0042-6989(82)90143-2
56. Zele AJ, Cao D. Vision under mesopic and scotopic illumination. *Front Psychol.* (2014) 5:1594. doi: 10.3389/fpsyg.2014.01594
57. Shapiro AG. Cone-specific mediation of rod sensitivity in trichromatic observers. *Invest Ophthalmol Vis Sci.* (2002) 43:898–905.
58. Alpern M, Campbell FW. The spectral sensitivity of the consensual light reflex. *J Physiol.* (1962) 164:478–507. doi: 10.1113/jphysiol.1962.sp007033
59. Saito M, Miyamoto K, Uchiyama Y, Murakami I. Invisible light inside the natural blind spot alters brightness at a remote location. *Sci Rep.* (2018) 8:7540. doi: 10.1038/s41598-018-25920-9
60. Miyamoto K, Murakami I. Pupillary light reflex to light inside the natural blind spot. *Sci Rep.* (2015) 5:11862. doi: 10.1038/srep11862
61. Bouma H. Size of the static pupil as a function of wavelength and luminosity of the light incident on the human eye. *Nature* (1962) 193:690–1. doi: 10.1038/193690a0

Permissions

All chapters in this book were first published by Frontiers; hereby published with permission under the Creative Commons Attribution License or equivalent. Every chapter published in this book has been scrutinized by our experts. Their significance has been extensively debated. The topics covered herein carry significant findings which will fuel the growth of the discipline. They may even be implemented as practical applications or may be referred to as a beginning point for another development.

The contributors of this book come from diverse backgrounds, making this book a truly international effort. This book will bring forth new frontiers with its revolutionizing research information and detailed analysis of the nascent developments around the world.

We would like to thank all the contributing authors for lending their expertise to make the book truly unique. They have played a crucial role in the development of this book. Without their invaluable contributions this book wouldn't have been possible. They have made vital efforts to compile up to date information on the varied aspects of this subject to make this book a valuable addition to the collection of many professionals and students.

This book was conceptualized with the vision of imparting up-to-date information and advanced data in this field. To ensure the same, a matchless editorial board was set up. Every individual on the board went through rigorous rounds of assessment to prove their worth. After which they invested a large part of their time researching and compiling the most relevant data for our readers.

The editorial board has been involved in producing this book since its inception. They have spent rigorous hours researching and exploring the diverse topics which have resulted in the successful publishing of this book. They have passed on their knowledge of decades through this book. To expedite this challenging task, the publisher supported the team at every step. A small team of assistant editors was also appointed to further simplify the editing procedure and attain best results for the readers.

Apart from the editorial board, the designing team has also invested a significant amount of their time in understanding the subject and creating the most relevant covers. They scrutinized every image to scout for the most suitable representation of the subject and create an appropriate cover for the book.

The publishing team has been an ardent support to the editorial, designing and production team. Their endless efforts to recruit the best for this project, has resulted in the accomplishment of this book. They are a veteran in the field of academics and their pool of knowledge is as vast as their experience in printing. Their expertise and guidance has proved useful at every step. Their uncompromising quality standards have made this book an exceptional effort. Their encouragement from time to time has been an inspiration for everyone.

The publisher and the editorial board hope that this book will prove to be a valuable piece of knowledge for researchers, students, practitioners and scholars across the globe.

List of Contributors

R. Becket Ebitz
Department of Neuroscience and Center for Magnetic Resonance Research, University of Minnesota, Minneapolis, MN, United States

Tirin Moore
Department of Neurobiology, Stanford University School of Medicine, Stanford, CA, United States
Howard Hughes Medical Institute, Seattle, WA, United States

A. V. Rukmini and Joshua J. Gooley
Programme in Neuroscience and Behavioural Disorders, Centre for Cognitive Neuroscience, Duke-NUS Medical School, Singapore

Inès Daguet and Claude Gronfier
Lyon Neuroscience Research Center, Waking Team, INSERM UMRS 1028, CNRS UMR 5292, Université Claude Bernard Lyon 1, Université de Lyon, Lyon, France

Didier Bouhassira
INSERM U987, Centre d'Evaluation et de Traitement de la Douleur, Hôpital Ambroise Paré, Boulogne-Billancourt, France

Carina Kelbsch, Torsten Strasser, Tobias Peters, Helmut Wilhelm and Barbara J. Wilhelm
Pupil Research Group, Centre for Ophthalmology, University Hospitals Tübingen, Tübingen, Germany

Kathryn A. Roecklein
Department of Psychology, University of Pittsburgh, Pittsburgh, PA, United States

Stuart R. Steinhauer
VA Pittsburgh Healthcare System, VISN 4 MIRECC, University Drive C, Pittsburgh, PA, United States
Department of Psychiatry, University of Pittsburgh School of Medicine, Pittsburgh, PA, United States

Yanjun Chen
Department of Ophthalmology and Visual Sciences, University of Wisconsin School of Medicine and Public Health, Madison, AL, United States

Randy Kardon
Neuro-Ophthalmology Division, University of Iowa and Iowa City VA Healthcare System, Iowa City, LA, United States

Rawan Omary and Klara Landau
Department of Ophthalmology, University Hospital Zurich, University of Zurich, Zurich, Switzerland

Christopher J. Bockisch
Department of Ophthalmology, University Hospital Zurich, University of Zurich, Zurich, Switzerland
Department of Neurology, University Hospital Zurich, University of Zurich, Zurich, Switzerland
Department of ENT, University Hospital Zurich, University of Zurich, Zurich, Switzerland

Randy H. Kardon
Department of Ophthalmology, University of Iowa and Veterans Medical Center, Iowa City, IA, United States

Konrad P. Weber
Department of Ophthalmology, University Hospital Zurich, University of Zurich, Zurich, Switzerland
Department of Neurology, University Hospital Zurich, University of Zurich, Zurich, Switzerland

Sylvain V. Crippa
Neuro-Ophthalmology Unit, Jules-Gonin Eye Hospital, University of Lausanne, Lausanne, Switzerland Group for Retinal Disorder Research, Jules-Gonin Eye Hospital, University of Lausanne, Lausanne, Switzerland
Group for Retinal Disorder Research, Department of Ophthalmology, Hôpital Ophtalmique Jules Gonin, University of Lausanne, Lausanne, Switzerland
Neuro-Ophtalmology, Department of Ophthalmology, Hôpital Ophtalmique Jules Gonin, University of Lausanne, Lausanne, Switzerland

Fatima Pedrosa Domellöf
Ophthalmology, Department of Clinical Science, Umeå University, Umeå, Sweden

Aki Kawasaki
Neuro-Ophthalmology Unit, Jules-Gonin Eye Hospital, University of Lausanne, Lausanne, Switzerland
Neuro-Ophtalmology, Department of Ophthalmology, Hôpital Ophtalmique Jules Gonin, University of Lausanne, Lausanne, Switzerland

Noémie Kircher, Catherine Martin and Corinne Kostic
Group for Retinal Disorder Research, Department of Ophthalmology, Hôpital Ophtalmique Jules Gonin, University of Lausanne, Lausanne, Switzerland

Irene Sperandio and Nikki Bond
The School of Psychology, University of East Anglia, Norwich, United Kingdom

Paola Binda
Department of Translational Research and New Technologies in Medicine and Surgery, University of Pisa, Pisa, Italy
Institute of Neuroscience, Consiglio Nazionale delle Ricerche (CNR), Pisa, Italy

Elemer Szabadi
Developmental Psychiatry, University of Nottingham, Nottingham, United Kingdom
Developmental Psychiatry, Queen's Medical Centre, University of Nottingham, Nottingham, United Kingdom

Pratik S. Chougule and Maxwell T. Finkelstein
Department of Visual Neurosciences, Singapore Eye Research Institute, Singapore

Raymond P. Najjar
Department of Visual Neurosciences, Singapore Eye Research Institute, Singapore
The Ophthalmology & Visual Sciences ACP, Duke-National University of Singapore (NUS) Medical School, Singapore

Nagaendran Kandiah
Department of Neurology, National Neuroscience Institute, Singapore
Duke-National University of Singapore (NUS), Singapore

Dan Milea
Department of Visual Neurosciences, Singapore Eye Research Institute, Singapore
The Ophthalmology & Visual Sciences ACP, Duke-National University of Singapore (NUS) Medical School, Singapore
Singapore National Eye Centre, Singapore Eye Research Institute, Singapore

Corinne Frances Carle
John Curtin School of Medical Research, Eccles Institute of Neuroscience, The Australian National University, Canberra, ACT, Australia
ANU Medical School, The Australian National University, Canberra, ACT, Australia

Andrew Charles James and Ted Maddess
John Curtin School of Medical Research, Eccles Institute of Neuroscience, The Australian National University, Canberra, ACT, Australia

Yanti Rosli
Diagnostic and Applied Health Sciences, Biomedical Science Program, Faculty of Health Science, Universiti Kebangsaan Malaysia, Kuala Lumpur, Malaysia

Maria A. Bonmati-Carrion, Juan A. Madrid and Maria A. Rol
Chronobiology Laboratory, Department of Physiology, IMIB-Arrixaca, University of Murcia, Murcia, Spain
Ciber Fragilidad y Envejecimiento Saludable, Madrid, Spain

Konstanze Hild and Stephen J. Sweeney
Advanced Technology Institute and Department of Physics, University of Surrey, Guildford, United Kingdom

Cheryl M. Isherwood and Debra J. Skene
Chronobiology, Faculty of Health and Medical Sciences, University of Surrey, Guildford, United Kingdom

Victoria L. Revell
Surrey Clinical Research Centre, Faculty of Health and Medical Sciences, University of Surrey, Guildford, United Kingdom

Chin-An Wang
Centre for Neuroscience Studies, Queen's University, Kingston, ON, Canada
Graduate Institute of Humanities in Medicine, Taipei Medical University, Taipei, Taiwan
Research Center of Brain and Consciousness, Taipei Medical University, Shuang Ho Hospital, New Taipei City, Taiwan

Talia Baird, Jeff Huang, Jonathan D. Coutinho, Donald C. Brien and Douglas P. Munoz
Centre for Neuroscience Studies, Queen's University, Kingston, ON, Canada

Carey D. Balaban
Departments of Otolaryngology, Neurobiology, Communication Sciences and Disorders, and Bioengineering, University of Pittsburgh, Pittsburgh, PA, United States

Alex Kiderman and Robin C. Ashmore
Neuro Kinetics Inc., Pittsburgh, PA, United States

Mikhaylo Szczupak
Department of Otolaryngology, University of Miami Hospital, Miami, FL, United States

Michael E. Hoffer
Department of Otolaryngology, University of Miami Hospital, Miami, FL, United States
Neurological Surgery, University of Miami Hospital, Miami, FL, United States
Sports Performance and Wellness Institute, University of Miami Hospital, Miami, FL, United States

Pablo Alejandro Barrionuevo
Instituto de Investigación en Luz, Ambiente y Visión, Consejo Nacional de Investigaciones Científicas y Técnicas–Universidad Nacional de Tucumán, San Miguel de Tucumán, Argentina

J. Jason McAnany and Dingcai Cao
Department of Ophthalmology and Visual Sciences, University of Illinois at Chicago, Chicago, IL, United States

Andrew J. Zele
Visual Science Laboratory, School of Optometry and Vision Science & Institute of Health and Biomedical Innovation, Queensland University of Technology, Brisbane, QLD, Australia
School of Optometry and Vision Science, Queensland University of Technology, Brisbane, QLD, Australia
Institute of Health and Biomedical Innovation, Queensland University of Technology (QUT), Brisbane, QLD, Australia

Chiara La Morgia and Valerio Carelli
Unità Operativa Complessa Clinica Neurologica, IRCCS Istituto delle Scienze Neurologiche di Bologna, Ospedale Bellaria, Bologna, Italy

Michele Carbonelli
Dipartimento di Scienze Biomediche e Neuromotorie, Università di Bologna, Bologna, Italy

Prakash Adhikari
Institute of Health and Biomedical Innovation, Queensland University of Technology (QUT), Brisbane, QLD, Australia
School of Optometry and Vision Science, Queensland University of Technology (QUT), Brisbane, QLD, Australia

Beatrix Feigl
Institute of Health and Biomedical Innovation, Queensland University of Technology (QUT), Brisbane, QLD, Australia
School of Biomedical Sciences, Queensland University of Technology (QUT), Brisbane, QLD, Australia
Queensland Eye Institute, Brisbane, QLD, Australia

Manuel Spitschan
Department of Experimental Psychology, University of Oxford, Oxford, United Kingdom

Tom Woelders
Chronobiology Unit, Groningen Institute for Evolutionary Life Sciences, University of Groningen, Groningen, Netherlands

Index

www.ingramcontent.com/pod-product-compliance
Lightning Source LLC
LaVergne TN
LVHW081015210926
848485LV00004B/870